Core Textbook of
PEDIATRICS

Core Textbook of PEDIATRICS

Robert Kaye, M.D.

Professor and Chairman
Department of Pediatrics
Hahnemann Medical College and Hospital
Philadelphia, Pennsylvania

Frank A. Oski, M.D.

Professor and Chairman
Department of Pediatrics
State University of New York
Upstate Medical Center
Syracuse, New York

Lewis A. Barness, M.D.

Professor and Chairman
Department of Pediatrics
University of South Florida
Tampa, Florida

with 24 Additional Contributors

J. B. Lippincott Company

Philadephia • Toronto

Aquisitions Editor: William Burgower
Sponsoring Editor: Sanford J. Robinson
Manuscript Editor: Delois Patterson
Indexer: Alexandra Weir
Art Director: Maria S. Karkucinski

Designer: Larry Didona
Production Supervisor: N. Carol Kerr
Production Assistant: Susan A. Caldwell
Compositor: General Graphic Services, Inc.
Printer/Binder: R.R. Donnelley & Sons Company

2nd Edition

For information write J. B. Lippincott Company, East Washington Square, Philadelphia, Pennsylvania 19105

3 5 6 4 2

Library of Congress Cataloging in Publication Data
Main entry under title:

Core textbook of pediatrics.

Bibliography
Includes index
1. Pediatrics. I. Kaye, Robert. II. Oski, Frank A. III. Barness, Lewis A.
RJ45.C78 1982 618.92 81-18625
ISBN 0-397-52097-2 AACR2

The authors and publisher have exerted every effort to ensure that drug selection and dosage set forth in this text are in accord with current recommendations and practice at the time of publication. However, in view of ongoing research, changes in government regulations, and the constant flow of information relating to drug therapy and drug reactions, the reader is urged to check the package insert for each drug for any change in indications and dosage and for added warnings and precautions. This is particularly important when the recommended agent is a new or infrequently employed drug.

To

Edwards A. Park, Joseph Stokes, Jr., Paul Gyorgy, Louis K. Diamond, Charles A. Janeway, all Howland Awardees of the American Pediatric Society who have been our most significant teachers and sources of inspiration, and to the medical students who will become the pediatricians of the future.

Contents

Contributors

David Baker, M.D.
Associate Professor of Pediatrics
Hahnemann Medical College and Hospital
Philadelphia, Pennsylvania

Lewis A. Barness, M.D.
Professor and Chairman
Department of Pediatrics
University of South Florida
Tampa, Florida

Herman S. Belmont, M.D.
Professor and Deputy Chairman for Child and Adolescent Mental Health Sciences
Hahnemann Medical College and Hospital
Philadelphia, Pennsylvania

Charles B. Brill, M.D.
Associate Professor of Pediatrics
Director, Section of Pediatric Neurology
Hahnemann Medical College and Hospital
Philadelphia, Pennsylvania

John S. Curran, M.D.
Professor of Pediatrics
University of South Florida
Tampa, Florida

Eliot H. Dunsky, M.D.
Associate Professor of Pediatrics and Internal Medicine
Director, Section of Allergy and Immunology
Hahnemann Medical College and Hospital
Philadelphia, Pennsylvania

Sidney Friedman, M.D.
Professor of Pediatrics
University of Pennsylvania School of Medicine
Chief Cardiologist
The Children's Hospital of Philadelphia
Philadelphia, Pennsylvania

Ian S. E. Gibbons, M.D.
Professor of Pediatrics and Medicine
Chief, Division of Pediatric and Adolescent Gastroenterology
Thomas Jefferson University School of Medicine
Medical Director, Children's Heart Hospital
Philadelphia, Pennsylvania

James A. Hallock, M.D.
Professor of Pediatrics
University of South Florida
Tampa, Florida

Douglas S. Holsclaw, M.D.
Professor of Pediatrics
Director, Cystic Fibrosis and Pediatric Pulmonary Centers
Hahnemann Medical College and Hospital
Philadelphia, Pennsylvania

Paul J. Honig, M.D.
Associate Professor of Pediatrics in Dermatology
University of Pennsylvania School of Medicine
Director of Dermatology
The Children's Hospital of Philadelphia
Philadelphia, Pennsylvania

J. Martin Kaplan, M.D.
Associate Professor of Pediatrics
Hahnemann Medical College and Hospital
Philadelphia, Pennsylvania

Robert Kaye, M.D.
Professor and Chairman
Department of Pediatrics
Hahnemann Medical College and Hospital
Philadelphia, Pennsylvania

John I. Malone, M.D.
Professor of Pediatrics
University of South Florida
Tampa, Florida

Julia A. McMillan, M.D.
Assistant Professor of Pediatrics
Division of Infectious Diseases
Department of Pediatrics
State University of New York
Upstate Medical Center
Syracuse, New York

Michael H. Mitchell, M.D.
Chief, Pediatric Neurology
Letterman Army Medical Center
Clinical Assistant Professor
Department of Neurology
University of California
San Francisco, California
Affiliated Assistant Professor
Pediatrics and Neurology
Uniformed Services University of the Health Sciences School of Medicine
Bethesda, Maryland

Frank A. Oski, M.D.
Professor and Chairman
Department of Pediatrics
State University of New York
Upstate Medical Center
Syracuse, New York

Edward O. Reiter, M.D.
Associate Professor of Pediatrics
University of Massachusetts Medical School
Worchester, Massachusetts
Acting Chairman
Department of Pediatrics
Baystate Medical Center
Springfield, Massachusetts

Allen W. Root, M.D.
Professor of Pediatrics
University of South Florida
Tampa, Florida
Director of University Service
All Children's Hospital
St. Petersburg, Florida

Edward R. Root, M.D.
Assistant Professor of Pediatrics
University of South Florida College of Medicine
Tampa, Florida

Thomas F. McNair Scott, M.D.
Professor of Pediatrics
Director, Pediatric Ambulatory Clinic
Hahnemann Medical College and Hospital
Philadelphia, Pennsylvania

Walter W. Tunnessen, Jr., M.D.
Professor of Pediatrics
Director, Diagnostic Referral Center
Upstate Medical Center
State University of New York
Syracuse, New York

Peter W. Vanace, M.D.
Associate Professor of Pediatrics
Director, Division of Pediatric Rehabilitation
Hahnemann Medical College and Hospital
Philadelphia, Pennsylvania

Mary L. Voorhess, M.D.
Professor of Pediatrics
State University of New York at Buffalo School of Medicine
Co-Director, Division of Endocrinology
Buffalo Children's Hospital
Buffalo, New York

Howard L. Weinberger, M.D.
Professor of Pediatrics
Director, Ambulatory Services
Upstate Medical Center
State University of New York
Syracuse, New York

Margaret L. Williams, M.D.
Professor of Pediatrics
State University of New York
Upstate Medical Center
Chief, Division of Neonatology
Director of Nurseries
Crouse-Irving Memorial Hospital
Syracuse, New York

Elaine H. Zackai, M.D.
Assistant Professor of Pediatrics and Human Genetics
University of Pennsylvania School of Medicine
Associate Physician
The Children's Hospital of Philadelphia
Philadelphia, Pennsylvania

Preface

In the preface to the first edition of *Core Textbook of Pediatrics*, the editors stated their objective of providing a text that would be most useful to the medical student in his initial contact with pediatric medicine. To this end, we have presented material encompassing the major topics related to the health needs of children. We have attempted to provide a readable book in a size that could be read during the limited time allocated to the pediatrics rotation.

We believe that the material should also be of value to students of nursing, physicians' assistants, nurse practitioners, and other health care professionals. Physicians who deal with children may also find the material valuable in providing current information on the variety of topics addressed.

As in the first edition, we have not attempted to supplant the major textbooks in pediatrics that provide rich sources of supplemental information.

In keeping with our desire to provide a readable book that does not overwhelm the student and still attempts to address most major pediatric topics, we have shortened some of the original chapters to make room for topics not previously discussed. Therefore, additional chapters have been included that deal with "Child Abuse and Neglect," "The Child with a Limp," and "The Skin."

The editors would be gratified if our book serves to arouse an interest in medical students and other health professionals leading them to a career dedicated to meeting the health needs of children.

ROBERT KAYE, M.D.
FRANK A. OSKI, M.D.
LEWIS A. BARNESS, M.D.

From the Preface to the First Edition

Each of the editors of *Core Textbook of Pediatrics* has had the responsibility of organizing and presenting the introductory course in pediatrics to medical students. We undertook the preparation of this volume in the belief that there was an unmet need for a book that would help students to acquire a beginning familiarity with the major topics in the health needs of children, and we intended that the book be of a size that could be read during the limited time alloted to the pediatrics rotation.

A problem-oriented presentation was used whenever appropriate, since parents usually seek medical care for their children because of the appearance of a worrisome symptom or sign rather than for treatment of a specific disease. We hope that this approach assists the students in developing competence and satisfaction in the decision-making process, leading from the identification of the patient's problems to diagnosis.

This book is not intended to supplant the major textbooks in pediatrics . . . those books should serve as sources of supplemental information to the reader. We hope that *Core Textbook of Pediatrics* will help students enjoy their first professional contacts with children, while sparing them dismay at the multitude and variation of illnesses with which the complete pediatrician is faced.

ROBERT KAYE, M.D.
FRANK A. OSKI, M.D.
LEWIS A. BARNESS, M.D.

Acknowledgments

We are pleased that the first edition of *Core Textbook of Pediatrics* achieved sufficient readership to warrant a new edition. We appreciate the support and encouragement of J. Stuart Freeman, Jr. and the editorial assistance of Delois Patterson of the J.B. Lippincott Company.

It has given the authors great pleasure to see medical students carrying *Core Textbook of Pediatrics* and even more to learn that reading it has been profitable to them.

We are grateful to the original group of contributors, who have been so effective in updating their material, and to those who have submitted new chapters. We believe the new material will add to the usefulness of our book.

Core Textbook of
PEDIATRICS

History and Physical Examination

1

Lewis A. Barness

HISTORY

Taking an adequate history is essential to making a diagnosis of pediatric diseases. Since most infants and children are unable to give good histories, an adequate history can be formulated by first taking a history, then interpreting the remarks of an observer, and synthesizing these into a relatively accurate data base.

Until the novitiate learns the significance of signs and symptoms, it is reasonable to ask all questions in an orderly fashion. As the student learns the different diseases, lines of questions may be pursued to make or eliminate specific diagnoses. Even then, it is important not to miss negative historical information which may be significant to a future date or future illness.

Interest in the well-being of the child as well as in the illness should be conveyed to the parent. The informant should be allowed to talk freely at first about the child's problem; further information is then obtained by direct questioning. A service will be performed for your patient if this information can be transcribed into a meaningful medical record, which aids and complements the medical care to be delivered.

The medical record is the basis for medical care, and every effort should be made to organize the record and include all pertinent information. The following guidelines aid in organizing the history and physical data.

ELEMENTS OF A COMPLETE HISTORY

General Information

A complete history includes the name, age and birth date, sex, race, admission date, referral source (*e.g.*, a clinic or physician), and relation of informant to the child, including a statement of the reliability of the informant.

Chief Complaint

The chief complaint (CC) is a brief statement, in the informant's or patient's own words, of the reason the child was brought to the hospital or clinic. The duration of the problem should also be noted.

History of the Present Illness

The history of the present illness (HPI) is the portion of the history that tells, in chronologic sequence, the problem or problems for which the child is being seen. It should begin with a statement of the child's general status and onset of illness, such as "This is the first admission of this 5-year-old white boy who was well until 3 days prior to admission . . ." Each problem defined in the history should include the following information:

1. Date of onset
2. Chronologic development of symptoms and duration of symptoms
3. Treatment and response to treatment
4. Change or changes in condition (course of the illness)

If the medical history is significant to the development of the current illness, a brief summary may be included. Old charts may be used for this information, and they may be included in this section or in the review of the medical history. However, this information need not be recorded in both places. Pertinent negative findings should be included in this section.

Medical History

Prenatal History. The informant should supply information about the pregnancy such as number of previous pregnancies and the health of the mother during pregnancy; these data include any infections, illnesses, vaginal bleeding, or toxemia. If radiographs were taken or medications given, this information should also be included. The results of serology tests as well as the blood types of the mother and baby should be recorded. Details of the baby's movement in the uterus should also be recorded.

Birth History. The examiner should ascertain the duration of pregnancy, the ease or difficulty of labor, and the duration of labor. Whether the delivery was spontaneous, forceps-assisted, or by cesarean-section should be recorded, as well as the type of anesthesia used during delivery. The place and date of birth and the birth weight are also pertinent.

Neonatal History. Inquire about the condition of the baby after birth, recording such information as difficulty in starting to breathe, and the presence of cyanosis or convulsions. If the baby was jaundiced during the neonatal period, ascertain the date of onset, duration, and need for treatment. The baby's length of stay in the nursery and need for special care, such as an incubator, transfusions, medications, should be included.

Feeding History. It should be noted whether the baby was breast- or bottle-fed and how well the baby took the first feeding. If the infant has been bottle-fed, the type of formula, amounts of components used, and total amount of formula taken in a 24-hour period must be recorded. Details of the introduction of solid food and the use of vitamins and fluorides are pertinent. Problems with food intolerance or vomiting should be included in this section.

For an older child, the diet history may be ascertained by asking the informant to supply sample breakfast, lunch, and supper menus.

In any child with feeding difficulties or a nutritional problem, the following information should be detailed: the onset of the problem, methods of feeding, types of formula used, reasons for changes, interval between feedings, amount taken per feeding, vomiting, crying, and weight change.

Developmental History. The progression of weight gain is important in a developmental assessment. Therefore, birth weight, weight at 6 months, weight at 1 year, and weight at 2 years should be ascertained. Any sudden gain or loss of weight should be listed first. The informant should compare the child's general growth with that of his siblings. In all instances, and in older children with a developmental problem, the dates of the following developmental milestones should be included in the history: followed person with eyes, held head erect, transferred objects, walked with support, spoke first words and sentences, sat alone, smiled responsively, reached for objects, and walked alone. For children 2 years of age and older, pertinent developmental landmarks should be recorded. For a school age child, his grade and marks received in school should be ascertained and compared with those of his siblings.

Behavior History. The informant should supply information as to whether the child is happy or is difficult to manage. The child's response to other children and to new situations, strangers, and school are clues to behavior problems. If the child manifests successive demands for attention such as showing off, nagging, temper tantrums, and crying, these should be recorded. Problems with bowel or bladder training and habits such as thumb-sucking, nail-biting, and masturbation are important. The examiner should discover if the child has nightmares and whether he suffers from pica, particularly for paint or plaster.

Immunization History. The types of immunization, the number and dates given and the child's reactions, if any, should be recorded.

History of Past Illnesses. A statement should be made here as to the health of the patient before this illness. Specific inquiry should be made as to the child's having had: roseola, rubeola, rubella, pertussis, mumps, varicella, scarlet fever, tuberculosis, anemia, recurrent tonsillitis, otitis media, pneumonia, meningitis, encephalitis or other nervous system disease, gastrointestinal tract disease, and any other disease. The history of each past illness should include the date of onset, symptoms, and course, termination, and whether there were complications or sequelae. If the child was hospitalized or had surgery in the past, the diagnoses for these events should be stated. The results of surgery should be ascertained. Details of allergy include: the occurrence and type of drug reactions, and the presence of food allergies, hay fever, and asthma. All accidents, injuries, and poisonings should be included.

Review of Systems

Review of systems (ROS) should supplement the history of present illness, and information included there need not be repeated, but merely referred to as "See PI."

Head. Injuries, headache

Eyes. Visual changes, crossed or tendency to cross, discharge, redness, puffiness, injuries, glasses

Ears. Difficulty in hearing, pain, discharge, history of ear infections

Nose. Discharge (watery or purulent), difficulty in breathing through nose, epistaxis

Mouth and Throat. Sore throat or tongue, difficulty in swallowing, dental trouble

Lungs. Difficulty in breathing, cough (time and character), hoarseness, wheezing, hemoptysis, pain in chest

Heart. Cyanosis, edema, history of heart murmurs or "heart trouble," ability to keep up with other children in active play, shortness of breath, chest pains

Gastrointestinal. Appetite, nausea, vomiting (relation to feeding, amount, character), bowel movements (number and character), abdominal pain, distention, jaundice

Genitourinary. Frequency, dysuria, hematuria, character of urinary stream, bedwetting, urethral or vaginal discharge, menstrual history

Extremities. Weaknesses, deformities, difficulty in moving extremities or in walking, joint pains or swelling

Neurologic. Headaches, dizziness, incoordination, convulsions

Skin. Rashes, hives

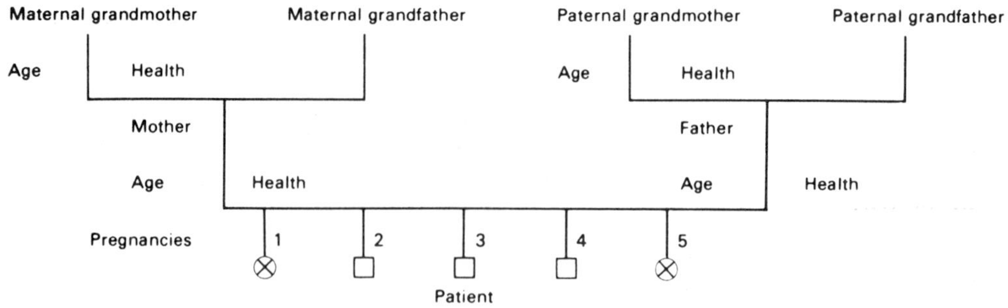

Fig. 1-1. Genetic chart.

Family History

A genetic chart (Fig. 1-1) may be used in the family history (FH) and should include parents, siblings, and grandparents, with their ages, health, and cause of death.

When problems with genetic implications exist, inquiry should be made about other relatives. If a genetic chart is used, the pregnancies should be listed in a series, and include the health of the siblings, for example:

1. 1964—stillbirth at . . . month of gestation
2. 1966—boy with hay fever
3. 1968—boy (the patient)
4. 1970—a boy who is well
5. 1976—girl who died at age 2 days with hyaline membrane disease

Inquiries should be made about a family history of allergy, blood disease, heart disease, lung disease, kidney disease, tuberculosis, diabetes, rheumatic fever, convulsions or mental disorders, skin or gastrointestinal disorders, cancer, venereal disease or behavioral disorders, and any other diseases in the family.

Social History

Record details of the family unit in the social history section. Include information on the presence of grandparents and the marital status of the parents (living together, separated, divorced). Data on home living conditions should include details as whether the family lives in a house or an apartment, whether the mother works and if so who looks after the patient when she is working, and the father's employment. If pertinent to the child's problem, detailed inquiry should be made about the family's attitudes toward each other and toward the child. A typical day in the child's life may be outlined.

PHYSICAL EXAMINATION

The physical examination of a child cannot be approached in the same manner as that of an adult, that is, starting with the head and ending with the feet. The child is in a new situation and may be apprehensive. An attempt should be made to befriend the child before examining him, and the order of the examination should fit the child and the circumstances. In general, it is wise to make no sudden movements, and to first complete those parts of the examination for which the child's cooperation is needed. All painful or disagreeable procedures should be deferred until the end of the examination, and the child should be warned before the start of these procedures. Thoroughness is essential. The child should be completely undressed, but not necessarily all at once. In recording findings of physical examination, descriptions should be exact as to size, color, and so forth.

Although the physical examination may not necessarily be conducted in this order, the recorded information should follow the outline below.

Measurements. Measurements should include height, weight, head circumference (all given with percentile for age), temperature (oral or rectal), pulse, respiration, blood pressure (site used and position in which taken, *e.g.*, left arm supine position; skin folds, arm circumferences).

General Appearance. A statement should be included about the child's general development and nutrition, any unusual positions he assumes, his mental status, activity, and evidence of how the child apparently feels. The apparent degree and acuteness of illness and the presence of any distress should be noted.

Skin. Include color, the presence of cyanosis, jaundice, eruptions, edema, skin turgor, amount of subcutaneous tissue, and evidence of recent weight loss.

Lymph Nodes. Location and size of lymph nodes and the presence of tenderness should be recorded.

Head. The head should be examined for shape, symmetry, sutures, bone defects, and size and tension of fontanels (posterior fontanel usually closed by 2 months, anterior fontanel usually closed by 12 to 18 months, but occasionally as early as 9 months). The hair and scalp should also be examined, with pertinent findings recorded.

Eyes. Make a gross test of vision. Visual fields should be tested in all children old enough to cooperate. The eyes should be evaluated for strabismus by position of the light reflex in both eyes, and the cover test. The range of eye movements should be evaluated. The presence of nystagmus should be noted. Other structures to be examined around the eyes include the conjunctivae and sclerae, the cornea for haziness and opacities, the pupils for size and shape, and the iris and lens. The reaction to light (direct and consensual) and accommodation should be noted. A funduscopic examination should be performed, noting the presence of the red reflex, the condition of the veins and arteries (they should be of almost equal caliber or veins slightly larger than arteries), the presence of hemorrhages or pigmented or depigmented areas. Visualization of the disk should reveal sharp or blurred borders. The macula is examined to detect possible degenerative changes. Testing of the corneal reflex may also be part of the examination.

Ears. Evaluate hearing and the condition of the external ear (deformity or unusual shape, pain with movement of the ear), the canal wall, the drum, and the mastoid.

Nose. The nasal examination is performed to detect deformities, condition of the airway, color and state of the mucosa and turbinates, discharge (amount and character), sinus tenderness and swelling. At birth, the maxillary antrum, anterior and posterior ethmoid cells and sphenoid sinus are present. However, the latter does not assume clinical significance until the child is approximately 5 years of age. At 2 to 4 years of age, pneumatization of the frontal sinus occurs, but it is rarely a site of infection until after ages 6 to 10.

Mouth and Throat. Examination of the mouth and throat should include the number and condition of the teeth, condition of the gums, buccal mucosa, the tongue, palate, tonsils, and posterior pharynx. Listening to the voice reveals the presence of hoarseness, the quality of the cry, and the presence of stridor.

Neck. Examination of the neck may reveal rigidity or swelling, abnormalities in the lymph nodes, salivary glands, and thyroid, and in the position of the trachea.

Chest. The general shape of the chest and the presence of any deformities should be noted. In infancy, the chest is almost round. As the child grows, the chest normally expands in the transverse diameter. Abnormal signs to look for are beading, asymmetry of expansion, and suprasternal, intercostal, and subcostal retractions.

Lungs. The type of breathing (regular, Cheyne-Stokes) and rate of respiration should be recorded.

Auscultation. Breath sounds are usually bronchovesicular in children. To be noted are whether they are increased or decreased. Rales, rhonchi, friction rub, and inspiratory or expiratory wheezes are abnormal findings. Also listen for vocal resonance.

Palpation. Chest palpation detects tactile fremitus and masses on the chest wall.

Percussion. Percussion is done to detect areas of dullness or hyperresonance. Normally the top of the liver is percussed anteriorly at about the level of the sixth rib from the midaxillary line to the sternum. The lower edge of the lung or the top of the diaphragm is usually percussed to the level of the 8th to 10th ribs posteriorly on both sides.

Heart and Cardiovascular System. A thorough examination of the heart and cardiovascular system should include the following:

Inspection. The presence of cyanosis, edema, clubbing of fingers, and respiratory distress suggest a cardiac etiology.

Palpation. Part of the cardiac examination is locating the apex beat. The apex beat is normally felt in the fourth interspace just to the left of the midclavicular line in children under 7 years of age. After 7 years, it is felt in the fifth intercostal space in the midclavicular line. Thrills at the apex are best felt with the child lying on the left side; basal thrills are felt with the child sitting up.

Percussion. An attempt should be made to percuss the heart borders. Learn scratch percussion which is accurate in normal as well as in crying children and children with thick pectoralis muscles or heavy breasts.

Auscultation. Heart rate and rhythm are detected and auscultation is performed over the entire chest, anteriorly and posteriorly, with particular attention at the listening posts of the four valve areas. The quality of the heart sounds is normally sharp and clear; splitting of the first or second heart sounds may be heard.

Murmurs. The presence of heart murmurs must be documented by noting location, intensity (I to VI), quality, duration, and transmission. Also note the effect of change of position and excerise.

Radial and Femoral Pulses. Radial and femoral pulses are palpated and the blood pressure taken. The blood pressure should be taken in both arms and one leg if the child has a cardiac problem or hypertension or if only weak femoral pulses are palpated.

Abdomen. In the abdominal examination, look for shape (distended or flat), tenderness (include costovertebral), rigidity, palpable organs or masses, hernia, visible peristalisis, ascites, and bowel sounds.

Back. By employing both observations and palpation, the spinal shape and posture (lordosis, kyphosis, scoliosis), masses, tenderness, limitation of motion, spina bifida, and pilonidal dimples or cysts may be detected.

Genitalia. In the male, descent of the testes, presence of hydrocele, state of the foreskin, adequacy of urethral meatal orifice, and malformations such as hypospadia should be recorded. In the female, abnormalities such as fused labia minora or imperforate hymen, urethral or vaginal inflammation or discharge, pubic and axillary hair are recorded. A vaginal examination is not done routinely.

Anus. The anus should be examined for patency, presence of fissures, fistulae, or hemorrhoids, and for the state of the sphincter. Rectal examination is performed whenever the child has an abdominal problem.

Extremities. All extremities are observed for asymmetry, anomalies, unusual length, pain and tenderness, temperature, swelling deformities, and shape (genu varum, genu valgum, tibial torsion, metatarsus varus). The presence of a limp should be recorded. Abnormal findings of the joints include heat, tenderness, swelling, effusion, redness, and limitation or pain on motion. In infants, the examiner must always test for congenital dislocation of the hips.

Muscles. Muscle development and tone are noted, as is the presence of tenderness, spasm, paresis (weakness) or paralysis, flaccidity, spasticity, rigidity, and muscle atrophy.

Neurologic Examination. The mental status and orientation are recorded, stating how this was determined.

Abnormal Movements. Tremors, twitchings, choreiform movements and athetosis should be noted.

Coordination. The gait is observed and the Romberg and finger-to-nose tests are performed.

Cranial Nerves. All of the cranial nerves are tested: I (olfactory), II (optic), III (oculomotor), IV (trochlear), V (trigeminal), VI (abducens), VII (facial), VIII (auditory and vestibular divisions), IX (glossopharyngeal), X (vagus), XI (accessory), XII (hypoglossal).

Reflexes. The biceps, triceps, radial, finger flexion, patellar, Achilles tendon, plantar, abdominal, and cremasteric reflexes are recorded after evaluation on both the right and left sides. Other reflexes in a young infant include sucking, rooting, and Moro reflex. In cases of suspected meningeal irritation, the Brudzinski and Kernig signs must also be checked.

Sensory Examination. Includes evaluation of the senses of touch, pain, vibration, and position.

Muscle Strength. If not done during the examination of the extremities, muscle strength may be evaluated here.

SUMMARY

A thorough history and physical examination aid in making a differential diagnosis and in delineating problems. A problem list is then drawn up, based on the history and physical examination. The problems are numbered and subjective findings (see symptoms), objective signs (physical) and laboratory results, assessment and plan are included. Progress notes should be kept for each problem until it is resolved.

BIBLIOGRAPHY

Barness LA: Manual of Pediatric Physical Diagnosis, 5th ed. Chicago, Year Book Medical Publishers, 1981

This is a manual detailing how to perform and record a complete physical examination with suggestions for approaching the patient at various ages. Differential diagnosis of significant signs is given.

Weed LL: Medical Records, Medical Education and Patient Care. Chicago, Year Book Medical Publishers, 1971

This short book delineates the method and value of obtaining a problem-oriented history and the usefulness of a problem-oriented record in following the course of a patient in health or disease.

Genetic Disorders

2

Elaine H. Zackai

Recent studies indicate that 25% to 30% of hospitalized children have genetic conditions. Genetics is particularly important in pediatric practice when an infant or child is malformed with or without serious developmental problems. The parents of such patients want to learn not only about cause and treatment, but risks to other children in their present and future family. Genetic screening is an expanding form of preventive medicine, a traditional concern of the pediatrician. In order to decide who should be screened, the physician needs to understand the genetic risks of specific population groups. We now realize that many people with relatively high risk of bearing children with specific genetic diseases may not have an affected relative.

Counseling the families of children affected with heritable diseases should involve the pediatrician or family physician primarily responsible for the care of such patients. Their intimate knowledge of and continuing relationship with these families are unique assets of this type of health care.

Categories of Clinical Genetic Problems

Mendelian—Autosomal or X-linked
Chromosomal—Sex (X or Y) chromosome or autosome
Polygenic
Non-genetic

GENETIC COUNSELING OF PATIENTS WITH BIRTH DEFECTS

Genetic counseling is an attempt to help the family understand a disease problem or malformation present in the family and the risk of recurrence of that particular disorder. To do this effectively requires an accurate and specific diagnosis, as well as the ability to place this condition into one of the categories of clinical genetic problems listed below. Some problems may be easy to categorize, for example, when a chromosomal syndrome (Down's syndrome, or mongolism) is recognized and the chromosome analysis (trisomy 21) is confirmatory, or when a mendelian trait is diagnosed both clinically and by the appropriate biochemical analysis (Lesch-Nyhan syndrome with hypoxanthine-guanine phosphoribosyl-transferase [HGPRT] deficiency in the patient's red cells), or the pedigree and pathology support a mendelian mechanism (aqueduct stenosis in X-linked hydrocephalus). More often than not the problem is rare and may not be immediately obvious; if this is the case, all the tools listed below should be used in making the diagnosis.

CLINICAL EVALUATION

(The geneticist refers to the patient as "index case," "proband," or "propositus.") A thorough physical examination should include a dissection of the dysmorphic features of the patient—head shape, evidence of hypo- or hypertelorism, shape and position of ears (see Feingold, 1974, for normative values of these physical parameters), dermatoglyphics of hands and feet. Physical features should be carefully compared with first-degree relatives (both parents and sibs), since many anomalies are dominant traits (*e.g.*, syndactyly, polydactyly, ear lobe anomalies, missing teeth, etc.) and can be diagnostic "red herrings." Appropriate radiologic and pathologic analyses are often required.

Tools Available for Diagnosis of Genetic Conditions

1. Clinical evaluation
2. Pedigree analysis
3. Literature search
4. Special laboratory procedures

Family Analysis

Family history should include a complete pedigree with a record of abortions (and the length of gestation of abortions), both normal and abnormal persons in the generations of the index case, the parents and grandparents. Evidence of consanguinity should be specifically asked for as well as the ethnic origin of parents. Rare genetic disorders are more common in certain population groups (*e.g.*, Ellis-van Creveld syndrome in the Amish). Rare autosomal traits are more likely to be homozygous if there is a common ancestor.

Literature Search

Armed with information obtained by physical examination and family analysis, the literature must be screened for evidence that similar malformations have been observed in other index cases. A number of compendia of malformation syndromes is now available in both book and computerized forms (see Bibliography at end of chapter). The latter method produces a differential diagnosis for a particular constellation of physical findings with references to pertinent literature for the various diagnostic entities.

Laboratory Studies

Although specific entities may be suggested by the above analysis of the problem with appropriate laboratory analysis (*e.g.*, a specific enzyme analysis), more often the laboratory must be used as a screening activity. Chromosomal analysis, biochemical screening (urine and blood amino acid, organic acid, urine mucopolysaccharides, etc.) may produce evidence of a diagnosis that was not specifically suggested by the clinical presentation. However, the type of laboratory study most likely to be informative can be predicted from the history or history of multiple spontaneous abortions in the first trimester and physical examination (*e.g.*, retardation and 3 or more physical malformations suggest a chromosomal abnormality), while a family history of consanguinity suggests an inborn error of metabolism (autosomal recessive gene disorder).

GENETIC PRINCIPLES APPLIED TO CLINICAL PROBLEMS

The following discussion illustrates how genetics is applied to clinical problems included under the various categories listed previously.

Mendelian Traits

See McKusick's *Mendelian Inheritance in Man* for a compendium of the more than 2000 identified human traits believed to be determined by single genes.

Autosomal. An autosomal trait may be manifested when only one dose of a mutant gene (in the *heterozygous* state) is present. This is referred to as a *dominant trait.* If a disease occurs only when the patient has two doses of the mutant gene (*homozygous* state), it is considered a *recessive disorder.* Both heterozygous and homozygous states may be expressed, but the clinical picture may be different. The homozygote may have a more severe disease than the heterozygote. An example is familial hypercholesterolemia that is associated with lipid-containing skin tumors (xanthomas) and is caused by a defect in a gene that affects the control of cholesterol biosynthesis. The following outline contrasts the manifestations of those who are heterozygous for the defective gene and those who are homozygous for the same mutant gene.

Familial Hypercholesterolemia

Disease in Heterozygotes
- Hypercholesterolemia
  - 300–600 mg/dl in adults
  - 230–500 mg/dl<20 years
- Tendon xanthomas
  - lipid-containing skin tumors
- Coronary heart disease
  - 3rd–6th decade

Disease in Homozygotes
- Profound hypercholesterolemia
  - >500 mg/dl
- Cutaneous planar xanthomas
  - appear before age 10—palms, buttocks, knees, and tendon xanthomas
- Progesssive coronary heart disease
  - death often by 20 years

In contrast to familial hypercholesterolemia, most inborn errors of metabolism in man are caused by autosomal recessive genes. For example, phenylketonuria (PKU) is a defect in the conversion of phenylalanine to tyrosine (phenylalanine hydroxylase). Children with PKU are usually mentally retarded unless phenylalanine is sharply restricted from early infancy. They are homozygous (have a double dose of the mutant gene). Heterozygotes are found to be phenylalanine intolerant: for example, when a load of phenylalanine is administered, it disappears at a slower rate from the blood than it does in persons who do not carry this gene.

Dominant traits are frequently puzzling in terms of pedigree analysis because of their variation in clinical expression. *Penetrance* refers to the situation in which the gene is not expressed at all in the person, but is certainly present by virtue of the transmission of the disease to offspring who manifest (express) the disorder. Single dominant traits often have several forms of expression, referred to as *pleiotrophy*. Waardenburg's syndrome illustrates these principles. Families with this dominant trait usually come to clinical attention because of congenital deafness in several members of the family. Figure 2-1 is the pedigree of a family with this gene disorder; deafness is not expressed in many members of this family who are carrying the gene. However, it is clear that they are carrying the gene because they have children who are deaf. The gene might be considered "nonpenetrant" in those persons who are not deaf, if deafness were the only expression of the gene. However, the gene results in a syndrome the expressions of which are listed in Table 2-1. The various expressions are the *pleiotrophic traits* of this gene and nearly all persons carrying the gene have at least one expression—broad nasal bridge, lateral displacement of the inner canthus, and so forth.

Diagnosis of this particular syndrome demands clinical skill; it does little good to look at a child and comment on his "odd" or "funny-looking" or "dysmorphic" appearance. However, a description of a widened nasal root and lateral displacement of the inner canthus, along with a test of hearing,

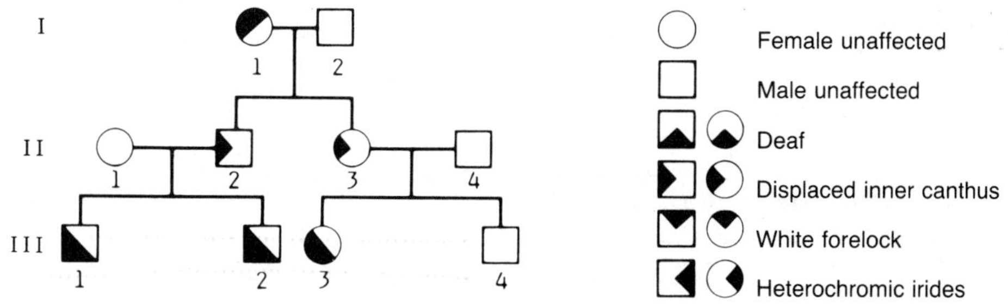

Fig. 2-1. Waardenburg's syndrome.

can prove diagnostic *if* the parents and siblings are also carefully examined. The father may well have the same facies, for example, anomalies of the midface, but normal hearing (II-2, Fig. 2-1), or he may have other expressions of Waardenburg's syndrome such as heterochromia of the irides. With this information about the syndrome, it is clear how to counsel this family in terms of explaining the mechanism of inheritance and the risk of recurrence. The pediatrician with an epidemiologic orientation would advise the parents how other children such as first cousins might also be affected by the disorder. (A first cousin, III-3, of the index case in Fig. 2-1 was labeled mentally retarded until the diagnosis in the index case led to the realization that deafness was responsible for that child's "retardation.")

X-linked Traits. An X-linked trait is transmitted from an unaffected carrier mother to her son when the trait is recessive. A number of pathologically important genes has been localized to the X-chromosome (*e.g.*, those for coagulation factors, deficiencies of which lead to hemophilia A and B, respectively; HGPRT [hypoxanthine-guanine phosphoribosyl transferase] deficiency that leads to the Lesch-Nyhan syndrome [ataxia, self-mutilation, and overproduction of uric acid], and ornithine carbamyl synthetase deficiency, a fatal liver dysfunction with hyperammonemia.) With the exception of the last example, where the female heterozygous for the mutant gene is affected (although she may not have a fatal disease), the other conditions are only expressed in the hemizygous male whose one X-chromosome carries the mutant gene. The heterozygous female is clinically unaffected, even though specific biochemical analysis often can reveal a partial defect.

An example of an X-linked recessive trait that is expressed as a congenital malformation is a particular form of hydrocephalus. Most hydrocephalus is unexplained, while noncommunicating hydrocephalus due to stenosis of the aqueduct of Sylvius occurs in families with the pattern of an X-linked recessive trait (Fig. 2-2). Infants with this disorder often devolop such massive head

TABLE 2-1. Waardenburg's Syndrome: Frequency of Clinical Features

Clinical Features	Percentage
Lateral displacement of inner canthi	99
Broad and high nasal bridge	78
Medial hyperplasia eyebrows	45
White forelock	17
Partial or complete loss of pigment in the iris	25
Congenital deafness	20

enlargement before birth that vaginal delivery is not possible.

There is a form of X-linked mental retardation in which affected males have been noted to have an X-chromosome marker. It is estimated that one-third of families with X-linked retardation are affected with fragile X syndrome. The X-chromosome marker has been described as a constriction near the end of the long arm resulting in a small knob separated by a thin stalk from the main portion of the chromosome. It is detectable when partially deficient growth media is used in chromosome culture.

Some males with the fragile X syndrome have a few subtle phenotypic features, the most characteristic being enlargement of the testes to several times the normal size. Next to trisomy 21, the fragile X syndrome is thought to be the most common of the causes of mental retardation that can be specifically diagnosed.

Chromosomal Disorders

Chromosomal *aneuploidy* usually refers to the state when the chromosome number is greater or less than the *euploid* number of 46. The chromosome involved may be one of the 22 pairs of autosomes or the sex chromosome pair (XX in the female and XY in the male). Structural rearrangements also occur that may alter the amount of genetic information without changing the chromosome number.

The chromosomes of a large number of newborn infants have been examined in recent years. Studies performed in several centers throughout the world have obtained similar results, which are summarized in Table 2-2. Approximately 1/200 newborns have chromosomal abnormalities and about half involve sex chromosomes. A newborn with physical anomalies has about a 4% chance of having a chromosome aberration.

The autosomal trisomies that are

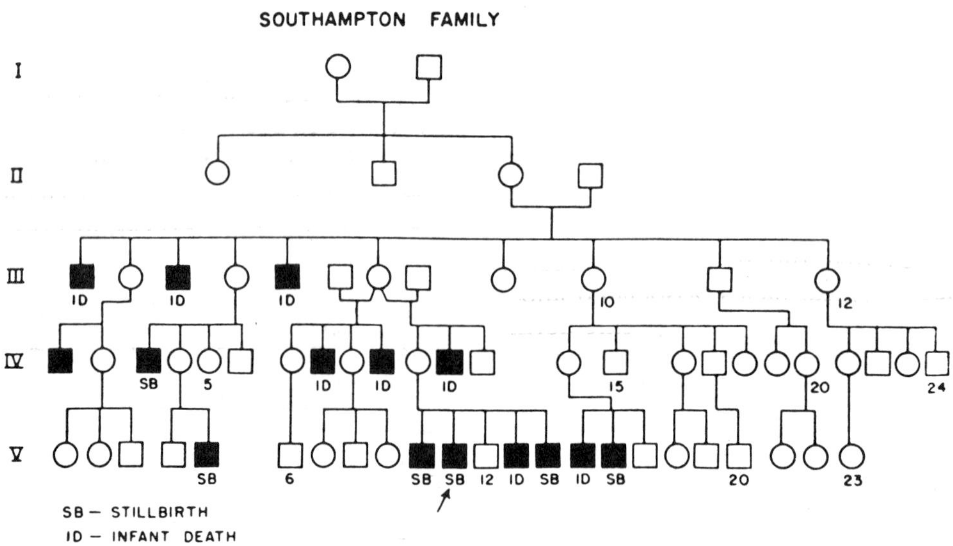

Fig. 2-2. X-linked hydrocephalus. (Darkened boxes denote hydrocephalus, ID denotes infant death, and SB denotes stillbirth.) (Edwards JH, Norman RM, Roberts JM: Sex linked hydrocephalus. Report of a family with 15 affected members. Arch Dis Child *36*:481, 1961)

TABLE 2-2. Newborn Surveys

Sex Chromosome Abnormality		Number	Frequency (%)
Females	XO	2	
	XXX	13	
	Other	5	
Total		20	.13
Males	XYY	26	
	XXY	30	
	Other	17	
Total		73	.26
Autosomal Abnormality			
Structural rearrangements			
Euploid		81	.19
Aneuploid		21	.05
Total		102	
Trisomies			
13		3	
18		4	
21		45	
Other		2	
Total		54	.12
Total		249	.57

Total: 43,558 (28,582 males, 14,976 females)

found regularly among liveborn infants are trisomy 13,18, and 21. Syndromes ascribed to the various autosomal trisomies are reasonably specific. Table 2-3 lists their features. The clinical diagnosis of these trisomies requires that the physician be able to recognize a typical facies, associated anomalies of the extremities, and specific dermatoglyphic features (particularly with trisomies 18 and 21).

Trisomy 21 is the most common autosomal disorder in clinical medicine. It is responsible for the syndrome currently called Down's syndrome, known for over a century as mongolism. Down's syndrome is usually a sporadic error in gametogenesis that causes trisomy 21 in a single affected fetus of the involved couple. Occasionally the extra chromosome is present as part of a compound or "translocated chromosome" (3.5% of all patients), most commonly translocated with another small acrocentric (G group) chromosome (56% of translocations) or a large acrocentric (D group) chromosome (44% of translocations). Such "translocation mongols" have 46 chromosomes, yet have the extra chromosomal material to account for the trisomy 21 syndrome. Some translocation trisomies are the consequence of the carrier state in one of the parents (for DG translocations, 49% are inherited, for G/G—5.6%). In such cases, there is a significant recurrence risk to that particular couple and their relatives who might also be carriers of the translocation. (D/G father = 2.4% risk of affected offspring.)

Trisomy 21 (as well as other trisomies, XXY and XXX) occurs more frequently

TABLE 2-3. Features of Autosomal Trisomies 13, 18, and 21

Disorder	Clinical Manifestations	
Trisomy 13	Developmental retardation	
	Facies	
	Microcephaly—sloping forehead (holoprosencephaly type brain defect)	
	Microphthalmia	
	Cleft lip and palate	
	Low-set malformed ears	
	Extremities	
	Polydactyly of hands and feet	
	Rocker bottom feet	
	Position anomaly of fingers—flexed with overlapping index over third	
	Cardiac	
	Abnormality in 80%	
	Renal	
	Polycystic kidneys in 31% (and other malformations—hydronephrosis, horseshoe kidney, duplicated ureters)	
Trisomy 18	Developmental retardation—difficulty feeding, poor suck, low birth weight	
	Facies	
	Prominent occiput	
	Low-set malformed ears	
	Small mouth	
	Micrognathia	
	Extremities	
	Rocker-bottom feet	
	Position anomaly of fingers—flexed with overlapping index over third	
	Dermatoglyphics	
	Simple arches on 6 or more digits >80%	
	Cardiac	
	VSD, PDA >95%	
	Renal	
	Renal malformation—horseshoe kidney, hydronephrosis, hydroureter	
Trisomy 21	Developmental retardation, hypotonia	
	Facies	
	Flattened facies	
	Flat occiput	
	Oblique palpebral fissures	
	Epicanthal folds	
	Brushfield spots	
	Protruding tongue	
	Excess skin nape of neck (infants)	
	Three fontanels (infants)	
	Ears—small, boxlike configuration	
	Extremities	
	Short broad fingers	hands
	Clinodactyly	hands
	Transverse palmar crease	hands
	Increased space 1st & 2nd toes	
	Dermatoglyphics	
	Distal axial triradii—palm	
	Ulnar loops—digits	
	Open field—hallucal area	
	Heart	
	Cardiac abnormality in 35% of cases (most common—endocardial cushion defect)	

in the offspring of women of advanced child-bearing age. Figure 2-3 indicated the relative risk at varying maternal ages for trisomy 21. Even though the relative risks are significantly greater for women over 35, the absolute number of pregnancies are distributed by maternal age in such a way that more than half the infants with trisomy 21 are born to women under 35. Translocation trisomies are less common among the offspring of women over 35 years. *Mosaicism* refers to the situation in which there are two (or more) populations of cells with different chromosome compositions. *Mosaic mongolism* usually refers to patients who have a proportion of cells with trisomy 21 and a proportion with the normal number of chromosomes.

The clinical expression of trisomy 21 is highly variable in terms of physical and mental development. Adults with trisomy 21 have a wide range of IQs, although the range is considerably below that of a normal population. The distribution of IQs of mosaic mongols tends to be closer to that of the general population, even though it is rare for persons in this group to have a "normal IQ."

Dermatoglyphics. The dermal ridge patterns that are formed in early embryonic life vary considerably owing to differences that are inherited, disturbances in

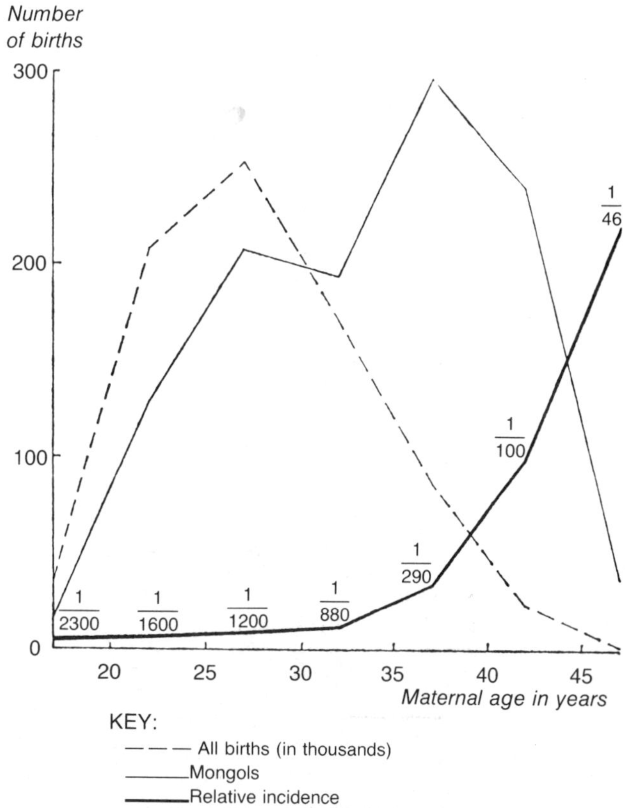

Fig. 2-3. Incidence at birth. (Colman RD, Staller A: Am J Public Health *52*:813, 1962)

the normal differentiation of the peripheral limb buds (such as the influences of intrauterine infections like rubella), and chromosome abnormalities. The *distal phalanges* have a variety of dermal ridge patterns that can be classified into three major patterns—arches, whorls, and loops (Fig. 2-4). The occurrence of *arches* on eight or more digits would be a rare event, yet in trisomy 18 this is the usual finding. The *palmar* patterns usually are absent or small in the hypothenar area, the ulnar portion of the proximal palm. When the pattern is large, a junction pattern (triradius or delta) formed by the hypothenar, thenar, and distal palmar patterns occurs in the middle third of the palm along an axis that passes through the fourth digit and the middle of the wrist. This *distal palmar axial triradius* (Fig. 2-5) is found in 75% of patients with trisomy 21 and in less than 3.5% of control subjects. In the foot there is a pattern in the dermal pad at the base of the great toe. In 50% of patients with trisomy 21 there is a simple arch pattern in the hallucal region (Fig. 2-6) that is found in less than 1% of control subjects. This unusual dermal pattern in the foot of patients with trisomy 21 is associated with hypoplasia of the hallucal pad and a wide space between the great and second toes.

Sex Chromosome Aneuploidy. Even though sex chromosome aneuploidy occurs more frequently than trisomy 21, it is less appreciated as a clinical problem. XXY and XYY occur in male newborns at a combined incidence of about 1/400; XXX and XO occur in female newborns at a com-

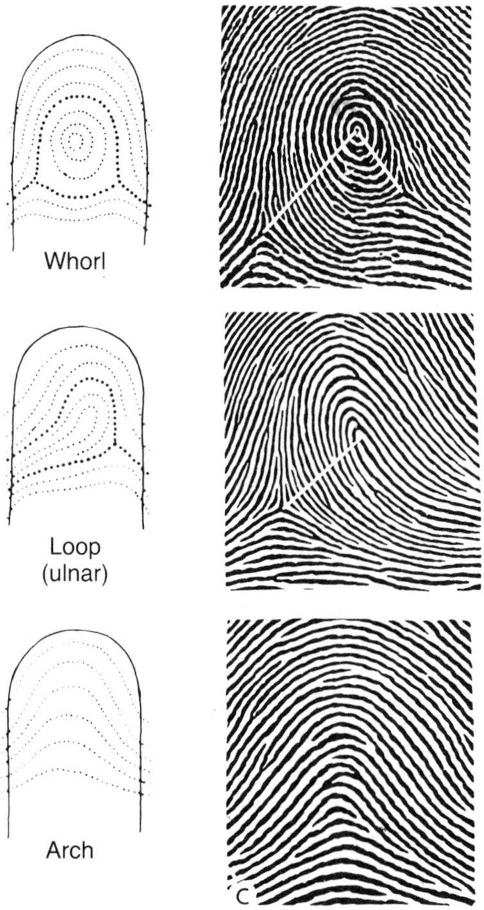

Fig. 2-4. The three dermal ridge patterns—whorl, loop, and arch. (Holt S: The genetics of dermal ridges. Br Med Bull *17*:247, 1961)

bined incidence of 1/800. The clinical significance of XYY and XXX is still poorly defined, but appear to be associated with learning and perhaps behavioral disorders.

Klinefelter's (XXY) and Turner's (XO) syndromes are summarized in Table 2-4. Both syndromes should be recognized so that appropriate hormonal therapy can be instituted. For the former there is still controversy as to when and how androgen therapy should be administered, and its influence on the general psychological and social mal-

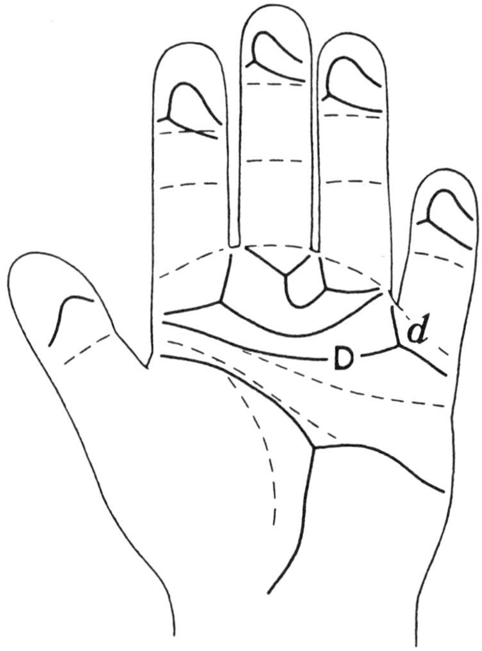

Fig. 2-5. Distal palmar axial triradius. (Holt S: The Genetics of Dermal Ridges. Springfield, Ill, Charles C Thomas, 1968)

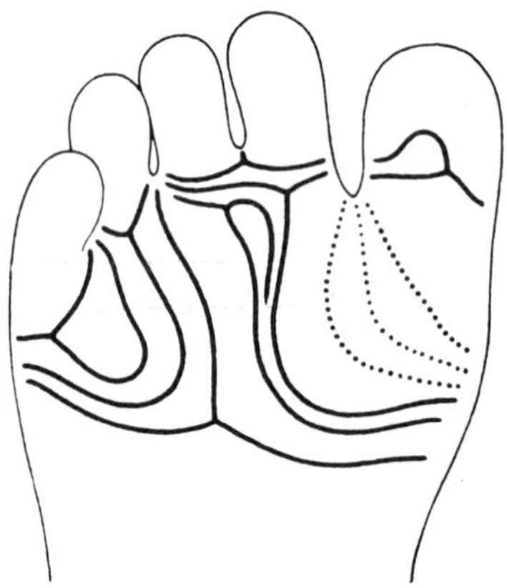

Fig. 2-6. Hallucal area—simple arch pattern (open fields). (Holt S: The Genetics of Dermal Ridges. Springfield, Ill, Charles C Thomas, 1968)

adjustments commonly found with XXY. Turner's syndrome patients need estrogen therapy to artificially stimulate sexual maturation and menarche. Because of the slow linear growth of these patients from infancy, early diagnosis is important to avoid unnecessary anxiety and diagnostic activity. Infertility is a manifestation of both syndromes.

TABLE 2-4. Differentiating Features of Klinefelter's and Turner's Syndromes

Syndrome	Clinical Features

XXY (Klinefelter)	Buccal smear chromatin positive
	Phenotype
	  External and internal male ductal system
	Hypogonadism (<2 cm diameter postpubertal testes)
	  Firm to palpation
	  Biopsy—hyalinization and hypoplasia of seminiferous tubules
	Azospermia (90%)
	Gynecomastia (25–40%)
	  Secondary development—variable (completely normal to infantile)
	Height
	  Taller than average
	  Decreased U/L segment ratio
	Intelligence
	  Variable (normal to moderate retardation)
	Behavioral abnormalities
	  Lack of goal orientation
	  Social ineptness
	  Poor school performance
	  Speech difficulty

XO (Turner)	Buccal smear chromatin negative
	Phenotype
	  Female
	  Absence of definitive gonad ("streak ovaries")
	  Infantile uterus in presence of female external genitalia
	Lack of secondary sex characteristics
	Primary amenorrhea
	Height
	  Short stature (mean adult height 55 in.)
	  Birth length below 18.5 in.
	Normal intelligence
	Variable findings
	  Shield chest
	  Congenital lymphedema
	  Low posterior hairline
	  High arched palate
	  Hyperconvex nails
	  Cubitus valgus
	  Webbed neck
	  Pigmented nevi
	  Small mandible
	  Short 4th metacarpal
	  Renal anomaly
	  Cardiac anomaly (coarctation of aorta most frequent)

Polygenic Inheritance

Polygenic inheritance is perhaps the most difficult category of inherited disorders to explain mechanistically. Since a significant proportion of inherited congenital malformations is included in this class of disorders, it cannot be neglected. The genetic principles involved are based solidly on scientific evidence in both humans and experimentally bred animals. There are several genetic factors that determine an individual fetus's susceptibility to a number of specific malformations (*e.g.*, cleft lip, neural tube defects, congenital hip dislocation, hypertrophic pyloric stenosis). This susceptibility has a continuous distribution in the general population and the factors involved determine this susceptibility. Persons with certain hereditary endowments may exceed the "threshold" of susceptibility, but this threshold may also be exceeded by environmental influences that shift an individual's position in the susceptibility distribution. Relatives of affected persons also have a range of susceptibility similar to the general population but the mean susceptibility is greater than that of the general population. The more distantly related a peson is to an affected subject, the more his risk approaches that of the general population (see Fig. 2-7). This same theory of polygenic inheritance also applies to height and IQ (*e.g.*, relatives of tall or very intelligent persons have a greater "risk" than the general population of being tall or very intelligent; the converse is true for shortness

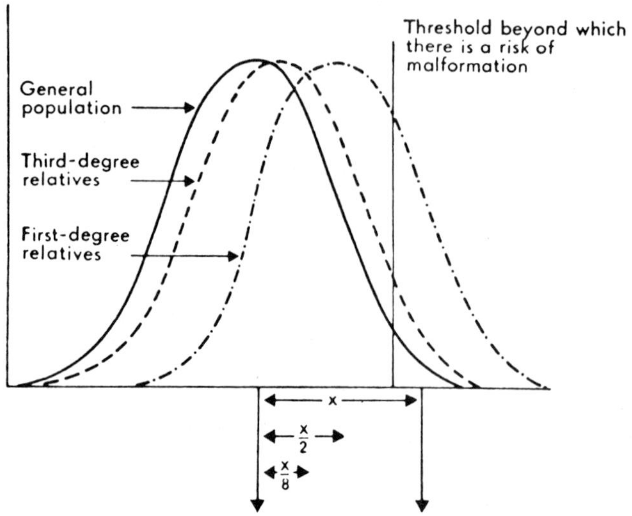

Fig. 2-7. Model for polygenic inheritance of cleft lip, with or without cleft palate. (Carter CO: Genetics of common disorders. Br Med Bull *25*:52, 1969)

and lower intelligence). This "threshold theory" can account for the observed risks to relatives of different degrees—grandparents, aunts, and uncles—and to malformations believed to be polygenically inherited. (See Table 2-5 for empiric risk of cleft lip and cleft palate to various degrees of relatives.)

Although most occurrences of cleft lip are based on a polygenically inherited mechanism with 3% to 5% risk of recurrence to parents of an affected child, cleft lip can be one of the findings in a child with multiple malformations. Careful classification of these multiple malformations may lead to a previously described syndrome. A syndrome is a grouping of congenital malformations that show a "tendency to run together" and have a uniform etiology. Once a syndrome has been identified it should be examined in terms of the principles outlined under catagories of Clinical Genetic Problems (mendelian trait, chromosomal disorders, polygenic disorder, nongenetic). The family can then be properly counseled with information based on previously reported cases and, when available, etiologic factors.

Nongenetic Causes of Congenital Anomalies

Nongenetic congenital anomalies are almost certainly manifold even though the identified ones are few; included are congenital infections (rubella, cytomegaloinclusion disease, syphilis, toxoplasmosis) and teratogenic drugs (aminopterin, thalidomide). Other drugs inspire less confidence. Anticonvulsant drugs are currently highly suspected (diphenylhydantoin, trimethadione). There are problems in incriminating drugs as teratogens: two are the relatively high incidence of malformations in random pregnancies (Table 2-6) and the near certainty that teratogenic drugs only cause problems in a proportion of fetuses. These differences in susceptibility to potential teratogens may well be genetic, either at the maternal or fetal level of response to the drug. As pharmacogeneticists develop more data on individual responses to drugs and other environmental agents, there may well be an improved understanding of why one fetus is damaged by certain drugs taken by the

TABLE 2-5. Risk of Cleft Lip and Cleft Palate

Risk in	Cleft Lip with or without Cleft Palate
General Population	0.001
Monozygotic twins	×400
First-degree relatives (siblings, parents, offspring)	× 40
Second-degree relatives (aunts, uncles, nieces, nephews, grandchildren)	× 7
Third-degree relatives (first cousins)	× 3

mother, while another is unaffected by the same agents. With such insights, the category of "nongenetic" may well be changed to "environmental with genetic predisposition."

Alcohol in heavy usage is now thought of as a teratogen. It has been estimated that the risk of a problem to offspring (full or partial fetal alcohol syndrome) of chronic alcoholics is 30% to 50%. The strongest relationship between maternal drinking and fetal outcome seems to exist in the month preceding recognition of pregnancy.

Fetal alcohol syndrome is made up of a triad of diagnostic findings: facial abnormalities, growth deficiency, and mental retardation. Facial findings include small head circumference, low nasal bridge, epicanthal folds, short palpebral fissures, short nose, small midface, indistinct philtrum, and thin upper lip. There is prenatal growth deficiency with little postnatal catch-up growth. Most children have had significant mental handicaps in the mild-to-moderate range.

The effect of social drinking or binge drinking on the fetus is not clear at this time.

RECURRENCE RISKS

Once a patient's condition has been diagnosed and classified accurately, parents can be provided with specific risk rates for certain disorders, for example, 25% for autosomal recessive disorders, 50% for males when the mother carries an X-linked recessive trait, 50% for autosomal dominant disorders with an affected parent, 3% to 5% for cleft lip and palate, anencephaly, meningomyelocele, and other polygenic disorders when sib is affected, 10% for offspring of women with a D/G translocation, 2.5% for offspring of men with the same translocation. Often specific risk cannot be ascribed. In other situations, there may be no specific risks to the family seeking counsel (*e.g.*, "sporadic" translocation mongolism with chromosomally normal parents and achondroplasia with normal parents; therefore, the index case is the result of a fresh dominant mutation). Risks may be those of the general population (1/100 for a woman of 39 who is concerned that her infant may be born with trisomy 21 and who bore a child with this condition at age 35).

TABLE 2-6. Malformations in Random Pregnancies

Genetic Problem	Newborns Afflicted (%)
Congenital malformations (polygenic disorders)	2–2.5
Chromosomal abnormalities	2.5
Single gene disorders	< .1
	2.5–3

Prenatal diagnosis can now be used to identify some disorders of an affected or unaffected fetus by removing amniotic fluid after the 14th week of gestation. Conditions that can be diagnosed from amniotic fluid study's are listed below (biochemical assay, chromosome analysis, α-fetoprotein determination). In addition, maternal serum fetoprotein is a useful screening test for neural tube defects in low-risk population.

Amniotic Fluid Study for Prenatal Diagnosis

Chromosome disorders
- Indications
  - Familial translocation
  - Advanced maternal age
  - Previous trisomy

Biochemical disorders
- Inborn errors—specific biochemical diagnosis is possible in over 60 disorders
- Hemoglobinopathies—detectable using recombinant DNA methodology
- Hemophilia—detectable through Factor VIII/Factor VIII antigen (measured in blood, obtained through fetoscopy)

Neural tube defects (anencephaly, meningomyelocele)

X-linked disorders—determination of sex of the fetus by chromosome analysis.
The male has a 50% chance of being affected.
Not a diagnostic test for a specific X-linked disorder in most cases (exception—hemophilia; see above)

SCREENING THE FAMILIES OF PATIENTS WITH GENETIC DISORDERS

Thus far we have been dealing with the propositus (affected patient) and the risk of recurrence in his future siblings. The scope of the pediatrician should extend beyond the nuclear family to include other relatives who may have a greater risk of bearing affected offspring than the general population.

Chromosome Translocations

Many people with mental retardation and dysmorphic features have been identified as having unbalanced translocations, that is extra or missing portions of the chromosomes involved in the translocation. With the advent of specialized chromosome banding techniques (Giemsa and fluorescent banding), the specificity of these anomalies has improved dramatically, and, therefore, many new "partial trisomy" syndromes are being described. In most instances, one parent of a patient is then detected as the balanced carrier. The transmission of translocations in the balanced form may resemble that of a dominant trait. Siblings and cousins of a translocation-bearing parent may be carriers also and susceptible to the production of a chromosomally abnormal fetus. Once these "at risk" carrier individuals have been identified, prenatal diagnosis of the chromosomally unbalanced fetus can be offered. For example, a severely retarded dysmorphic proband was identified as trisomic for the distal part of long arm of chromosome 10 (46, XY, −17, +t) (17p:10q) (see Fig. 2-8A). His mother is a balanced carrier for the translocation which involved the short arm of chromosome 17 and long arm of chromosome 10 (17p:10q−) (Fig. 2-8B and C). This balanced translocation was traced through three generations of this family (Fig. 2-9). The proband's fourth cousin, also severely retarded with a strikingly similar dysmorphia, had the same unbalanced translocation.

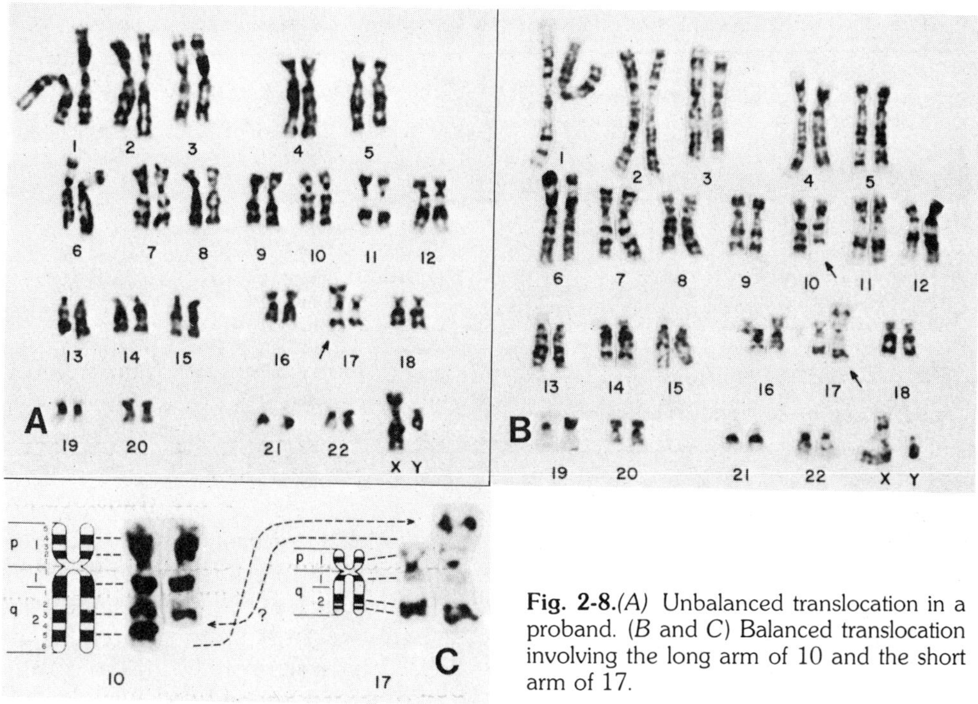

Fig. 2-8. *(A)* Unbalanced translocation in a proband. (*B* and *C*) Balanced translocation involving the long arm of 10 and the short arm of 17.

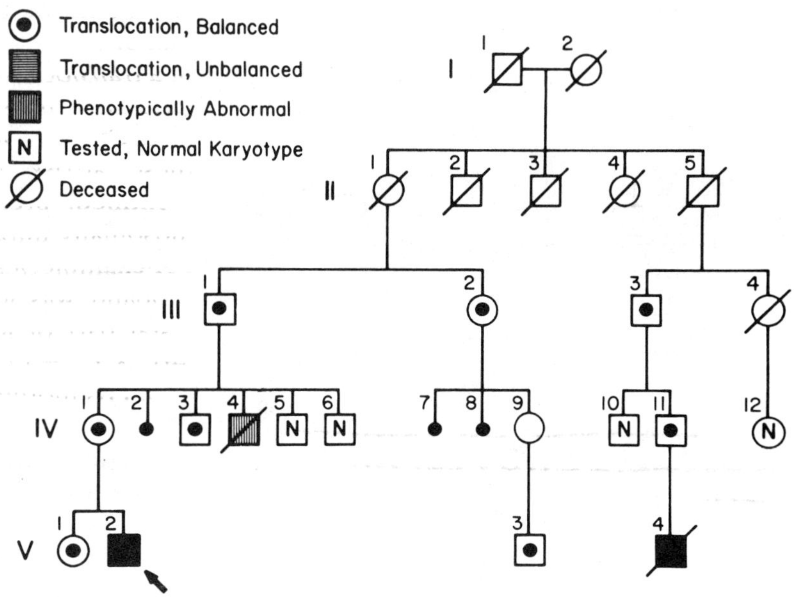

Fig. 2-9. Familial translocation 10q:17p. Note unbalanced 4th cousins V2 & V4.

TABLE 2-7. Frequency of Disease with Gene and Carrier Frequency

Disease and Ethnic Group	Estimated Incidence of Homozygotes Among Newborns	Population Gene Frequency	Population Carrier Frequency
Cystic fibrosis (Northern Europeans)	1:2500	1 in 50	1 in 25
Sickle-cell anemia (Blacks)	1:600	1 in 25	1 in 12
Tay-Sachs (Ashkenazic Jews)	1:3600	1 in 60	1 in 30
β thalassemia (Greeks, Italians)	1:3600	1 in 60	1 in 30
Phenylketonuria	1:11,500	1 in 100	1 in 50
Maple syrup urine disease	1:200,000	1 in 450	1 in 225
Homocystinuria	1:230,000	1 in 480	1 in 240
Galactosemia	1:187,171	1 in 435	1 in 218

Family Risks for Autosomal Recessive Disorders

The special risk for families in which the proband has a rare autosomal recessive disease should be considered when caring for a diseased patient. The gene frequency of a rare trait in the population is surprisingly common. It can be calculated by estimating the frequency of the disease (persons homozygous for the gene) and determining its square root. Carrier frequency is twice the gene frequency since, for autosomal genes, two loci are involved. Table 2-7 compares the frequency of some diseases with their gene and carrier frequencies in the population. The parents are almost certainly carriers of rare diseases. Their siblings have a 50% risk of also being carriers; uncles and aunts 25%, and first cousins, 12½%. Spouses of these relatives, unless related by blood (consanguinous), have the same probability of being carriers as the general population. Based on these probabilities, the risk of close relatives producing offspring diseased with rare recessive conditions is usually small but often more likely than in the general population (see Table 2-8). This information demonstrates why physicians with an epidemiologic orientation to health care should be able to estimate the risk and be alert to the diagnosis in relatives other than the siblings of an affected person (*e.g.*, first cousins of patients with phenylketonuria, Tay-Sach's disease, sickle-cell anemia are much more likely to be affected with these diseases than random persons in the population).

TABLE 2-8. Risk to Offspring for Phenylketonuria

Population at Risk	Risk Ratio
General population	~1:10,000
Parents of affected	1:4
Siblings of carriers	1:400
Uncles and aunts of carrier	1:800
First cousins of carrier	1:1600

SPECIAL POPULATIONS AT RISK OTHER THAN RELATIVES OF AFFECTED PATIENTS

In addition to being "proband-oriented," the pediatrician must realize that he may be dealing with many people who do not have an affected relative yet are at a relatively high risk of bearing children with specific genetic diseases. Genetic screening or preproband identification of the at-risk person or family is an expanding form of preventive medicine. This involves the identification and screening of high-risk subpopulations. One such subpopulation discussed earlier is women over the age of 35 who have a substantially greater risk relative to younger women of bearing children with nondisjunctional chromosomal aberrations (especially Down's syndrome; Fig. 2-3). The counseling of this population as to risk and availability of prenatal diagnosis is a key in the prevention of such disease.

Various subpopulations have high carrier frequencies of specific recessive traits that are rare in the general population (see Table 2-7 for ethnic group) and high frequencies of specific gene abnormalities. The identification of carriers within these high-risk subpopulations, identification of at-risk couples, genetic counseling, and in some instances prenatal diagnosis (Tay-Sachs disease) is another aspect of preventive medicine within the scope of the genetically oriented physician.

BIBLIOGRAPHY

Bergsma D: Birth Defects: Atlas and Compendium, 2nd ed. Baltimore, Williams & Wilkins, 1979

Carter CO: Multifactorial genetic disease. In McKusick VA, Claiborne R (eds): Medical Genetics, p 199. New York, Hospital Practice, 1973

Feingold M, Bassert W: Normal values for selected physical parameters. An aid to syndrome delineation. In Birth Defects—Original Article Series Vol. Y, No. 13, 1974

Gerald P: X-linked mental retardation and an X chromosome marker. N Engl J Med 303:696, 1980

Holt S: The Genetics of Dermal Ridges. Springfield, Ill, Charles C Thomas, 1968

Lewandowski RC, Yunis J: New chromosomal syndromes. Am J Dis Child 129:515, 1975

McKusick VA: Mendelian Inheritance in Man, 5th ed. Baltimore, Johns Hopkins Press, 1975

A useful catalogue from which one is able to learn the pattern of inheritance of all known genetic disorders. In addition, it gives a summary of the disease entity with pertinent references.

Polin R, Mennuti M: Genetic disease in the neonate. In Fanaroff A, Martin R (eds): Behrman's Neonatal-Perinatal Medicine 2nd ed. St. Louis, CV Mosby, 1977

The section on Prenatal Genetic Disease is an excellent overview of the subject.

Rimoin DL, Schimke RN: Genetic Forms of Hypogonadism in Phenotypic Males. Genetic Disorders of the Endocrine Glands. St Louis, CV Mosby, 1971

Smith DW: Recognizable Patterns of Human Malformation; Genetic Embryologic and Clinical Aspects, 2nd ed, Philadelphia, WB Saunders, 1976

Stanbury JB, Wyngaarden JB, Fredrickson DS (eds): Metabolic Basis of Inherited Disease, 4th ed. New York, McGraw-Hill, 1978

Excellent coverage of all inborn errors of metabolism from a biochemical and genetic viewpoint.

Streissguth A, Landesman-Dwyer S *et al*: Teratogenic effect of alcohol in humans and laboratory animals. Science 209:353, 1980

Thompson JS, Thompson MW: Genetics in Medicine, 3rd ed. Philadelphia, WB Saunders, 1980

Written for the student in medicine with a brief discussion of genetics and emphasis on clinical problems.

Warkany J: Congenital Malformations. Chicago, Year Book Medical Publishers, 1971

Complete discussion of all birth defects from historical, embryologic, and etiologic viewpoints. Good discussions of familial patterns and risk of recurrence.

Warkany J: Syndromes. Am J Dis Child 121:365, 1971

Motor and Intellectual Development

3

David Baker
Peter W. Vanace

PRINCIPLES OF CHILD DEVELOPMENT

Development is a dynamic process that begins with fertilization and is molded by the interaction of genetic and environmental influences. Although genetic factors may be viewed as setting upper limits to development, bioenvironmental factors figure powerfully in the expression of genetic influences and also may cause injury to the central nervous system and to somatic systems as well. In addition to these biologic factors, socioenvironmental and emotional factors play a major role in determining the outcome of development.

Development follows a dynamic sequential pattern with the timetable varying not only in normal versus abnormal persons, but also reflecting individual differences among children. The newborn, equipped with innate instinctive reflex responses, develops in a pattern of cephalocaudal and proximodistal progression of function. The massive diffuse responses of the newborn become more differentiated with progressive myelination and inhibition from higher centers. Intersensory and sensorimotor integration emerge while synaptic connections are elaborated in the association cortex.

Genetic Factors

Genetic factors that influence development operate through a wide continuum including, on one extreme, conditions in which environmental factors are minimally involved and, on the other extreme, conditions in which environmental factors are necessary to produce clinically evident alterations. Furthermore, because of variable penetrance and expressiveness, a wide spectrum of clinical manifestations may be seen. For example, in a child with neurofibromatosis, severe mental retardation, convulsions, and sensorimotor signs may be seen as one extreme, while other members of the family may have cutaneous lesions only.

There are four types of genetic disorders: (1) single gene defects transmitted by recessive or dominant inheritance (recessive disorders are related to inborn errors of metabolism [enzyme defects], and may be autosomal or sex-linked; dominant genetic conditions are related to structural malformations); (2) polygenic defects resulting in familial retardation; (3) chromosome defects transmitted on autosomal or sex chromosomes; and (4) congenital malformations in which there is an empirical high risk of recurrence. These include meningomyelocele (neural tube defects) and some cases of hydrocephalus. Some genetic disorders become clinically evident only after birth (such as PKU), when the maternal metabolism is no longer available to metabolize the neurotoxic substance.

A careful family history, noting consanguinity especially, is of extreme importance. Laboratory tests necessary to ascertain genetic disorders are: (1) metabolic screening tests, (2) buccal smears and karyotypes,

(3) enzyme studies, (4) dermatoglyphics, and (5) amniocentesis and examination of amniotic fluid for specific risk situations.

Environmental Factors

The environment exerts an influence that extends from preconception through pregnancy (intrauterine environment) and continues postnatally. The infant who has an intact central nervous system and is exposed to a nurturing, stimulating environment should grow and develop normally. Defects in development, then, may be caused by impairment of the primary neural apparatus, to maturational lag, or to an unfavorable environment. The normal infant reaches out to explore his environment and thus develops a sense of reality and mastery of tasks. Motility plays a vital part in development of the learning process.

Environmental stimulation as well as parental goals and expectations play a powerful role in shaping linguistic, intellectual, emotional, and social functions in preparing the child for school experience (learning readiness). On the other hand, sensory and emotional deprivation (deprivation not only in terms of quantitative reduction of stimuli, but also in the qualitative sense or disordered, chaotic stimulation) may induce varying degrees of retardation which, if sustained early and for a prolonged period, may be irreversible. The child with a *pre-existing* visual, auditory, or neurologic handicap may suffer compounding increments of retardation with still further loss of developmental

TABLE 3-1. Infantile Reflexes and Automatisms

Response	New-born	Age in Months 1	2	3	4	5	6	9	12
Primitive Responses									
Moro	+	+	+	70%	+	±	0	0	0
Rooting and sucking	+	+	+	+	+	+	+	0	0
Palmar grasp	+	+	+	+	+	0	0	0	0
Asymmetric tonic neck	+	+	+	50%	±	±	±	0	0
Plantar grasp	+	+	+	+	+	+	+	0	0
Pacing	+	+	+	+	+	+	+	decreased but persists to 24 months	
Stepping	+	+	+	+	+	0	0	0	0
Supporting reaction	±	50%	+	+	+	+	66% true supporting	100%	
Secondary Responses									
Neck righting reactions									
Head	0	0	+	+	+	+	+	+	+
Body	0	0	0	+	+	+	+	+	+
Body derotative	0	0	0	0	+	+	+	+	+
Body rotative	0	0	0	0	0	0	0	+	+
Parachute reaction									
Downward	0	0	0	0	+	+	+	+	+
Sideways (propping)	0	0	0	0	0	0	+	+	+
Forward	0	0	0	0	0	0	0	+ (at 7 months)	+
Backward	0	0	0	0	0	0	0	+	+
Landau	0	0	0	0	0	0	42%	+	+ to 24 months

TABLE 3-2. Events in Postural and Motor Development

Response	Newborn	Age in Months 1	2	3	4	5
Gross Motor						
Ventral suspension						
Head	hangs down		in plane of body	above body plane		
Extremities	flexor tone		extensor tone			
Prone position						
Head	to one side	lifts chin	midline	chin to 45° and shoulder up	head up 90°; chest up	rolls over prone to supine
Extremities	knees under abdomen			pelvis flat	extension	up on forearms
Sitting; traction from supine	head lag complete			slight head lag		no head lag
Standing and walking	automatic walk; legs flexed	diminished	absent	astasia	legs extend	legs straight
Fine Motor						
Manipulation of hands	grasp reflex; hands closed	grasp reflex	grasp reflex; hands open	diminished grasp reflex;	diminished grasp reflex; reaching	voluntary grasp; puts objects in mouth; bidextrous approach

potential. Hence, this child's handicap should be detected early and he should be stimulated at the earliest possible age.

Normal Development

The traditional treatment, after Gesell, divides development into five basic sectors: (1) gross motor, (2) fine motor, (3) adaptive, (4) speech and language, and (5) personal-social.

This discussion will emphasize selected basic concepts. In the infant, assessment of development is dependent on motor and reflex parameters. Later, language and visual motor perception assume greater relative importance.

Motor Development

Motor development begins *in utero* and proceeds in a predetermined phylogenetic sequence. Although refinement of motor performance and skills continues through and probably beyond adolescence, by approximately 15 months of age all the basic motor movements necessary for the rest of life are established.

Age in Months					
6	9	12	15	18	24
pushes up on hands	crawls backward	bear walk	walking; kneeling		
lifts head from supine; sits propped; rolls over supine to prone at 7 months	sits without support	pivots	seats self in chair		
initial weight bearing	bears full weight; pulls to stand	walks with support at 11 months	walks without support at 13 months	up and down stairs; jumping	backward; runs; kicks ball
palmar grasp radial at 8 months; transfer objects to opposite hand at 7 months	finger to thumb (pincer) grasp releases ± 10 months; unidextrous approach	throws	tower 2-3 cubes	tower 3-4 cubes; removes pellet from bottle; draw a stroke	tower 6-7 cubes; imitates circular stroke

The sequential age range of related motor landmarks from birth to 5 years of age are outlined in Tables 3-1, 3-2, and 3-3. Because of the rapid and extensive process of motor development in the first year, the major emphasis will be focused on this period, and the student is referred to the bibliography for discussion beyond this age.

A full appreciation of normal and dysfunctioning motor development can be acquired from a knowledge of the longitudinal sequence of motor development and understanding the neurophysiologic basis for this orderly sequence of events. The discussion will start with descriptions of development as observed in different positions and be followed by review of the neurophysiologic basis for normal motor development.

In Figure 3-1, motor development from birth through the first year in the prone position is depicted. As the infant develops during the first year of life normal motor development can be determined by careful observation of head-chest, shoulder-elbow, pelvis-hip, and knee positions.

At birth and through the first month of life, the head is held to one side (not extended); the pelvis is held with the knees drawn under the abdomen. The shoulders and elbows are tucked under the chest with a cubital angle of less than 90 degrees.

By the time the infant is 2 months

TABLE 3-3. Developmental Milestones: 2 to 5 Years

Response	Age in Months: 24	36	48	60
Gross Motor	Runs, walks backward Kicks large ball	Steps: Up: alternates feet Balances one foot 2–5 sec	Alternates feet up and down	Skips both feet, alternating
			4–8	8–10
			Hops 2–8 times	9–12
				Skips alternating feet
		Throws ball one hand	Overhand throw	
		Rides tricycle	Catches ball	
Fine Motor	Cubes: tower of 6–7	9–10	Copies bridge	Copies gate
		Imitates bridge	Imitates gate	Serial finger to thumb sequencing movements; holds pencil in mature fashion
Adaptive	Inserts square block in performance board	Repeats 3 digits Matches 3 colors	Counts 3 objects	Counts to 10
	Imitates vertical stroke	Copies circle Imitates cross	Copies a cross	Copies square Knows morning, afternoon
Language:				
Vocabulary	200-300 words	900	1500 words	2000
Sentence Length	2 words	3 words	4 words	5 words
Articulation	Repetitions	90% intelligible		100% initelligible
Comprehension & syntax	Obeys one directional preposition* and 2 commands Identifies familiar objects	Uses we, us, you, I; 3 prepositions; names objects	Size labels. Numbers 1,2,3, and all; obeys 3 commands	4 prepositions Describes a picture
Personal-social	Improved feeding; pulls on simple garment; mimics domestic tasks	Knows own name & sex; feeds self; unbuttons	Washes and dries face; brushes teeth, laces shoes	Dressing self-sufficient
	Parallel play	Associative play	Cooperative play	Tells fanciful tales; plays games
Vision	Convergence-accommodation weak; may develop esotropia	V.A. 20/40. Test with Sjogren Hand Card, Illiterate E chart, STYCAR or Allen picture card test; Denver eye screening test	20/30	True stereopsis & color perception Tests with + lens for hyperopia
Developmental Neurologic Signs				After 5, spooning of outstretched fingers is abnormal; can identify bilateral simultaneous visual stimuli

*"On" or "under".

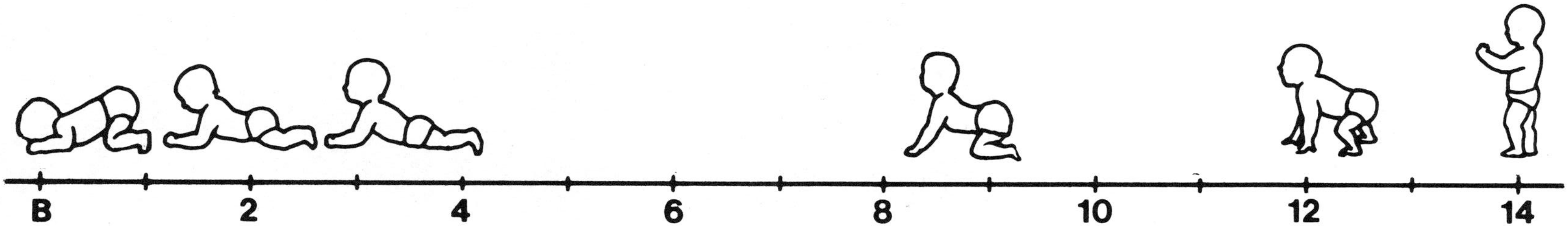

Fig. 3-1. Motor development in the prone position.

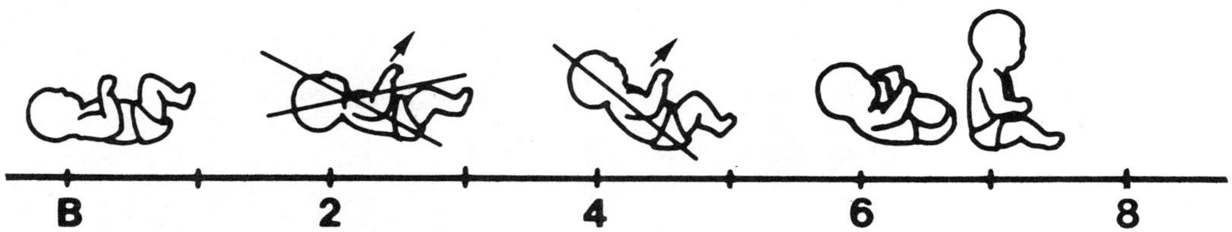

Fig. 3-2. The supine-sitting position.

of age, the head is extended off the table in line with the body, the pelvis is beginning to drop, with increasing extension of the hips and knees out from under the abdomen, and the shoulders and forearms are beginning to move forward with a resultant cubital angle of approximately 90 degrees.

By 3 months of age, the infant's head and neck extend so that the face makes a 45-degree angle with the examining surface; the pelvis is flat, with the hips and knees nearly fully extended. The shoulders and arms are forward with increasing cubital angle greater than 90 degrees and support on the forearms.

At 4 months of age, the infant's head is extended up to 90 degrees and the chest is off the examining surface. The hips and knees remain fully extended and body weight support is definitely forward on the forearms.

By 5 months, the plane of the infant's face is 90 degrees to the examining surface with the chest off the surface; the arms are fully extended in front of the body with the elbows fully extended (180 degrees), and weight is on the hands. At this time, the child can roll from prone to supine.

At 7 months of age, the child can momentarily bear weight on one hand, by 9 months, he can bear weight on hands and knees, and by 10 months, on hands and feet. Crawling on the abdomen occurs at about this time, followed by creeping (with abdomen off the surface) on hands and knees (11 months) and subsequently on hands and feet (typical bear walk) by 12 months. Erect standing and walking are established by 14 to 15 months.

In summation of *prone* development, the infant by *1 month* of age holds his head to the side with beginning extension of hips and knees, and the elbow cubital angle is less than 90 degrees. By *3 months* of age, the head is raised so that the face makes an angle of 45 degrees, the pelvis is flat with the hips and knees fully extended, and the cubital angle is greater than 90 degrees with beginning support of weight on the elbows. By *5 months*, the plane of the face with the surface is 90 degrees with the chest completely raised. The hips and knees are fully extended and the arms are forward with full extension of the elbows and weight on the hands. Over the next 6 to 9 months, the infant finally overcomes gravity in this position by the gradual attainment of hand-knee, hand-feet, crawling, creeping, and walking.

Figure 3-2 diagrams motor development during the first year of life in the supine-sitting development.

At birth, the infant in supine position lies with arms and hips and knees flexed and, when pulled to the sitting position, the head lags or bobs forward and the back is rounded in a slumped position. This head lag and slumped position usually persist to about 4 months of age. (Contrast this with head-body alignment in the prone position.)

Between 4 and 6 months of age, the infant's head balance and back support improve so that there is no head lag when he is pulled up from the supine position and the back begins to straighten up to the level of L3. The knees are flexed with a popliteal angle of 90 degrees.

By 5 months of age, the infant can begin to lift his head and assist in pulling himself to a sitting position.

By 6 months the infant can spontaneously lift his head in the supine position and in pulling up to sitting, he demonstrates a forward flexion, or lead of the head before the chest. This ability to spontaneously flex the head, combined with development of the abdominal flexor muscles allows the infant to play with his feet while lying supine. By this age, the upper and lower back is straight and the infant can sit with forward propping if his hands and knees are fully extended (popliteal angle of 180 degrees).

By 7 months of age, the infant can sit without support. By 9 months he can go from the sitting to prone position, and by 11 months of age he can pivot into the sitting position.

A summary of supine-sitting position development indicates that by 4 months there is a gradual development of head support and no head lag in pulling from the supine to sitting positions. By 6 months of age, the child can spontaneously lift his head in supine position, and actively assist the examiner in the pulling-up maneuver with a forward lead of the head. He plays with his feet. Head bobbing and a slumped position of the back persist until approximately 4 months of age; full head support and straight back in sitting appear by 6 months. Full sitting without propping occurs at about 7 months and pivoting at about 11 months of age. The initial knee flexion with a popliteal angle of approximately 90 degrees in the sitting position changes at about 4 to 5 months to full knee extension and a popliteal angle of 180 degrees by 6 to 7 months of age.

Walking Development

The newborn infant has a primitive walking reflex pattern which is probably integrated by a few months of age. (See Fig. 3-3 for developmental chart.)

Between 1 month and 4 months, the infant's lower extremities bear only slight weight when held upright. This is probably due to the presence of a positive supporting reaction. At about 3 to 4 months of age, the infant develops a posture of astasia (failure of extension) of the lower extremities when held supported, and at about 5 months of age the lower extremities extend and begin to support weight. By 9 to 10 months, the infant pulls to a standing position and can stand holding onto furniture. By 10 to 12 months, he walks holding onto furniture, and by 12 to 14 months, he walks holding on by one hand after which independent walking develops.

The immature pattern of walking at this time can be described as the arms held in a "high guard" position with the shoulders slightly abducted, the elbows flexed, and no reciprocal movement related to the lower extremities. The gait is wide-based and flat-footed (not heel-toe). The high guard posture of the upper extremities gradually changes to a medium and no guard position, and reciprocation with the lower extremities develops. This is combined with narrowing of the stance and a heel-toe gait over the next 6 to 12 months.

Upper Extremity Development

During the first 6 weeks of the infant's life, the upper extremities demonstrate primarily windmill movements. The hands are held predominantly fisted, the thumbs are adducted, and a palmar grasp reflex can be elicited. At about 2 months of age, the infant's hands are often open; by 3 months, they are mostly held open and the first poorly directly reaching responses begin.

By 4 months of age, conscious grasp rather than reflex begins, and objects are held between the palm and ulnar fingers. Both hands can be brought together in the midline.

By 6 months, eye-hand coordination is developing and the infant looks at what he is trying to grasp; he reaches purposefully with forearm pronation using a midpalmar grasp and transfers objects from hand to hand.

Between 6 to 10 months, grasp develops radially from a 3-jaw chuck grasp (thumb, index, and middle fingers) to thumb, index adduction, and finally distal thumb-index finger pincer grasp. At about the time good pincer grasp develops, release is beginning.

In summation, upper extremity development starts with fist and windmill movements. Hand opening starts at about 6 weeks of age and is persistent by 3 months.

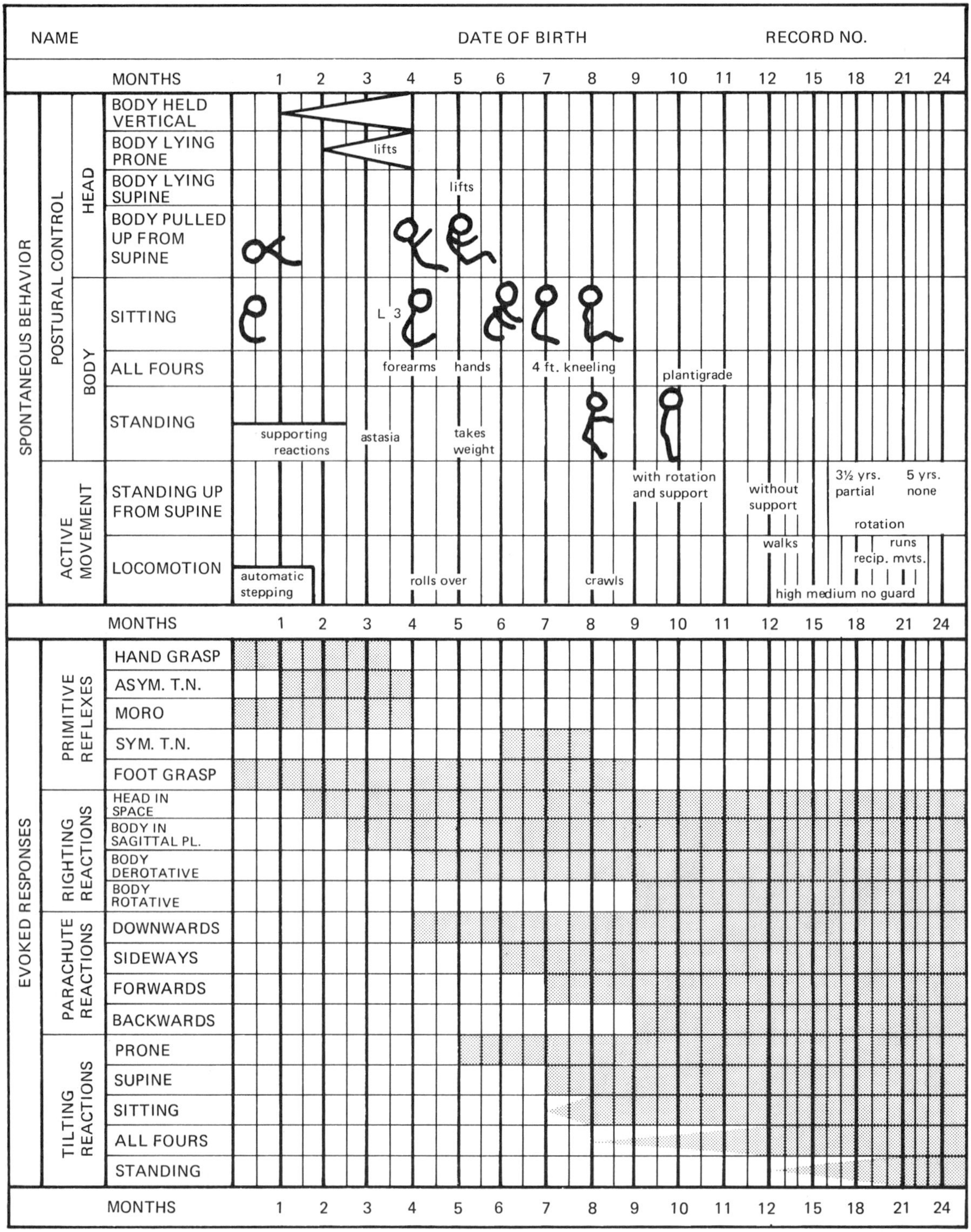

Fig. 3-3. The Developmental Chart, used as a profile of a child's motor development. (Milani-Comparetti A, Gidoni EA: Dev Med Child Neurol 9:766, 1967)

By 6 months, bimanual hand activity has developed, along with purposeful reaching and transfers. Grasp is initially palmar-ulnar and gradually develops radially to a thumb-index pincer grasp with beginning release by 10 months of age.

NEUROPHYSIOLOGIC BASIS OF NORMAL MOTOR DEVELOPMENT

The orderly acquisition of voluntary movement and motor skills depends on a complex neurophysiologic, organizational, developmental scheme. A conceptual approach to this organizational process includes a description of three interrelated developmental components: phylogenetic pattern, postural tone, and postural reflex.

The *phylogenetic cephalocaudal antigravity pattern* of motor development relates to a predetermined order of development from head to feet and from the proximal to the distal parts of the body. The infant develops head control, followed by sitting and then standing. Proximal control of the extremities is attained before distal fine motor control. Head and neck extensors develop before the head and neck flexors. This is followed by development of the hip extensors and then hip and abdominal flexors.

The phylogenetic sequence of muscle development is observable in the prone developmental pattern of infants. The sequence of head extension beginning quite early in the first 6 weeks of life followed by hip extension during this interval of time is characteristic. In the supine position, head flexion occurs later than head extension and isolated head and neck flexion takes approximately 6 months. Around 6 months when active head and neck flexion is occurring, the hip flexors and abdominal flexors are coming in after the hip extensors. This allows the youngster to accomplish the task of playing with his toes.

The second process is neurodevelopmental organization closely associated with antigravity muscle development of *postural tone. Muscle tone* is the constant tension in resting muscle activated by muscle stretch through the proprioceptive system and regulated by postural reflexes. For approximately the first 6 weeks of life, flexor tone predominates. This is followed by a gradual development of extensor body tone. A period of astasia at about 3 months when muscle tone tends to decrease is followed over the next few months by an equalization of flexor-extensor tone (by 6 months of age). Muscle tone is not synonymous with muscle strength, and examination techniques and description of muscle tone including evaluation of the stretch reflex are listed under the assessment techniques of the neurodevelopmental examination.

A substrate of *reflex patterns* is the third prerequisite for orderly normal motor development. Developmentally, this can be divided into two general groups of responses: the primary reflexes or primary motor patterns which develop *in utero* and are usually integrated by 6 months of age, and the postural reflexes which are responsible for maintaining the orientation of the body in space and in relation to body parts. The postural responses are not present at birth and develop gradually around 4 months of age and persist throughout life.

The names, age of appearance, and age span of evolution of the primary motor patterns and postural reflexes are listed in Table 3-1 and Figure 3-4. The description of these reflexes and techniques for demonstration are listed under assessment techniques in the neurodevelopmental examination.

It is important to understand the timetable of appearance and integration of reflexes and how an orderly sequence of reflex maturation makes possible attainment

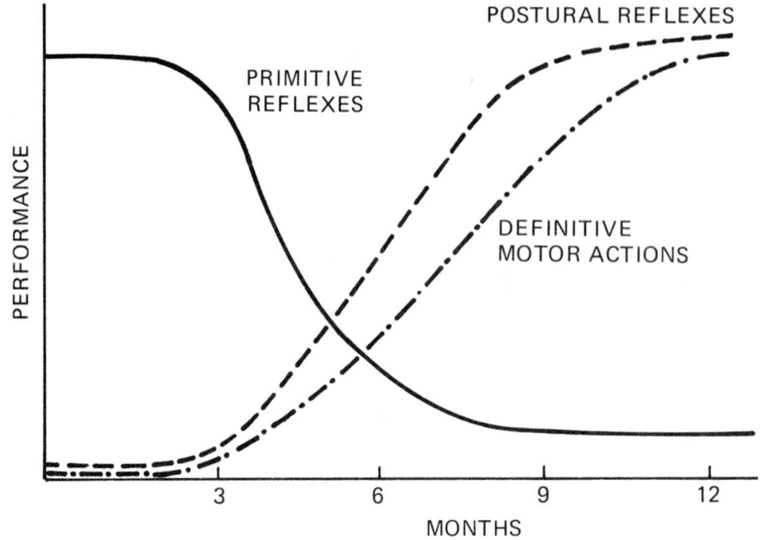

Fig. 3-4. The declining intensity of primitive reflexes and the increasing strength of postural reflexes represent at least permissive, and possibly necessary, conditions for the development of definitive motor actions. (A reflex substrate would never be sufficient to account for the achievement of voluntary motor acts.) The specific combinations of primitive and postural reflexes differ for each motor skill as does the point of intersection of the curves with reverse slopes. (Capute AJ, Accardo PJ, Vining EPG *et al*: Primitive Reflex Profile. Baltimore, University Park Press, 1978)

of normal gross motor landmarks and skills. A careful review of the data in Table 3-1 and the graphic representation of these reflex developmental patterns in Figure 3-4 show that at approximately 6 months of age, there is full integration of the primary motor patterns and emergence of the basic postural responses. This is the age when head balance, proximal and beginning distal arm and hand control, and beginning sitting balance have been attained. Further development of the gross motor landmarks of standing and walking and fine motor control of the hands occurs between 6 and 12 months of age concurrent with the rapid development of these postural reflexes. The acquisition of equilibrium responses begins during the latter part of the first year and continues for the next few years; it is associated with fine tuning of gross motor behavior related to the control of balance in space.

In summation, the normal, integrated, sequential timetable of motor development of infants is related to the fine phasing in of the processes of a phylogenetic cephalocaudal timetable, the development of antigravity postural tone and the smooth integration of the primary motor patterns with the acquisition of postural reflexes. Normal sequential motor development can be interrupted and an infant classified as dysfunctional due to central nervous system injury. The sequelae of this injury inevitably appear as a delay or abnormal motor development which can be discovered by careful clinical assessment of muscle tone and reflex behavior.

Cognitive Development

The major milestones are noted on Tables 3-2 and 3-3.

Intellectual development involves conceptualization based on nonverbal learning and language. The nonverbal aspect concerns visual input, visual perception of forms and *spatial* relationships, and the output of visual-motor integration (drawing, writing) and fine motor manipulation and construction. In contrast, language involves auditory input and processing, the essential qualities of which are *temporal* relationships and orderly sequencing. The output involves speech, gestures (pantomine, sign language), and writing/spelling. Reading is a language-related function involving auditory-visual integration and comprehension of concepts.

The sequential pattern of visual-motor integration can be demonstrated by imitating and copying standard geometric forms.* Imitation of an act, after observation of the examiner performing it, precedes direct copying. The child imitates a vertical and circular stroke at 2 years of age, a horizontal line at 2½ years; he will copy a circle and imitate a cross at 3, copy a cross at 4, a square at 4½ to 5, a triangle at 5 to 6, a diamond at 6 to 7, and a cylinder and cube at 12 years of age.

That the spatial concepts develop in the order of vertical, horizontal, diagonal is paralleled in the child's manipulation of cubes: building a tower (vertical)—15 months to 2 years, imitation of a train (horizontal)—2 years, adding a chimney—2½ years, imitation of a bridge (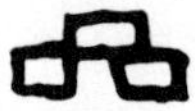)—3 years, copying it—3½ years, imitation of a gate (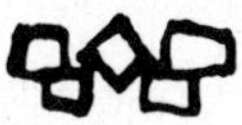)—4 years, and copying it—4½ years. The child may construct steps at age 6 years.

The preschool child draws a circle starting at the bottom, but by 5 to 6 years he will start at the top. Drawings of a person (body concept) has its own sequence of maturation and is described in the section on evaluation.

Language development depends on intact hearing and central auditory processing. The latter includes attention (selection of focus, concentration, avoiding distraction by extraneous stimuli), localization, discrimination, blending and closure of sounds, sequencing, memory, and auditory-visual integration.

Key norms for language and general understanding of concepts are presented in Table 3-4.

The following outline lists age-related norms for articulation of speech:

Age, years	
3½	p—peach, jump
	b—bird, tub
	m—mouth, game
	w—wet, now
	h—house
4½	t—tub, wet
	d—dish, red
	n—new, pin
	g—game, leg
	k—car, kick
	ng—sing
	y—you
5½	f—feet, knife
	v—van
	s—see
	z—zoo
6½	sh—ship
	zh—rouge
	l—leg
	th—the
to 8	ch—church
	r—red, bird, car
	wh—white

NEURODEVELOPMENTAL EVALUATION

Clinical Assessment

The *history* follows a traditional format, but focuses on specific issues related to development. It begins with the reason for

* Imitation means the performance of a task after observation of the *process* of someone doing it; copying, on the other hand, is the duplication of the completed product.

TABLE 3-4. Development of Language and Concepts

Age	Expressive	Receptive	Concepts & Memory
Birth	Reflexive cry	Transiently attends to voice	
4 weeks	Coos, sighs, grunts	Attends to voice	
16 weeks	Babbles, laughs aloud	Turns to voice deliberately and searches for source	
28 weeks	Raspberry (20 weeks), syllables, lalling speech (la la)	Responds to name	
40 weeks	Echolalia; ma-ma, da-da and one word with meaning	Comprehends no, da-da, pat-a-cake, bye-bye (gestures)	
1 year	2–3 words; tries to imitate words	Understands phrase	Knows name (13–14 months). Interest in environmental noises or new situations
18 months	Jargon, 10 + words	Responds to simple commands, points to 3 body parts	
2 years	Meaningful speech; 2 word phrases; names 5 pictures; nouns, verbs, prepositions	Identifies pictures; understands short sentences, carries out 4 directions with a ball	
3 years	Asks questions: what? where? who? Uses plurals; pronouns	Comprehends more complex sentences	Repeats 3 digits; beginning concepts of time: past, future
4 years	Asks questions: why? how?	Answers simple questions; comprehends cold, tired, hungry; comprehends directions under, on, in front of, behind	Names 1 + colors; 4 digits at 4½. Counts 3 objects by pointing
5 years	Uses basic structures of sentences; conjunctions; future tense	Opposite analogies	4 + colors; age and address; names 3 coins; counts 10 objects with pointing. Understands morning, afternoon
6 years	Asks meaning of words; defines words	Comprehends composition of objects	Beginning reading and writing 5 digits; abstracting and categorizing
7 years	Fluent syntax		Symbolic language; understands time, seasons, days of the week

referral or the presenting complaints (perhaps the parents or the staff of the school noticed that the child was not developing normally). The plan of workup depends upon the age of the child.

The prenatal and perinatal history should stress high-risk factors associated with developmental disabilities. This includes the social environment (age and marital status of parents, living conditions), the prenatal environment (circumstances of this pregnancy, nature of prenatal care, mother's health). The perinatal history includes complications and progress of labor and delivery. The neonatal history includes an account of neonatal and maternal complications such as separation from a sick baby or postpartum depression.

A postnatal history is taken to elicit evidence of impaired development, such as poor feeding, hyper- or hypoactivity, and convulsions. Delayed developmental milestones may be manifestations of developmental impairment, especially when the child does not sit alone before 9 months, does not walk or speak before 18 months, and does not form sentences before 3 years. A history of trauma, poisoning, or meningitis, encephalitis, or other severe infections should be noted. Some behavior patterns seen in retarded, deprived, or disturbed children are rocking, head-banging, pica, breath-holding, temper tantrums, and unusual approaches to the environment, such as touching, tasting, or smelling objects (use of proximal sensory receptors rather than distal). These should be noted if they extend beyond the normal age.

Family history includes the age and health of all family members, and genetic aspects, and also the environmental background. Environmental stresses and the observed impact on the child should be noted.

Social history should include peer interaction and the ages of playmates (often younger or older than the patient).

Physical Examination

A complete physical examination is performed, noting special points that may be related to the development of the child. Attempts should be made to examine the child before using instruments that might frighten him. The developmental examination may be done best prior to the general physical examination. The head, eyes, ears, nose, and throat should be examined last.

The special points to be observed are: (1) general growth failure and (2) morphologic stigmata of congenital defects and mental retardation.

Neurological Examination

Accurate examination of the nervous system in infants and children is dependent upon the degree of relaxation and cooperation of the child. Thus, the first task of the examiner is to avoid frightening the child. It is best to make general observations and to observe how the child reacts to the parents, siblings, and other children.

The general habitus and posture of the child can be observed. Weakness and hypotonia may also be evident during the child's spontaneous behavior. The examiner should note the activity of the child and his ability to shift and adjust to a change in stimulation (habituation and perseveration). Is the child alert, does he have an ability to focus, concentrate, and maintain attention span, or is he overly distractible? How does the child react to people? Does he withdraw, is he shy, does he have appropriate affect, does he maintain eye contact? Does he show an interest in his surroundings, does he show curiosity? On the other hand, does he appear to be unresponsive and indifferent to external stimuli? Many retarded, neurologically impaired, or severely emotionally disturbed children have ritualistic, repetitive mannerisms. Occasionally there may be evidence of seizure activity, and it should be noted whether the child is responsive to external stimuli during seizure activity. In the child suspected of *petit mal* seizures, a 3- to 5-minute period of hyperventilation may evoke an absence spell.

The child's speech and communication skills, including nonverbal communication, should be observed. Is the child's thinking concrete; can he abstract and conceptualize?

Visual and hearing acuity should be assessed carefully. In the assessment of the cranial nerves, the visual fields should be checked by confrontation. Eye tracking movements should be noted. The immature response is for the head and eyes to move synchronously, but later, as the child matures, he initially moves his eyes and the head follows after a brief interval.

Examination of the motor system includes assessment of muscle tone, bulk, and strength. Changes in muscle tone may be elicited by changes in position. Subtle spasticity in the adductors of the hips and gastrocnemii becomes more evident when the child is held upright in vertical suspension. The muscles should be palpated for abnormal consistency, a condition seen in myopathies. Fasciculations and fibrillations should be noted, especially in the tongue. The examiner should also check for easy fatigability, myotonic phenomena, and percussion myotonia.

Observe gross motor behavior, including the gait with normal walking, walking on tiptoes, and walking on heels. Children with spastic diplegia, myopathies and autistic children may prefer toe-walking. Heel-walking is difficult for the child with spastic paresis or any condition that produces contractures of the ankles in plantar flexion. Ataxia should be noted. Associated arm-swinging movements should be observed, as they may give a clue to a subtle hemiparesis. In addition to walking on heels, many children with extrapyramidal involvement may show abnormal posturing. The child should be observed while standing.

Gross movements such as running, hopping on either foot, and skipping should be observed. For the older boy who finds it embarrassing to skip, jumping jacks, with which school-age children are familiar, afford an opportunity to observe synchronized movements of the upper and lower extremities.

Fine motor activities can be observed while watching the child dress and undress. Buttoning and tying shoelaces may be extremely difficult for the child with subtle impairment of fine motor function.

Cerebellar signs such as rebound phenomenon, pendular reflexes, intention tremors, dysmetria, and tandem walking should be observed.

The child should be observed while standing with feet together, arms outstretched in front, to the side, and upward to observe for jerking choreiform movements, abnormal posturing, motor impersistence, and dystonia.

Visual motor coordination can be observed while the child copies geometric figures, writes, and performs manual construction skills.

Sensory examination includes not only assessment of primary sensory modalities, but also tests of higher sensory integration such as stereognosis, graphesthesia, and finger agnosia. One should note the preferred eye, hand, and foot. This may give a clue to a subtle hemiparesis or amblyopia. In addition, the child's sense of direction should be tested by having him point to his left ear with his right hand; with an older child, have him identify the right hand of the examiner when the examiner is facing the child.

"Soft" neurologic signs are those that are truly indicators of development in that they are normal at a certain age, but disappear with maturation. They are not to be confused with "hard" neurologic signs such as hemiparesis, cranial nerve palsy, sensory deficits, and asymmetric and pathologic reflexes which are abnormal at any age. The soft neurologic signs include the synkinesias (associated movements) and overflow movements, including choreiformlike movements of the upper extremities. The presence of these phenomena at an age when they should have disappeared suggests developmental immaturity of the nervous system and may be seen in children with so-called minimal brain dysfunction and children with learning disabilities.

Associated or synkinetic movements are those which involve automatic movements of one part of the body in response to voluntary movements of other parts. They can be ipsilateral or symmetric. These associated movements may be seen physiologically in infants in whom movements of one limb are accompanied by similar ("mirror") involuntary movements of the opposite limb. These gradually disappear with maturity (about age 9). They appear when learning new patterns of movements or during excessive physical or mental effort.

Developmental Evaluation

The developmental phase of the evaluation assesses the level of maturity of the patient. It differs from the standard neurologic examination because it is concerned with quantitive ("neurometric") rather than qualitative or localizing signs.

Assessment of the Newborn and Young Infant

Assessment of the newborn should include observations of the baby's cry, measurement of the head circumference and any abnormal cranial features, transillumination of the head, the character of spontaneous and provoked movements, the waking and sleeping pattern, estimations of alertness and abnormal muscle tone, and especially asymmetry in muscle tone.

The *primitive responses* include general reactions (Moro response and asymmetric tonic neck reflex) and local responses (righting response of the head, primitive grasp of the fingers, and forward movement of the arms when the baby is placed in the prone position). In the lower limbs, the local responses are the primitive grasp reflex of the toes, placing response of the lower limbs, and supporting and primary stepping responses. Asymmetry in the grasp reflex, in the placing and stepping reactions and in the Moro response may be of value in detecting or localizing an early hemiparesis (See Fig. 3-4.)

The *Moro reflex* traditionally is elicited by lifting the infant's head 30 to 45 degrees and allowing it to fall gently; it may also be elicited by lifting the baby slightly by the hands and releasing or by causing sudden jarring movements of the examining table and sudden auditory stimuli. The Moro reflex consists of two phases, the first of which is sudden symmetric abduction and extension of all extremities. The second phase consists of a more gradual flexion and adduction movement of the extremities, with slight shaking movements. In addition to hemiparesis, injuries of the brachial plexus and various orthopedic disorders may cause an asymmetric Moro response.

The asymmetric tonic reflex is elicited by rotating the head to one side. The ipsilateral (chin) arm will extend and the contralateral (occipital) arm will flex. An obligatory response, in which the infant is unable to change posture during elicitation of the reflex, is abnormal.

By the time the infant is 6 to 12 weeks, it should be possible to elicit all deep reflexes. A few beats of ankle clonus is permissible if present bilaterally, but unilateral sustained responses are abnormal. The plantar reflex is one of withdrawal, simulating the Babinski reflex; there is extension of the great toe and there may be extension and fanning of the other toes as well. This response is normal up to age 2 years, but if present unilaterally in association with marked ankle clonus, spasticity or asymmetric reflexes it may be indicative of brain damage.

Other reflexes which reflect immature development of the pyramidal pathways are palmar and plantar grasp reflexes, adductor spread of the knee reflex, and crossed extension and automatic walking reflexes. These are basically spinal automatisms, or spinal defense reflexes.

The avoidance response is prepotent in early infancy and childhood. In the course of normal maturation, the avoidance response becomes integrated with the grasping automatisms to permit control of voluntary prehension. It may persist in the child with brain damage and produce abnormal postures and movements.

Another group of special reflexes of the newborn and young infant are the postural and righting reflexes. One group of reflexes of posture and movement are independent of gravity. This includes the Moro reflex, the compensatory ("doll's eye") movements of the eyes when the head is shifted in position, postural reflexes including the tonic neck reflex, spinal or trunk incurvation reflex, and righting reflexes of the neck on the body and of the body on the head.

Postural reflexes dependent upon gravity include the labyrinthine reflexes of the head, which orient the head with respect to the gravitational field and ultimately allow the infant to assume an upright position (bipedal) with arms free to explore his surroundings. His head is held upright by 4 to 6 months of age and, subsequently, chain reflexes are involved in sitting and standing. Gravity-stimulated reflexes of station and gait are seen in the readiness to stand at 4 to 6 months; the infant extends his legs when the soles touch the horizontal surface and after 6 months has true supporting reactions of the legs.

The *secondary responses*, which appear at 4 to 7 months of age and persist to some degree, include the rolling, balancing, and protective reactions.

The rolling response permits the infant to roll from supine to prone position. After the fourth month, the supine infant whose head is turned exhibits the body-on-head and head-on-body righting response requisite for rolling over. The balancing (righting) reactions serve to right the head with respect to gravity and can be elicited by tilting the infant to one side.

Protective reactions include the propping or parachute reactions; these are reactions to acceleration forces. When the prone infant is thrust toward the examining table he extends both arms and fingers toward the table. The lateral propping reaction is elicited by suddenly tilting the baby (in a sitting position) to one side. The arm on that side will extend. It is necessary for the child to develop balancing and protective reactions in order to walk.

The *Landau reflex*, which is seen from about 8 months to 24 months, is based on the otolith and tonic neck reflexes. When the infant is held in a prone position parallel with the floor, he will dorsiflex his head and extend his spine so that the curve of the spine is convexly downward. If the head is ventriflexed, the vertebral column and extremities will flex, producing an upward convexity of the spine.

The newborn can register and discriminate sensory input in all modalities including responses to visual, auditory, and tactile stimuli. Neonatal visual testing by studying visual fixation responses to patterned stimuli correlated better with subsequent development than the standard neurologic evaluation.

Estimation of oculomotor function in the newborn can be obtained by rotating the baby; this should produce deviation of the eyes in the direction of movement followed by nystagmus in the opposite direction when the movement ceases. Photic stimulation evokes eye-blink and pupillary reflexes. Opticokinetic nystagmus can be elicited by moving a striped cloth or a revolving drum. The baby can fix, follow, and be alert to the stimulus of a bright red ball 2 inches in diameter suspended 6 to 10 inches from his face. Responses to thermal stimuli and olfactory discrimination have been established. Certain innate reflexes, such as the rooting reflex, not only facilitate feeding, but also evoke responses from the mother and are important in mediating the earliest interactions between the newborn and his mother. The development of facial movements toward a social smile serves a similar purpose.

Variations among newborns are found in their response to exciting stimuli. Brazelton has devised a behavioral examination and rating scale to assess individual characteristics in the newborn (see biblio.).

INFANT AND PRESCHOOL CHILD

Assessment of developmental progress should be incorporated into the timetable of child care, but special notes should be made at certain key ages: 4, 16, 28, 40, and 52 weeks and 18, 24, 36, 48, and 60 months (Tables 3-1 to 3-4).

SCHOOL-AGE CHILD

Developmental assessment of school-age children involves assessment of cognitive abilities, and testing is usually performed by psychologists. Developmental abnormalities are often related to problems of minimal brain dysfunction and learning disabilities, the typical presenting complaint being poor school performance despite intelligence within the normal range.

In childhood, many central nervous system abnormalities are diffuse or global and do not produce focal abnormalities but rather are signs of immature development in various spheres. Associated movements normally present in 3- to 4-year-old children decrease with age and should disappear by 9 years. Mirror movements may be present until age 10. After age 3, the width of the gait should not exceed 11 cm to 20 cm. In children up to age 4 to 5, the plantar response may reveal inconsistent dorsiflexion and also fanning or spreading of the small toes.

TESTS USED IN DEVELOPMENTAL ASSESSMENT

The Denver Developmental Screening Test (DDST) is most widely used by pediatricians. It is made up of 105 test items culled from 12 developmental and preschool intelligence tests. It is not an "intelligence" test, however, and it does not establish a diagnosis. Its purpose is to screen children for detection of deviation from normal development and to provide a baseline for further investigation of the problem.

Adherence to the instructions and interpretation of the DDST is necessary. The child must be retested in one month if the initial findings are abnormal, and suitable referral consistent with the overall clinical picture must be followed.

Other commonly used developmental tests are the Peabody Picture Vocabulary test (for receptive language) and the Draw-a-Man test.

The pediatrician should be familiar with the Goodenough Draw-a-Man test. The child is asked to draw a picture of a person which can be scored and converted into a "mental age equivalent." A great deal can be learned from the administration of this test in addition to the score for mental age. The drawing reflects visual motor and perceptual functions and occasionally in a very severely disturbed child reflects bizarre, inappropriate perception. The following criteria are used in scoring the test:

1. Head present
2. Legs present
3. Arms present
4. Trunk present
5. Length of trunk greater than breadth
6. Shoulder indicated
7. Both arms and legs attached to trunk
8. Legs attached to trunk and arms to trunk at correct point
9. Neck present
10. Outline of neck continuous with that of head or trunk or both
11. Eyes present
12. Nose present
13. Mouth present
14. Both nose and mouth in two dimensions; two lips shown
15. Nostrils indicated
16. Hair shown
17. Hair on more than circumference of head, nontransparent, better than scribble
18. Clothing present
19. Two articles of clothing, nontransparent
20. Entire drawing, with sleeves and trousers shown, free from transparency
21. Four or more articles of clothing definitely indicated
22. Costume complete without incongruities
23. Fingers shown
24. Correct number of fingers shown

25. Fingers in two dimensions; length greater than breadth; angle subtended not greater than 180 degrees
26. Opposition of thumbs down
27. Hand shown as distinct from fingers or arms
28. Arm joint shown—either elbow, shoulder or both

The test is scored by adding to a basal age of 3 years, $\frac{1}{4}$ year for each item present in the drawing to obtain a mental age equivalent. $MA = 3 + \frac{\text{no. items}}{4}$

In the Gesell Incomplete Man Test*, the child is asked to identify this figure and to finish the drawing.

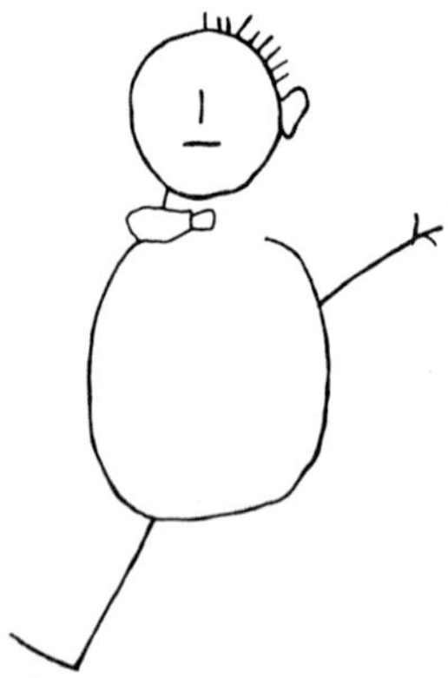

Age	*Response*
3 yr	Names picture as man or snowman; adds 1-2 parts
4 yr	Adds 3 parts
$4\frac{1}{2}$ yr	Adds 6 parts
5 yr	Adds 6-7 parts
6 yr	Adds 8 parts

For the school-age child, achievement tests such as the Wide Range Achievement Test, the Gray Oral Reading Test, and tests of word recognition such as those devised by Glaser and Boder are useful. One should assess word recognition (decoding), comprehension, spelling (encoding), and writing a dictated word.

Reversals in reading and writing may be present up to the middle of first grade in normal children. These may be static reversals with confusion of b/d, p/q (horizontal), and n/u, w/m (vertical) or kinetic, that is, reading from right to left as "on" for "no" and "saw" for "was." The spelling pattern of words correctly read and those which the child cannot read gives information regarding the nature of the reading disorder. The problem may involve recognition of visual symbols, phonetic analysis, sound symbol association, or multiple impairment of these basic modalities.

DEVELOPMENTAL DISABILITIES

Deviations from normal development may be classified under the following broad categories:

I. Major Chronic Brain Syndromes (Chronic Static Encephalopathy)
   A. Mental retardation (see chap. 31)
   B. Motor disorders
      Cerebral palsy
      Diseases of the peripheral motor unit
      Myopathies
   C. Convulsive disorders (see chap. 32)
II. Minor Chronic Brain Syndromes (Minimal Brain Dysfunction)
   A. Attention deficit syndrome with or without hyperactivity
   B. Learning disorders
   C. Language disorders
III. Psychiatric Disorders

The *Diagnostic and Statistical Manual of Mental Disorders (DSM-III)* classifies disorders of infancy, childhood, and adolescence into five major groups.†

* Ilg FC, Ames LB, Haines J: School Readiness, 4th rev ed, p 209. Copyright © 1978 by Gesell Institute of Child Development Inc. By permission of Harper & Row.

† R.L. Spitzer, Diagnostic and Statistical Manual of Mental Disorders, pp. 481–482.

I. Mental retardation
II. Behavioral reactions
  A. Attention deficit disorder
  B. Conduct disorder
III. Emotional disorders
IV. Physical
V. Development disorders
  A. Pervasive developmental disorders
  B. Specific developmental disorders (corresponding to learning and language disorders)

LEARNING DISABILITY

Learning disabilities include disorders of language (speaking, reading, spelling, writing) and mathematics. A child may have a normal capacity or potential to perform but may be learning at reduced efficiency and, hence, underachieving. This may be due to factors involving general health, specific sensory disorders, or reactive disorders related to the situation at home or in school. The child may have a central nervous system problem that can result in global mental retardation, or he may have specific deficits interfering with learning, as in the case of the child with minimal brain dysfunction or with a learning disability. The examination may disclose hints of a seizure disorder or a neuromotor disorder.

DIFFERENTIAL DIAGNOSIS OF LEARNING DISABILITY

There are many factors to consider when determining whether a child has a learning disability. Low overall intelligence or psychiatric disorders may be responsible. On the other hand, a child of normal intelligence might be reacting to unreasonable demands and expectations of parents or teachers. Culturally different children and those with difficult temperament may appear to have a learning disability when confronted with a new school or learning situation.

A learning disability may be the result of a physical disability—systemic or neurologic including epilepsy—including defects of special senses.

The diagnosis of *minimal brain dysfunction* depends upon criteria related to (1) behavior (hyperactivity, attention deficit, impulsivity), (2) neurologic "soft" signs, and (3) psychological evaluation showing an uneven distribution of subtest scores.

The behavioral characteristics overlap those of the child with "different temperament" including low adaptability, low persistence, high activity, and more negative responses. Therefore, the diagnosis of minimal brain dysfunction should not be based on behavior alone.

Diagnostic labels become the *sine qua non* for educational placement of children. Often these are oversimplified (such as "brain damage," which covers a multitude of problems) and stigmatizing.

A more rational but empiric approach would be to construct a profile for each child that includes (1) general physical status, (2) neurologic findings, (3) language development, (4) information processing abilities, (5) temporal-sequential organization, (6) visual and auditory processing, (7) psychomotor maturation, (8) cognitive ability, (9) temperament, and (10) psychological adjustment in the context of environmental stress. From these data, an individualized program for each child can be prescribed.

LANGUAGE DISABILITY

The language pathways begin at the peripheral receptive organ, and receptive language disorders occur when there is pathology of the peripheral auditory apparatus including the middle ear (conductive hearing loss) or the inner ear and cochlear nerve (sensorineural loss) or its central connections. This may be very difficult to assess in the newborn or young infant. A history of maternal exposure to rubella or a family history of hearing disorder mandates consultation with an experienced audiologist. The cortical-evoked response to sound stimuli and assessment of auditory reflexes may be useful.

Many children seem to have more difficulty with expressive than with receptive language; this group includes those with articulation difficulties and those who are immature in their syntactic construction of sentences. Children with simple delays in expressive language respond better to speech and language therapy than children who appear to have a central auditory imperception. Any child not using a few intelligible phrases or sentences by 30 months should be of concern to his physician.

In the differential diagnosis of the child who is not talking appropriately, the following must be considered:

1. Hearing loss, which may be due to conduction defects or sensorineural involvement and which may vary from mild to profound. The child who has a high frequency hearing loss may omit consonants.
2. Mental retardation. Although it is true that delayed speech and language development is seen uniformly in children who prove to be mentally retarded, there are children with delayed speech and language development who develop normal intellect.
3. Specific impairments of speech and language, either developmental or acquired
4. Situational disorders, including multilingualism in the home, cultural differences, "private language of twins," and social and environmental deprivation
5. Severe emotionally disturbance, including autism
6. Inborn error, histidinemia

In summation, the child who fails to respond to sound should be referred for audiologic evaluation. By 6 months of age this should clearly be ascertained; congenitally deaf children make cooing and babbling sounds initially but then cease to make progress.

It is extremely important to have a hearing and speech evaluation of any child who is not developing properly. Often children may be misdiagnosed as having mental retardation or autism who, in reality, have an underlying hearing or language disturbance.

Since there is no satisfactory technique for routine hearing screening of all newborns, certain infants at risk for hearing impairment should be tested within two months after discharge from the nursery and at regular intervals thereafter. These infants include those with a genetic history of hearing impairment, rubella, or other nonbacterial intrauterine fetal infections, congenital defects of the ears, nose, and throat, birthweight less than 1500 g, exposure to ototoxic drugs, and a bilirubin concentration that is potentially toxic.

Assuming that the integrity of the auditory pathway is intact, one should look into the environment to see whether adequate stimulation and nurture are provided including assessment of maternal-infant interaction. Development of speech and language needs to be related to other aspects of development to give clues about whether one is dealing with a specific deficit in this area or whether it is part of a global retardation. Early intervention, including infant stimulation programs and speech therapy, should be considered. It would be better to "over-refer" such children to competent centers than the reverse.

Mechanical speech problems are not truly included in the group of language disorders but deserve early recognition and appropriate therapy. Disorders of articulation and phonation and anatomic disturbances such as cleft palate and severe malocclusions are commonly seen. *Functional speech problems* such as stuttering, stammering, and cluttered speech (other than the repetitions seen normally in the $2\frac{1}{2}$- to 3-year-old) are characterized as dysfluency or disturbance in rhythm. Aberrations in intonation and regional variations (accent) are readily recognized.

Neuromotor Speech Problems

Impairment of cranial nerve motor functions produces *dysarthric speech*.

Dyspraxia is impairment of voluntary motor patterns with no loss of involuntary function of oral, facial lingual muscles, as in swallowing.

The prognosis for children with *developmental language disabilities* depends on the cause of the problem. The group with delayed speech but adequate comprehension may have a prognosis favorable for the later development of speech, but these children may have language learning disabilities involving higher order processing of concepts. On the other hand, the child with language retardation who has difficulty understanding language and, therefore, cannot develop expressive speech has a poor prognosis. This child may have structural abnormalities of the central auditory pathways and no neurologic substrate for decoding language symbols.

Acquired language disturbance is a concept implying that the child who was developing normally in the language area sustained an insult to the central nervous system, as a result of which he suffered a loss of these skills.

The term *aphasia* refers to central language disorders (expressive, receptive, central). In children, these are often mixed disorders and are rarely present in pure form.

Mention of the so-called plasticity of the nervous system is appropriate here. The left hemisphere is dominant for speech and language in most right-handed and a substantial number of left-handed people. The cerebral hemispheres are equipotential for language development in the infant. If damage is sustained early in life to the dominant hemisphere, there is the possibility of recovery with the nondominant hemisphere subserving language function. This may occur up to age 3 and perhaps to age 8 or more.

If the child sustains damage with retrograde amnesia, he will also suffer a loss of memory of previously learned material. Bilateral focal lesions involving the limbic system may cause this type of memory loss.

BIBLIOGRAPHY

General

Holt KS: Developmental Paediatrics. London, Butterworth & Co, 1977

Illingworth RS: The Development of the Infant and Young Children, Normal and Abnormal. Baltimore, Williams & Wilkins, 1972

The author, a colleague and student of Gesell, discusses theoretical and practical issues in detail. Enjoyable and indispensable reading for anyone concerned with the care of children.

Knobloch H, Pasamanick B (eds): Gesell and Amatruda's Developmental Diagnosis, 3rd ed. Hagerstown, Md, Harper & Row, 1975

Meir J: Developmental and Learning Disabilities: Evaluation, Management and Prevention in Children. Baltimore, University Park Press, 1976

A remarkable compendium of basic developmental psychology and a concise overview of the subject with a complete bibliography.

Spitzer, RL (Chairperson Task Force): Diagnostic and Statistical Manual of Mental Disorders, 3rd ed. Washington, DC, American Psychological Association, 1980

Neurologic Examination

Capute AJ, Accardo PJ, Vining EPG, Rubinstein JE, Harryman S: Primitive Reflex Profile. Baltimore, University Park Press, 1978

Milani-Comparetti A, Gidoni EA: Routine developmental examination in normal and retarded children. Dev Med Child Neurol 9:631, 1967

Milani-Comparetti A, Gidoni EA: Pattern analysis of motor development and its disorders. Dev Med Child Neurol 9:625, 1967

Paine RS, Oppe TE: Neurological examination of children. In Clinics in Developmental Medicine (Vol 20/21). London, Spastics Society and William Heinemann, 1966

Prechtl H, Beintema D: The Neurological Examination of the Full-Term Infant. London, William Heinemann, 1964

Thomas A, Chesni Y, Dargassies S: The Neurologic Examination of the Infant. London, National Spastics Society, 1960

Touwen CL, Prechtl HGR: The neurological examination of the child with minor nervous dysfunction. In Clinics in Developmental Medicine, No. 38. London, Spastics International Publications and London, William Heinemann, 1970

These publications are unique in setting up criteria for systematic and standardized neurologic examinations.

Developmental Screening

Brazleton TB: Neonatal Behavioral Assessment Scale. London, William Heinemann, 1973

Frankenberg, WK: Pediatric Screening Tests. Springfield, Ill, Charles C Thomas, 1976

Frankenberg, WK *et al*: The revised Denver Developmental Screening Test. J Pediatr 79:988, 1971

Authoritative discussion of the rationale and practical applications of screening tests by the mentor of the Denver Screening Test.

Gottlieb MI, Zinkus PW, Thompson A: Chronic middle ear disease and auditory perceptual defects. Clin Pediatr 18:725, 1979

Schwartz AH, Murphy MW: Cues for screening language disorders in pre-school children. Pediatrics 55:712, 1975

A useful summary and check-list for early detection of language disorders.

Minimal Brain Dysfunction

Carey WB, McDeavitt SC, Baker D: Differentiating minimal brain dysfunction and temperament. Dev Med Child Neurol 21:765, 1979

Clements SD, Peters JE: Minimal brain dysfunction in the school age child. Arch Gen Psychiatry 6:185, 1962

This paper represents a milestone in formulating and popularizing the concept of MBD.

De La Cruz FF, Fox BH, Robert RH: Minimal brain dysfunction. Ann NY Acad Sci 205:1, 1973

An excellent compilation of background papers with an exhaustive bibliography.

Gardner RA: The Objective Diagnosis of Minimal Brain Dysfunction. Creskill, NJ, Creative Therapeutics, 1979

Learning Disorders

Boder E: Developmental dyslexia: a diagnostic approach based on three atypical reading-spelling patterns. Dev Med Child Neurol 15:663, 1973

Denhoff E, Tarnapol L: Medical responsibilities in learning disorders. In Tarnapol L (ed): Learning Disorders in Children, pp 65-118. Boston, Little, Brown, 1971

The author spells out procedures for evaluation and management of the child with a learning disorder.

Glazer K, Clemmens RL: School failure. Pediatrics 35:128, 1965

Goldberg HK, Schiffman GB: Dyslexia. New York, Grune & Stratton, 1971

Illuminates a very confusing field with factual material and clear thinking. A joint collaboration by an ophthalmologist and an educator.

Kinsbourne M: School problems. Pediatrics 52:697, 1973

Provocative and exciting in terms of the keen insights the author conveys. Highly recommended for those who are skeptical about the role of the physician in this area.

Kinsbourne M, Caplan PJ: Children's Learning and Attention Problems. Boston, Little, Brown, 1979

Levine MD, Brooks R, Shonkoff JP: A Pediatric Approach to Learning Disorders. New York, John Wiley & Sons, 1980

Oberkaid F, Levine MD: Precursors of school failure. Pediatr Rev 2:5, 1980

Shain RJ: Neurology of Childhood Learning Disorders, 2nd ed. Baltimore, Williams & Wilkins, 1977

A "hard" neurologic look at a "soft" subject and a monograph well worth reading.

Principles of Immunization

4

Julia A. McMillan

Immunization can be defined as an effort to prevent or modify natural infection by administration of antibody or antigen. Passive immunization is defined as the administration of antibody, either by intramuscular injection or by intravenous infusion. This temporary protection lasts as long as the antibody survives (half-life about 3 to 4 weeks).

Active immunization is defined as the administration of antigen as a killed microorganism, a component of a microorganism, or a live, attenuated microorganism. Active immunization should provide permanent immunity by stimulation of the host to produce its own antibody and other components of immunity.

ANTIBODY PREPARATIONS

Human Convalescent Plasma

Human convalescent plasma is obtained from persons recovering from a naturally occurring illness. For example, plasma obtained from an adult recovering from chickenpox may be useful in modifying or preventing chickenpox in a child with leukemia, if given shortly after the child is exposed.

Animal Hyperimmune Serum

Animal hyperimmune serum is obtained after active immunization of animals. For example, diphtheria antitoxin is produced by immunization of a horse with diphtheria toxoid. Animal hyperimmune sera, such as for rabies, have a high risk of serum sickness and anaphylactoid reactions; human hyperimmune serum is always preferable if it is available.

Immune Serum Globulin

Immune serum globulin is the gamma globulin fraction obtained from unselected blood donors. It also has been called "gamma" globulin or "immune human" globulin. The type and quantity of antibodies present are variable, and depend on the past infections or immunizations of the donors. In past years, it could be assumed that ordinary gamma globulin contained antibodies protective against poliovirus, measles, and infectious hepatitis. In recent years, the preparations available usually have been titered to standardize the antibody content against measles.

Human Hyperimmune Globulin

Human hyperimmune globulin is obtained from humans who have a very high titer of antibody. The source of these preparations can be persons who have recovered from the natural illness (zoster immune globulin) or who have been immunized with a live virus (vaccinia immune globulin), a killed bacteria or virus (pertussis immune globulin or rabies immune globulin), or a toxoid (tetanus immune globulin).

Passive Immunity from Transplacental Antibodies

The very young infant is often protected by maternal antibodies which pass transplacentally from the pregnant woman to the fetus before bith. Only the smaller antibodies (IgG) pass the placental barrier. The duration of protection by transplacentally acquired antibodies depends on the initial concentration (titer) of antibodies of the mother. The antibody titer of transplacentally acquired antibodies then decreases gradually during the first year of the infant's life. Measles, tetanus, and polio are examples of diseases from which the infant is often protected for a variable period in the first year of life, usually about 6 months. Maternal antibodies can also prevent immunization of the infant by live vaccines, such as attenuated measles vaccine, until as late as 13 months of age.

ACTIVE IMMUNIZATION

The decision to use a vaccine should depend on a balance between the need for the vaccine and the risk of the vaccine (Fig. 4-1). These general principles are particularly important in the evaluation of the indications for use of new vaccines. The balance between need and risk may be shifted by changes in these factors, so that routine use of a vaccine may be discontinued, as in the case of smallpox vaccine. The balance between need and risk factors is a useful concept when explaining immunization of children to the parents.

NEED FACTORS

Severity of the Natural Disease

The severity is best defined in terms of the mortality rate or the damage done by the naturally occurring disease. Rabies is the most severe disease for which immunization is used, since it is virtually always fatal. In children, mumps and rubella are the least severe diseases for which live virus vaccines are available. However, the possible complications of orchitis in adult males and congenital rubella syndrome in the infant born to a pregnant woman with rubella make immunization desirable at some time before adulthood is reached.

Probability of Exposure

The probability of exposure depends on the degree to which the agent is contagious and the age, occupation, and geographic exposures of the patient. For example, there is a relatively high risk of

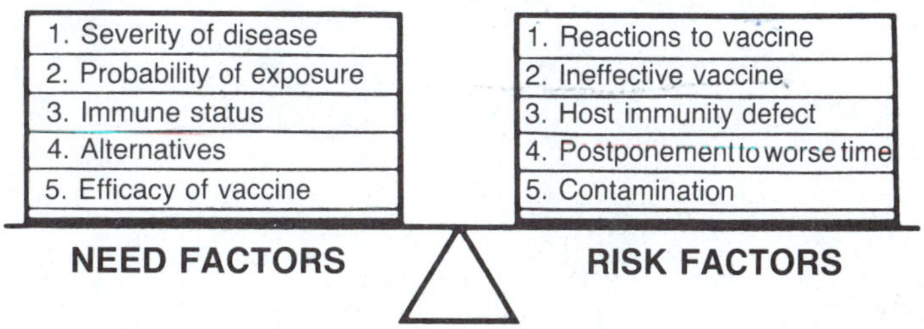

Fig. 4-1. Need and risk factors in immunization. (Moffet HL: Pediatric Infectious Diseases, p. 409. Philadelphia, JB Lippincott, 1975)

exposure to measles in the United States, especially in areas where many children have not received adequate immunization.

Immune Status

Although determination of a person's immune status is usually not convenient, it may be useful in several situations. For example, rubella antibodies should be measured before giving rubella vaccine to a woman of childbearing age because the vaccine is not necessary if antibodies indicate past natural infection. In addition, natural infection requires no boosters, and rubella vaccine possibly may require boosters if long-term studies indicate the need.

Alternatives to Immunization

Immunization is not the only method available to prevent infections, although few of the alternatives are superior.

Avoidance of Exposure. Some infections can be prevented by education of people to avoid unnecessary exposures. Measles is an example of the importance of the exposure factor. Measles may occur in infants between 6 months and 1 year of age, at a time when they have lost some or most of their transplacentally acquired maternal antibodies. If exposure to measles can be avoided, measles vaccine is usually postponed until 15 months of age when all maternal antibodies are gone; these antibodies may prevent infection and immunization by the vaccine.

Chemoprophylaxis. Antibiotics or other drugs can be given to persons in advance of any exposure and can effectively prevent infections, if directed at a specific pathogen. Chemoprophylaxis with erythromycin to prevent pertussis in an exposed susceptible sibling is an example.

Deliberate Exposure to Natural Disease. Controlled exposure is a possible method of protecting the person from a more severe form of infection. Examples include the past practice of deliberate exposure of susceptible persons to rubella or mumps during childhood to avoid complications which may occur if these diseases are acquired as an adult. Deliberate exposure is not used now for these diseases, since the vaccine is less likely to produce complications in children than is the natural disease.

Effectiveness of the Available Vaccine

Sometimes a vaccine has limited effectiveness and may be used only for special needs. Typhoid vaccine is an example of a vaccine with a limited need because of limited effectiveness.

RISK FACTORS

Contamination

Bacterial contamination is extremely unlikely in modern commercial vaccines, but viral contamination can occur. Administration of yellow fever vaccine stabilized with human serum contaminated with hepatitis virus resulted in an outbreak of viral hepatitis. There were about 28,000 cases and 62 fatalities in 1942, during World War II.

In 1973, 17 of 71 tested lots of live virus vaccines for polio, measles, mumps, and rubella contained bacteriophage. These viruses that infect bacteria usually come from the fetal calf serum used to support the growth of the cell cultures in which the vaccine viruses are grown. There has been no evidence that these bacteriophages have a harmful effect on humans. Endotoxin also has been detected in small quantities in some viral vaccines.

Virulent Vaccine

In 1969, an attenuated live measles virus vaccine used in Great Britain was withdrawn due to some cases of measles encephalitis which occurred immediately following administration of the vaccine.

Worsened Natural Disease

Early field trials of a killed respiratory syncytial virus vaccine indicated that more severe bronchiolitis occurred in immunized infants than in unimmunized. This was attributed to an antigen-antibody reaction between natural wild virus and serum antibodies.

Lack of Protection

This can be an unexpected risk. Use of live measles vaccine in the first year of life may not result in infection by the attenuated virus because of residual transplacentally acquired maternal antibodies. This may leave the infant unprotected against measles, and when the infant is exposed, unmodified measles may occur.

Postponement of Natural Disease to a Worse Time

This risk is largely theoretical. It has been suggested that mumps or rubella immunization in early childhood may postpone the natural disease until adulthood, at which time the complications of orchitis (mumps) or fetal infection (rubella) may occur. However, postponement of natural disease has not yet been observed.

Host Defects and Pregnancy

Existing disease in the host may result in complications from immunization. For example, eczema is a contraindication to smallpox vaccination because the affected skin may become extensively infected by the vaccinia virus. In addition, smallpox vaccination may produce progressive, and even fatal, disease in persons with a defect of cellular immunity.

No live vaccine should be given during pregnancy. Immunosuppressive drugs or diseases are also important contraindications to immunization. Known or suspected hypersensitivity to a vaccine or one of its components is also a contraindication to the use of the vaccine.

Vaccine Reactions, Complications, or Side-Effects

All vaccines contain small to moderate amounts of antigens other than the agent being immunized against. Most killed vaccines or toxoids are given in multiple doses; this can result in the development of hypersensitivity, with subsequent local or anaphylactoid reactions.

Some complications of attenuated virus vaccines are similar to effects of the wild virus but occur much less frequently than after the natural disease. These include the extremely rare complication of flaccid paralysis after poliovaccine, which may sometimes be related to an immunologic problem of the host. Rubella vaccine may produce arthritis, but with current vaccines this occurs less frequently than the arthritis after the natural disease.

Contagion

Some vaccines have a risk because the vaccine virus can be contagious. Vaccinia virus can be transmitted by direct contact with the inoculation site, so a child with eczema must be protected from exposure to another person with a recent smallpox vaccination.

EFFICACY

Efficacy of a vaccine can be quantitated by comparing the frequency of the illness in immunized and unimmunized persons during an outbreak.

Indirect Efficacy (Herd Immunity)

Herd immunity refers to protection of a patient indirectly by reduction or prevention of exposure by immunization of the patient's contacts. If a very high percentage of a "herd" is immune, some diseases may not be transmitted to the susceptible individuals. This concept was used to predict that there should be significant protection of pregnant women; they are protected from exposure to rubella by immunization of children. However, recent observations have indicated that rubella spreads rapidly through exposed susceptibles even if 85% of the group is immune. Furthermore, the concept of protection by herd immunity assumes random contacts, and does not apply to the nonrandom interaction that occurs between the many small groups in most societies.

Vaccine Failure

Vaccine failure can be defined as the occurrence of unmodified natural disease in vaccinated persons. It can be a result of failure to include all important antigens in the vaccine, as has been observed in pertussis and influenza. It can be caused by inadequate preservation of the vaccine by deficient refrigeration or freezing, as has been observed for measles and smallpox vaccines. It can be caused by failure of the vaccine virus to infect the subject because of the presence of antibodies in the person being immunized, as has been observed after measles immunization in the first year of life.

Overattenuation

Some investigational vaccines have not been released because they have been overattenuated by too many passages in tissue culture and fail to produce an adequate frequency of infection in subjects. In the case of rubella vaccine, the vaccine has been attenuated enough to be noncontagious, but is not so overattenuated that it fails to infect the subject. It is possible that this desired degree of attenuation found in the final vaccines available may be appropriate for most hosts, but it may represent overattenuation for a few.

PRACTICAL PROBLEMS

Availability of Vaccine

The first vaccine available usually gets the most early use. Killed virus vaccines usually have been available before live vaccines, as in measles, poliovirus, and mumps vaccines. The first vaccine tends to get a safety record established and continues to be used more often until the newest vaccine has been proved better in some way.

Cooperation of Susceptible Groups

Social factors are extremely important in immunization. Some socioeconomic or ethnic groups are notoriously underimmunized, either because the vaccine is not available or because the person will not accept immunization, even when offered without charge. The physician should always be alert for the opportunity to immunize susceptible children; this often can be done when the child is seen during convalescence from another illness. Minor respiratory symptoms should not be used as a reason to defer immunizations in infancy if the physician knows that the child is usually not seen for supervisory health care. Unfortunately, any immunization given during a prodrome of a serious illness is likely to be blamed for the illness. Viral interference between vaccines is not a practical problem.

The major emphasis of immunization programs in the United States should now be the identification and immunization of susceptible subgroups. An immunization program directed at susceptible people is more important than mass programs which may give repeated immunization to cooperative people who may already have had the vaccines. Recent antibody surveys indicate that many young children in lower socioeconomic groups have no protective antibodies against polio or measles; increased efforts are necessary to reach these children.

Immunization Schedules

Often used by physicians, particularly for infants (Tables 4-1 and 4-2), these schedules need to be revised every few years because of the introduction of new vaccines or modified vaccines, or newly recognized side-effects of vaccines. Unfortunately, the complexity of such schedules tends to make the physician overlook the general principles involved. It is important to be aware of the principles of immunization and avoid the rigidity of schedules if they become outdated.

The most important single principle in the immunization of any person is to adapt the schedule to the person's particular needs and risks.

Immunization Records

Records kept by the patient or parent are extremely important and in the past have been greatly neglected by many physicians and patients. Such records are useful in reminding the patient of the need for immunizations, and in preventing unnecessary treatment; they can be used as a record of allergies, chronic illnesses, or medications.

Excessive Immunization

The risks of excessive immunization are primarily related to allergic reactions, although any *unnecessary* immunization producing an untoward reaction can be regarded as excessive. Several vaccines and situations are often unnecessary. Paratyphoid vaccine is not indicated in the United States. Typhoid vaccine has no indications in the United States, except in a household with exposure to known typhoid fever, or in travel to an area where there is an outbreak of typhoid fever. It is unnecessary for people in flooded areas or for those taking camping trips.

Tetanus toxoid boosters should not be given routinely each year for the convenience of summer camps. Rabies vaccine is seldom if ever indicated for rodent bites. Skunks (which are not rodents), however, have a high risk of transmitting rabies. Combinations of live virus vaccines, such as rubella and measles, should not be given if the patient needs only one of the vaccines.

VACCINES COMMONLY USED

DPT

DPT vaccine contains diphtheria and tetanus toxoids and killed pertussis bacteria. Pertussis is the most likely component to produce hypersensitivity reactions such as fever, local pain, and swelling. Encephalopathy is a very rare complication of pertussis immunization. Pertussis vaccine is not rec-

TABLE 4-1. Recommended Schedule for Active Immunization of Normal Infants and Children

Age		
2 mo	DTP[1]	TOPV[2a]
4 mo	DTP	TOPV
6 mo	DTP	[2b]
1 yr		Tuberculin Test[3]
15 mo	Measles,[4] Rubella[4]	Mumps[4]
1½ yr	DTP	TOPV
4–6 yr	DTP	TOPV
14–16 yr	Td[5]—repeat every 10 years	

[1] DTP—diphtheria and tetanus toxoids combined with pertussis vaccine.
[2a]TOPV—trivalent oral poliovirus vaccine. This recommendation is suitable for breast-fed as well as bottle-fed infants.
[2b]A third dose of TOPV is optional but may be given in areas of high endemicity of poliomyelitis.
[3] Frequency of repeated tuberculin tests depends on risk of exposure of the child and on the prevalence of tuberculosis in the population group. For the pediatrician's office or outpatient clinic, an annual or biennial tuberculin test, unless local circumstances clearly indicate otherwise, is appropriate. The initial test should be at the time of, or preceding, the measles immunization.
[4] May be given at 15 months as measles-rubella or measles-mumps-rubella combined vaccines (see Rubella, section 9, and Mumps, section 9, for further discussion of age of administration).
[5] Td—combined tetanus and diphtheria toxoids (adult type) for those more than 6 years of age, in contrast to diphtheria and tetanus (DT) toxoids which contain a larger amount of diphtheria antigen. *Tetanus toxoid at time of injury*: For clean, minor wounds no booster dose is needed by a fully immunized child unless more than 10 years have elapsed since the last dose. For contaminated wounds, a booster dose should be given if more than 5 years have elapsed since the last dose.

Concentration and Storage of Vaccines

Because the concentration of antigen varies in different products, the manufacturer's package insert should be consulted regarding the volume of individual doses of immunizing agents.

Because biologics are of varying stability, the manufacturer's recommendations for optimal storage conditions (e.g., temperature, light) should be carefully followed. Failure to observe these precautions may significantly reduce the potency and effectiveness of the vaccines.

(Report of the Committee on Infectious Diseases, American Academy of Pediatrics, 1977.)

TABLE 4-2. Primary Immunization for Children not Immunized in Early Infancy*

Under 6 Years of Age	
First visit	DTP, TOPV, Tuberculin Test
Interval after first visit	
1 mo	Measles,† Mumps, Rubella
2 mo	DTP, TOPV
3 mo	DTP, TOPV‡
4 mo	DTP, TOPV
10 to 16 mo or preschool	Td–repeat every 10 yr
Age, 14–16 yr	
6 Years of Age and Over	
First visit	Td, TOPV, Tuberculin Test
Interval after first visit	
1 mo	Measles, Mumps, Rubella
2 mo	Td, TOPV
8 to 14 mo	Td, TOPV
Age, 14–16 yr	Td–repeat every 10 years

*Physicians may choose to alter the sequence of these schedules if specific infections are prevalent at the time. For example, measles vaccine might be given on the first visit if an epidemic is underway in the community.
†Measles vaccine is not routinely given before 15 months of age (see Table 4-1).
‡Optional.
(Report of the Committee on Infectious Diseases, American Academy of Pediatrics, 1977)

ommended for use after 6 years of age, because then the risks of hypersensitivity reactions are thought to exceed the need for protection against pertussis (which can produce serious disease or even death in infants and young children).

Routine tetanus toxoid boosters are given every 10 years after the initial series of five injections with DPT. Whether an "emergency" tetanus toxoid booster is recommended after injury depends on the severity and contamination of the wound and the number and timing of past doses of tetanus toxoid. In equivocal situations, a dose of 0.1 ml of toxoid is as effective as the usual 0.5 ml and is less likely to produce a local reaction. Human tetanus immune globulin should be given if the patient has had no previous toxoid, and has a deep puncture or other significant wound.

Poliovaccine

Poliovaccine provides excellent protection against one of the dread diseases of the past. The live attenuated vaccine virus is excreted in the feces of immunized children and can infect exposed susceptible contacts. Paralytic disease is very rarely caused by the vaccine virus and sometimes an immunologic defect can be detected in persons who develop paralysis. Whether this risk of paralysis is greater than the need for the vaccine depends on the risk of exposure to wild poliovirus. Very likely the severity of the natural disease would be much worse than paralysis from the vaccine, if the susceptible person were exposed to the wild virus.

Measles

Measles is a very important vaccine, because the risk of naturally occurring measles virus infection is significant and often results in brain damage or death. Because the disease is very contagious, exposed children will contract measles if they are not immunized by past infection or immunization. Very rarely will a child who has received measles vaccine develop a progressive fatal encephalitis 2 to 10 years later. This subacute sclerosing panencephalitis is a rare late complication of naturally occurring measles. It is possible that children who develop this complication after vaccine do so because of naturally occurring measles in the first year of life that was made milder by maternal antibodies and was not recognized as measles.

Rubella

Rubella vaccine is used to prevent fetal damage by direct administration to susceptible but nonpregnant females. It also is given to male children so they will not be a source of wild rubella exposure to susceptible pregnant women (who should have been immunized but have not been). Immunization of male children also protects them against complications of rubella infection, such as arthritis and the rare complication of encephalitis.

Mumps

Mumps vaccine appears to produce minimal discomfort and no serious complications. Although the need to protect children from naturally occurring mumps virus infection is limited to prevention of aseptic meningitis and perhaps a few rare complications, this need appears to exceed the very low risk of the vaccine. The skin test is not useful as a guide to susceptibility of adults.

Rabies

The availability of duck embryo vaccine and human rabies immune globulin has made rabies immunization much less of a risk than when horse serum and nervous system (Semple) vaccine were used. The decision to use rabies vaccine or globulin is quite complicated; current guidelines should be consulted for most situations.

Vaccines for Foreign Travel

The Center for Disease Control guidelines should be consulted for most recent recommendations for specific countries.

BIBLIOGRAPHY

Center for Disease Control: Health information for international travel. Morbidity Mortality Weekly Report 26 (Suppl):1-97, 1977

Very useful guide for travellers. It is revised each year.

Harrison HR, Fulginiti VA: Bacterial immunizations. Am J Dis Child 134:184, 1980

A recent review.

Levine MM, Edsall G, Bruce-Chwatt LJ: Live-virus vaccines in pregnancy. Risks and recommendations. Lancet 2:34, 1974

A review of data on vaccines in pregnancy.

Moffet HL: Pediatric Infectious Diseases: A Problem-Oriented Approach (Chapter on Immunization). Philadelphia, J B Lippincott, 1975.

A detailed discussion of general principles and specific need and risk factors for each vaccine.

Report of the Committee on Infectious Diseases. Evanston, Illinois, American Academy of Pediatrics, 1974, 1977

The "Redbook." Authoritative recommendations, revised about every 3 years.

Wilson GS: The Hazards of Immunization. University of London, Athlone Press, 1967

A broad and historical approach to complications of immunization.

5

Feeding

Lewis A. Barness

A limited number of guidelines is necessary for the feeding of low birth weight infants, term infants, and older children. A few principles of infant nutrition help to determine how these have been formulated.

The natural food of term infants is human milk. Although certain formulas have been developed that can lead to more rapid growth in infants than those breast-fed, no formula has ever been shown to be superior to human milk for the human infant. Most of the newer formulas have been developed to simulate human milk.

Certain aspects of breast-feeding have not yet been approached by artificial feeds. Among these are the low incidence of allergy, the presence of antibodies to common viruses, the high biologic value of the protein, the low eletrolyte content, the favorable calcium:phosphorus ratio to produce high calcium absorption, and probably other factors not yet delineated. Nursing in the postpartum period helps to contract the mother's uterus.

Aspects of artificial feeding that have been developed to approach human milk include lowering of the saturated fat in artificial milks, increasing the unsaturated fat, lowering of the protein and salt content to approach human milk, providing the carbohydrate almost entirely as lactose, and in some, adjusting the calcium:phosphorus ratio.

Most term infants gain satisfactorily for the first half-year if they consume 90–120 cal/kg and 150–200 ml/kg/day. Thus, the caloric and water requirements are both met with 150–200 ml/kg/day of breast milk or formula. (See Table 5-1).

Wide variation in the requirements of infants may be due not only to the variability of infants and their families but also to metabolic factors that are not well defined.

BREAST-FEEDING

Breast-feeding can be successfully accomplished by most mothers if support is given during the first weeks. Mothers are encouraged to feed from both breasts during the first week, 10 minutes on each side, and then to alternate breasts. The baby should be fed if crying or hungry; intervals should be 3 to 5 hours with 6 feedings a day for the first month. Generally, during the second month, the 2 AM feeding can be stopped, and by the fifth month, the 10 PM can cease so that the baby is fed four times a day. The back should be patted every 10 minutes during the feeding to burp the baby, helping him to get rid of swallowed air.

Vitamins are not necessary if the mother is well nourished. If the mother is not exposed to sunlight 400 IU of vitamin D should be given. In areas where the water supply is not flouridated, 0.25 mg of flouride per day should be given.

TABLE 5-1. Composition of Human Milk, Simulated Human Milk, and Cow's Milk Formulas

Nutrient (per dl.)	Human Milk	Simulated	Cow's Milk
Calories	67	67	65
Protein	0.8–1.1	1.5	3.5
Carbohydrate (Lactose)	7	7	4.5
Fat	3.5	3.5	3.5
Minerals	0.2	0.3–0.7	0.7–0.9

Solid feedings may be begun at 4 to 6 months of age. Because they may have increased caloric density, the likelihood of early obesity is increased. The baby's extrusion reflex, the reflex which causes the baby to push out any material on the anterior third of the tongue, normally disappears at about 6 weeks to 3 months of age.

No more than one new food should be introduced a week. If reaction occurs, the food should not be offered again for 3 months. Foods with the least allergenicity should be offered first. Although the infant is born with apparently normal intestinal trypsin and lipase and deficient amylase, customarily cereal is introduced first.

A typical feeding schedule is:

6:00 AM	breast
10:00 AM	breast
2:00 PM	breast
6:00 PM	breast
10:00 PM	breast
2:00 AM	breast

Offer water twice daily and add vitamins at five days if necessary.

At 1 month, omit the 2 AM feeding. At 4 to 6 months add rice cereal, 2 tablespoons in diluted form at 10 AM and 6 PM. Add fruits, 1/3 to 1/2 jar or equivalent at 2 PM (apples, pears, peaches) when the baby is 5 to 7 months old. At 6 to 8 months add meats, 1/3 to 1/2 jar or equivalent at 2 PM (beef, lamb, liver). Vegetables can be added at 7 to 9 months: 1/3 to 1/2 jar or equivalent at 6 PM (peas, beans, carrots). Omit the 10 PM feeding. Add an egg yolk at the 10 AM feeding when the baby is 7 to 10 months old. At 8 months, "chewy" foods (*e.g.*, Zwieback, cottage cheese) can be added. Change to junior foods and wean to a cup at 9 months. An egg white can be added at 12 months.

BOTTLE FEEDINGS

At present, available evidence indicates that breast-feeding remains the superior feeding for human infants. Although evaporated milk formulas are somewhat cheaper than the simulated formulas, the next most desirable form of infant feeding, according to current information, is a simulated human milk formula. The more nearly it approaches the composition of human milk, the better. Life and growth are, at present, measurements of a baby's well-being; in developed countries there does not seem to be a difference among those fed human milk, cow's milk, or simulated human milk formulas. However, as measurement techniques improve other more subtle differences, such as those below, indicate that one or another feeding is more desirable. These include: decreased infections, repair of injury, avoiding special disease states, imprinting for high-sodium diets, allergies, mental status, learning ability, hyperkinesis, onset of degenerative diseases.

Simulated human milks are diluted to contain 67 cal/100 ml and are fed as human milk to provide 150 to 200 ml/kg/day in divided feedings. These formulas contain sufficient vitamins that no vitamin supplements are given. If fluoridated water is not used for diluting the formula, give the baby fluoride drops daily.

Satisfactory evaporated milk formulas can be made with one ounce of evaporated milk per lb/day. Sugar is added to make a 5% addition, for example:

10 lb (5 kg)		cal	13 lb (6.5 kg)		cal
EM	10 oz	400	EM	13 oz	520
Sugar	1½ oz	180	Sugar	1 oz	120
Water	20 oz	0	Water	17 oz	0
		580			640

Formulas should be sterilized and kept in the refrigerator.

OLDER INFANTS AND CHILDREN

Calories

The daily caloric requirement decreases to 80 to 120 cal at 1 year. A simple estimate for the caloric requirement past 1 year is:

1000 cal + age in years × 100 cal

This is only an estimate and most children adjust caloric requirements to need. The doctor should check that weight gain is satisfactory but not excessive.

Much has been written about the kinds of foods a child should eat. Presently, factual dietary advice goes no further than providing a balanced diet which includes:

4 daily servings of colored vegetables, fruits
2 or more daily servings of meat, eggs, fish, liver
4 or more daily servings of cereal, bread
not more than 1 pt daily from the milk group

These diets should provide sufficient calories, and contain sufficient known vitamins if the foods are not overcooked. Excess milk may decrease intake of necessary foods, decrease iron absorption, and provide a high saturated fatty acid diet.

Vitamins and Minerals

The Recommended Daily Dietary Allowances of the NAS-NRC (1980) are found in Table 5-2. Vitamins are necessary for a number of biochemical and biologic effects. (See Tables 5-3 and 5-4).

Minerals are also required; these minerals, with their major function and manifestations, are listed in Table 5-5.

DEFICIENCY AND EXCESS STATES

Calories

Caloric deficiency, a form of starvation, is probably the leading cause of failure to thrive in young children. In severe states it is known as marasmus. Causes include emotional problems and educational defects in the family.

In addition, calorie requirements may be elevated or calories may be lost. If these increased requirements are not met, signs of deficiency become obvious: failure to gain, weight loss, failure to grow, failure of chest circumference to increase, wasting of buttocks, cheeks, and fat pads, failure of head circumference to increase.

TABLE 5-2. Food and Nutrition Board, National Academy of Sciences National Research Council Recommended Daily Dietary Allowances,[a] Revised 1980

Designed for the Maintenance of Good Nutrition of Practically All Healthy People in the U.S.A.

		Weight		Height			Fat-Soluble Vitamins			Water-Soluble Vitamins							Minerals					
	Age (years)	(kg)	(lb)	(cm)	(in)	Protein (g)	Vitamin A (μg RE)[b]	Vitamin D (μg)[c]	Vitamin E (mg α-TE)[d]	Vitamin C (mg)	Thiamin (mg)	Riboflavin (mg)	Niacin (mg NE)[e]	Vitamin B-6 (mg)	Folacin[f] (μg)	Vitamin B-12 (μg)	Calcium (mg)	Phosphorus (mg)	Magnesium (mg)	Iron (mg)	Zinc (mg)	Iodine (μg)
Infants	0.0–0.5	6	13	60	24	kg × 2.2	420	10	3	35	0.3	0.4	6	0.3	30	0.5[g]	360	240	50	10	3	40
	0.5–1.0	9	20	71	28	kg × 2.0	400	10	4	35	0.5	0.6	8	0.6	45	1.5	540	360	70	15	5	50
Children	1–3	13	29	90	35	23	400	10	5	45	0.7	0.8	9	0.9	100	2.0	800	800	150	15	10	70
	4–6	20	44	112	44	30	500	10	6	45	0.9	1.0	11	1.3	200	2.5	800	800	200	10	10	90
	7–10	28	62	132	52	34	700	10	7	45	1.2	1.4	16	1.6	300	3.0	800	800	250	10	10	120
Males	11–14	45	99	157	62	45	1000	10	8	50	1.4	1.6	18	1.8	400	3.0	1200	1200	350	18	15	150
	15–18	66	145	176	69	56	1000	10	10	60	1.4	1.7	18	2.0	400	3.0	1200	1200	400	18	15	150
	19–22	70	154	177	70	56	1000	7.5	10	60	1.5	1.7	19	2.2	400	3.0	800	800	350	10	15	150
	23–50	70	154	178	70	56	1000	5	10	60	1.4	1.6	18	2.2	400	3.0	800	800	350	10	15	150
	51+	70	154	178	70	56	1000	5	10	60	1.2	1.4	16	2.2	400	3.0	800	800	350	10	15	150
Females	11–14	46	101	157	62	46	800	10	8	50	1.1	1.3	15	1.8	400	3.0	1200	1200	300	18	15	150
	15–18	55	120	163	64	46	800	10	8	60	1.1	1.3	14	2.0	400	3.0	1200	1200	300	18	15	150
	19–22	55	120	163	64	44	800	7.5	8	60	1.1	1.3	14	2.0	400	3.0	800	800	300	18	15	150
	23–50	55	120	163	64	44	800	5	8	60	1.0	1.2	13	2.0	400	3.0	800	800	300	18	15	150
	51+	55	120	163	64	44	800	5	8	60	1.0	1.2	13	2.0	400	3.0	800	800	300	10	15	150
Pregnant						+30	+200	+5	+2	+20	+0.4	+0.3	+2	+0.6	+400	+1.0	+400	+400	+150	*h*	+5	+25
Lactating						+20	+400	+5	+3	+40	+0.5	+0.5	+5	+0.5	+100	+1.0	+400	+400	+150	*h*	+10	+50

[a] The allowances are intended to provide for individual variations among most normal persons as they live in the United States under usual environmental stresses. Diets should be based on a variety of common foods in order to provide other nutrients for which human requirements have been less well defined. See text for detailed discussion of allowances and of nutrients not tabulated. See Table 1 (p. 20) for weights and heights by individual year of age. See Table 3 (p. 23) for suggested average energy intakes.

[b] Retinol equivalents. 1 retinol equivalent = 1 μg retinol or 6 μg β carotene. See test for calculation of vitamin A activity of diets as retinol equivalents.

[c] As cholecalciferol. 10 μg cholecalciferol = 400 IU of vitamin D.

[d] α-tocopherol equivalents. 1 mg d-α tocopherol = 1 α-TE. See text for variation in allowances and calculation of vitamin E activity of the diet as α-tocopherol equivalents.

[e] 1 NE (niacin equivalent) is equal to 1 mg of niacin or 60 mg of dietary tryptophan.

[f] The folacin allowances refer to dietary sources as determined by *Lactobacillus casei* assay after treatment with enzymes (conjugases) to make polyglutamyl forms of the vitamin available to the test organism.

[g] The recommended dietary allowance for vitamin B-12 in infants is based on average concentration of the vitamin in human milk. The allowances after weaning are based on energy intake (as recommended by the American Academy of Pediatrics) and consideration of other factors, such as intestinal absorption; see text.

[h] The increased requirement during pregnancy cannot be met by the iron content of habitual American diets nor by the existing iron stores of many women; therefore the use of 30–60 mg of supplemental iron is recommended. Iron needs during lactation are not substantially diferent from those of nonpregnant women, but continued supplementation of the mother for 2–3 months after parturition is advisable in order to replenish stores depleted by pregnancy.

TABLE 5-3. Summary of Vitamins in Nutrition

Vitamin	Manifestation	Function	Source	Test
A		Rhodopsin formation Epithelialization Lysomal instability	Fish liver oil Carotene containing vegetables	
Deficiency	Failure to gain, vaginitis, bronchitis, etc. Bitot's spots, xerophthalmia, Night blindness, keratinization			Blood level Flicker fusion
Excess	Carotenemia, hepatosplenomegaly, anemia, coarse hair, periosteal swelling, pseudo-tumor cerebri, hypercalcemia			
B_1 (Thiamine) deficiency	Beriberi, neuritis, edema, cardiomegaly	Cocarboxylase	Cereals, meats, legumes	Lactate-pyruvate ratio, urine excretion
B_2 (Riboflavin) deficiency	Conjunctivitis, glossitis, cheilosis, dermatitis, keratitis	Coenzymes, flavin enzymes	Eggs, milk, yeast	Excretion
Niacin deficiency Toxicity-vascular dilatation	Pellegra, diarrhea, dermatitis, dementia	Coenzymes: NAD, NADP	Liver, meat, eggs	Therapeutic
Panthothenic acid	?	Coenzyme A	Liver	
Pyridoxine (B_6) deficiency	Anemia, polyneuritis, seizures, dermatitis	Coenzyme Transaminases	Yeast, meat, cereal	Therapeutic, blood
Biotin deficiency	? Dermatitis, ? neuritis	CO_2 fixation	Liver	Blood propionate
Inositol	? Fatty liver	Phospholipid formation	Grain	
Folic acid	Macrocytic anemia	Purine precursor	Yeast, vegetables	Blood, formimino glutamic acid excretion
B_{12} deficiency	Pernicious anemia, B_{12} neuropathy	Methylation	Liver, animal protein	Methylmalonic acid excretion
Choline deficiency	Fatty liver	Methylation	Yeast	
C deficiency	Scurvy, hemorrhage, irritability, pseudoparalysis, spongy gums, rosary	Collagen formation	Fruit juice	Blood level, radiograph Tourniquet
D deficiency	Rickets, craniotabes, rosary, large fontanel, tetany	Mineralization, calcium absorption	Fish liver oil, sunlight	Radiograph, blood phosphorus, phosphatase
Excess	Calcification of soft tissues, kidneys, pallor weakness, anorexia			Calcinuria, albuminuria
E	Hemolysis in premature	? Respiratory enzyme	Vegetables	
K deficiency	Hemorrhagic disease	Prothrombin formation	Fish meal	Prothrombin time

TABLE 5-4. Estimated Safe and Adequate Daily Dietary Intakes of Additional Selected Vitamins and Minerals*

		Vitamins			Trace Elements†						Electrolytes		
	Age (yr)	Vitamin K (μg)	Biotin (μg)	Pantothenic Acid (mg)	Copper (mg)	Manganese (mg)	Fluoride (mg)	Chromium (mg)	Selenium (mg)	Molybdenum (mg)	Sodium (mg)	Potassium (mg)	Chloride (mg)
Infants	0–0.5	12	35	2	0.5–0.7	0.5–0.7	0.1–0.5	0.01–0.04	0.01–0.04	0.03–0.06	115–350	350–925	275–700
	0.5–1	10–20	50	3	0.7–1.0	0.7–1.0	0.2–1.0	0.02–0.06	0.02–0.06	0.04–0.08	250–750	425–1,275	400–1,200
Children and adolescents	1–3	15–30	65	3	1.0–1.5	1.0–1.5	0.5–1.5	0.02–0.08	0.02–0.08	0.05–0.1	325–975	550–1,650	500–1,500
	4–6	20–40	85	3–4	1.5–2.0	1.5–2.0	1.0–2.5	0.03–0.12	0.03–0.12	0.06–0.15	450–1,350	775–2,325	700–2,100
	7–10	30–60	120	4–5	2.0–2.5	2.0–3.0	1.5–2.5	0.05–0.2	0.05–0.2	0.1 –0.3	600–1,800	1,000–3,000	925–2,775
	11+	50–100	100–200	4–7	2.0–3.0	2.5–5.0	1.5–2.5	0.05–0.2	0.05–0.2	0.15–0.5	900–2,700	1,525–4,575	1,400–4,200
Adults		70–140	100–200	4–7	2.0–3.0	2.5–5.0	1.5–4.0	0.05–0.2	0.05–0.2	0.15–0.5	1,100–3,300	1,875–5,625	1,700–5,100

*Because there is less information on which to base allowances, these figures are not given in the main table of the RDA and are provided here in the form of ranges of recommended intakes.

†Since the toxic levels for many trace elements may be only several times usual intakes, the upper levels for the trace elements given in this table should not be habitually exceeded.

Reproduced from Recommended Dietary Allowances, 9th. ed. with the permission of the National Academy of Science, Washington, D.C.

TABLE 5-5. Minerals and Their Functions

Mineral	Major function	Clinical Manifestations Deficiency	Excess
Sodium	Osmotic regulation	Weakness Hypotension Convulsions	Edema Hypertension Intracranial bleed
Potassium	Intracellular enzyme activity	Weakness Heart failure Alkalosis	Paralysis Heart block Alkalosis
Chloride	Osmotic regulation	Similar to sodium	
Calcium	Bone metabolism Nerve conduction	Tetany Seizures	Renal failure Aberrant ossification
Phosphorus	Bone metabolism Energy transfer enzymes	Weakness Bone pain	Hyperparathyroidism Hypocalcemia
Magnesium	Electric potential Intracellular enzymes	Seizures Neuritis	Catharsis Paralysis
Iron	Hemoglobin formation	Anemia	Hemosiderosis
Copper	Enzymes, collagen formation	Anemia Skeletal defects	
Iodine	Thyroid function	Hypothyroidism	Hyperthyroidism? Skin lesions
Fluorine		Caries	Hypoglycemia Bone lesions
Zinc	Major metabolic enzymes	Hypogonadism Failure of wound Healing	
Chromium	Glucose metabolism	Diabetes?	
Cobalt	Vitamin B_{12}	Anemia	
Manganese	Enzymes	Bone defects	
Molybdenum	Xanthine oxidase		

Increased caloric requirements are seen in hypermetabolic states: fever, emotional distress, infection, hyperthyroidism, renal disease, heart disease, hypothalamic lesions, ectodermal dysplasia, hemolytic anemia, other anemia states, drug ingestion.

Wasting of calories occurs with: celiac disease, cystic fibrosis, renal disease, antibiotic administration, ulcerative colitis, regional enteritis, diarrheal states, iron deficiency, diabetes.

Calorie excess occurs when caloric intake is greater than calorie utilization and waste. Excessive calorie intake can result in vomiting, diarrhea, or obesity.

Causes of excessive calorie intake and obesity are not well understood. Some causes include: familial patterns, habit, genetics, hypothalamic lesions, rapid growth *in utero*, rapid growth in first few months, familial emotional problems, patient emotional problems, infections (resulting in bed rest), social factors, hypothyroidism, sedation.

Protein Deficiency

When caloric requirement is almost sufficient but protein intake is low, weight loss may not be prominent. In severe protein deficiency, kwashiorkor occurs. Symptoms and signs include: lethargy, hyperactivity, distended abdomen, skin rash, decreased hair coloration, low-serum proteins, anemia, edema, diarrhea, frequent infections.

Children consuming a high-carbohydrate, low-protein diet exhibit multiple deficiencies.

Essential Fatty Acids

Small amounts of long-chain polyunsaturated fats cannot be formed in humans. Deficiency results in seborrhealike skin rash and failure to grow (probably due to inefficient utilization of calories).

Fat and Carbohydrate

Since fat and carbohydrates are the main sources of usable calories, deficiency signs may be restricted to those of calorie deficiency or, if calories are supplied as protein, of protein intoxication. These signs include: lethargy, hyperammonemia, abnormal liver function tests, asterixis, failure to gain, diarrhea. Signs of excess are those of calorie excess.

Water

Although man may be able to live 40 days without food, he cannot live more than 2 to 3 days without water. Dehydration in infants is always a critical problem, requiring immediate attention.

Excessive water ingestion results in water intoxication. Signs include: weight gain, edema, decreased serum electrolytes, seizures, anuria-oliguria, heart failure, signs of increased intracranial pressure.

Causes of increased water intake may be: iatrogenic—excessive or improper parenteral fluids, psychogenic, or heat induced.

PROBLEMS RELATED TO FEEDING

Colic

The symptoms of colic are paroxysmal crying and drawing up of the legs—symptoms apparently associated with pain. The cause is unknown, but factors which produce this complex include: overfeeding, underfeeding, tension or other psychological factors, food allergy or intolerance, peritonitis, incarcerated umbilical or inguinal hernia, eyelash in the eye.

Holding the infant or placing warmth over the abdomen may relieve symptoms. Medications or formula changes do not help. The condition usually disappears by the time the infant is 3 months old.

Constipation

Constipation refers to hard stools. Stools can be softened by increasing dietary carbohydrates. However, rectal examination may reveal tight anal sphincter or megacolon. Tests for hypothyroidism and observation for dehydration or underfeeding may be indicated.

BIBLIOGRAPHY

Fomon S: Infant Nutrition, 2nd ed. Philadelphia, WB Saunders, 1974

One of the few available books on infant nutrition which gives some of the bases of current feeding practices.

Pediatric Nutrition Handbook. Evanston, Illinois, American Academy of Pediatrics on Nutrition, 1979

Many nutritional problems and recommendations are discussed.

Fever

6

J. Martin Kaplan
Thomas F. McNair Scott

CLINICAL PROBLEM

Often a parent brings a child to the physician because "he has a fever." First, the physician should ascertain what the parent considers as fever. Then, he should make sure that the parent understands what is "normal" for the three common methods of determining body temperature.

For children over the age of 5, the *oral* route of determining temperature is usually preferred. The thermometer is placed under the tongue for 4 minutes while the lips are closed; "normal" is 37° ± 0.3°C (98.6° ± 0.5°F). The *rectal* route is used for younger children. The lubricated thermometer is placed in the rectum for 4 minutes; "normal" equals 37.6° ± 0.3°C (99.6° ± 0.5°F). *Axillary* temperatures are taken only when the rectal route is impractical (*e.g.*, imperforate anus, diarrhea). Parents sometimes use it when they are hesitant to try the rectal method. The thermometer is placed under the arm which is held close to the trunk; "normal" is 36.5° ± 0.3°C (97.6° ± 0.5°F).

Deviations from normal occur for various reasons and require an understanding of the physiology of temperature control. These deviations will be discussed later in the chapter.

Temperature Control

The naked human body is able to maintain its temperature at or about 37° ± 0.6°C in environmental temperatures ranging from 16°–55°C (61°–131°F). This stability is maintained by cells in the anterior hypothalamus which constitute a thermo regularity set point or thermostat influenced by a complex feedback mechanism. In the hypothalamus, there appears to be separate but closely interrelated centers for heat loss mainly through skin and lungs and for heat production by muscles and liver.

With a change in thermostat setting imposed by various mechanisms, either heat loss or heat production is initiated.

Heat Loss

Twenty-five percent of heat generated is normally dissipated by evaporation of water from the body surface and lungs; the remainder is lost by radiation (60%), convection (12%), and conduction (3%). Any rise in temperature above 37°C (98.6°F) sets the mechanism of heat loss in motion. Centrally, in the hypothalamus, there is a simultaneous inhibition of vasoconstriction and activation of the sympathetic innervation to the sweat glands. This leads to dilatation of the peripheral vessels and increased moisture from sweat. With the increment in vapor pressure from heat generated by peripheral vasodilatation, there is a rise in insensible loss (1°C elevation in temperature increases insensible losses by 10%); a further dissipation of body heat takes place by evaporation of sweat.

Heat Conservation and Generation

Heat conservation or generation starts after a drop of temperature below 37°C (98.6°F). The body responds either by decreasing heat loss or by activating heat production.

Decrease in heat loss is accomplished in either of two ways: (1) by allowing peripheral vasoconstriction to occur under the influence of the sympathetic areas in the hypothalamus by turning off the previously mentioned active inhibition of this mechanism or (2) by concurrently diminishing cholinergic stimulation of sweat glands, thus decreasing water evaporation from the skin. Heat production is activated by shivering or chemical thermogenesis. Shivering can increase heat production by 500%; it results when the inhibition of the primary motor center in the dorsomedial area of the posterior hypothalamus is shut off, leaving the motor center to be driven by signals from cold sensors in the skin and spinal cord. Chemical thermogenesis accounts for a 50% increase in heat production and is the result of increased cell metabolism in the muscles and liver initiated by the action of centrally released norepinephrine. The thyroid makes a small contribution, secondary to an increase of thyroid-releasing factor.

Modification of Normal Temperature

Modification of normal temperature may come about because of (1) age, (2) transient physiologic factors, (3) disease states.

Age. Neonates exposed to a cold environment will experience a drop in core temperature more rapidly than a 2- or 3-month old infant. A chilled newborn becomes restless but cannot shiver; heat production is not regulated by increased metabolism of muscles and liver but by the breakdown of "brown fat." This tissue begins to form at about 26 to 30 weeks of gestation and reaches its peak 3 to 5 weeks postpartum. Though a major collection is found between the scapulae, there are deposits along the major blood vessels and the perinephric region. The thermolability of the neonate is enhanced by the facility for heat loss provided by the large surface area/weight (sa/wt) ratio and the small amount of subcutaneous (yellow) fat. For the premature, these factors are exaggerated, because of less "brown fat," less subcutaneous fat and greater sa/wt ratio.

In the older infant and child, the importance of brown fat and sa/wt ratio decreases with the increase of subcutaneous fat, and control of temperature gradually approaches that of the adult as normal growth proceeds.

Transient Physiologic Factors. (Diurnal Variation). Depending on age, there is a normal temperature fluctuation between a low at 4:00 AM and a peak at 6:00 PM. This variation is very slight under the age of 2 but may reach a maximum of 1.2°C (2°F) by the time the child is 6 years old. It remains at this level through adolescence, decreasing to 0.8°C (1.4°F) in adulthood. The "normal" temperature range is between 35.5° and 38.4°C (96.0°–101.1°F).

Activity. After strenuous exercise, athletes experience a rise in temperature of several degrees. An active child probably outdoes the athlete, so that an increase in temperature can be expected after vigorous activity.

Emotion. A sudden rise in temperature of several degrees is not an uncommon accompaniment of acute anxiety. This disappears rapidly as the anxiety is dissipated. The mechanism may be that vasoconstriction, resulting from the sudden catecholamine production caused by the emotional outburst, activates cold sensors to initiate heat production.

Disease States. Disease states can modify temperature in two ways:

1. by raising the set point of the thermostat
2. by altering heat production or heat loss with a normal set point

1. If the first mechanism is involved, the body responds by conserving heat through peripheral vasoconstriction. Symptomatically, this is felt as a "chill"; shivering is also experienced because of the body's demand for more heat through increased muscle contraction. As the new level of temperature is reached, any excess heat is given off by vasodilatation and sweating, and the patient feels "feverish." There are two ways in which this change in setpoint is initiated.

(a) Pyrogenic material is contained in the walls of some organisms including group A streptococcus and gram-negative bacilli which can cause an elevation of body temperature. Most of the fevers we experience, however, are not generated by bacterial products but through the production and release of endogenous pyrogens (EP). These small molecular weight proteins (15,000 daltons) are produced and released either by phagocytes after contact with the invading etiologic agent (*e.g.*, bacteria), as occurs in infection or possibly by release of lymphokines induced by malignancy, steroids, allergy, or connective-tissue disease. The EP circulate in the blood and affect the central thermostat through some intermediary product. The most likely candidate for this role is prostaglandin E, because injection in animals of nanogram amounts of this substance into the anterior hypothalamus produces fever after a short latent period. The antipyretic drug, aspirin, is a prostaglandin inhibitor. Other candidates are cyclic adenosine monophosphate (cAMP), epinephrine, and norepinephrine.

(b) The same effects on the center can be initiated directly without mediation of EP by such agents as drugs, for example, epinephrine overdosage, by radiation, CNS lesions or poisons, for example, DDT and scorpion venom.

2. Changes in heat production with normal setpoint exceeding the capabilities of heat loss can be caused by hyperthyroidism, malignant hyperpyrexia, aspirin overdosage, or environmental temperatures, for example, sauna. Fever can also occur when heat loss mechanisms are disturbed, as in, ectodermal dysplasia, burns, heat stroke, and atropine poisoning.

Approach to the Problem

Parents' Interpretation. Many parents suffer from what has been appropriately named "fever phobia." They look on any deviation from the commonly accepted norm of 37°C (98.6°F) with anxiety and assume that this "fever" indicates illness. A responsibility of the physician is to modify this perception. This can be done by discussion of how the temperature was taken, the possible physiologic variations as discussed above, and the adaptive nature of moderate fever.

Evidence continues to accumulate that the defense mechanisms of the body are enhanced by fever probably as high as 41°C (106°F). This evidence comes from animal experiments in which, following inoculation of infectious agents, animals survived when the temperature was allowed to rise but died when the temperature was artificially maintained at a normal level.

In humans, fever enhances leukocyte mobility, bactericidal activity, and the production of leukocyte migration inhibition factor (LIF). There is also a stimulation of lymphocyte transformation and the effect of interferon. EP have been found to increase acute phase globulins, stimulate release of leukocytes from the bone marrow, and decrease iron, required for growth by some pathogenic bacteria.

Diagnosis and Therapy

In certain children, the mother's anxiety may be fully justified, and it is the physician's responsibility to decide which child is sick enough to require further management. One of the criteria is evidence of toxicity; this demands skilled judgment.

Overestimation of toxicity can result in unnecessary investigation or admission to the hospital, while failure to recognize it may seriously jeopardize the child's life or health. An assessment of the child's functional capacity is therefore essential, regardless of the height of the fever. There may be a lack of correlation of the height of the temperature and its depressant effect on functioning.

Infants less than 1 month of age with systemic infection frequently do not have a febrile response. However, in this age group an elevated temperature is more often indicative of serious disease than in the older child. Therefore, in early infancy, fever is usually an indication for admission and further investigation.

Some children tolerate high temperatures without serious consequences. Their parents may state that the child "always runs a high temperature" with apparently trivial infections. These children can have documented temperatures of 39.5°C (103°F) and above without appearing sick, while others manifest symptoms of marked toxicity at these levels. Even in these temperature-prone children, extreme elevations should be an indication for therapy, as temperatures of approximately 41.3°C (106°F) may cause neuronal damage from denaturation of cellular proteins.

When the parent reports that fever continues in the absence of toxicity, it is important to remember two points: (1) recognize that parental anxiety heightens with uncertainty. This may increase the focus on temperature taking, which however justifiable at the onset of the illness, may now lead to misinterpretation of physiologic variations as indications of disease. (2) The child may perceive secondary gains from the constant attention and may support by appropriate complaints the parental interpretation of illness. Clarification of these points with the parents often allows them to put aside the thermometer and minimize the child's complaints. If the parents' anxiety cannot be sufficiently allayed, further evaluation of the parent/child relationship is in order and admission probably will be necessary.

If the clinical evidence points to a definite illness, the advisability of reducing the fever should be considered. This is at present a controversial matter, and many physicians routinely prescribe antipyretics for fever of 38°C (101°F). Others recognizing the adaptive nature of fever, withhold therapy for temperatures less than 39.5°C (103°F). From the above discussion on the mechanisms of fever production, an attempt should be made to distinguish between fever resulting from a change in the setpoint and fever resulting from a disturbance of production/loss balance with normal setpoint. For the former, antipyretic drugs are essential. The two most commonly used antipyretics are aspirin and acetaminophen given in doses of 10mg/kg every 4 hours up to a total of 60mg/kg/24 hrs. Table 6-1 compares their advantages and disadvantages. Since both drugs appear to act by inhibiting prostaglandin synthetase, only one should be used. Also, there is no advantage in using the drugs alternately, and it is possible to induce toxicity by doing this.

If the fever continues unabated and no cause can be found after physical examination, the physician should order appropriate diagnostic studies including a CBC, urinalysis, and chest x-ray study. These tests are usually obtained before considering hospitalization. If the results of these examinations are normal or do not suggest an etiology and the fever has continued for two or

TABLE 6-1. Antipyretic Drugs

	Aspirin	Acetaminophen
Available as liquid	No	Yes
Safety/efficacy ratio	Low	High
Antipyretic effect	Good	Good
Antiinflammatory effect	+	–
Common side-effect	gastrointestinal	None
Cumulative potential	High	Low

more weeks, the child requires hospitalization for investigation of fever of unknown origin (FUO).

After hospital admission, the steps taken must reflect the clinical status of the patient. A toxic child requires expeditious initiation of appropriate diagnostic procedures. The preferred management of the nontoxic patient is to delay initiation of extensive laboratory evaluation. This allows observation of the fever during hospitalization, and may suggest the following two important causes of fever.

1. *Emotional Fever.* A child who at home has had documented fever as high as 39.5°–40°C (103°–104°F) may, in the neutral atmosphere of the hospital, have temperatures within the normal range. Such an occurrence requires a search for a source of stress in the home environment. As Apley points out, "recurrent pyrexia" is one of several recurrent symptoms associated with emotional stress, such as "recurrent abdominal pain" and "recurrent limb pain."

2. *Factitious Fever.* In 10% of 200 patients admitted for FUO of greater than 1 year's duration, the fever was factitious (self-induced) or caused by a parent. An older child can achieve this by various means. Sometimes self-inflicted infections are used to produce a true fever, but more often manipulation of the thermometer is the mechanism employed. Such "factitious fever" can be confusing unless its possibility is considered early in hospitalization. Diagnosis rests on the recognition that the temperature elevations are noted only when the nurse leaves the room during their determination. No child with an FUO should be left alone while his temperature is being taken. In suspicious circumstances, it is usually wise to take simultaneous oral and rectal measurements on several occasions. Even the presence of an observer, which precludes use of the radiator or hot water bottle, cannot prevent manipulation of oral temperatures by a prior mouthful of hot water or rapid rubbing of the end of the thermometer by the tongue. A diagnosis of "factitious fever" should be considered a "cry for help," and appropriate steps should be taken to understand the factors troubling the patient. In the absence of either of these possibilities, there are three major categories of disease that include most of the entities causing fever of unknown origin. A partial list includes the following:

INFECTIOUS DISEASE

1. Subacute bacterial endocarditis
2. Urinary tract infection
3. Prolonged viral infection
4. Salmonella infections
5. Tuberculosis

MALIGNANCY

1. Leukemia
2. Lymphoma
3. Neuroblastoma

③ CONNECTIVE-TISSUE DISEASE

1. Juvenile rheumatoid arthritis
2. Systemic lupus erythematosus
3. Polyarteritis nodosa

SUMMARY

Fever is a symptom; it is usually caused by the production of endogenous pyrogens but may also represent a disorder of the heat production or loss mechanisms. Elevation of the body's temperature serves as a protective function. Therefore, it deserves treatment only when the undesirable effects outweigh the protective ones. Treatment should be directed against the mechanisms responsible for the fever.

BIBLIOGRAPHY

Apley J, MacKeith R: The Child and His Symptoms, 2nd ed. Philadelphia, F. A. Davis, 1968

Atkins E, Bodel P: Fever. N Engl J Med 286:27, 1972

A review of the pathophysiology of fever.

Pizzo PA, *et al*: Prolonged fever in children. Review of 100 cases. Pediatrics 55:468, 1975

A clinical article reviewing the final diagnosis of pediatric patients with FUO. The authors point out those laboratory procedures that were particularly helpful.

Steele RW, *et al*: Evaluation of sponging and of oral antipyretic therapy to reduce fever. J Pediatr 77:824, 1970

Vane JR: The mode of action of aspirin and similar compounds. J Allergy Clin Immunol, 58:691, 1976

This article discusses the recent work on the pyrogenic action of prostaglandins and the mechanism of the antipyretic effect of aspirin and like drugs.

Pallor

7

Frank A. Oski

Pallor does not necessarily indicate that an infant or child is anemic. A child may appear pale due to lack of sufficient exposure to sunlight, chronic illness, edema, or asphyxia. Observation of the color of the mucous membranes of the mouth, the conjunctiva, and the creases in the hyperextended palm of the hand, are all far better indicators of anemia than the color of the skin. Even these observations may fail to reveal the presence of anemia when the hemoglobin value is above 8 g/dl.

Because physical examination alone will fail to reveal the presence of mild anemia, a laboratory test such as the hemoglobin or hematocrit should be performed on all infants at some time during their nursery stay and again at 6 months, 12 months, and 2 years of age.

The normal hemoglobin value and the definition of anemia change with the age of the patient. Failure to appreciate this developmental fact generally results in underdiagnosis of anemia in the newborn period and overdiagnosis of anemia during the period from 3 months to 2 years of age. Normal values for hemoglobin as a function of age are listed in Table 7-1.

Once it has been established that the infant or child is anemic, an orderly approach to the diagnosis of the disease should begin with an examination of the peripheral blood smear, a reticulocyte count, and a measurement of the red cell indices. The interpretation of these results is facilitated by an understanding of the more probable causes of anemia at the varying stages of infancy and childhood.

This knowledge together with the information obtained from the history and physical examination will generally enable the physician to make a correct presumptive diagnosis that can be confirmed by a minimum of additional laboratory tests.

In the physical examination, attention should be paid to the color of the mucous membranes, the presence of lymphadenopathy, the size of the liver and spleen, the presence of bruises or petechiae, and the presence of jaundice.

The history should include information regarding the patient's racial background, information concerning the presence of anemia, jaundice, or gallstones in other family members, a detailed dietary history, inquiries regarding the frequency and color of the child's stools, the presence of pica, drug ingestion, previous episodes of jaundice, and the frequency of infections.

ANEMIA IN EARLY INFANCY

The diagnosis of anemia in early infancy is a far more complicated process than it is at any other time of life. During the first 3 months of extrauterine existence, continuous changes produced by growth and

TABLE 7-1. Red Blood Cell Values at Various Ages: Mean and Lower Limit of Normal (−2 SD)

Age	Hemoglobin (g/dl)		Hematocrit (%)		Red Cell Count (10^{12}/liter)		MCV (fl)		MCH (pg)		MCHC (g/dl)	
	Mean	−2 SD	Mean	−2 SD	Mean	−2 SD	Mean	−2 SD	Mean	−2 SD	Mean	−2 SD
Birth (cord blood)	16.5	13.5	51	42	4.7	3.9	108	98	34	31	33	30
1 to 3 days (capillary)	18.5	14.5	56	45	5.3	4.0	108	95	34	31	33	29
1 week	17.5	13.5	54	42	5.1	3.9	107	88	34	28	33	28
2 weeks	16.5	12.5	51	39	4.9	3.6	105	86	34	28	33	28
1 month	14.0	10.0	43	31	4.2	3.0	104	85	34	28	33	29
2 months	11.5	9.0	35	28	3.8	2.7	96	77	30	26	33	29
3 to 6 months	11.5	9.5	35	29	3.8	3.1	91	74	30	25	33	30
0.5 to 2 years	12.0	11.0	36	33	4.5	3.7	78	70	27	23	33	30
2 to 6 years	12.5	11.5	37	34	4.6	3.9	81	75	27	24	34	31
6 to 12 years	13.5	11.5	40	35	4.6	4.0	86	77	29	25	34	31
12 to 18 years—female	14.0	12.0	41	36	4.6	4.1	90	78	30	25	34	31
male	14.5	13.0	43	37	4.9	4.5	88	78	30	25	34	31
18 to 49 years—female	14.0	12.0	41	36	4.6	4.0	90	80	30	26	34	31
male	15.5	13.5	47	41	5.2	4.5	90	80	30	26	34	31

(Dallman PR, Siimes MA: Percentile curves for hemoglobin and red cell volume in infancy and childhood. Pediatr 94:26, 1979)

TABLE 7-2. Serial Hemoglobin Values (g %) in Low Birth Weight Infants

Birth weight (g)	Age (in weeks) 2	4	6	8	10
800–1000	16.0 ± 0.6	10.0 ± 3.2	8.7 ± 1.5	8.0 ± 0.9	8.0 ± 1.1
1001–1200	16.4 ± 2.3	12.8 ± 2.5	10.5 ± 1.8	9.1 ± 1.3	8.5 ± 1.5
1201–1400	16.2 ± 1.3	13.4 ± 2.8	10.9 ± 1.2	9.9 ± 1.9	—
1401–1500	15.6 ± 2.2	11.7 ± 1.0	10.5 ± 0.7	9.8 ± 1.4	—

development result in week-to-week variations in what may be regarded as the normal hemoglobin value. In addition, unique pathologic processes are operative at this age that also contribute to diagnostic confusion. These unique processes are a consequence of maternal-fetal interactions, the rapidity of growth with its attendant nutritional requirements, and the proclivity of newborns to acquire a variety of infections.

After the 34th to 35th week of gestation, the mean cord blood hemoglobin value is approximately 17.0 g/dl. Values of less than 13.5 g/dl at birth may be regarded as abnormal. During the first hours of life, the hemoglobin value may rise by as much as 20% in infants whose umbilical cords were not clamped immediately at birth. During the first week of life in both the term and premature infant, there is very little change in the hemoglobin concentration, and values at 7 days of age are very similar to those values present at birth.

Beyond the first week of life, the hemoglobin values begin to decline rapidly. In the term infant, the hemoglobin value reaches its lowest level at 8 to 9 weeks of age (Table 7-1). At this time, hemoglobin values as low as 9.5 g/dl can be viewed as normal. Hemoglobin values tend to fall more rapidly and reach lower levels in apparently healthy premature infants (Table 7-2). At 6 to 8 weeks of age, the hemoglobin value of infants weighing 1200 g or less at birth averages about 8.0 g/dl and values of 7.0 g/dl are frequently observed in the absence of any recognizable pathologic process.

Regulation of Erythropoiesis

This fall in hemoglobin levels appears to be a normal physiologic process that is influenced by both the oxygen requirements of the infant and the mechanisms governing oxygen release to the tissues. Although it seems clear that the regulation of erythropoiesis in the adult is under the influence of erythropoietin, the modulation of fetal and newborn erythropoiesis has been more difficult to understand because of the many complex factors affecting red cell formation during this stage of development. These factors include the influence of maternal erythropoiesis, variations in placental function, multiple sites of red cell production in the fetus, changes in arterial oxygenation at birth, the gradual replacement of fetal hemoglobin by adult hemoglobin, and alterations in the concentration and effects of red cell 2,3-diphosphoglycerate.

Red cell formation *in utero* begins at approximately day 14 of gestation and occurs successively in the yolk sac, liver, and bone marrow. Erythropoietin is produced by the fetus and appears to be responsive to the usual factors stimulating its production. Both term and preterm infants have normal or elevated erythropoietin levels when compared with normal adults. Infants with erythroblastosis fetalis increase erythropoietin production in the presence of anemia. Infants with polycythemia at birth also demonstrate elevations in erythropoietin levels. This is seen in infants who are small for gestational age or who are postmature, and is associated with placental insufficiency and presumed intrauterine hypoxia.

The erythropoietin present in the plasma of the newborn appears to be produced endogenously and under fetal control. Although maternal plasma erythropoietin levels are slightly elevated during pregnancy, the cord blood samples from anemic infants with erythroblastosis show even greater erythropoietin activity.

The normal or elevated plasma erythropoietin level present at birth declines to undetectable levels within several days of birth and rises again between 60 and 90 days of life. During this period, the hemoglobin level falls progressively, accompanied by a decreased rate of erythropoiesis. The bone marrow at this time is capable of increased erythropoiesis mediated by means of erythropoietin if appropriate stimulation is present such as that observed with anemia or the hypoxemia of cyanotic heart disease. Thus, it appears that the fall in hemoglobin level that is observed during the first 2 to 3 months of life occurs as a result of increased oxygen delivery to the tissues with removal of the stimulation to erythropoietin production. At birth, arterial oxygen saturation promptly rises from the intrauterine value of 45% to 95%. During the next several months of life, the position of the oxygen-hemoglobin dissociation curve gradually shifts to the right as the hemoglobin falls. This gradual shift in the curve facilitates oxygen release to the tissues. As a result, the term infant at 3 months is capable of releasing as much oxygen to his tissues, at a mixed venous oxygen tension of 40 mm Hg, as the normal newborn infant despite a pronounced fall in the oxygen-carrying capacity of the blood. This shift in the position of the curve to the right is mediated by the replacement of fetal by adult hemoglobin and its interaction with red cell 2,3-diphosphoglycerate.

The causes of true anemia both at birth and during the first several months of life can be considered against this background of normal developmental changes.

Anemia at Birth

Anemia at birth or during the first week of life is generally the result of hemolysis or hemorrhage. Hemolytic anemias occurring during this early period of life are of multiple etiologies and generally are associated with serum bilirubin levels in excess of 6 to 8 mg/dl. Hemolytic disease in the newborn can be broadly classified into three large categories: isoimmunization, inherited defects of the red cell, and acquired defects of the red cell. In most parts of the world, isoimmunization as a result of maternal-fetal incompatibilities in either the Rh or ABO blood group systems is the leading cause of hemolytic disease. Of the inherited defects of the red cell, red cell glucose-6-phosphate dehydrogenase deficiency appears to be the abnormality most commonly associated with both anemia and hyperbilirubinemia. Virtually all of the red cell enzyme deficiencies described to date have been associated with anemia and hyperbilirubinemia during the early days of life. The red cell membrane disorders, which include hereditary spherocytosis, elliptocytosis, and stomatocytosis, may also be associated with anemia in early life. Approximately 50% of patients with hereditary spherocytosis experience hyperbilirubinemia during the first week of life.

Anemia and jaundice frequently accompany profound acidosis and hypoxemia in the young infant. In many instances, this hemolytic anemia may be a consequence of the associated pathologic process of disseminated intravascular coagulation. Infections, most notably those produced by congenital cytomegalovirus, toxoplasmosis, rubella, syphilis, herpes, group B hemolytic streptococcus, and gram-negative bacteria, are other causes of anemia during this period. Red cell hypoplasia (Blackfan-Diamond syndrome) may also manifest itself at the time of birth as anemia and reticulocytopenia.

Other inherited abnormalities that may result in anemia during the first several days of life include defects in alpha-chain synthesis (alpha-thalassemia trait) or gamma-chain synthesis (gamma-thalassemia).

Hemorrhage leading to anemia at birth or in the first few days of life may be broadly grouped into three major etiologic categories. These include hemorrhage associated with obstetric accidents or malformations of the placenta and cord, occult hemorrhage from the fetus into the maternal circulation or from twin to twin, and internal hemorrhages (Table 7-3). In these situations, pallor and signs of circulatory collapse are prominent clinical features and jaundice is generally absent.

Anemia at 1 to 3 Months of Life

Anemia that is first detected at 1 to 3 months of life may represent the sequel of previously undiagnosed events in the immediate newborn period. Most frequently, these include mild isoimmunization, fetal to maternal hemorrhage, or chronic congenital infections.

By this period of life, hemoglobinopathies involving defects of the beta chain become clinically apparent. Both thalassemia major and sickle-cell anemia produce anemia by 3 months of age.

In the rapidly growing premature infant, both folic acid deficiency and vitamin E deficiency also may produce true anemia by 8 to 10 weeks of life. Folic acid deficiency is most commonly observed in those infants whose clinical course has been complicated by diarrhea and infections. Vitamin E deficiency occurs almost exclusively in infants with birth weights less than 1500 g. The anemia is primarily the result of excessive hemolysis and is accompanied by reticulocytosis, poikilocytosis, red cell fragmentation, mild spherocytosis, thrombocytosis, and in the more severely deficient infants, edema may be observed.

Vitamin E deficiency results from a combination of factors which include: low Vitamin E stores at birth, inadequate dietary intake, and poor absorption of this fat-soluble vitamin. If the low birth weight infant is fed a diet rich in polyunsaturated fatty acids, is not provided with adequate amounts of Vitamin E, and then given medicinal quantities of iron, a hemolytic anemia may be initiated. Iron, in such circumstances, acts as an oxidant compound.

In Table 7-3, the more common cause of anemia during the first 3 months of life are listed. Because of the plethora of diagnostic possibilities, the physician must approach this challenging problem with a clear understanding of what "true" anemia is, diligently collect relevant information concerning family history, obstetric history, the early neonatal course of events, and dietary history before instituting a myriad of unnecessary and ill-suited diagnostic procedures.

ANEMIA AFTER 3 MONTHS OF AGE

The rational approach to diagnosis at this age again begins with an attempt to classify the anemia based on its morphologic characteristics. A simple flow diagram for this purpose is depicted in Figure 7-1. The anemias are subdivided into those in which the red cells are small in size (microcytic), normal in size (normocytic), or large in size (macrocytic). In addition, the anemias that are generally normocytic are further subdivided into those anemias that are primarily a result of accelerated red cell destruction as contrasted with those that are primarily a result of impaired red cell production.

Between 3 months and 2 years of age, and particularly between 9 months and 2 years of age, iron deficiency is the leading cause of anemia. During this period of life, an infant outgrows his iron endowment. Normal newborns are born with an iron endowment of approximately 75 mg/kg.

TABLE 7-3. Common Causes of Anemia in Early Infancy

Age	Diagnosis	Supporting data
At birth	Hemorrhage	
	Obstetric accidents (placenta previa, abruptio placenta, incision of placenta, rupture of cord, rupture of anomalous placental vessel)	History and visual inspection of placenta and cord
	Occult hemorrhage	
	Fetomaternal	Demonstration of fetal cells in maternal circulation
	Twin-to-twin	Demonstration of significant difference in hemoglobin values of identical twins
	Internal hemorrhage (intracranial, retroperitoneal, intrahepatic, intrasplenic, cephalohematoma)	Physical examination CT scan Ultrasonography
	Isoimmunization	Blood groups of mother and infant, evidence of antibody on infant's red cells
	Inherited defect of red cell (includes G-6-PD deficiency, pyruvate kinase deficiency, hereditary spherocytosis, elliptocytosis, stomatocytosis, etc.)	Red cell morphology, family history, and appropriate screening tests
	Acquired defect (generally in association with hypoxemia, acidosis, or infection)	Physical findings, red cell morphology, coagulation disturbance, blood and urine cultures, and serologic studies and Gamma M determination
	Red cell hypoplasia (Blackfan-Diamond syndrome, congenital leukemia, osteopetrosis)	Rare disorders. Bone marrow aspirate
2–3 months	Iron deficiency as a consequence of previous hemorrhage	Obstetric history when available
	Late manifestation of previous isoimmunization	Blood types of mother and infant; maternal and infant antibody titers
	Hereditary defects of the red cell	Persistence of hemolytic anemia. Red cell morphology and laboratory tests
	Thalassemia major	Red cell morphology, splenomegaly, persistence of fetal hemoglobin elevation, family studies (see Table 7-4)
	Sickle-cell anemia	Red cell morphology, hemoglobin electrophoresis (see Table 7-5)
	Vitamin E deficiency	Infant of low birth weight. Red cell morphology, low serum E level, positive hydrogen peroxide hemolysis test
	Folic acid deficiency	Premature infant, history of infections or diarrhea, red cell and marrow morphology, response to folic acid
	Persistent infection	Elevated titers to rubella, cytomegalovirus, toxoplasmosis
	Renal tubular acidosis	Acidosis, hypochloremia, mild azotemia, urine pH of 6.0 or greater in presence of acidosis

Almost two-thirds of this iron endowment is present in the infant's red cell hemoglobin. Very little iron is normally lost from the body so that the infant can increase his birth weight approximately 2½-fold before his iron stores are depleted and iron deficiency begins to limit the rate of hemoglobin synthesis. For this reason, nutritional iron deficiency is rarely observed during the first 6 months of life. Only in infants who are growing rapidly (*e.g.*, infants born of low birth weights who may quadruple their birth weights within the first 6 months of life) will nutritional causes of iron deficiency occur early in life.

Other causes of microcytic anemias that may be confused with iron deficiency are listed in Figure 7-1.

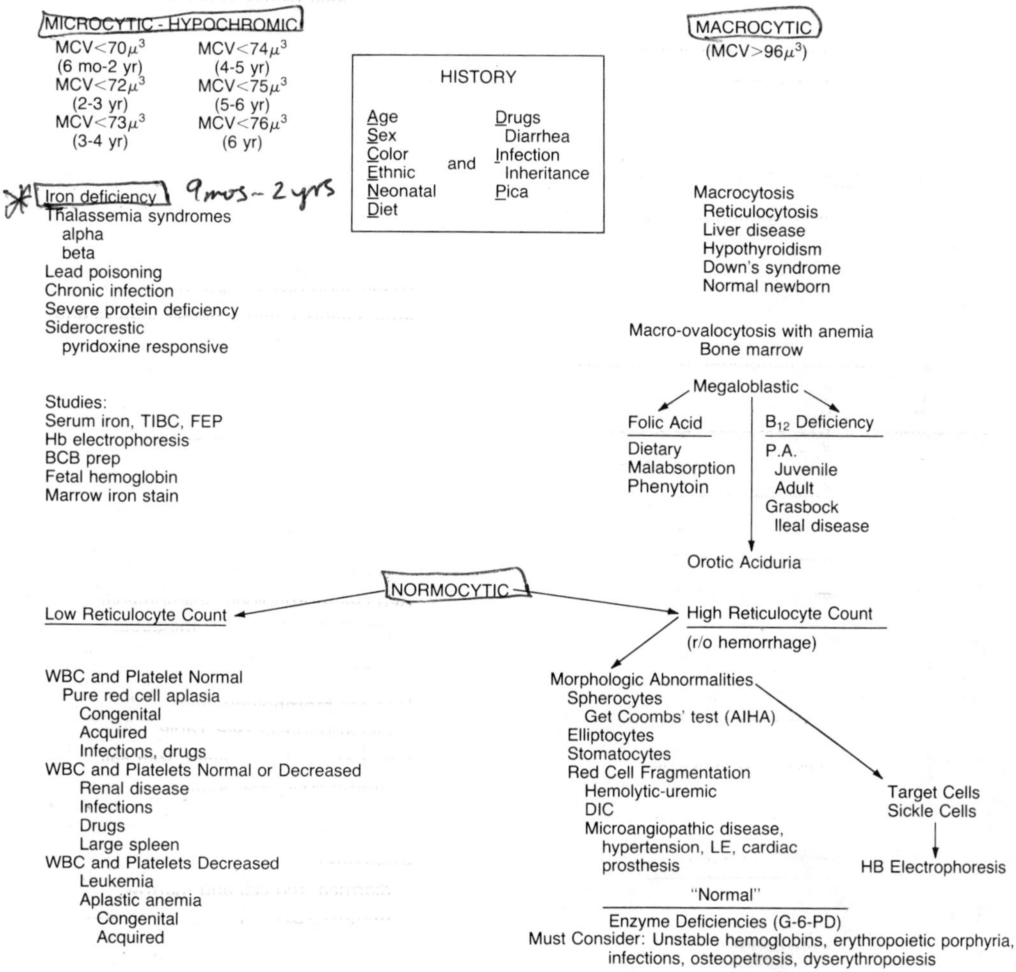

Fig. 7-1. A diagnostic approach to anemia. (Must get red cell indices, reticulocyte count and smear.)
TIBC = total iron binding capacity
FEP = free erythrocyte protoporphyrin
BCB prep = brilliant cresyl blue preparation
AIHA = autoimmune hemolytic anemia

TABLE 7-4. Differential Diagnosis of Thalassemia Syndromes

Disorder	HgB A_2 (%)	HgB F (%)	MCV (fl)	HgB (g/dl)	Morphology
α-Thalassemia					
Silent carrier	Normal	Normal	Normal	Normal	Normal
Heterozygous	Normal	Normal	Low/normal	Low/normal	Normal or microcytic target cells
HbH (~5%)	Low/normal	Normal	Low	Low/normal	Supravital stain of peripheral blood inclusion (Heinz) bodies
Homozygous α-thal (Hydrops Fetalis)					Marked abnormality of RBC, pronounced erythroblastemia anisopoikilocytosis
β-Thalassemia					
Heterozygous β^0 or β^+	3.5 – 8.0	2 – 4	64 ± 4	Low/normal	Microcytosis, anisocytosis, poikilocytosis, hypochromia, target cells, basophilic stippling
Homozygous					
β^0/β^0 (no HbA)	1 – 6	95	Low	Very low	Severe anemia, reticulocytosis, nucleated RBC, basophilic stippling, target cells, extreme poikilocytosis, anisocytosis
β^+/β^+ (variable)	2 – 8	Variable			
β^+/β^0 (amount of HbA present)	1 – 3	Variable			Supravital stain–bone marrow–inclusions in RBC precursors
Lepore heterozygous 5–15%	Low/normal	2 – 4	Low	Low/normal	Poikilocytosis, hypochromia, anisocytosis, microcytic target cells
Lepore homozygous 10–20%					
HPFH					
Greek	1 – 3	10 – 20	Normal	Normal	Hypochromia, microcytosis, anisocytosis, and poikilocytosis
Swiss		3 – 13			Normal, few target cells
Black		17 – 33	Low/normal	Low/normal	

SS—Homozygous sickle cell disease
S—Sickle trait
C—Chemoglobin
B^0/B^+—β-Thalassemias
HPFH—Hereditary persistence of fetal hemoglobin
(Lubin, B *et al:* Differential diagnosis of thalassemia syndromes. Lab Manage 18:38, 1980)

TABLE 7-5. Differential Diagnosis of Common Hemoglobinopathies

Diagnosis	Frequency	Clinical Severity	HGB (g/dl)	HCT (%)	MCV (μ^3)	% Retic	RBC Morphology	Solubility Test	Electro-phoresis	Distribution HbF
SS	1:625	Moderate/ Severe	7.5 (6–10)	22 (18–30)	93	11 (4–30)	Many ISC's, target cells, nucleated red cells	Positive	80–90%S 2–20%F <3.6%A_2	Uneven
SC	1:833	Mild/ Moderate	10 (9–14)	30 (26–40)	80	3 (1.5–6)	Many target cells, rare ISC's	Positive	45–55%S 45–55%C . 2–8%F	Uneven
S/B^0 Thal		Moderate/ Severe	8.1 (7–12)	25 (20–36)	69	8 (3–18)	Marked hypochromia, microcytosis & target cells, variable ISC's	Positive	50–85%S 2–30%A >3.6%A_2	Uneven
S/B + Thal	1:1667	Mild/ Moderate	11 (8–13)	32 (25–40)	76	3 (1.5–6)	Mild microcytosis, hypochromia rare ISC's	Positive	55–75%S 15–30%A 1–20%F >3.6%A_2	Uneven
S/HPFH	1:25000	Asymptomatic	14 (11–15)	40 (32–48)	84	1.5 (.5–3)	No ISC's, occasional target cells, and mild hypochromia	Positive	60–80%S 16–35%F 1–3%A_2	Even
AS	1:17	Asymptomatic	Normal	Normal	Normal	Normal	Normal	Positive	38–45%S 60–55%A 1–3%A_2	Uneven
ASα-Thal	1:300	Asymptomatic	Low/ normal	Low/ normal	70	Normal	Microcytic	Positive	29–35%S 71–75%A	Uneven

SS—Homozygous sickle cell disease
S—Sickle trait
C—Chemoglobin
B^0,B^+—β-Thalassemias
HPFH—Hereditary persistence of fetal hemoglobin
(Lubin B *et al:* Lab Manage 18:38, 1980)

Another major subdivision of anemia is the macrocytic and megaloblastic anemias. Macrocytes in and of themselves are not diagnostic of a megaloblastic anemia. Macrocytes are large erythrocytes and may be seen in anyone with reticulocytosis. As young cells are larger cells, they may be seen in patients with hemolytic diseases. They may also be seen in patients with hypothyroidism, liver disease, and in the normal newborn. The hallmark of a macrocytic-megaloblastic anemia is the presence of macro-ovalocytes in the peripheral blood smear. In addition, changes in white cell morphology are extremely important in substantiating the diagnosis of megaloblastic anemia. The normal person has a mean neutrophil lobe count of approximately 3.2. In general, a normal person may have as many as three, 5-lobed polymorphonuclear leukocytes in a peripheral smear when 100 cells are counted. The presence of more than this number of 5-lobed polys or the presence of polys with six or more lobes should alert the physician to the possibility that the patient may have a megaloblastic anemia.

Dietary folic acid deficiency can occur in young infants, particularly those raised on goat's milk, which is very low in this vitamin. It is more commonly seen in patients with malabsorptive states. Folic acid is absorbed primarily in the jejunum and vitamin B_{12} is absorbed primarily in the ileum. Diseases in these portions of the gastrointestinal tract can result in the appearance of a deficiency of these vitamins. In patients with macro-ovalocytes or white cell changes suggestive of a megaloblastic anemia, bone marrow studies should be performed to confirm the fact that megaloblastic erythropoiesis is present. Once this is established, attention should be directed to the cause of the deficiency.

The normocytic anemias are a heterogenous group of disorders. Although every anemic patient should have a reticulocyte count performed, it is particularly important in facilitating a diagnosis in patients in this category. When anemia is associated with a low reticulocyte count, one must seriously suspect some form of bone marrow dysfunction. Attention should be paid to the white cell and platelet count in an effort to determine if all the formed elements are involved in the bone marrow failure. Both congenital and acquired diseases may produce disburbances in erythropoiesis. Many of these diagnostic possibilities are listed in Figure 7-1. Confirmation requires bone marrow examination coupled with other appropriate laboratory studies.

Another large group of patients with normocytic anemias is associated with reticulocytosis and a shortened red cell life span. Here, the morphology of the red cells provides an important clue as to etiology. Based on the appearance of the red cells, the physician may decide to request additional confirmatory studies such as hemoglobin electrophoresis, enzyme assays, and study of other possibly affected family members. Tables 7-4 and 7-5 provide additional information to assist in the differential diagnosis of the thalassemia syndromes and common hemoglobinopathies.

It must be realized that anemia is never a diagnosis. It is only evidence of the presence of a disease whose cause must be ascertained. Through a series of generally simple and logical steps, a diagnosis can be established in most patients. Treatment can then be directed in an appropriate fashion.

BIBLIOGRAPHY

Baehner RL: Symposium on pediatric hematology. Pediatr Clin North Am 27:215, 1980

Includes chapters dealing with aplastic anemia, nutritional anemias, hereditary hemolytic anemias, and autoimmune hemolytic anemias. An excellent reference source.

Dallman PR, Siimes MA: Percentile curves for hemoglobin and red cell volume in infancy and childhood. J Pediatr 94:26, 1979

Oski FA: Anemia in children. Hosp Prac, 11:63, 1976

A review of the causes and diagnosis of anemia in infants and children.

Oski FA: Differential diagnosis of anemia. In Nathan DG, Oski FA (eds): Hematology of Infancy and Childhood, 2nd ed. Philadelphia, WB Saunders, 1981

8

Bruising and Bleeding

Frank A. Oski

Parents of young toddlers commonly remark that their child bruises easily. Children with recurrent epistaxis are frequently referred for evaluation of a possible bleeding disorder. An accurate and detailed history often discloses justification for suspecting an underlying inherited or acquired bleeding disturbance. A history and a careful physical examination generally eliminate the need for further laboratory investigation.

The parents and family should be specifically questioned about all past injuries including needle punctures, minor cuts in the mouth and skin, and all instances of surgery including dental extractions, tonsillectomy, and circumcision. The absence of excessive bleeding after dental extractions, tonsillectomy, surgical incisions, and major trauma eliminates the possibility of a longstanding or inherited defect in coagulation.

Excessive bruising and bleeding can be the result of: (1) a deficiency of one of the coagulation factors, (2) a quantitative deficiency of platelets, (3) a qualitative abnormality of platelets, or (4) an abnormality of the vessels—either excessive capillary fragility or the presence of vasculitis.

Some features of the history and physical examination allow you to categorize the suspected bleeding disturbance into either (1) a defect of the fluid phase of coagulation or (2) an abnormality of platelets or vessel wall. The distinguishing characteristics are described in Table 8-1. The steps in the coagulation pathway are illustrated in Figure 8-1.

When one suspects a bleeding disorder, initial laboratory studies should include a partial thromboplastin time, a prothrombin time, a platelet count, a smear to examine platelet morphology, and a standardized Ivy Bleeding Time. This battery of tests allows a presumptive diagnosis of a bleeding disturbance. The only defect not detected by one of these procedures is an inherited deficiency of Factor XIII (fibrin-stabilizing factor). The use of such tests in arriving at a presumptive diagnosis is illustrated in Table 8-2. Once a provisional diagnosis has been made, it can be confirmed by assay of specific clotting factors. The mode of transmission of the inherited defects of coagulation is listed below.

Mode of Transmission of the Hereditary Coagulation Disorders

Sex-linked recessive (disorders primarily of males)
- Factor VIII (AHF) deficiency
- Factor IX (PTC) deficiency

Autosomal dominant (disorders of both sexes; one parent affected)
- Factor XI (PTA) deficiency
- von Willebrand's disease

Autosomal recessive (disorders of both sexes; parents appear normal)
- Prothrombin deficiency
- Factor V (proaccelerin) deficiency

TABLE 8-1. Clinical Features That Serve to Distinguish Bleeding as a Result of a Defect in the Fluid Phase of Coagulation from a Platelet or Capillary Defect

Clinical Features	Coagulation Defects	Platelet and Capillary Defects
Bleeding from superficial cuts and abrasions	Usually not excessive	Often profuse and prolonged
Spontaneous bruises and hematomas	Often deep and spreading hematoma Only a few at any one time	Usually small, superficial, and multiple
Hemarthroses	Common in severe cases	Very rare
Bleeding from deep cuts and tooth extractions	Onset often delayed for minutes or hours. Not permanently controlled by local pressure	Onset usually immediate. Frequently permanently arrested by local pressure
Most common bleeding manifestations	Deep tissue hemorrhages, often involves joints and muscle. Prolonged bleeding after injury	Epistaxis, menorrhagia, and gastrointestinal bleeding
Petechiae	Rare	Common

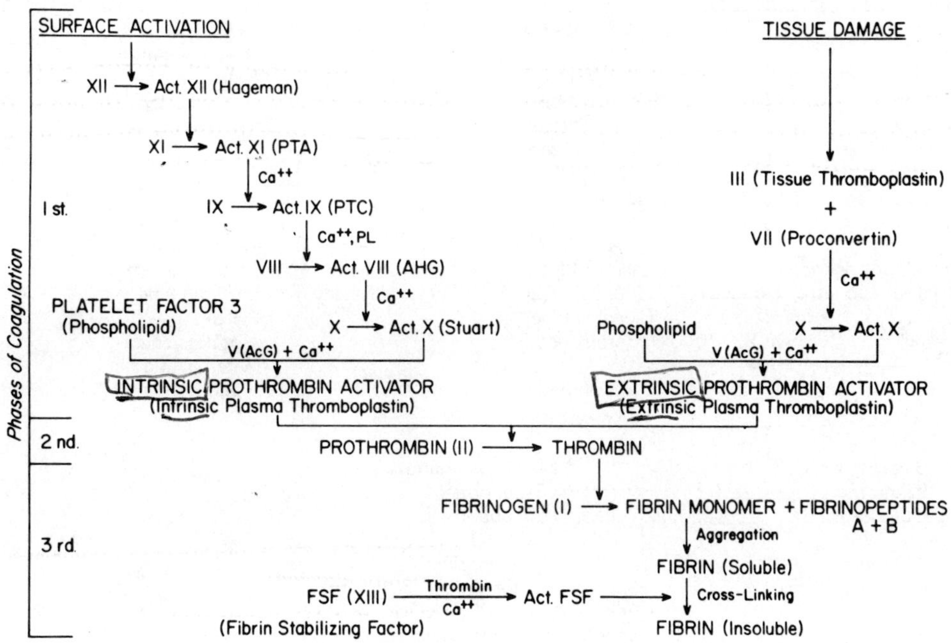

Fig. 8-1. The coagulation scheme.

Factor VII (proconvertin) deficiency
Factor X (Stuart-Prower) deficiency
Factor XII (Hageman) deficiency—no bleeding associated with this disorder
Factor XIII (fibrin-stabilizing factor) deficiency
Afibrinogenemia, congenital
von Willebrand's disease (severe form)

If the patient is found to be thrombocytopenic, it must be determined whether the low platelet count is the result of inadequate platelet production or accelerated platelet destruction. Simple studies that assist the physician in this determination include a bone marrow examination to determine the adequacy of megakaryocyte number, and an examination of the peripheral smear. Young platelets tend to be large (greater than 2.5 μm in diameter). In patients with destructive thrombocytopenias, young platelets are usually evident on the blood

TABLE 8-2. A Diagnostic Approach to the Bleeding Patient

Platelets decreased PT prolonged PTT prolonged	Platelets normal PT prolonged PTT prolonged	Platelets normal PT normal PTT prolonged	Platelets normal PT prolonged PTT normal	Platelets normal PT normal PTT normal	Platelets decreased PT and PTT normal
Consider: disseminated intravascular coagulation, particularly in patients with sepsis or hypoxia. ↓	*Consider:* Vitamin K deficiency. ↓	*Consider:* Congenital Factor VIII deficiency Congenital Factor IX deficiency Congenital Factor XI deficiency Congenital Factor XII deficiency von Willebrand's disease Heparin treatment ↓	*Consider:* Congenital Factor II deficiency Congenital Factor VII deficiency ↓	*Consider:* Factor XIII deficiency Platelet dysfunction von Willebrand's disease ↓	Determine cause of thrombocytopenia
Tests to confirm: Thrombin time Fibrin split products Factor V assay Red cell fragmentation	If vitamin K has not been given, administer vitamin K_1, 2.0 mg I.V. Repeat PT and PTT in 4 hours	*Tests to confirm:* Factor VIII, IX, XI, XII assay Bleeding time (prolonged in von Willebrand's disease)	*Tests to confirm:* Factor II assay Factor VII assay	*Tests to confirm:* Factor XIII assay Bleeding time Platelet adhesiveness Maternal and infant drug history	

(Repeat PT and PTT in 4 hours →)

Bleeding stops
PT normal
PTT normal
↓
Diagnosis:
Vitamin K deficiency

Bleeding continues
PT abnormal
PTT abnormal
↓
Consider:
Congential Factor V deficiency
Congential Factor X deficiency
Congenital fibrinogen deficiency
Severe liver disease
↓
Tests to confirm:
Factor V assay
Factor X assay
Fibrinogen assay

film. If the results of the bone marrow examination and peripheral smear are indecisive, the patient can be administered platelets and their survival determined.

Causes of thrombocytopenia are listed below. In addition to these more common causes of bleeding, a large variety of rare disorders of platelet function have now been described.

Causes of Thrombocytopenia

Decreased rate of production
- Leukemia
- Aplastic anemia (inherited and acquired)
- Drug-induced
- Prolonged steroid therapy

Increased rate of destruction
- Idiopathic thrombocytopenic purpura
- Disseminated intravascular coagulation
- Hypersplenism
- Systemic lupus erythematosus
- Wiskott-Aldrich syndrome
- Inherited platelet defects
- Evan's syndrome
  (thrombocytopenia in association with autoimmune hemolytic anemia)

Bleeding in the newborn infant presents some unique problems of interpretation and management. With the prolongation of life in small and desperately ill premature infants, the incidence of clinical coagulation problems appears to be increasing.

The bleeding problems of the newborn can be conveniently divided into the following broad categories: (1) inherited defects of the coagulation mechanism, (2) accentuation of the normally occurring transitory deficiencies of the coagulation mechanism characteristic of this period of life, (3) transitory disturbances secondary to an associated disease process, (4) quantitative or qualitative abnormalities of the platelets.

Many of the coagulation factors are not present in normal concentrations in the blood of the newborn infant. These deviations from normal adult values are particularly marked in the premature infant. The typical values encountered in the term and preterm infant are summarized in Table 8-3. It should be noted that the vitamin K-dependent factors (Factors II, VII, IX, and X) and Factors XI, XII, and XIII are gen-

TABLE 8-3. Coagulation Factors and Test Values in Term and Premature Infants

Factor	Normal	Term Infant (cord blood)	Premature Infant (cord blood)
Fibrinogen (mg/dl)	200–400	200–250	200–250
Factor II (%)	50–150	40	25
Factor V (%)	75–125	90	60–75
Factor VII (%)	75–125	50	35
Factor VIII (%)	50–150	100	80–100
Factor IX (%)	50–150	25–40	25–40
Factor X (%)	50–150	50–60	25–40
Factor XI (%)	75–125	30–40	—
Factor XII (%)	75–125	50–100	50–100
Factor XIII (titer)	1:16	1:8	1:8
Partial thromboplastin time (sec)	30–50	70	80–90
Prothrombin time (sec)	10–12	12–18	14–20
Thrombin time (sec)	10–12	12–16	13–20

erally decreased while the levels of fibrinogen (Factors V and VIII) and platelets are in, or near, the normal adult range.

Despite deficiencies of many of these factors, the whole blood of the newborn infant is hypercoagulable. This hypercoagulability appears related most closely to a deficiency of antithrombin-III in infants who developed the respiratory distress syndrome.

INHERITED DEFECTS OF THE COAGULATION MECHANISM

Although the majority of infants with congenital deficiencies of the coagulation factors do not bleed during the first weeks of life, all the congenital defects can manifest themselves with hemorrhage in the newborn period.

It is not clear why hemorrhage does not occur more frequently. None of the coagulation factors crosses the placenta, so infants with hemophilia can be diagnosed at birth and are presumably at risk from hemorrhage.

From studies of patients with Factor VIII deficiency (classic hemophilia), it appears that only the most severely affected persons bled during the newborn period. When bleeding occurs in the newborn, it is most frequently a result of a circumcision. More serious bleeding may take the form of giant cephalohematoma, intracranial hemorrhages, hemarthroses, and intramuscular hematomas. Petechiae and flat ecchymotic areas are uncommon isolated manifestions of hemophilia.

VITAMIN K DEFICIENCY

Vitamin K deficiency, or true "hemorrhagic disease of the newborn," is caused by an accentuation of the normally occurring transient deficiencies of the coagulation mechanism that characterize this period of life. Biochemical and immunologic studies have provided new insights into the chemistry of Factors II, VII, IX, and X and the mechanism of action of vitamin K. The coagulation factors are synthesized in the liver in a precursor form that is biologically inactive. Conversion of the inactive precursor to the active protein requires a carboxylase enzyme, oxygen, carbon dioxide, and vitamin K. Accumulated evidence suggests that the initially decreased activity of the vitamin K-dependent factors observed in healthy infants is primarily a result of inadequate synthesis of the precursor proteins. Only after several days of life will the major consequences of vitamin K deficiency be responsible for the measured coagulation abnormalities. Term infants with complications of labor and delivery, however, have laboratory findings suggestive of vitamin K deficiency within the early hours of life.

Bleeding due to vitamin K deficiency can occur on the first day of life but is more commonly observed on the second or third day of life. Bleeding from the gastrointestinal tract, umbilical cord, circumcision site, nose, and into the scalp, as well as generalized ecchymosis, are the most frequent external manifestations of the disease. Internal hemorrhages can also occur. Prolonged oozing from capillary punctures may be the first clue to its presence.

The laboratory features of the disease are summarized in Table 8-4 and contrasted with those observed in neonates with disseminated intravascular coagulation. Vitamin K deficiency is characterized by a marked prolongation in the prothrombin time and partial thromboplastin time. Slight prolongations of either of these tests should not be used as an explanation for serious hemorrhages.

Treatment of bleeding due to vitamin K deficiency consists of the intravenous administration of 1 mg vitamin K_1. If this deficiency is responsible for the abnormal

TABLE 8-4. Differential Features of Hemorrhagic Disease of the Newborn

Features	Vitamin K Deficiency	Disseminated Intravascular Coagulation
Uniformity of clotting defect	Constant	Variable
Capillary fragility	Normal	Usually abnormal
Bleeding time	Normal	Often prolonged
Clotting time	Prolonged	Variable
One-stage prothrombin	Very prolonged (5% or less)	Moderately prolonged
Partial thromboplastin time	Prolonged	Prolonged
Thrombin time	Normal for age	Usually prolonged
Fibrin degradation products	Not present	Present
Factor V	Normal	Decreased
Fibrinogen	Normal	Often decreased
Platelets	Normal	Often decreased
Red cell fragmentation	Not present	Usually present
Response to vitamin K	Spectacular	Diminished or absent
Associated disease	Usually trivial (trauma may be precipitating factor)	Severe. May include sepsis, hypoxia, acidosis, or obstetric accident
Previous history	No vitamin K given or mother receiving barbiturates or anticonvulsants	Above illnesses Vitamin K given

test results, dramatic correction may be observed in a period as short as 2 hours. Maximal correction may be observed in 24 hours. It is important to remember that neither the prothrombin time, the partial thromboplastin time, nor the level of Factor II may reach the expected adult normal values for a period of several weeks to months. The response to vitamin K is less marked in the premature infant, but even in these infants, if otherwise well, a therapeutic response can be anticipated.

DISSEMINATED INTRAVASCULAR COAGULATION

Disseminated intravascular coagulation (DIC) is an acquired pathophysiologic process characterized by the intravascular consumption of platelets and plasma clotting factors, most notably Factors II, V, VIII, XIII, and fibrinogen. This widespread coagulation within the circulation results in the deposition of fibrin thrombi in small vessels and the production of a hemorrhagic state when the level of platelets and clotting factors drop to values that are insufficient to maintain hemostasis. The accumulation of fibrin in the microcirculation also produces mechanical injury to the red cells, leading to erythrocyte fragmentation and a hemolytic anemia.

Disseminated intravascular coagulation is recognized with increasing frequency as an associated event in a variety of disorders. Clinical conditions in the newborn period that may be accompanied by DIC are summarized in Table 8-5. Gram-negative septicemia, acidosis, hypoxia, and hypotension appear to be the most common initiating events during the first several days of life. Coagulation disturbances characteristic of disseminated intravascular coagulation are seen in many of the sickest infants with the respiratory distress syndrome. The disturbance in coagulation reflects the severity of the disease process and in no way is responsible for the idiopathic respiratory distress syndrome. Hemorrhage, however, may be

TABLE 8-5. Conditions Associated with Disseminated Intravascular Coagulation in the Newborn

Obstetric Complications	Neonatal Infections	Miscellaneous Conditions
Abruptio placentae	Bacterial, both gram-negative and gram-positive	Respiratory disease syndrome
Preeclampsia and eclampsia	Disseminated herpes simplex	Severe erythroblastosis fetalis
Dead twin fetus	Cytomegalovirus infections	Giant hemangioma
Fetal distress during delivery	Rubella	Renal vein thrombosis
Amniotic fluid embolism	Toxoplasmosis	Severe acidosis and hypoxemia
Breech delivery	Syphilis	Indwelling catheters

a terminal event in many of these sick infants.

The clinical manifestations of disseminated intravascular coagulation are variable, and are determined in part by the associated disease process, in part by the severity of the coagulation disturbance. In a typical case, oozing at puncture sites is noted in a sick infant. Closer examination usually reveals the presence of petechiae and scattered purpura. Clinical manifestations may include pulmonary, cerebral, and intraventricular hemorrhages. Also observed are bleeding from the umbilical stump and body orifices, and thrombosis of peripheral or central vessels with tissue necrosis and gangrene.

Laboratory abnormalities include the presence of a hemolytic anemia with red cell fragmentation visible on the peripheral smear, variable degrees of thrombocytopenia, and a prolongation of the prothrombin, partial thromboplastin, and thrombin time. The level of Factor V and fibrinogen are most commonly decreased in the sickest infants. This decrease may reflect impaired hepatic synthesis in a very sick, immature infant and does not establish the presence of disseminated intravascular coagulation. The presence of elevated levels of fibrin-split products occurs invariably in older infants, children, and adults with disseminated intravascular coagulation, but may not always be present in the neonate. This can be a result of a relative deficiency of plasminogen and plasminogen activators during this period of life. The laboratory features characteristic of disseminated intravascular coagulation are described in Table 8-4.

Treatment must be directed at both the underlying disease process and the coagulation abnormality. Success, in general, depends on the ability to correct the condition that initiated the process of disseminated intravascular coagulation rather than merely on the management of the hematologic abnormalities.

PLATELET DISTURBANCES

A platelet count of less than $100{,}000/mm^3$ is abnormal in either the term or premature infant. The level of platelets in the blood reflects a balance between their production and destruction. Platelet production is evaluated chiefly by inspection of the number and appearance of megakaryocytes in a carefully collected sample of bone marrow. This is not always easy to accomplish in a small infant. Platelet destruction may be evaluated by determination of the platelet survival, using platelets labeled with isotopes such as chromium-51 or by merely monitoring the disappearance rate of platelets following a transfusion of unlabeled platelets. An additional clue to the mechanism of thrombocytopenia may be obtained from an evaluation of platelet size. Young platelets are larger than old platelets. The predominance of large platelets in a peripheral smear of blood collected in EDTA, to prevent platelet aggregation, suggests that the thrombocytopenia is a result of peripheral platelet destruction with a compensatory increase in young platelets from the bone marrow.

There are many causes of thrombocytopenia in the newborn. The most common of these disorders are outlined below.

Etiologic Classification of Neonatal Thrombocytopenia

Immune disorders
- Passive (acquired from mother)—ITP, drug-induced thrombocytopenia, systemic lupus erythematosus
- Active
  - Isoimmune—platelet group incompatibility
  - Associated with erythroblastosis fetalis—due to the disease or to exchange transfusion

Infections (? mediated in part by intravascular coagulation)
- Bacterial—generalized sepsis, congenital syphilis
- Viral—cytomegalic inclusion disease, disseminated herpes simplex, rubella syndrome
- Protozoal—congenital toxoplasmosis

Drugs (administered to mother)—nonimmune mechanism (*e.g.*, thiazide diuretics, tolbutamide)

Congenital megakaryocytic hypoplasia
- Isolated—congenital hypoplastic thrombocytopenia
- Associated with: absent radii, microcephaly; rubella syndrome; pancytopenia and congenital anomalies (Fanconi's anemia)
- Associated with pancytopenia but no congenital anomalies
- Associated with trisomy syndromes—D_1 (13, E 18)

Bone marrow disease
- Congenital leukemia

Disseminated intravascular coagulation (DIC)
- Sepsis
- Obstetrical complications—abruptio placentae, eclampsia, amniotic fluid embolism, dead twin fetus
- Anoxia
- Stasis—giant hemangioma (including placental chorangioma), renal vein thrombosis, polycythemia

Inherited (chronic) thrombocytopenia
- Sex-linked:
  - Pure
  - Aldrich's syndrome
- Autosomal:
  - Pure—dominant or recessive
  - May-Hegglin anomaly—dominant

Miscellaneous
- Thrombotic thrombocytopenic purpura
- Inherited metabolic disorders—glycinemia, methylmalonic acidemia, isovaleric acidemia
- Congenital thyrotoxicosis

Immune Thrombocytopenia

A variety of conditions are associated with the passage of antibody from the mother across the placenta to the infant that result in immunologic destruction of the infant's platelets. The antibody may be formed against an antigen on the mother's platelets (autoimmune) or those of the infant (isoimmune).

The maternal disorders in which thrombocytopenia may occur in both the mother and infant include idiopathic thrombocytopenic purpura, drug-induced thrombocytopenia, and systemic lupus erythematosus.

In isoimmune thrombocytopenia, the thrombocytopenia is confined to the infant. In this condition, the infant possesses a platelet antigen lacking in the mother and the infant's platelets cross the placenta into the maternal circulation, resulting in the formation of antibodies by the mother against the foreign platelet antigen. This immunologic mechanism is analogous to that of red cell sensitization that occurs in erythroblastosis fetalis.

Infants born with immune thrombocytopenia have a wide variety of clinical manifestations, although bleeding manifestations appear to be more severe in the isoimmune form of the disease. Infants tend to show maximal signs of bruising and bleeding shortly after birth as a consequence of the mechanical trauma of the birth process. The most common type of bleeding consists of generalized petechiae and purpuric spots. Bleeding from other sites may be observed (*e.g.*, oozing from the cord, epistaxis, hematuria, melena, and bleeding from needle punctures). Intracranial hemorrhages may also occur.

Jaundice may develop as a consequence of the increased breakdown of red cells within entrapped hemorrhages. Hepatosplenomegaly is absent in these conditions. Bone marrow examination usually reveals the presence of normal to increased numbers of megakaryocytes.

It has been estimated that approximately 10% of infants born to mothers with autoimmune thrombocytopenia die in the neonatal period as a consequence of hemorrhage, while 15% of infants with isoimmune thrombocytopenia succumb. These figures appear excessive. The thrombocytopenia of passively acquired thrombocytopenia may persist for 1 to 4 months, while the course of isoimmune thrombocytopenia is generally only 1 to 6 weeks' duration.

Treatment is generally reserved for the infant with bleeding. In infants with passive forms of thrombocytopenia, exchange transfusion, followed by platelet transfusion, appears to be most effective in management. In infants with isoimmune thrombocytopenia, transfusions of platelets obtained from the mother will normalize the platelet count and produce a cessation of bleeding. Neither steroids nor splenectomy has been demonstrated to be of benefit, and splenectomy should never be considered in management of the newborn.

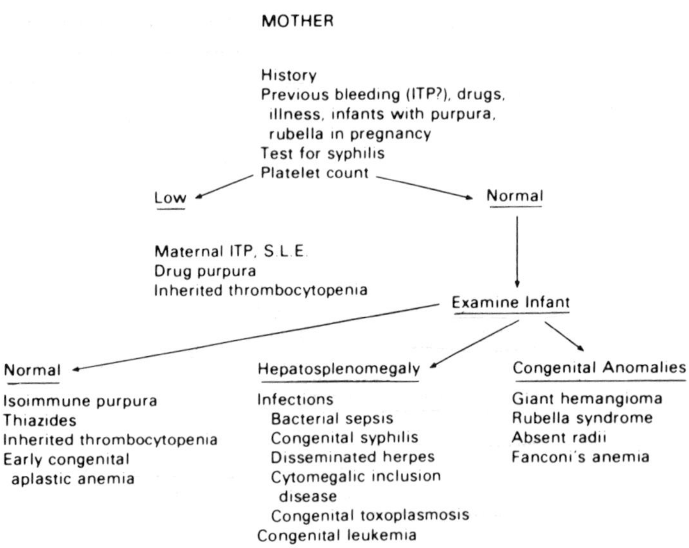

Fig. 8-2. Approach to the diagnosis of the thrombocytopenic newborn.

In pregnancies complicated by isoimmune thrombocytopenia, it would be advantageous to reduce the hazards of bleeding in subsequent children by delivering the infant by cesarean section.

Other Forms of Thrombocytopenia

As already indicated, a variety of other disorders may produce a reduction in platelet count. Infections are a common cause of thrombocytopenia. Inherited defects in platelet production or platelet function may also manifest themselves at this period of life. An approach to the multiple diagnostic possibilities is outlined in Figure 8-2.

In this scheme, it is as important to study the mother as it is to study the infant. Points requiring specific inquiry include: (1) a history of previous bleeding in the form of purpura, bruising, or nosebleeds that might suggest a diagnosis of maternal ITP at some time in the past; (2) ingestion of drugs that might cause thrombocytopenia in the mother and infant (*e.g.*, quinidine and quinine) or in the infant alone (thiazide diuretics, tolbutamide); (3) previous infants affected with purpura, suggesting either one of the immune or inherited thrombocytopenias; (4) skin rash or exposure to rubella in the first 8 weeks of pregnancy. The results of the routine test for syphilis should be sought and recorded rather than left buried among the other routine laboratory results performed earlier in pregnancy. Finally, an accurate platelet count should be performed on the mother as soon as possible after delivery to separate immune neonatal thrombocytopenia due to maternal ITP from that due to platelet isoimmunization (in which case the mother's platelet count is normal).

Important physical findings in differential diagnosis in the affected newborn include the presence or absence of hepatosplenomegaly and congenital anomalies. Hepatosplenomegaly is often accompanied by jaundice and suggests an infectious process as the most likely cause of thrombocytopenia. In some cases, congenital leukemia may also have to be considered. Among the congenital anomalies associated with neonatal thrombocytopenia, the most common group recognizable at birth is that occurring in the rubella syndrome (congenital heart defects, cataracts, and microcephaly). Deformity and shortening of the forearms should suggest bilateral absence of the radii with associated megakaryocytic thrombocytopenia. A single large hemangioma or multiple smaller hemangiomas point to these tumors as the problem site of platelet trapping leading to thrombocytopenia.

TABLE 8-6. Differential Features of ITP in Childhood

Acute	Chronic
Onset at under 10 years of age	Over 10 years
Onset acute with preceding viral illness	Insidious
Male: female equal	More common in females
Platelet count less than 20,000/mm³	20,000 to 75,000/mm³
Immunoglobulins normal	IgA often decreased
No other immunologic abnormalities	Other immunologic abnormalities present in both propositus and other family members
Platelet-associated IgG antibody markedly elevated	Modestly increased
No common pattern in HLA typing	Increase in A3, B7, or A26,W16 haplotypes

Idiopathic Thrombocytopenic Purpura in Childhood

Idiopathic thrombocytopenic purpura (ITP) is a relatively common cause of petechiae and purpura in children. It is usually an acute self-limited disorder often precipitated by an antecedent viral illness (see Table 8-6). From a review of almost 1400 patients, the clinical manifestations at the time of presentation include: skin bleeding (100%), epistaxis (25%), minimal splenomegaly (10%), oral bleeding (7%), gastrointestinal bleeding (5%), hematuria (5%), and intracranial hemorrhage (1%).

The platelet count is less than 40,000/mm^3 in most patients. Large platelets and atypical lymphocytes are often present in the peripheral smear. Since leukemia is commonly associated with thrombocytopenia, a bone marrow examination should be performed in most patients to confirm the diagnosis and to reassure the parents.

In 80% to 90% of children who develop ITP, uneventful recovery will ensue within 3 weeks to 6 months. Listed below are those features which help to distinguish the acute, self-limited disorder from that which is more likely to result in chronic disease.

It seems reasonable to use corticosteroids in the treatment of children with ITP when the platelet count is less than 20,000/mm^3. They should be given initially for a period of no longer than 3 weeks. Steroid therapy does not improve the eventual outcome but can produce a more rapid return to normal in the platelet count. Platelet transfusions are generally of no benefit because the transfused platelets are rapidly destroyed. In children who develop chronic ITP, removal of the spleen will produce a return of the platelet count to normal in approximately 75% of instances.

BIBLIOGRAPHY

Buchanan GR: Neonatal coagulation: normal physiology and pathophysiology. Clin Haematol 7:85, 1978.

Lightsey AL, Jr: Thrombocytopenia in children. Pediatr Clin North Am 27:293, 1980.

Montgomery RR, Hathaway WE: Acute bleeding emergencies. Pediatr Clin North Am 27:327, 1980.

Stuart MJ: Inherited defects of platelet function. Semin Hematol 12:233, 1975.

Lymphadenopathy

9

Frank A. Oski

The presence of lymphadenopathy, either localized or generalized, is often greeted with fear and apprehension both by parent and physician. This is due to the mistaken impression that lymph node enlargement generally signifies the presence of a malignant process.

It must be appreciated that the lymphatic tissue forms a larger percentage of the total body weight during infancy and childhood than in adult life, and as a result lymphoid tissue is easily palpable in many areas of the body. The relative abundance of lymphoid tissue is reflected by the size of the pharyngeal tonsillar tissue. The tonsils generally reach their maximal size when the child is about 7 years of age and gradually atrophy. Cervical, axillary, and inguinal nodes are palpable in almost all infants and children. Occipital nodes may be palpable in about 5% of children less than 12 years of age. Enlargement of postauricular, supraclavicular, epitrochlear, popliteal, mediastinal, and abdominal nodes is uncommon and suggests the presence of an associated pathologic process.

Lymph node enlargement results from one of two basic processes. These processes are *proliferation* of cells intrinsic to the lymph node and *infiltration* by extrinsic cells. Cells intrinsic to the lymph node that may undergo proliferation include lymphocytes, plasma cells, and histiocytes. This form of proliferation occurs in response to antigenic stimulation. Infiltration of a lymph node involves invasion by malignant cells or by polymorphonuclear leukocytes in response to a local infection.

In attempting to determine the significance of lymphadenopathy, a number of facts should be ascertained which will facilitate a decision as to what should be done next in reaching a diagnosis and instituting appropriate therapy.

The following questions should be answered:

1. Is the lymphadenopathy generalized (enlargement of more than two noncontiguous lymph node regions), or is it localized? Generalized lymphadenopathy is caused by generalized disease.
2. If the lymphadenopathy is localized, is it accompanied by signs of infection in the involved node? Is the node tender, is the skin over the node warm or red?
3. If the lymphadenopathy is localized, is there evidence of infection in the drainage area of the lymph node or a history of recent antigenic introduction in the drainage area?
4. Which lymph nodes are involved in the process?
5. If the lymphadenopathy is generalized, what are the associated symptoms and signs? Of importance in the physical examination are the presence of hepatic and splenic enlargement, the size of the thyroid gland, and the presence of disease involving the heart, lungs, or joints. Is there any evidence of pallor and easy bruising?

GENERALIZED LYMPHADENOPATHY

Generalized lymphadenopathy does not usually present the same diagnostic dilemma to the physician as local lymphadenopathy. Generalized lymphadenopathy is usually associated with other abnormalities in the history, physical examination, or initial laboratory tests and thus enables the physician to reach a probable diagnosis.

The more common causes of generalized lymphadenopathy are listed below.

Causes of Generalized Lymphadenopathy

Infections
- Pyogenic infections
- Tuberculosis
- Syphilis
- Toxoplasmosis
- Brucellosis
- Histoplasmosis
- Malaria
- Typhoid fever
- Cytomegalovirus infection
- Infectious mononucleosis
- Exanthems (scarlet fever, rubella, rubeola)
- Infectious hepatitis

Collagen vascular diseases
- Lupus erythematosus
- Rheumatoid arthritis

Immunologic reactions
- Serum sickness
- Drug reactions
- Granulomatous diseases (sarcoid)

Drug-induced
- Phenytoin, antithyroid medication, hydralazine, allopurinol

Storage diseases
- Gaucher's disease
- Niemann-Pick's disease

Malignancies
- Leukemia
- Neuroblastoma, metastatic
- Lymphomas
- Histiocytosis

Infections must always be seriously considered in patients with generalized lymphadenopathy. Viral infections are probably the most common group of infections responsible for such a response. Viral infections associated with an exanthem such as rubella and rubeola should produce no diagnostic confusion. Infants and children with acquired cytomegalovirus infections or infectious mononucleosis may have nonspecific eruptions. The presence of more than 10% atypical lymphocytes in the peripheral blood smear should alert you to this diagnostic possibility.

With acute overwhelming infections, the presence of fever, leukocytosis, signs of toxicity, and perhaps evidence of a focal lesion responsible for the dissemination process will generally alert the physician to the nature of the underlying disease.

Chronic infections with tuberculosis or syphilis may be causes of generalized lymphadenopathy. This is a very unusual manifestation of these disorders in children.

In patients with rheumatoid arthritis or lupus erythematosus, the history is characterized by the presence of chronic, intermittent fever, evanescent rashes, and arthralgia and arthritis. Physical examination and laboratory tests may indicate the presence of disease involving the joints, kidney, lungs, liver, myocardium, and pericardium.

In patients with storage disorders that are associated with lymphadenopathy, the spleen and liver will also be enlarged. In young infants and children with these generalized disorders, evidence of cerebral involvement may dominate the clinical picture.

Although it is estimated that as many as 70% of pediatric patients with acute lymphoblastic leukemia will have generalized lymphadenopathy, this finding is rarely the initial manifestation of the disease. The clinical picture in these patients is dominated by a history of unexplained fever, general malaise, pallor, and easy bruising. With generalized lymphadenopathy, splenomegaly is invariably present.

The patient with histiocytosis frequently has associated skin involvement, a history of chronic otitis media, and evidence of disease involving the lungs, liver, and spleen.

REGIONAL LYMPHADENOPATHY

Regional lymphadenopathy, and most particularly lymphadenopathy in the cervical area, produces the greatest diagnostic dilemma to the physician. The physician must decide if the lump is malignant or not and how long he can observe the patient before resorting to a biopsy or lymph node excision.

The area of involvement and the associated findings will facilitate a logical decision. For example, isolated supraclavicular lymph node involvement should always suggest the presence of malignancy. This is usually accompanied by signs of mediastinal disease and is generally a result of Hodgkin's disease or nonHodgkin's lymphoma.

Cervical Lymph Node Enlargement

Isolated enlargement of the cervical nodes is generally the result of localized infection. The most common agents producing adenitis in this region are staphylococcus and streptococcus. Often a history of a recent upper respiratory infection will be elicited. The major causes of cervical adenopathy and their distinguishing characteristics are described in Table 9-1.

A systematic approach to patients with cervical adenitis is extremely important and a timetable that may ultimately lead to biopsy should be established.

When the cervical nodes are warm and tender and evidence of overlying infection is present in the overlying skin, then diagnosis is relatively simple. These nodes should be aspirated for purposes of bacterial culture and smear for bacteriologic identification. In addition, a search should be made for a primary focus of infection in the scalp, mouth, pharynx, and sinuses. The submandibular nodes are most frequently enlarged in patients with infections in the ethmoid and maxillary sinuses. A history of cat scratch should also be elicited.

When the cervical node enlargement is nontender and not associated with signs of infection, other diagnostic procedures should accompany the initial evaluation. The following should be included: a complete blood count and smear to detect evidence of atypical lymphocytes, a heterophile test

---

Guidelines for Diagnosis of Localized Noncervical Lymphadenopathy

Supraclavicular
- Always consider mediastinal disease (tuberculosis, histoplasmosis, coccidiomycosis, sarcoidosis).
- Always consider lymphoma. In absence of evidence of pulmonary infection, early node biopsy indicated.

Axillary
- Secondary to infections in the hand, arm, lateral chest wall or lateral portion of the breast. May be result of recently administered immunizations in the arm. Very common with BCG innoculations.

Epitrochlear
- Secondary to infections on ulnar side of hand and forearm. Observed in tularemia when bite occurs on finger. Also observed in secondary syphilis.

Inguinal
- Look for evidence of infection in the lower extremity, scrotum, and penis in the male, vulva and vagina in the female, the skin of the lower abdomen, perineum, gluteal region, or anal canal.
- May be manifestation of lymphogranuloma venereum.
- May represent metastatic disease from testicular tumors or bony tumors of the leg.

---

or a titer to detect the presence of Epstein-Barr virus antibodies, skin tests for both mycobacteria tuberculosis and atypical mycobacteria, and a chest film.

If the cervical enlargement is accompanied by supraclavicular enlargement or if splenomegaly is present in the absence of evidence of a viral illness, recent immunization, or signs of drug allergy, then an early lymph node biopsy should be obtained.

If all studies are not diagnostic, the patient can be treated safely for several weeks on the presumption that an undiagnosed, deep-seated bacterial infection is present in the node. Treatment should be with penicillin or a penicillin derivative in large doses. Careful measurements of the node should be performed. If at the end of 2 to 4 weeks of observation, the node has not changed in size or character or has grown painlessly larger, then node biopsy or excision should be performed.

It must be remembered that not all masses in the neck are of lymphoid origin. Palpable lumps in the neck may represent a cervical rib, thyroglossal cysts, branchial cleft cysts, cystic hygromas, goiters, and thyroid carcinomas.

LYMPHADENOPATHY ELSEWHERE IN THE BODY

The presence of localized lymphadenopathy in noncervical regions does not generally produce the same diagnostic di-

TABLE 9-1. Causes of Cervical Adenitis

Cause	Comment
Viral upper respiratory infections	Most common cause. Nodes soft, minimally tender, and not associated with evidence of redness and warmth of overlying skin.
Bacterial infection	Streptococcus and staphylococcus most common etiologic agents. Usually secondary to previous or associated infection in drainage area of node. More frequently unilateral. Signs of infection—tenderness, warmth and redness—generally present.
Tuberculosis	Mycobacteria tuberculosis infections generally bilateral, involve multiple nodes. Associated with evidence of chest disease and systemic signs. Atypical mycobacteria infections more commonly unilateral initially. Not associated, in general, with other foci of disease. With either agent, evidence of local warmth and redness uncommon.
Infectious mononucleosis	Fever, malaise, preceding upper respiratory infection often noted. Splenomegaly common. Atypical lymphocytes present. Epstein-Barr virus titers required for diagnosis in younger children.
Cytomegalovirus Toxoplasmosis	Clinically indistinguishable from Epstein-Barr virus infections. Requires serologic studies to make the diagnosis.
Cat scratch disease	History of contact with young cat. May be preceded by history of fever and malaise. Adenopathy restricted to area drained by initial cat scratch.
Sarcoidosis	Disease bilateral. Chest film almost always abnormal. May have keratitis, iritis, and evidence of bone disease.
Hodgkin's disease	Common presenting symptom. Frequently unilateral at time of initial manifestation. Node is rubbery, nontender, and not associated with signs of inflammation. Make certain that supraclavicular involvement is not present. When present, strongly suspect lymphoma.
NonHodgkin's lymphoma	Bilateral at time of initial presentation in approximately 40% of patients. Cervical and submaxillary nodes commonly involved together.

lemma. Usually this reflects infection or the introduction of an antigen into the area drained by the nodes. The principal causes of localized noncervical lymphadenopathy are described on page 95. Management of this form of lymphadenopathy is dictated by the associated findings.

BIBLIOGRAPHY

Barton LL, Feigin RD: Childhood cervical lymphadenitis: a reappraisal. J Pediatr 84:846, 1974

A study of the infectious agents that produce lymphadenopathy in children and a guide to their diagnosis and management.

Bedros AA, Mann JP: Lymphadenopathy in children. Adv Pediatr 28:341, 1981.

A thorough review of all causes of lymphadenopathy accompanied by a very helpful algorithm to assist in diagnosis.

Jones PG: Swellings in the neck in children. Med J Aust 1:212, 1963

Snapper I: The bedside diagnosis of cervical lymphadenopathies. Med Clin North Am 51:627, 1962

A review of the most common form of adenopathy in children—cervical adenopathy.

Zeulzer WW, Kaplan J: The child with lymphadenopathy. Semin Hematol 12:323, 1975

A comprehensive discussion of the causes of lymphadenopathy in infants and children with suggestions regarding diagnosis and management.

Splenomegaly

10

Frank A. Oski

The spleen is one of the major components of the reticuloendothelial system. It is comprised of two distinct but closely related elements: the white pulp and the red pulp. The *white pulp* represents histiocytic macrophages, lymphocytes, and plasma cells, while the *red pulp* is composed of the Billroth cords and splenic sinuses. As a consequence of its dual anatomic construction, the spleen serves dual functions. The two primary functions are the filtration of particulate matter and formed elements from the blood and the production of humoral factors required for the opsonization of infectious organisms. Splenic enlargement can be observed in disease states in which either the clearing function of the spleen is excessive or in circumstances in which antigenic stimulation is either massive or prolonged. During fetal life and early infancy, the spleen is also the site of erythropoiesis. In response to needs for augmented red cell production, the spleen may continue to serve as a site for erythrocyte production, and this also is reflected by the presence of splenomegaly.

The spleen is normally palpable as a soft organ in most infants born prior to 40 weeks' gestation. In this circumstance, the spleen can be felt 1 to 2 cm below the left costal margin in the midclavicular line. The spleen can be palpated in approximately 30% of normal term infants and in 10% of healthy infants at 1 year of age. By age 12, about 1% of normal children still have a spleen that is palpable approximately 1 cm below the left costal margin. In healthy infants and children, the spleen, when palpable, is soft and nontender and feels much like a normal lymph node.

There are many diseases in which the spleen may be palpable. It is useless to try to memorize lengthy lists of this sort in an attempt to reach a diagnosis of splenomegaly. It is far more helpful to visualize the different processes that result in splenomegaly by using the letters in the word SPLEEN.

SEQUESTRATION

The spleen sequesters effete red cells at the end of their normal 120-day lifespan. Abnormal red cells are also retained within the red pulp of this organ. Two main mechanisms are operative under conditions that result in splenic sequestration of erythrocytes. The first is an alteration in the surface properties of the red cell. The presence of immunoglobulins or complement on the surface of the red cell results in their recognition, detention, and ultimate phagocytosis by the monocytes and macrophages within the endothelial lining of the spleen. Diseases accompanied by antibody coating of red cells are generally associated with some degree of splenomegaly. Examples of such diseases include Rh and ABO isoimmunization during the newborn period and "autoimmune" hemolytic anemias later in life.

Splenic sequestration causes a loss of the normal deformability of the erythrocyte. Red cells may lose their normal deformability as a result of alterations in membrane proteins, intracellular deposition of precipitated or aggregated hemoglobin, or as a result of alterations in cell water, cations, or metabolic intermediates such as adenosine triphosphate.

Hereditary hemolytic anemias that are accompanied by alterations in red cell deformability include sickle-cell anemia, hemoglobin C disease, thalassemia major, many of the unstable hemoglobins, some of the enzyme deficiencies such as pyruvate kinase deficiency, hereditary spherocytosis, hereditary elliptocytosis, and hereditary stomatocytosis.

The enlargement of the spleen should not be accompanied by generalized lymphadenopathy in patients in whom splenomegaly is produced by sequestration of red cells. A history of anemia or jaundice may be present in the patient or in other family members. Examination of the well-prepared peripheral blood smear and a determination of the patient's hemoglobin, red cell indices, and reticulocyte count should enable the physician to make a preliminary decision that the patient's splenomegaly is primarily a result of an alteration of the red cell.

PROLIFERATION

Many viral and bacterial infections result in a proliferation of the white pulp of the spleen. Chronic immunologic stimulation from any cause can also result in splenomegaly.

Examples of viral infections that commonly result in splenic enlargement in pediatric patients include infectious mononucleosis (Epstein-Barr virus) and cytomegalovirus infections. Splenic enlargement in these diseases is usually accompanied by lymphadenopathy, a history of fever and sore throat, a nonspecific rash in some instances, laboratory evidence of hepatic dysfunction, and the presence of atypical lymphocytes in the peripheral blood smear.

Bacterial infections frequently accompanied by splenic enlargement include severe pneumonias, typhoid fever, bacterial endocarditis, and indolent septicemias. The other manifestations of the disease usually dominate the clinical picture and isolated splenomegaly is rarely present as a diagnostic enigma.

LIPID

The large and heterogenous group of disorders in which "foam cells" or lipid-laden macrophages accumulate within the spleen and bone marrow result in splenomegaly. Lipids appear to accumulate in the spleen in these disorders because of defects in catabolism of sphingolipids or other related metabolic intermediates. Many of these disturbances have sufficiently distinct clinical manifestations which may lead to a presumptive diagnosis. Tables 10-1 to 10-5 summarize their salient features.

ENGORGEMENT

Engorgement of the spleen may produce splenomegaly; leukopenia and thrombocytopenia are also common findings in patients with splenic engorgement. Localized engorgement can result from splenic trauma and the accumulation of blood within

TABLE 10-1. Characteristics of Niemann-Pick Disease

	Niemann-Pick Disease Type A	Niemann-Pick Disease Type B	Niemann-Pick Disease Type C	Niemann-Pick Disease Type D
Clinical onset (yrs.)	½	2–4	3–5	3–5
Life expectancy (yrs.)	<4	Unknown	<15	<20
Earliest manifestations	FTT* HSmegaly, PM† deterioration	HSmegaly	PM deterioration, HSmegaly	PM deterioration, HSmegaly
Additional abnormalities				
Cherry red spot	+	–	–	–
Foam cells	+	+	+	+
Unique features	Reticular pulmonary infiltrates, vacuolated lymphocytes	Reticular pulmonary infiltrates		
Inheritance	Autosomal recessive	Autosomal recessive	Autosomal recessive	Autosomal recessive
Ethnic extraction	Often Jewish			Nova Scotian
Lipids accumulated	Sphingomyelin, cholesterol	Sphingomyelin, cholesterol	Sphingomyelin, cholesterol	Sphingomyelin, cholesterol
Enzyme deficiency	Sphingo-myelinase	Sphingo-myelinase	?	?

*FTT: Failure to thrive.
†PM deterioration: progressive mental deterioration.
(Sloan HR, Breslow JL: Foam cells. *In* Nathan D, Oski F (eds): Hematology of infancy and Childhood. Philadelphia, W B Saunders, 1974)

TABLE 10-2. Characteristics of Gaucher's Disease

	Gaucher's Disease Type I	Gaucher's Disease Type II	Gaucher's Disease Type III
Clinical onset (yrs.)	0–91	½	1–3
Life expectancy (yrs.)	Variable	<2	<30
Earliest manifestations	HSmegaly, thrombocytopenia & bleeding	PM deterioration, HSmegaly	PM deterioration, HSmegaly
Additional abnormalities			
Cherry red spot	–	–	–
Foam cells	+	+	+
Unique features	Bony lesions, reticular pulmonary infiltrates	Head retroflexion, coughing, trismus, laryngospasm, abnormal facies, nystagmus	
Inheritance	Autosomal recessive	Autosomal recessive	Autosomal recessive
Ethinic extraction	Often Jewish		
Lipids accumulated	Glucosyl ceramide (GLla)	Glucosyl ceramide (GLla)	Glucosyl ceramide (GLla)
Enzyme deficiency	GLla-β-glucosidase	GLla-β-glucosidase	?

(Sloan HR, Breslow JL: Foam cells. *In* Nathan D, Oski F, (eds): Hematology of Infancy and Childhood. Philadelphia, WB Saunders, 1974)

TABLE 10-3. Characteristics of G_M Gangliosidosis and Other Storage Disorders

	G_{M1} Gangliosidosis Type I	G_{M1} Gangliosidosis Type II	Lactosyl Ceramidosis	Fabry's Disease	Krabbe's Disease
Clinical onset (yrs.)	Birth	1–2	1	5–20	¼–½
Life expectancy (yrs.)	<2	<10	<4	Variable	<2
Earliest manifestations	PM deterioration, FTT, HSmegaly	PM deterioration	FTT, PM deterioration, HSmegaly	Fever, joint swelling, peripheral pain and edema, telangiectasias	PM deterioration
Additional abnormalities					
Cherry red spot	+	–	–	–	–
Foam cells	+	Variable	+	Variable	–
Unique features	Bony lesions, abnormal facies, vacuolated lymphocytes, acid mucopolysaccharides in urine			Renal involvement	Optic atrophy
Inheritance	Autosomal recessive	Autosomal recessive	Unknown	Sex-linked	Autosomal recessive
Ethnic extraction				Often Scandinavian	
Lipids accumulated	Ganglioside G_{M1}	Ganglioside G_{M1}	Lactosyl ceramide (GL2a)	Trihexosyl ceramide (GL3), dihexosyl ceramide (GL2b)	Galactosyl* ceramide (GL1b)
Enzyme deficiency	G_{M1}-β-galactosidase	G_{M1}-β-galactosidase	GL2a-β-galactosidase	GL3-α-galactosidase	GL1b-β-galactosidase

*Extensive demyelination with relative increase of GL1b.
(Sloan HR, Breslow JL: Foam Cells. *In* Nathan D, Oski F (eds): Hematology of Infancy and Childhood. Philadelphia, WB Saunders, 1974)

the splenic capsule. Splenic engorgement can be observed in children with portal hypertension that is a consequence of hepatic disease, with primary disease in the portal vein or splenic vein, or with congestive heart failure.

Portal hypertension secondary to liver disease has many causes in pediatric patients. Diseases to consider in such circumstances include chronic hepatitis, cystic fibrosis, Wilson's disease, cirrhosis secondary to intrahepatic biliary atresia, and the consequences of ascending infection by way of the umbilical vein following catheterization in the neonatal period. In patients with portal hypertension; hepatomegaly, ascites, esophageal varices, internal hemorrhoids, and historical features of liver disease may be found. In patients with congestive splenomegaly as a result of portal vein thrombosis or obstruction to the splenic vein, diagnosis often may be made only with contrast studies of the portal circulation.

Acute splenic engorgement, the so-

TABLE 10-4. Characteristics of Metachromatic Leukodystrophies

	Infantile Metachromatic Leukodystrophy	Juvenile Metachromatic Leukodystrophy	Adult Metachromatic Leukodystrophy	Metachromatic Leukodystrophy, Multiple Sulfatase Deficiency Form
Clinical onset (yrs.)	1–2	5–10	19–46	1–2
Life expectancy (yrs.)	<10	<20	Variable	<12
Earliest manifestations	PM deterioration	PM deterioration	Dementia	PM deterioration
Additional abnormalities				
Cherry red spots	–	–	–	–
Foam cells	–	–	–	–
Unique features	Nonfunctioning gallbladder, optic atrophy	Optic atrophy		Acid mucopolysaccharides in urine, bony lesions, granulated lymphocytes
Inheritance	Autosomal recessive	Autosomal recessive	Autosomal recessive	Unknown
Ethnic extraction				
Lipids accumulated	Sulfatide	Sulfatide	Sulfatide	Sulfatide
Enzyme deficiency	Sulfatidase (arylsulfatase A)	Sulfatidase (arylsulfatase A)	Sulfatidase (arylsulfatase A) Arylsulfatase A, B, C	

(Sloan HR, Breslow JL: Foam cells. *In* Nathan D, Oski F (eds): Hematology of Infancy and Childhood. Philadelphia, WB Saunders, 1974)

TABLE 10-5. Characteristics of Tay-Sachs Disease

	Tay-Sachs Disease Type I	Tay-Sachs Disease Type II	Tay-Sachs Disease Type III
Clinical onset (yrs.)	¼–½	¼–½	1–2
Life expectancy (yrs.)	<5	<4	<15
Earliest manifestations	PM deterioration, hypotonia, "hyperacusis"	PM deterioration, hypotonia, "hyperacusis"	PM deterioration
Additional abnormalities			
Cherry red spots	+	+	–
Foam cells	–	–	–
Unique features	Macrocephaly	Macrocephaly	
Inheritance	Autosomal recessive	Autosomal recessive	Unknown
Ethnic extraction	Usually Jewish		
Lipids accumulated	Ganglioside G_{M2}	GL4, ganglioside G_{M2}	Cholesterol, cholestanol
Enzyme deficiency	Hexosaminidase A	Hexosaminidase A & B	?

(Sloan HR, Breslow JL: Foam cells. *In* Nathan D, Oski F (eds): Hematology of Infancy and Childhood. Philadelphia, WB Saunders, 1974) called "sequestration crisis," may also be observed in patients with sickle-cell anemia. In this circumstance, for unknown reasons, the spleen rapidly fills with blood and the patient literally bleeds within himself. These patients, usually under the age of 5 years, may present with signs of profound hypovolemia and anemia. This complication of sickle-cell anemia is one of the primary causes of early death.

ENDOWMENT

Abnormalities in this category of endowment are rare causes of splenomegaly. Among congenital causes of splenomegaly may be included splenic hemangiomas, splenic cysts, and splenic cystic hygromas.

INVASION

Splenomegaly may accompany a variety of malignant processes. Fifty to sixty percent of children with leukemia may have splenomegaly at the time of diagnosis. Splenomegaly tends to be more common and of greater size in patients with myelogenous rather than lymphatic leukemia. Other manifestations of the disease tend to dominate the clinical picture, and it is extremely rare for isolated splenomegaly to be the sole historical or physical finding in a child with leukemia.

Lymphomas may also be associated with splenomegaly. In this circumstance, isolated splenomegaly may prove to be a source of real diagnostic confusion.

Splenomegaly is generally present in patients with histiocytosis, but this is rarely an isolated finding.

The spleen may be the site of metastatic disease. The most common pediatric tumor associated with metastases to the spleen is neuroblastoma.

The spleen may be the site of granuloma formation in diseases such as sarcoidosis, tuberculosis, and some of the systemic fungal infections.

CONCLUSION

Because the causes of splenomegaly are so numerous, it is essential that an attempt be made to fit the patient into one of the six categories just described before undertaking extensive diagnostic procedures. Usually a careful history, physical examination, routine blood count, and, on occasion, a bone marrow examination, are all that is necessary to reach a tentative assignment to a major pathophysiologic cause for the splenomegaly. After that decision has been reached, more specific tests can be employed to reach a precise diagnosis. Let the SPLEEN guide your thinking.

BIBLIOGRAPHY

Boles ET Jr, Baxter CF, Newton WA Jr: Evaluation of splenomegaly in childhood. Clin Pediatr 2:161, 1963

A review of the causes and diagnostic approach to splenic enlargement in the pediatric patient.

Sloan HR, Breslow JL: Foam cells. In Nathan D, Oski F (eds): Hematology of Infancy and Childhood. Philadelphia, WB Saunders, 1974

An extensive discussion of the biochemistry and clinical manifestations of the lipid storage disorders.

Abdominal Masses

11

Frank A. Oski

The discovery of an abdominal mass requires an immediate orderly investigation to determine its precise nature. As is true with many signs and symptoms in pediatrics, the etiology of abdominal masses differs among infants and children of various ages.

In the immediate neonatal period, the presence of an abdominal mass is generally a sign of a congenital malformation, and in approximately one-half of all patients it reflects an abnormality of the genitourinary system. In older infants and children, neoplasms and complications of infectious processes are the more common causes of the presence of a palpable mass.

Beyond the newborn period, most masses are discovered by parents rather than physicians. The single most important part of the physical examination of an apparently healthy infant is a careful palpation of the abdomen. After the initial examination of the newborn and that performed at 6 weeks of age, the routine physical examination of an asymptomatic, healthy infant generally discloses few or no abnormalities except for those that may be found in the abdomen. All too often, this portion of the examination may be cursory.

The diagnostic considerations that accompany the finding of a mass are largely determined by the age of the patient, associated symptoms, and physical findings.

Often abdominal masses detected in routine physical examination ultimately prove to be fecal material, a distended urinary bladder or the abdominal aorta.

Fecal material in the colon is usually freely movable and easily compressed. If one suspects that the mass is fecal in nature and it cannot be confirmed by rectal examination, an enema should be given. Following the enema, the patient should be reexamined before proceeding to further diagnostic studies.

A distended bladder may be palpated in the newborn infant who has not voided within the first 24 hours of life. This may signify the presence of abnormalities of the urethra such as posterior urethral valves. Other causes of bladder distention include the use of anticholinergic drugs, spinal cord tumors, and abnormalities of the spinal cord. Bladder distention may also be observed in the comatose patient, during the immediate postoperative period, and as a result of bladder irritation produced by inflammatory lesions in the pelvis such as an appendiceal abscess. In these situations, the mass appears to originate at a point below the symphysis pubis and may extend as high as the umbilicus. Rectal examination usually confirms the presence of a distended bladder. If the child cannot be induced to void, catheterization may be required to confirm the diagnosis.

ABDOMINAL MASSES IN THE NEWBORN

The finding of an abdominal mass in the newborn commonly signifies the presence of an abnormality of the genitourinary system. The major abnormalities detected during this period of life are listed below.

Abdominal Masses in the Newborn

Kidney
- Hypoplastic multicystic kidney, unilateral or bilateral
- Hydronephrosis secondary to distal obstruction
- Mesoblastic nephroma
- Solitary cyst
- Renal vein thrombosis

Liver and biliary tract
- Hematoma of the liver
- Hemangioma of the liver
- Solitary cyst of the liver
- Hepatoma
- Choledochal cyst
- Distended gallbladder secondary to cystic fibrosis

Gastrointestinal tract
- Duplication of the duodenum, jejunum, or ileum
- Mesenteric cyst
- Volvulus secondary to meconium ileus
- Leiomyosarcoma of the intestine

Female genital tract
- Ovarian cyst
- Hydro- and hematocolpos

Retroperitoneal teratomas

Adrenal hemorrhage

Neuroblastoma

Malignant tumors are uncommon at birth. Although Wilms' tumor was previously believed to occur with some frequency during this period of life, it is now realized that most of these tumors are mesoblastic nephromas. A mesoblastic nephroma is histologically distinct in its fibroblastic appearance and shows only minimal nuclear polymorphism and mitotic activity. Even though this tumor may grow large and show evidence of local extension, it does not appear to metastasize, and cure may be achieved with surgery alone. Mesoblastic nephromas may constitute as many as 50% of the renal tumors of early infancy and may be responsible for the previous observation that children with Wilms' tumor under the age of 2 had a better prognosis than that observed in older children.

The nature of the mass, cystic or solid, as well as its location often can be initially determined by the use of ultrasound. Contrast studies, such as the intravenous pyelogram or isotope scans, can be used to accurately define the abnormality. Almost all infants ultimately require exploration by a pediatric surgeon.

ABDOMINAL MASSES IN OLDER INFANTS AND CHILDREN

Gastrointestinal Masses

In the infant 3 to 6 weeks of age, the most commonly palpated mass is the "tumor" of *pyloric stenosis*. A history of vomiting, often projectile, of several weeks' duration should alert the physician to this diagnostic possibility. This mass is best felt immediately after the infant has vomited. The mass is felt on deep palpation and is generally 1 to 2 cm in diameter. It is usually located at the end of the stomach somewhere along the edge of the liver from the costal margin in the midline to the underside of the right lobe of the liver.

Another mass that is generally accompanied by symptoms of intestinal obstruction is that produced by the presence of a *duplication* of the alimentary tract. Symptoms may include pain, vomiting, and hemorrhage. Most duplications occur in the small bowel. Some of these cysts are of neuroenteric origin and may be associated with defects in the vertebral column. The mucosa of the cyst is usually well preserved but need not correspond to that part of the gastrointestinal tract from which the duplication arises. Gastric mucosa is commonly present and occasionally these cysts may also contain pancreatic tissue.

In the infant 6 months to 3 years of age, symptoms of intermittent abdominal pain, often associated with vomiting, may indicate the presence of an *intussusception.* An intussusception may be initiated by enlarged mesenteric lymph nodes. In the young infant and child, the enlarged nodes are generally the result of an associated viral illness. In the child over 6 years of age, the enlarged lymph nodes should strongly suggest the presence of a lymphatic neoplasm.

Polyps, Meckel's diverticulum, and other anatomic abnormalities of the gastrointestinal tract may also serve as the leading point or initiator of the intussusception. Intussusception is also a well-recognized complication of Henoch-Schönlein purpura. Edema and hemorrhage of the bowel wall are responsible for the process. Although the cutaneous manifestations of this disorder are usually present at the time of the intussusception, this abdominal complication may precede the rash and thus produce diagnostic confusion.

The intussusception is a sausage-shaped tender mass that is usually palpable on the right side of the abdomen. On occasion, the mass may travel up into the upper right quadrant leaving an empty right lower abdomen where no bowel is palpable (Dance's sign). An intussusception is usually accompanied by the presence of high-pitched peristaltic sounds indicative of intestinal obstruction.

Painless abdominal enlargement, sometimes of several years' duration, should suggest the presence of a *mesenteric cyst.* The mass is freely movable in a lateral direction and sometimes a fluid wave or shifting dullness may be detected.

Inflammatory processes may be accompanied by abdominal masses. These include appendiceal abscesses and abscesses associated with fistulas in patients with granulomatous colitis. A history of fever, vomiting, irritability, diarrhea, and anorexia should arouse suspicion of this diagnostic possibility. The mass is tender and the white count is generally elevated.

Neoplasms

The most common abdominal tumors of childhood are *Wilms' tumor* and *neuroblastoma.*

Approximately three-fourths of Wilms' tumors appear before the age of 5 years, and they are slightly more common in females. The presenting complaint is usually that of a palpable abdominal mass or asymptomatic abdominal enlargement. Fever, abdominal pain, and hypertension may also be present. Hematuria, considered a poor prognostic sign, may be present in approximately 20% of children at the time of diagnosis.

The mass is generally large, firm, and nontender. It may be palpable in either hypochondrium, and may extend to the midline and down into the iliac fossa. When present on the left, it may be confused with an enlarged spleen. Radiographic studies usually reveal a soft-tissue mass that displaces the intestine to the opposite side. Calcification is uncommon in this tumor in contrast to the frequently speckled calcifications observed in neuroblastomas. Intravenous pyelograms may fail to reveal the affected kidney or may merely demonstrate the presence of an intrarenal mass. On occasion, the tumor may be bilateral at the time of initial diagnosis.

Wilms' tumor tends to spread locally but may also metastasize to liver, lung, brain, and, most uncommonly, to bone. The current prognosis for children with Wilms' tumor appears to be better than for any other malignancy of childhood. With surgery, radiation, and chemotherapy, as many as 90% of children may be cured.

Wilms' tumor occurs with increased frequency in children with sporadic (in contrast to familial) aniridia. It also occurs with increased frequency in children with congenital hemihypertrophy or with congenital macrosomia (Beckwith's syndrome).

Neuroblastoma is the second most common solid tumor of childhood (brain tumors are the most common). About 50% of neuroblastomas manifest themselves during the first 2 years of life. In approximately one-half of the patients, the tumor arises in the abdomen, and in one-third, the neuroblastoma arises from the adrenal gland. In an additional 13% to 20% of the patients, it arises from nonadrenal intraabdominal sites. The mass is usually firm, irregular in outline, and nontender, and frequently crosses the midline. Although the most common initial presentation is that of a mass in the abdomen, the patient may also manifest symptoms and signs as a result of compression of other structures by the primary tumor or its metastatic deposits. Unfortunately, up to 70% of patients may have signs of metastasis at the time of diagnosis. Skeletal lesions are common. Metastatic spread to the lung is very rare. Invasion of the retrobulbar soft-tissues causes proptosis of the eye, as well as periorbital swelling and ecchymosis of the upper eyelid. Skin and nodal involvement may also be present.

Less commonly, the initial signs and symptoms are related to catecholamine or vasoactive substance production of the tumor. These symptoms and signs may include skin flushing, perspiration, tachycardia, hypertension, paroxysmal headaches, and intractable diarrhea. Uncommon initial manifestations may include signs of encephalopathy or opsoclonus.

The prognosis for this tumor is very poor except for patients with well-encapsulated tumors or for patients under 1 to 2 years of age in whom the metastatic process is confined to skin, liver, and bone marrow.

Other tumors of intraabdominal origin that may present as a mass include both Hodgkin's and nonHodgkin's lymphoma, teratomas, ovarian neoplasms, hepatic tumors, and rhabdomyosarcoma originating from the muscles in the retroperitoneal area.

Kidney Masses

Renal enlargement as a result of multicystic or polycystic kidneys, multilocular cysts, and hydronephrosis may all present as abdominal masses. Frequently the signs of a urinary tract infection accompany the process.

Liver Masses

Cystic disease of the liver, hepatic abscesses, hemangiomas, and hepatomas may all initially manifest themselves by abdominal enlargement and the detection of an abdominal mass.

DIAGNOSTIC APPROACH TO THE PATIENT WITH AN ABDOMINAL MASS

As previously indicated, the diagnostic approach to an infant or child with an abdominal mass is generally dictated by the age of the patient, the location of the mass, and the associated physical findings and history. A list of the more common abdominal masses is presented below.

Abdominal Masses in the Older Infant and Child

Renal malformations
Hydronephrosis
Duplication cysts of the intestine
Volvulus of the gut
Intussusception
Periappendiceal abscess
Mesenteric abscess
Mesenteric cyst

Hepatic cyst or abscess
Choledochal cyst
Hepatoma
Hemangioma of the liver or spleen
Wilms' tumor
Neuroblastoma
Lymphoma
Ovarian cyst
Ovarian tumor

In general, initial evaluation should include a careful rectal examination, urinalysis, complete blood count, and flat plate of the abdomen. More precise studies will be dictated by these preliminary studies. Contrast studies of the kidneys are frequently performed first and then may be followed by radiologic examination of the bowel, scans of the liver and spleen, sonography, and computerized axial tomography.

BIBLIOGRAPHY

Arey JB: Abdominal masses in infants and children. Pediatr Clin North Am 10:665, 1963

An overview of abdominal masses in infants and children by an experienced pathologist.

Longino LA, Martin LW: Abdominal masses in the newborn infant. Pediatrics 21:596, 1958

A surgeon's approach to the problem of masses in the abdomen of the neonate.

Sutow W, Vietti TJ, Fernbach DJ: Clinical Pediatric Oncology. St. Louis, CV Mosby, 1973

A comprehensive review of malignancies that may be encountered in pediatrics.

Jaundice and the Liver

12

Robert Kaye

Disease of the liver may be suspected by noting in the history or the physical or laboratory examinations any abnormality suggesting functional or structural pathology. These findings are grouped logically on the basis of their pathogenesis: impairment in the normal metabolic functions of the liver, circulatory abnormalities, response to infections, generalized metabolic disease or structural malformation involving the liver or its excretory ductal system. The principal abnormalities are presented in Table 12-1.

PHYSICAL EXAMINATION OF THE LIVER

In normal infants up to the age of 1 year, the liver edge may be palpable as much as 2 cm below the costal margin in the midclavicular line. After this age, the liver edge is usually felt no more than 1 cm below the costal margin. In children it is almost always possible to palpate the liver edge and thus know the position of its lower margin. Evaluation of liver size and span requires estimation of the position of its upper border by percussion, differentiating the resonance of the air-containing lung above and the liver dullness below. This will identify the liver that is pushed down below its normal position by overinflation of the lungs due to airway obstruction. The liver span approximates 6 to 9 cm at age 5 and 7 to 11 cm at age 12. The consistency of the normal liver on palpation is comparable to that noted in the relaxed biceps muscle of the adult. A malignant or cirrhotic process may impart a "stony-hard" consistency resembling that noted when pressing the fingers against the dorsum of the wrist. Markedly enlarged livers are usually harder than normal. The chief exception to this is the hugely enlarged liver of glycogen storage disease which is felt to be of normal consistency.

EVALUATION OF THE PATIENT

For evaluation of the patient suspected of liver disease, a variety of biochemical, histologic, radiographic, and isotopic techniques are available (Table 12-2). Because of its major role in metabolism, the damaged liver will yield alterations reflecting impairment of one or more of its physiologic functions. Histologic material obtained by open or needle biopsy often provides useful information bearing on diagnosis and prognosis. Radiographic studies are of particular importance in delineating anatomic abnormalities of the extrahepatic biliary system and the hepatic vascular pattern which may yield evidence of an infectious or neoplastic mass. Nuclear medicine procedures, angiog-

TABLE 12-1. Abnormalities Suggestive of Liver Disease

Abnormalities	Significance
I. Impaired metabolic function	
A. Jaundice (bilirubin > 1.0 mg/dl)	
1. Indirect hyperbilirubinemia	Hemolysis, defective uptake or conjugation
2. Direct hyperbilirubinemia	Hepatocellular injury, ductal obstruction, defective transport within liver cells
B. Steatorrhea and itching	Reduced bile acid excretion into gut and systemic retention
C. Edema	Decreased albumin synthesis
D. Bleeding	Reduced synthesis of coagulation Factors I, II, V, VII, XI, and XII
E. Nonglucose-reducing substance in urine	Impaired metabolism of galactose or fructose
F. Hypoglycemia	Decreased parenchymal mass or gluconeogenic enzyme deficiency
II. Enlarged or indurated liver	Hepatocellula inflammation, bile duct obstruction, congestive circulatory failure, cysts, tumors, storage diseases, systemic metabolic disease
III. Manifestations of portal hypertension	Intrahepatic portal obstruction: cirrhosis, fibrosis, cystic disease, storage diseases, systemic metabolic disease Extrahepatic portal obstruction: portal, splenic, hepatic vein thrombosis
A. Splenic enlargement	Impaired venous drainage
B. Hematemesis	Ruptured esophageal varix
C. Clubbing of nailbeds and spider nevi	Portal systemic shunting
D. Pancytopenia	Sequestration in engorged spleen

raphy, ultrasonography, and CT scans, yield information concerning the functioning mass of the liver, the presence of masses and the patency of the extrahepatic biliary system.

Serum measurements of hepatic enzymes are useful because they increase with hepatocellular injury and obstruction.

BILIRUBIN METABOLISM

Bilirubin is a linear tetrapyrrole formed by cleavage of the cyclic tetrapyrrole, protoporphyrin. Protoporphyrin in its iron complex (heme) is the prosthetic group of hemoglobin and other hemoproteins. Bilirubin is readily soluble in organic solvents, but only slightly soluble in aqueous solutions at physiologic pH. It can be determined by coupling with diazotized sulfanilic acid (diazo or van den Bergh reaction). Unconjugated bilirubin reacts in aqueous solution only in the presence of accelerator substances, methanol or ethanol (indirect reaction), which are unnecessary for the reaction of conjugated bilirubin (direct reaction). After the newborn period, the total bilirubin in plasma does not exceed 1.0 mg/dl with 0.2 mg/dl reacting directly.

The conversion of heme to bilirubin involves cleavage of the ferroprotoporphyrin ring by microsomal heme oxygenase yielding biliverdin. The latter compound is reduced to bilirubin by biliverdin reductase.

TABLE 12-2. Laboratory Aids in Evaluation of Liver Disease

	Normal Values	Significance
Bilirubin	0.2 direct, 1.0 total mg/dl	See text
Alkaline phosphatase	1–3 mo: 73–336 IU/l 3–10 yr: 57–151 IU/l Puberty: 57–258 IU/l 16 and older: 14–40	Increased: with complete or partial obstruction; biliary cirrhosis, tumors or inflammatory masses Decreased: with parenchymal injury; hepatitis
Transaminases	IU/l	
SGOT	Infants 67–118 Older children 3–27	Active hepatocellular injury; by infection or toxin
SGPT	0–54	SGPT more specific for liver
5′-nucleotidase	2.2–15 mIU/ml	Cholestasis
Sulfobromophthalein (BSP) excretion	95% clearance in 45 minutes of 5 mg/kg	Hepatic excretory capacity; Impaired by reduced parenchymal function or impaired hepatic blood flow
Blood proteins		
Albumin and haptoglobulin		Reduced with parenchymal cell impairment
Electrophoretic alterations α and β globulins		Increased with infection and obstruction Decreased with liver failure
IgG	240–1200 mg/dl	Increased with postnecrotic cirrhosis and chronic active hepatitis
Alpha$_1$-antitrypsin	200–400 mg/dl	Deficiency associated with acute and chronic liver disease
Coagulation Factors		See text
Alpha$_1$-fetoprotein		Associated with hepatoma
Bile acids and cholesterol		Elevated with obstruction and cholestasis
Hepatitis B surface antigen (HB_sAg)		Carrier stateor acute infection
Hepatitis B antibodies (anti-HB_s and anti-HB_c)		Past or current infection
IgM anti-HAV		Early hepatitis A infection
Anti-HAV (total IgM and IgG)		Positive in acute and past infections

The serum bilirubin concentration reflects an equilibrium between production and excretion. Bilirubin is derived from several sources. About 80% of daily bilirubin production results from breakdown of senescent red blood cells, aged approximately 120 days. Studies with labeled precursors of bilirubin have revealed the label in the fecal bilirubin (urobilinogen) within 1 to 2 days. This material, representing 10% to 20% of the daily bilirubin production, is referred to as the "early labeled" fraction. Its source is chromoproteins such as myoglobin, cytochromes, catalase, and peroxidases as well as hemoglobin which fails to be incorporated into red cells. Each of these represents a potential source of overproduction.

Understanding the metabolism of

bile pigments is facilitated by recognition of the fact that unconjugated bilirubin is a potentially toxic, end-stage metabolite requiring elimination from the body.

Essentially all of the bilirubin in the circulation is bound to albumin. In addition to conferring water solubility on bilirubin, the linkage with albumin restricts its transfer across cell membranes, thus protecting the cells from exposure to bilirubin toxicity. In competition with bilirubin for binding sites on albumin are free fatty acids, sulfonamides, thyroxine, and salicylates. The displacement of bilirubin from its albumin linkage by these substances is of particular importance in the icteric newborn in whom bilirubin concentrations may rise to levels saturating the total binding capacity of albumin.

Hepatic Uptake and Conjugation

There are mechanisms within the liver cell which establish gradients for the movement of unconjugated bilirubin from plasma to cell and facilitate its clearance into the bile. Lipid-soluble unconjugated bilirubin is able to cross the lipid-containing cell membrane. There are two hepatic cytoplasmic acceptor proteins, Y and Z, capable of binding unconjugated bilirubin, preventing its back-diffusion from the hepatocyte and fostering further transfer of pigment from the plasma.

Another mechanism providing the liver with its unique capacity to remove bilirubin from the plasma is the conversion of the intracytoplasmic pigment to water soluble conjugates of glucuronic acid. The ionic nature and increased molecular size of the conjugates limit back diffusion across the plasma membrane and foster their excretion into the bile.

Glucuronic acid conjugation of bilirubin requires uridine diphosphoglucuronic acid which donates its glucuronic acid to the propionic acid side chains of bilirubin. The reaction is catalyzed by the microsomal enzyme glucuronyl transferase which may be induced by phenobarbital and other compounds.

The bacterial flora of the lower bowel reduces conjugated bilirubin to a group of chromogens designated urobilinogen. Urobilinogen is poorly reabsorbed from the bowel, about 100 to 200 mg/day is excreted in the stool of adults. Of the small amount reabsorbed, most is excreted by the liver with approximately 4 mg/day eliminated in the urine.

Overproduction of bilirubin by hemolysis, impaired hepatic uptake, or glucuronide conjugation will result in increased concentrations of unconjugated (indirect reacting) bilirubin. Situations which permit bilirubin to gain access to the hepatocyte and undergo conjugation but interfere with its transport into the intestine (parenchymal cell injury, obstruction of the biliary tree or functional disorders of secretion into the bile) will lead to elevations of conjugated (direct-reacting) bilirubin.

Stool color yields important clues to the origin of jaundice. Acholic stools are commonly seen during the early stages of hepatitis and in complete extrahepatic biliary obstruction.

Bilirubin Excretion in the Newborn (Physiologic Jaundice)

In the fetus and newborn, special circumstances may modify the scheme of bilirubin metabolism just described. Unconjugated bilirubin formed by the fetus freely crosses the placenta and is excreted by the maternal liver. During the first week of extrauterine life, hepatic function is inadequate to prevent accumulation of bilirubin in plasma. This disability has been regarded as physiologic when limited to this age group and to a bilirubin concentration not in excess of 12 mg/dl. A pathologic process should be suspected and investigated when: (1) jaundice appears before 36 hours of age; (2)

serum bilirubin concentration exceeds 12 mg/dl; (3) jaundice persists beyond the eighth day of life; and (4) the direct-reacting bilirubin exceeds 1.5 mg/dl.

A transient deficiency of glucuronyl transferase observed in livers of newborn animals and recently expired premature infants was proposed as an explanation for the impaired clearance of unconjugated bilirubin characteristic of this age. Impaired hepatic uptake of unconjugated bilirubin is observed in newborn animals and suggests an important role of the cytoplasmic acceptor proteins in physiologic jaundice. The Z protein reaches full concentration during fetal life while the major binding protein Y is almost absent at birth reaching mature levels during the second week of life. Decreased effectiveness of the intestinal component of bilirubin elimination is also important in the hyperbilirubinemia of the newborn. This is dependent on reduction by the intestinal flora of conjugated bilirubin to urobilinogen. The newborn infant with a relatively sterile bowel is disadvantaged in this process. Furthermore, glucuronidases present in the intestinal epithelium of the infant at birth are capable of regenerating free bilirubin from its conjugated form. Unconjugated bilirubin can be freely absorbed into the circulation and subjects the neonatal infant to the superimposed burden of an enterohepatic recirculation of bilirubin. This phenomenon is exaggerated in infants with intestinal obstruction. As there is some bilirubin conjugation and excretion into the intestine beginning at 20 weeks of fetal life, this mechanism probably serves to protect the infant from accumulation of bilirubin within the intestinal lumen as a massive pigmented gallstone. Reabsorbed bilirubin traverses the placenta and is excreted by the maternal liver.

Also contributing to elevated levels of bilirubin in some newborns is continued patency of the ductus venosus which permits some portal blood to bypass the liver. Estrogens and progestins from maternal sources may play a role in physiologic jaundice through inhibiting bilirubin conjugation.

A variety of therapeutic approaches may increase the ability of the newborn to eliminate bile pigments. Early feeding of newborn infants serves to hasten bacterial colonization of the intestinal tract, thereby reducing the degree of unconjugated hyperbilirubinemia. Phenobarbital can enhance bilirubin glucuronyl transferase activity and increase the concentration of the Y acceptor protein, thus increasing both uptake and conjugation of the pigment. The sedative properties of phenobarbital limit its clinical application. Cholestyramine combines with bilirubin, and agar gels can sequester the pigment reducing the magnitude of the enterohepatic recirculation. Phototherapy based on the photolability of bilirubin has been used to reduce elevated plasma bilirubin levels. The simpler pyrrole derivatives produced by the action of light (wavelength 420–470 nm) can be excreted in the bile and urine without prior conjugation. Light therapy will reduce but not eliminate the need for exchange transfusions.

Disorders of Bilirubin Excretion

There are a number of disorders which involve impairment in one or more of the steps involved in the sequence from bilirubin production to its excretion in the stool. It is helpful to group these on the basis of whether elevation of unconjugated or conjugated bilirubin predominates (Table 12-3).

INFECTIONS

Neonatal Hepatitis

Hepatic inflammatory processes in the early weeks or months of life have several rather unique features. Chief among

TABLE 12-3. Disorders of Bilirubin Production, Hepatic Uptake, Conjugation, and Excretion

Abnormalities	Significance
I. Unconjugated hyperbilirubinemias	
A. Transient neonatal hyperbilirubinemia	
1. Delayed development of hepatic uptake and conjugating system	See above
a. Physiologic jaundice in full-term infant	
b. Physiologic jaundice in low-birth weight infant	More intense and prolonged
2. Inhibitors of conjugation	
a. Lucey-Driscoll syndrome	Serum inhibitors to conjugation of bilirubin
b. Breast-fed infant	Inhibitor, pregnanediol present in breast milk
3. Increased enterohepatic recirculation of bilirubin	Mechanical blockage or reduced hepatic blood flow with increased intraabdominal pressure and increased reabsorption of bilirubin from gut
a. Gastrointestinal obstruction	
B. Overproduction of bilirubin	
1. Hemolysis due to maternal-fetal blood group incompatibilities	
a. Rh and ABO systems	Antibody produced in mother to fetal red cell antigens leads to hemolysis in newborn
2. Deficiency of red cell enzymes	Glucose-6-phosphate dehydrogenase, fructokinase, glutathione peroxidase
3. Other hemolytic disorders	
a. Congenital	Spherocytosis, Cooley's anemia, sickle cell disease
b. Acquired	Drugs, autoimmune disease
4. Shunt hyperbilirubinemia	Increased erythrocyte destruction in bone marrow
5. Drugs and chemical agents	Vitamin K, toluene, phenacetin, lead
C. Mixed or undefined	
1. Septicemia	Hemolysis, toxic hepatitis
2. Hypothyroidism	Delayed maturation of glucuronyl transferase
3. Drugs and chemical agents	See B5, red cell and hepatic injury
D. Persistent jaundice with defective conjugation	
1. Crigler-Najjar syndrome	
a. Type I	Death in infancy, decreased transferase activity, phenobarbital unresponsive, recessive inheritance
b. Type II	Adult survival, phenobarbital responsive, autosomal dominant
2. Gilbert's syndrome	Onset late childhood, more frequent in males, constitutional and GI symptoms, jaundice, phenobarbital responsive
II. Conjugated hyperbilirubinemia due to impaired bilirubin excretion	
A. Transient neonatal hyperbilirubinemia	
1. Following Rh isoimmunization	Hepatic injury or bile duct plugging
B. Chronic non-hemolytic jaundice	
1. Dubin-Johnson syndrome	Pigment in hepatic cells
2. Rotor's syndrome	Without pigment in hepatic cells, both show decreased BSP and cholecystographic agent excretion and GI symptoms
C. Benign familial cholestasis	Recurrent jaundice with itching, increased alkaline phosphatase, cholestasis on biopsy, benign course

these, especially among familial cases, is a tendency to progress to postnecrotic cirrhosis and death with hepatic failure. The liver of the infant so affected responds to injury with the formation of multinucleated giant cells. This response may involve the entire hepatic parenchyma in a giant cell or syncytial transformation leading to use of the term "giant cell hepatitis" as a synonym for neonatal hepatitis.

Etiology. Among the viruses incriminated are those of hepatitis B, cytomegalic inclusion disease, herpes simplex, rubella, and Coxsackie infections.

Hepatitis B antigen (HB Ag) positivity during pregnancy entails little risk to the fetus of a maternal carrier. However, acute infection in the mother, particularly in the third trimester of pregnancy or within 2 months postpartum, leads to a high incidence of infection in offspring. A high incidence of neonatal hepatitis and biliary atresia has been noted in infants with the trisomy 17-18 syndrome. This association has led to the suggestion that an *in utero* viral infection may be the basis for the trisomy and the hepatic lesions. Also, in infants with intrauterine rubella, neonatal hepatitis and biliary atresia have been noted to occur at an increased rate. This coincidence supports the hypothesis that biliary atresia may be the consequence of an *in utero* viral infection in which the inflammatory reaction has been particularly localized in the biliary excretory apparatus.

The protozoan parasite toxoplasma has also been found in newborn infants with hepatomegaly and jaundice, usually as a part of a generalized infection involving the central nervous system, the eye, and the heart.

Hepatic involvement may be associated with such bacterial infections as septicemia, pneumonia, pyelonephritis, and listeriosis. Though syphilis may be responsible for neonatal hepatitis, significant clinical evidence of hepatic dysfunction is not common.

Alpha-1-antitrypsin deficiency has recently been found to be a major cause of the neonatal hepatitis syndrome.

Clinical Manifestation and Diagnosis. Infants affected with hepatitis are noted to have persistent jaundice due to increased conjugated bilirubin and often acholic stools suggesting complete interruption of the excretion of bile pigments. The clinical pattern consists of a history of onset of jaundice in the second to third weeks of life, of initially normal-colored stools which become acholic, persistent conjugated hyperbilirubinemia and positive tests for urobilinogen in urine and stool. These suggest the presence of an acquired disease with partial obstruction; however, similar clinical findings may occur in infants with extrahepatic biliary atresia.

The differentiation between hepatitis and biliary atresia is made difficult by the frequency with which hepatitis leads to prolonged, essentially complete obstruction to the passage of bile. Serial determinations of serum bilirubin in patients with hepatitis may be initially high levels with a tendency toward an irregular decline with time. The infant with biliary atresia initially has lower values with a gradual increase.

A combination of percutaneous liver biopsy and determination of the 72-hour fecal excretion of ^{131}I-rose bengal will provide a definitive diagnosis in most cases. In hepatitis, there is marked distortion of lobular architecture with transformation of hepatocytes into multinucleated giant cells. In contrast, in excretory duct anomalies (atresia, stenosis, hypoplasia, choledochal cyst), there is essentially normal lobular architecture with fibrosis and proliferation of bile ducts in the portal areas.

The rose bengal excretion test results in recovery of less than 10% of the dye in the feces of patients with excretory duct abnormalities, while 80% of patients with parenchymal lesions excrete larger amounts.

Persistence of HB Ag supports the diagnosis of neonatal hepatitis. If the studies suggest biliary atresia, operative intervention is undertaken promptly.

When a diagnosis of hepatitis is established and an additional period of a few weeks for observation shows no amelioration of jaundice, corticosteroid therapy is given for 4 to 6 weeks. Prognosis for recovery varies inversely with the duration of disease and is more favorable in sporadic rather than familial cases.

Viral Hepatitis

Clinical observations had suggested two types of viral hepatitis that were histologically alike. One, *infectious hepatitis* (hepatitis A, HA, short incubation period) appeared to be transmitted orally. Another, *serum hepatitis* (hepatitis B, HB, long incubation period) was thought to be transmitted only parenterally, by blood transfusion or contaminated instruments. The infectivity of serum of patients with HA was demonstrated in 1967 and virus shown in stools in 1973.

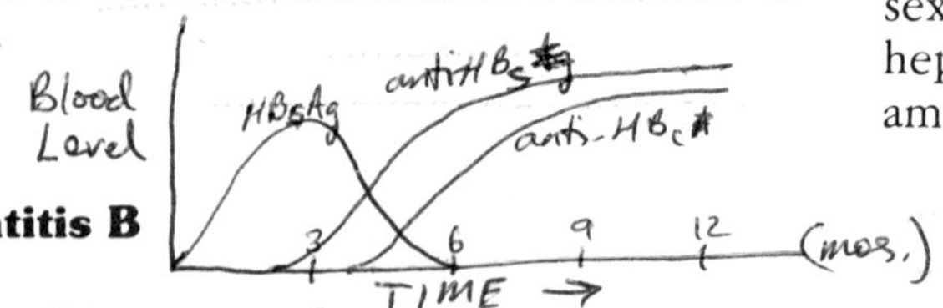

Hepatitis B

Discovery of the Australia antigen established the viral etiology of HB. Screening of donor blood for HB associated antigen reduced but did not eliminate post-transfusion hepatitis. Blood not positive for HA or HB may transmit a disease not distinguishable from HB. This non-A/non-B hepatitis virus (or probably viruses) now is responsible for the majority of cases of post-transfusion hepatitis.

Centrifugation of serum of persons whose blood contains the HB antigen yields spheres; the infective virus (Dane or core particles) and circular or filamentous forms which carry the surface antigen, (HB_sAg). An internal core particle contains the core antigen (HB_cAg) and an antigen HB_eAg, which correlates with infectivity. Anti-HB_e appears to protect against HB virus infection.

In HB infection, HB_sAg appears early and may persist for 3 to 6 months. Later, anti-HB_s and anti-HB_c appear and may persist indefinitely. Lymphocytes may become sensitized to HB antigens, and in patients with chronic active hepatitis may exhibit cytotoxic properties against hepatocytes *in vitro*. In most recovered patients with HB, antibody against HB virus permits clearance of virus from liver and blood.

Patients with chronic HB fail to achieve an effective antibody response and are unable to clear the virus. Presence of the virus may lead to faulty regulation of cellular immunity with attack against antigens in the liver cell resulting in chronic active hepatitis.

A vaccine derived from the plasma of HB carriers has shown effectiveness in controlled studies. It may be of great value in treatment of high risk groups such as dialysis patients and personnel, male homosexuals, and in reducing the frequency of hepatocellular carcinoma which is common among HB carriers.

Hepatitis A

Hepatitis A is usually a benign disease in contrast to HB, in which a small percentage of patients may progress to chronic liver disease. The HA virus and its antibody can be detected by immunologic techniques. A vaccine is under study. The HA virus can be detected in the blood about two weeks before and after the appearance of symptoms. A carrier state as seen with HB does not occur. HA virus is present in stools 2 to 3 weeks before and about 1 week after onset of jaundice.

Non-A/Non-B Hepatitis

About 90% of post-transfusion hepatitis is not due to HB virus. Screening for HB virus has reduced post-transfusion hepatitis by a factor of 4 and deaths 8-fold. This suggests that most cases of post-transfusion hepatitis are non-A/non-B and are less severe than the HB disorder. Transmission by blood suggests that a carrier state for these viruses exists. There is also evidence that they are more frequently associated with chronic active hepatitis than is HB.

Clinical Manifestations. The incubation period of type A hepatitis is approximately 14 to 40 days and 60 to 100 days for type B. Type A hepatitis infection is usually marked by an abrupt onset with fever, an autumn-winter incidence peak and a predilection for children and young adults. Type B hepatitis usually exhibits an insidious onset with little or no fever and a year-round incidence without age preference.

In the first phase (preicteric), symptoms usually begin 4 to 5 days before the appearance of jaundice. Prominent are fever, malaise, mild headache, chilliness, signs of mild upper respiratory tract infection, arthralgia, anorexia, nausea and vomiting, upper abdominal distress, and pain. Bile usually is present in the urine 1 to 3 days before the appearance of jaundice. Fever generally disappears with the onset of icterus, but anorexia continues, and severe prostration and vomiting may occur. Stools are light or clay-colored at this stage.

The second phase (icteric) usually continues 2 to 4 weeks with gradually increasing clinical and laboratory evidence of jaundice followed by a gradual diminution. There may be a further period of 1 to 2 months with malaise and fatigue.

The liver is commonly enlarged and tender. The spleen is palpable in up to 15% of patients, and other evidence of adenopathy including cervical adenopathy may be present.

Diagnosis. Serum bilirubin values, predominantly direct reacting, may be as high as 10 mg/dl or more. There is an increase in the urinary excretion of urobilinogen due to impaired hepatic clearance. With complete failure of bile to reach the intestine, urobilinogen disappears from the urine. With partial resolution of hepatic injury, there is resumption of excretion of bile into the intestine and urobilinogen is again formed and appears in the urine.

The serum glutamic oxaloacetic or glutamic pyruvic transaminases are elevated early in the course of the disease; their return to normal heralds the end of active disease and the beginning of recovery.

Differential Diagnosis. The diagnosis of viral hepatitis is dependent on the elimination of other causes of jaundice. The labial herpes, hemorrhagic exanthem, fever, leukocytosis, muscle pains, and albuminuria occurring in leptospirosis serve to distinguish it clinically. Involvement of the liver, which may mimic that in infectious hepatitis, is relatively common in infectious mononucleosis.

In the early preicteric phase, symptoms may be suggestive of influenza or gastroenteritis. Abdominal pain may resemble that of pneumonia or acute appendicitis. Drug-induced or toxic hepatitis must also be considered.

Pathology. Similar pathologic changes in the liver occur in all types of hepatitis. The hepatic lobules show varying degrees of cellular necrosis, autolysis, and thickening of the reticular fibers. Accompanying the hepatocellular necrosis is widespread infiltration with inflammatory cells. Proliferating bile ducts appear in the perilobular portal areas, and bile stasis is visible. With recovery, complete regeneration of the liver cells occurs without scarring. In fulminating and fatal cases, the hepatic changes are typical of yellow atrophy.

Mild Anicteric Hepatitis

Mild anicteric hepatitis is apparently more common among infants than the icteric form of the disease. The symptoms are those of a mild gastroenteritis with anorexia, diarrhea, and vomiting.

Chronic Hepatitis

Except in the very young infant, infectious hepatitis in childhood is usually a brief, self-limited illness. It is uncommon for children with an apparently typical bout of hepatitis to continue for months with hepatomegaly and biochemical evidence of continued hepatocellular injury. This type of course has been designated "prolonged or persistent hepatitis." Patients with this course may be expected to recover ultimately unless subacute hepatic necrosis progresses to postnecrotic cirrhosis. The unusual development of chronic active hepatitis is described below.

Treatment. Treatment of chronic hepatitis is symptomatic during the interval required for immunologic defenses to eradicate the virus. Maintenance of a reasonable state of nutrition during the illness is beneficial and requires intravenous alimentation when vomiting or anorexia is prominent.

Prevention. Isolation precautions appropriate for patients with intestinal infections are indicated during the period of hospitalization. Gamma-globulin prophylaxis is effective only in short incubation (or HB Ag-negative) hepatitis. The use of high-titer anti-B serum for patients exposed to B-positive hepatitis is promising.

Fulminant Hepatitis

Fulminant hepatitis, or acute massive necrosis, is usually fatal within a few weeks after onset. Particularly prominent are high fever, abdominal pain, and vomiting. Also indicative of an unfavorable outcome are rapid decrease in liver size, mental changes including lethargy, drowsiness and confusion, electroencephalographic changes of encephalopathy, and an increase in prothrombin time not corrected by parenteral administration of vitamin K. Transaminase levels may not be very high, reflecting failure of hepatic synthesis of the enzymes. Bleeding into the skin and mucous membranes, ascites, and deep coma are among the terminal manifestations.

Liver Failure in Hepatitis

In viral and toxic hepatitis and in chronic liver disease, sufficient functional alteration or reduction in parenchymal cell mass may result in the critical syndrome of liver failure. Fluid retention and ascites may occur as a consequence of obstruction to hepatic circulation with increased lymph exudation into the peritoneal cavity. Impaired hepatic synthesis of albumin may contribute to the accumulation of ascites. Loss of extracellular fluid as ascites initiates hormonal changes that result in increased renal tubular reabsorption of sodium. Therapy is designed to reverse the positive sodium balance and includes restriction of sodium intake combined with diuretics.

Decreased liver function and shunting of portal blood to the systemic circulation are the major underlying factors in hepatic encephalopathy. Gastrointestinal bleeding is a frequent precipitating factor because of the impairment in circulation and increased nitrogenous burden which accompany it. By reducing blood volume and depleting potassium stores, diuretics may also contribute to hepatic encephalopathy. Cerebral metabolism may be altered by accumulation of ammonia and other nitrogenous compounds. Increased brain serotonin and neural catecholamine depletion have also been implicated. To reduce the intestinal production of ammonia, protein should be eliminated from the diet. Adequate carbohydrate calories limit endogenous breakdown of protein. Bacterial breakdown of protein and ammonia formation are reduced by oral administration of a poorly absorbed antibiotic such as neomycin. Lactulose given orally converts ammonia to the less well-absorbed ammonium ion. Exchange transfusion may be indicated in patients with potentially reversible disease. The massive bleeding accompanying liver failure is best managed by the infusion of fresh frozen plasma.

CHRONIC LIVER DISEASE

Chronic liver disease may present as the principal clinical problem, for example, the cirrhosis secondary to biliary atresia, or as an associated disability of a systemic disturbance, such as cystic fibrosis.

The term "cirrhosis" implies extensive destruction of hepatic parenchyma, with replacement by diffuse fibrosis and distortion of lobular architecture. When hepatic cells are destroyed, new cells form from the cellular remnants. If cell death is confined to individual lobules, orderly restoration of histologic and functional relations is likely. Destruction of many adjacent lobules with collapse of intervening stroma leads to nodular regeneration. New blood vessels at the margins of growing nodules are compressed leading to dependence on hepatic arterial blood for nutrition as portal blood is shunted past. In conditions characterized chiefly by hepatic fibrosis, portal hypertension rather than parenchymal insufficiency may become the major clinical problem.

Postnecrotic Cirrhosis

In children, most instances of postnecrotic cirrhosis appear after recognized antecedent illness, for example, neonatal hepatitis and chronic active hepatitis. Children have fewer opportunities than adults to contact such hepatic toxic agents as carbon tetrachloride. Diagnostic efforts should be directed toward those diseases of childhood with which cirrhosis is associated, for example, cystic fibrosis, Wilson's disease, neonatal hepatitis or α-1-antitrypsin deficiency.

Clinical Features. The peak incidence occurs in the 10- to 20-year age group with female predominance. The onset may be abrupt or insidious with malaise, fatigue, weight loss, anorexia, and fever. Portal hypertension with bleeding esophageal varices or ascites usually occurs late. About 20% of patients have significant disease in other systems as the presenting complaint: hematuria, bloody diarrhea, acne, malar flush, or amenorrhea in females. Clinical study may reveal the presence of nephritis, thyroiditis, myositis, arthralgia, colitis, or hemolytic anemia. These multisystem symptoms may also develop during the course of the illness and suggest an "autoimmune" mechanism as etiologic or of importance in progression.

Laboratory Findings. Modest to marked elevations of bilirubin, serum transaminases, and gamma globulins are the typical biochemical changes in chronic active liver disease. Serologic abnormalities, including LE phenomena, antinuclear and smooth muscle antibodies, and positive Coomb's reaction are relatively common findings.

Pathology. Characteristically, the periolobular region shows degeneration and "piecemeal" necrosis of cells with lymphocytic and plasma cell infiltration. The limiting plate separating the portal tract and lobule is eroded. Varying degrees of fibrosis including features of multinodular cirrhosis can be seen as well.

Treatment. Over 80% of untreated patients with chronic liver disease die within 5 years. With treatment, improvement in early survival and quality of life is seen. The autoimmune mechanism hypothesis provides the rationale for corticosteroid and other immunosuppressive therapy which results in clinical, biochemical, and histologic improvement in the majority of patients. It is not proven that survival is favorably effected by therapy, although complete resolution has been described.

Biliary Cirrhosis

In children, biliary cirrhosis develops after prolonged obstruction of the biliary system by extrahepatic atresia, stenosis, or choledochal cyst. Less frequent causes in childhood are stones or sludge in the common bile duct, tumor, and recurrent attacks of pancreatitis.

Vascular Obstruction

Cardiac failure is the principal cause of passive congestion of the liver. Longstanding pulmonary vascular disease with stasis in the right side of the heart also engorges the liver. Constrictive pericarditis produces passive vascular congestion as does myocardial or valvular disease. With continuation of the hyperemia, the liver cells surrounding the central vein undergo degenerative changes due to hypoxia and become atrophic.

A number of hereditary disorders affecting the liver may lead to portal hypertension with or without cirrhosis (Table 12-4).

ACUTE ENCEPHALOPATHY AND HEPATOMEGALY WITH FATTY INFILTRATION: REYE'S SYNDROME (ENCEPHALOPATHY AND FATTY DEGENERATION OF THE VISCERA)

Reye's syndrome is acute and frequently fatal. There is usually a preceding mild viral illness which is followed by a rapid onset of vomiting and within hours by a change in the state of consciousness, which may progress through delirium to stupor and coma.

On examination, there is a mild-to-moderate hepatomegaly and central nervous system depression which may include signs of brain stem involvement, altered pupillary reflexes, and increased intracranial pressure. Marked increases in transaminases and ammonia are seen with little or no increase in the serum bilirubin. Bleeding may be a problem with reduction of liver-dependent coagulation factors. Hypoglycemia occurs commonly. Spinal fluid pressure is increased.

Liver tissue obtained by percutaneous biopsy is pale and at times white. Microscopically, diffuse fatty vacuolization of the enlarged hepatocytes is seen. Ultrastructurally, mitochondrial swelling and pleomorphism are seen. Lipid stains are positive, and chemical analysis of the liver tissue indicates large increases in triglyceride and fatty acid. Fatty degeneration of organs, such as the heart, pancreas, and kidney have been reported. The myocardial and renal tubular changes account for the occurrence of arrhythmias and aminoaciduria.

Etiology remains obscure. Evidence of infection with influenza B, herpes simplex, and varicella viruses have been found in some patients. Exogenous agents such as isopropyl alcohol, salicylates, and aflatoxins may be contributory.

Because the pathophysiology of this disease is poorly understood, specific ther-

TABLE 12-4. Developmental and Metabolic Liver Disease Leading to Portal Hypertension or Cirrhosis

Disorder	Transmission	Pathology
Developmental		
Polycystic liver disease	Autosomal recessive or Autosomal dominant	Multiple cysts in biopsy Usually with polycystic kidneys Wide bands of fibrotic tissue on biopsy
Congenital hepatic fibrosis	Autosomal recessive	Fibrous tissue in portal areas
Hereditary hemorrhagic telangiectasia (Osler-Weber-Rendu)	Autosomal dominant	Cirrhosis with immunologic impairment, discrete or massive hemangiomas
Metabolic		
Wilson's disease (Hepatolenticular degeneration)	Autosomal recessive	Increased hepatic copper, decreased serum ceruloplasmin, cirrhosis, basal ganglia symptoms Kayser-Fleischer ring in cornea, treatment with penicillamine
Galactosemia	Autosomal recessive	Nonglucose-reducing substance in urine, absent galactose-1-phosphate uridyltransferase, cirrhosis, cataracts, failure to thrive, treatment with galactose-free diet
Cystic fibrosis	Autosomal recessive	Increased sweat chloride concentration, focal cirrhosis
Fructose intolerance	Autosomal recessive	Absent-fructose-1-phosphate aldolase, cirrhosis, hypoglycemia
Sickle cell disease	Autosomal dominant	Cirrhosis, hemachromatosis, diagnosis by hemoglobin electrophoresis
Glycogen storage disease Type IV	Autosomal recessive	Cirrhosis, deficiency of branching enzyme
Sphyngolipid and mucopolysaccharide storage diseases (*e.g.*, Gaucher's, Niemann-Pick, Hurler's disease)	Autosomal recessive	Portal hypertension, deficiency of specific catabolic enzymes
Tyrosinosis	Autosomal recessive	Reduced p-OH phenylpyruvate oxidase, cirrhosis, rickets, renal tubular disorder, may present as neonatal hepatitis
Cystinosis	Autosomal recessive	Renal tubular dysfunction, rickets
Hepatic prophyria	Autosomal dominant	Abnormal prophyrins, postnecrotic cirrhosis
Hemachromatosis	Variable penetrance	Serum iron increased, saturation of iron binding protein
Progressive familial cholestasis	Autosomal recessive	Cirrhosis, steatorrhea, bile acid retention
α-1-antitrypsin deficiency	Autosomal recessive	May present as neonatal hepatitis decreased levels of α-l-antitrypsin in serum, cytoplasmic inclusions in liver

apy has not been found. The severe mitochondrial injury demonstrable by electron microscopy is accompanied by transient decreases in the levels of a number of mitochondrial enzymes with oxidative, gluconeogenic and urea cycle activities. First to be recognized were deficiencies of the urea cycle enzymes, carbamyl phosphate synthetase and ornithine transcarbamylase. Reduction in citrulline, the product of the enzymes, has been demonstrated and may account for the failure of conversion of ammonia to urea. Hypoglycemia is treated with infusions of glucose to support central nervous system metabolism and reconstitute glycogen stores. Acidosis should be corrected when present. Cerebral edema is managed by the infusion of mannitol A, intermediate acting barbiturates, and dexamethasone guided by intracranial pressure monitoring. The syndrome must be differentiated from carnitine deficiency which gives similar clinical symptoms and laboratory findings and may be treatable with oral l-carnitine. Exchange transfusion may improve the survival rates and reduce neurologic sequelae.

HEPATIC DRUG REACTIONS

The liver may be injured by a variety of chemical agents. Some of these are hepatotoxins, and the liver injury may be considered "predictable." With other compounds, hepatic damage is less frequent and may be considered "nonpredictable" or of immunologic, allergic, or idiosyncratic origin. Among the "predictable" agents are carbon tetrachloride, toluene and trichlorethylene in solvent "sniffers" and mitomycin in cancer therapy. These agents are generally toxic in animals, injurious after short exposure and produce characteristic hepatic lesions. In contrast, the "nonpredictable" hepatotoxins do not produce lesions in experimental animals and usually exhibit evidence of hepatic toxicity after relatively prolonged use. Withdrawal of the offending agent is usually associated with reduction of the hepatic injury. Prominent among this group are chlorpromazine, isoniazid, antithyroid drugs, erythromycin estolate, and oxyphenisatin, a component of some laxatives.

PORTAL HYPERTENSION

Etiology

In children, obstruction of the portal vein and cirrhosis are the leading causes of portal hypertension. Thrombosis may be secondary to neonatal omphalitis or to cannulation of the umbilical vein. Anomalies of the portal venous system are rare; obstructive valves, however, have been demonstrated. Obstruction of the portal vein by neoplastic invasion is uncommon.

Portal hypertension is a common sequel to cirrhosis secondary to extrahepatic biliary obstruction or to postnecrotic hepatocellular disease. Because of the poor prognosis, documentation of the presence of portal hypertension is often of only academic interest.

Clinical Manifestations

In portal vein thrombosis, hepatic function is usually normal and the presenting signs are those of portal hypertension. Hematemesis is common and is often accompanied by the passage of bright red blood by rectum. Collateral circulation between the portal and systemic vessels may be noted on inspection of the abdominal wall; such vessels radiating from the umbilical region are referred to as *caput medusae.* Of the varicosities accompanying portal hypertension, those arising in the esophagus and stomach are the most important because of their tendency to bleed massively. Pancytopenia (Banti's syndrome) related to the enlarged spleen is common.

Diagnosis

Radiographic demonstration of esophageal varices is the simplest and safest means of establishing the presence of collateral circulation secondary to portal hypertension. Esophagoscopy with small, flexible fiberoptic esophagoscopes is now possible. Celiac arteriography can localize the site of thrombosis and delineate collateral circulation. Obstruction to the main hepatic veins by cardiac failure or constrictive pericarditis results in postsinusoidal extrahepatic portal hypertension.

Treatment

In infants and children with portal hypertension secondary to cirrhosis, the prognosis of the underlying liver disease is often so poor that it contraindicates surgical treatment. The normal hepatic functions of patients with extrahepatic portal obstruction enable them to tolerate recurrent hemorrhages. Variceal bleeding may cease spontaneously after repeated episodes. Delay of surgical intervention until at least 4 to 6 years of age or older is a reasonable course in most instances. In emergency treatment of bleeding varices, transfusion of whole blood, preferably guided by measurement of central venous pressure, is indicated. Intravenous pitressin or esophageal tamponade with the Sengstaken-Blakemore tube usually controls bleeding.

CHOLECYSTITIS

Acute inflammation of the gallbladder is uncommon in childhood. It may accompany a variety of acute infections, including bacterial pneumonia, meningitis, peritonitis, and typhoid fever. The symptoms are nausea, vomiting, fever, abdominal distention, and pain in the right upper quadrant. The gallbladder may be palpable as a tense, excruciatingly tender mass. With advancing symptoms, surgery is advisable, although with treatment of the associated infection, symptoms and signs diminish rapidly.

CHOLELITHIASIS

Biliary calculi are infrequent in early life, but are more common than infection of the gallbladder. Cholelithiasis in childhood occurs frequently as a complication of the congenital hemolytic anemias and sickle-cell anemia. Calcium is deposited in some and a shadow may be visible radiographically. Pure pigment stones cast no shadow and are demonstrable only by the use of contrast medium. The treatment of symptomatic cholelithiasis is surgical. Dissolution of cholesterol gallstones by chenodeoxycholic acid in adults has been observed.

CHOLEDOCHUS CYST

Choledochus cyst, or cystic dilatation of the common bile duct, is generally considered to be of developmental origin. Cysts may grow to large dimensions; a capacity of 2 liters has been recorded. The clinical manifestations are upper abdominal pain, jaundice, and abdominal tumor. The liver may become enlarged and cirrhotic, and frequently there is cholangitis.

Prolonged obstructive jaundice associated with high serum alkaline phosphatase and cholesterol values is suggestive of choledochal cyst or other incomplete common bile duct obstruction by stenosis or tumor. Direct radiographic visualization by oral or intravenous cholangiography may be diagnostic. Demonstration of distortion or impression on the duodenal loop during barium contrast examination of the upper gastrointestinal tract are suggestive of obstruction of the common duct. Ultrasonography is helpful. Treatment is surgical by anastomosis between the biliary system and the intestinal tract. The results following operation are usually good, if cirrhosis has not developed and if cholangitis does not supervene.

ATRESIA OF THE EXTRAHEPATIC BILE DUCTS

Biliary atresia is generally thought to result from maldevelopment. In early fetal life the liver and its ductal system develop from a diverticulum of the ventral floor of the endodermal foregut. The ducts are initially patent, but become obliterated by epithelial proliferation to form solid cords. With further development, the cords are recanalized. Failure of this last phase may involve all or part of the extrahepatic biliary tree. Biliary atresia may also result from intrauterine or postnatal viral infection as described above.

Pathology

Histologically, there is little distortion of the normal architecture of the hepatic plates seen with biliary atresia. The outstanding feature is the extensive fibrosis within the portal triads, in which proliferating bile ducts are embedded. With increasing fibrosis and the development of cirrhosis, there is interference with hepatic circulation resulting in portal hypertension. The spleen becomes enlarged and during the second half of the first year of life esophageal varices, ascites, and the hematologic changes of hypersplenism may appear. Osteomalacia develops with prolonged malabsorption.

Clinical Manifestations

Jaundice and indurated hepatomegaly are the most striking signs of biliary atresia. The hyperbilirubinemia is predominantly conjugated and usually below 10 mg/dl during the first 6 to 8 weeks of life, after which it steadily increases. Growth is impaired. Portal hypertension, hypoproteinemic edema, bleeding secondary to prothrombin deficiency, and hyperammonemia occur during the latter part of the first year. The stools are pale and clay-colored. Small amounts of bile pigments on the surface of the stool are derived from intestinal secretions and epithelium. The urine is dark and contains large amounts of direct-reacting bilirubin. Urobilinogen is usually absent from the urine, but occasionally may be present in small amounts if bilirubin enters the bowel with intestinal secretions and desquamated cells and is subsequently absorbed and excreted in the urine.

There is moderate anemia and a steady increase in the conjugated hyperbilirubinemia. Transaminase values in the serum are elevated but usually remain below 400 units. Serum alkaline phosphatase is also moderately elevated. Prothrombin concentrations are maintained in the normal range in the early stages. When low values occur, correction is usually possible by parenteral administration of vitamin K until hepatic cellular failure has developed.

Diagnosis

Congenital malformation of the bile ducts must be differentiated from other causes of obstructive jaundice in early infancy. The principal problem is differentiation from neonatal hepatitis (see discussion above).

Treatment

When cholangiography determines that a portion of the extrahepatic biliary tree is patent, surgical correction of the obstruction is mandatory. A surgical procedure introduced by Kasai, involves resection of a cone of liver tissue in the hilar area of the liver, thus opening up many small bile ducts. This is followed by suture of an intestinal pouch to the site. The procedure is temporarily effective in approximately one-third of infants if carried out at about 2 months, prior to spontaneous obliteration of the lumen of the small bile ducts. Cholangitis or progressive sclerosis of the biliary ducts limits the long-term effectiveness of the procedure.

ATRESIA OF THE INTRAHEPATIC BILE DUCTS

Intrahepatic atresia of bile ducts may be partial or complete and has been observed most often in association with atresia of the extrahepatic biliary system, especially in infants with an unusually long survival time. It is likely that, in some instances, the intrahepatic atresia represents an atrophy of disuse of structures deprived of their normal function. Atresia of the intrahepatic biliary system coexisting with patency of the extrahepatic bile ducts is possible in view of the separate origin of the two portions of the biliary system from the cephalad and caudate portions of the foregut diverticulum, respectively. The outstanding clinical features are prolonged survival, often to the end of the first decade, and hyperlipidemia with prominent cutaneous xanthomas. Treatment is symptomatic, including that for pruritus. Cholestyramine increases the extrahepatic excretion of bile salts and decreases the serum lipids. Recently acquired forms of intra- and extrahepatic biliary atresia have been recognized. Alpha-1-antitrypsin deficiency may be associated with a paucity of intrahepatic bile ducts.

BIBLIOGRAPHY

Andres JM, Mathis RK, Walker WA: Liver disease in infants. Part I: Developmental hepatology and mechanisms of liver dysfunction. J Pediatr 90:686, 1977

Brown AK, McDonagh AF: Phototherapy for neonatal hyperbilirubinemia: efficacy, mechanism and toxicity. Adv Pediatr 27:431, 1980

Contains a detailed explanation of how and why phototherapy works in hyperbilirubinemia.

Bruce DA, Berman WA, Schut L: Cerebrospinal fluid pressure monitoring in children: physiology, pathology and clinical usefulness. Adv Pediatr 24:233, 1977

An excellent review of control and monitoring of cerebrospinal fluid pressure, particularly in Reyes syndrome.

Gartner LM, Arias IM: The liver. In Rudolph AM, Barnett HL, Einhorn AH (eds): Pediatrics, 16th ed. New York, Appleton-Century Crofts, 1977

Mathis RK, Andres JM, Walker WA: Liver disease in infants. Part II: Hepatic disease states. J. Pediatr 90:864, 1977

A comprehensive review of liver function and disease in infants. An excellent bibliography accompanies the articles.

Popper H, Schaffner F (eds): Progress in Liver Disease (vol 1–6). New York, Grune & Stratton, 1961–1979

This series offers excellent and complete reviews on selected topics related to liver physiology and disease. The fifth edition, 1976, includes chapters on "Neonatal Jaundice" by Gerard B Odell and "Cryptogenic Liver Disease in Young Infants" by M Michael Thaler. Both articles provide excellent summaries of these important areas of pediatric interest.

Schiff L: Diseases of the Liver, 4th ed. Philadelphia, JB Lippincott, 1975

Sherlock S: Diseases of the Liver and Biliary System, 5th ed. Oxford, Blackwell Scientific Publications, 1975.

These are general texts which provide authoritative and current discussions of the subject.

Watkins JB, Holtzapple PG, Shandling B: The Liver. In Vaughan VC, McKay JR, Behrman RE (eds): Nelson's Textbook of Pediatrics, 10th ed. Philadelphia, WB Saunders, 1979

Both Watkins *et al* and Gartner *et al* provide more extensive coverage of the subject and good bibliographies.

Abdominal Pain, Constipation and Melena

13

Ian S. E. Gibbons

ABDOMINAL PAIN

Pathophysiology

Abdominal pain may arise in any organ or tissue from the skin to the spine. The causes may range from an acute infection as in herpes zoster (shingles) to chronic degenerative change as in osteoarthritis of the spine with compression of nerves to the abdominal wall. The feature common to all is a disturbance of nerve fibers and end-organs giving rise to the sensation of pain. Pain from mild disease in many intra-abdominal organs may be referred to the periumbilical region; but when an organ is more severely involved, symptoms tend to localize accurately over it.

Abdominal pain may be acute or chronic. It becomes chronic when episodes recur over a period of 2 to 3 months or more. In general, the causes of acute pain are different from those causing chronic pain. This can be helpful in making an initial diagnosis and may influence the choice of the first steps taken in management of a patient's problem.

One way of approaching a diagnosis of pain is to consider various organ systems which may be involved. A knowledge of other symptoms and signs of disease together with examination of excreta will broaden the picture; extra help is obtained from the particular age group in which the problem presents. No attempt will be made to include all causes of abdominal pain, but listed are common disorders which should not be omitted in determining an initial diagnosis. Tables 13-1 and 13-2 contain some features of common disorders which may help in diagnosis, and include some of the rare causes of abdominal pain in childhood. Peptic ulcer is not a common cause of pain in children, as it is in adults.

When recording a history for abdominal pain, always determine what medications are being taken. Many substances prescribed by the physician, proprietary medicines bought by the patient, or food fads followed by the family may be causes of pain.

Techniques of Study

A careful history and physical examination are important parts of the study. Hematologic, chemical, and infective agents must be looked for. Radiographic studies are carried out according to the suspected diagnosis. If the focus is in the abdomen, a plain film may be most useful. If a cerebral tumor is suspected, a plain film of the skull may reveal calcification of a tumor. Other studies, including barium outline of the small and large bowel, may indicate abdominal masses, mucosal lesions, malrotation, and other conditions leading to intestinal pain such as duodenal bands and bowel atresias.

Radioisotope scan of specific organs provides relatively innocuous techniques to outline the liver, spleen, pancreas, and brain

TABLE 13-1. Acute Abdominal Pain: Differential Diagnosis and Symptoms

System	Disease	Other Major Symptoms	Signs	Excreta
Gastrointestinal				
	Gastroenteritis, viral or bacterial	Vomiting, diarrhea	General abdominal tenderness	Bilious vomitus, watery diarrhea
	Appendicitis	Fever, vomiting	Right-sided tenderness	Fecal vomiting, constipation or diarrhea
	Mesenteric lymphadenitis	Fever, vomiting	Right-sided or diffuse tenderness	
	Hernia (strangulated)	Vomiting	Distention	Fecal vomitus
	Volvulus	Vomiting	Distention	
	Intussusception	Vomiting	Sausage-shaped mass, obstruction	Blood-tinged mucus
	Intestinal atresias	Constipation	Obstruction	Bile-stained vomitus
	Infectious hepatitis	Nausea, poor appetite	Tender liver	Pale stools, diarrhea
	Infectious mononucleosis	Nausea, poor appetite	Tender liver and spleen	Usually normal
	Inflammatory bowel disease			
	Ulcerative colitis	Weight loss	Tender colon	Bloody stools
	Crohn's disease	Short stature	Tender mass	Loose and bloody stools
Iatrogenic and poisons				
	Lead poisoning, drugs (steroids, iron, imipramine) antibiotics (tetracycline, ampicillin, lincomycin, erythromycin, etc)			
Genitourinary				
	Infection	Dysuria, frequency	Tender renal angle	Urine may be cloudy or bloody
	Congenital abnormality	May be none	Abnormal facies or limbs	May be normal
	Stone renal or ureteric	Frequency, dysuria	Tender kidney, ureter	Bloody urine
	Acute glomerulonephritis	Elevated blood pressure	Edema	Smoky urine
	Torsion testis	Testicular pain	Swollen testis	Normal
	Twisted ovarian pedicle		Tender abdomen	Normal
Respiratory				
	Streptococcal adenitis	Sore throat	Generally tender abdomen	Normal
	Pleurisy or pneumonia	Cough, fever	Abdomen—no findings	Normal
	Cystic fibrosis of pancreas	Cough, sputum	Simulate appendicitis or obstruction	Stool, bulky and foul-smelling
Hematopoietic				
	Sickle-cell anemia	Joint pain	Rigid abdomen	Normal
	Acute leukemia	Joint, bone pain	Tender spleen	Blood in stool and urine

TABLE 13-1. Acute Abdominal Pain: Differential Diagnosis and Symptoms *(Continued)*

System	Disease	Other Major Symptoms	Signs	Excreta
	Infectious mononucleosis	Sore throat	Tender liver and spleen	Normal
	Septicemia	Weakness	Shock	Mostly normal
Metabolic				
	Diabetes	Vomiting, weight loss, diarrhea	Diffuse abdominal tenderness, dehydration, acidosis	Polyuria, glycosuria
	Hypoglycemia	Anxiety, irritability	Coma Convulsions	Normal
	Porphyria (rare)	Skin rash	Diffuse abdominal tenderness	
	Alkaptonuria (rare)			Urine black on standing
Reticuloendothelial				
	Rheumatic fever	Painful joints	Diffuse, nonspecific	Normal
	Henoch-Schönlein's purpura (rare)	Skin rash	Diffuse, nonspecific	Urine and stool may be bloody
Cardiovascular system				
	Myocardial infarction (rare)	Chest pain, arm pain	Arrhythmias	Normal

and may assist in diagnosis of lesions in these organs.

Biochemical Studies of Excreta. The stool may need to be examined for excessive fecal fat loss or for excessive stool sugars associated with disaccharidase deficiencies. It may also be examined for total nitrogen loss and pancreatic enzyme quantity and quality when pancreatic exocrine disease is suspected.

Stool Examination. Stools may carry ova or parasites associated with abdominal discomfort. Examination of two or three specimens of fresh stool may be helpful. Abnormal bacteria leading to invasive disease should be sought.

Ultrasound Techniques. Ultrasound is a useful adjunct in looking for masses and dilated ducts, particularly in the region of the liver, pancreas, and mesentery.

Computerized Axial Tomography. Computerized axial tomography is capable of producing a body scan showing a cross-section at various levels. Quite small masses or cysts may be detected.

Endoscopy. Various forms of endoscopy including sigmoidoscopy, colonoscopy, esophagogastroduodenoscopy, laparoscopy, and retrograde cannulation of pancreatic and biliary ducts may be important in evaluating causes of abdominal pain.

Biopsy Techniques. The distal colon, the major part of the small bowel, esophagus, and stomach are all accessible to biopsy techniques without surgical operation, using instruments with relative safety.

TABLE 13-2. Chronic Recurrent Abdominal Pain: Differential Diagnosis and Symptoms

System	Disease	Other Major Symptoms	Signs	Excreta
Gastrointestinal				
	Irritable bowel syndrome	Headache, vomiting, blurred vision	Tender over colon and small bowel	Pellet stools
	Constipation	Poor appetite, soiling	Masses of feces in colon	Hard or soft stool, usually not inspissated
	Infantile colic	Poor appetite	Soft abdomen (hard during pain)	Normal
	Peptic ulcer	Poor appetite, weakness	Epigastric tenderness	Black stools or coffee-ground vomitus
	Crohn's disease	Weight loss, short stature	Tenderness	Loose stools and blood
	Ulcerative colitis	Anorexia, weight loss	Tender intestines	Loose bloody stools
	Ascaris lumbricoides	Anemia	Abdominal distention	Worms in stool or vomitus
	Disaccharidase deficiency, congenital or acquired	Diarrhea, weight loss, vomiting	Abdominal distention	Reducing sugars in stools
	Cystic fibrosis of the pancreas	Cough, sputum	Palpable feces in right colon, enlarged liver and spleen	Fatty stools
	Peutz-Jeghers syndrome (rare)			
	Superior messenteric artery syndrome (rare)			
	Annular pancreas			
	Tumor gut or abdominal organs (Wilm's tumor) (rare)			
	Tuberculosis intestines (rare)			
	Pancreatitis (rare)			
	Meckel's diverticulitis (rare)			
	Cholecystitis and choledochal cyst (rare)			
Genitourinary (Accounts for half the "organic" causes of recurrent abdominal pain)				
	Recurrent urinary tract infection	Dysuria	Loin tenderness	Cloudy, foul-smelling urine
	Congenital anomalies and obstructions	Other visible anomalies	Enlarged kidneys or ectopic organs	Urine may be normal
Central nervous				
	Cerebral tumor	May be none	May be none or localizing cerebral signs	Normal
	Abdominal epilepsy	Transient impaired consciousness	None	Normal
Cardiovascular				
	Congenital heart disease with failure	Shortness of breath	Enlarged liver, cyanosis	Normal
	Coarctation of aorta	Cold feet	Diffuse nonspecific tenderness	Normal

Liver biopsy can be performed by a needle suction technique.

Manometrics. Pressure recordings of esophageal and sphincter function may be valuable in defining certain causes of abdominal pain. Spasm of the colon can be recorded by pressure-recording apparatus as well as by radiographic studies. These techniques are relatively simple, and cause little discomfort to the patient.

Electroencephalography. Electroencephalography may be important in looking for cerebral tumors or abdominal epilepsy. Computerized tomography has also been used in this area with success.

Examination of the Urine. Urinalysis is an important part of a search for the cause of abdominal pain. Infective and biochemical abnormalities may point to a diagnosis.

Intravenous Pyelography. Intravenous pyelography is an essential part of a search for organic causes of abdominal pain because genitourinary abnormalities account for half the organic causes of recurrent pain.

Principles of Management

Acute Abdominal Pain. In most cases, management of acute abdominal pain revolves around a diagnosis that is usually followed by therapeutic steps leading to cure or dramatic relief of symptoms. If the episode is short-lived (1 to 2 weeks), there is little effect upon the family or child, provided the end-result of the illness is satisfactory. If the end-result is not good or the acute episode leads to chronic illness, then management emphasis must change. The physician should always be aware, even in an acute illness, that certain children or their families may require in-depth studies and support, emotionally and physically, to help them through the crisis and to prevent an abnormal behavior developing on the way to recovery.

Chronic Abdominal Pain. Management of chronic abdominal pain also revolves around diagnosis, but the steps used in approaching this diagnosis are an important part of therapy and should be staged carefully. Usually, the disease has existed for 2 to 3 months or more, and is likely to be present longer. Frequently, the underlying disease is not amenable to curative procedures and the physician, family, and child are setting off together on a long road. Remember that therapy begins at the first sight of and with the first words spoken to the patient and family. The needs of emotional growth and development must be dealt with at the same time as diagnosis and therapy are started.

The struggle some children experience in developing emotional skills to cope with their environment may conveniently be called "adjustment reactions." These reactions to school, peers, family (including siblings and grandparents), and sexual awareness may sometimes be inappropriate. The persistence of an emotional struggle may lead to greatly increased abdominal symptoms; this is due to the well-known influence emotions have on the autonomic nervous system and intestinal motility. Treatment should include appropriate medications and, at times, surgery, as well as informed, supportive psychotherapy for adjustment reactions. The primary physician should bridge the gap between physical and emotional requirements; he can allay fears about ups and downs in bodily symptoms while working with emotions in a supportive way. If emotional needs are left to the psychologist or psychiatrist (except when serious problems are present), they are placed in a very difficult position during supportive therapy if severe abdominal pain occurs. Treatment is less effective if the patient is caught between two different physicians who, unknowingly may be giving conflicting advice.

Management Steps for Chronic Abdominal Pain. 1. Establish a good relationship with your patient. If he or she is old enough (3 to 4 years or older) and can separate easily from the family, explain carefully what a history and physical examination involves. Then ask the parents to leave while you talk with and examine your patient.

2. Don't do painful procedures such as blood tests or rectal examinations on your first encounter unless absolutely essential.

3. Ask the parents in and send your patient out of the room to wait or play while you take a thorough history from the parents. (Always try to have both parents together.) The history should include current details of the patient and how he reacts to peers, school, family, emotional growth, fears, likes, dislikes, and other attitudes. The parents' approach to and fear of the problem should be determined. When you have a well-rounded picture and have decided what you are going to do, invite your patient back in, explain the diagnosis in simple terms and indicate that you and the parents have agreed on a course of action. If the patient has irritable bowel syndrome, reassurance that the child is safe is often sufficient to reduce symptoms. Sometimes a radiograph of the large and small intestine may be necessary to assure you and the family that no serious intestinal problem is present. Many children with irritable bowel syndrome will settle completely with this treatment.

4. If symptoms persist or signs indicate a serious problem, admission to hospital for investigation and treatment may be necessary. This provides a chance to know your patient and family by gathering data from both parents and patient. You can observe your patient away from home and get him to undergo difficult investigations as he develops confidence in you.

5. When you have a diagnosis (on the way to which you have kept the family informed about every step), arrange a separate and lengthy meeting with the parents to discuss all of the studies done, outline the diagnosis, and plan therapy. This provides an opportunity for parents to ask questions, and especially allows them to express fears they may have. If you do not deal with these secret fears, therapy may not be effective.

6. Your patient should be interviewed separately at the time of discharge, his disease and therapy explained, and follow-up arranged. If necessary, you may have to contact school officials so they will be aware of treatment programs and will not unwittingly undermine any medical or supportive psychotherapy you have planned. Most school personnel are delighted to hear from a child's doctor and the teacher can be most helpful in keeping your patient in a normal school environment.

7. Sometimes an older brother or sister should be included in the understanding and counseling of your patient's disease.

8. Frequently repeated procedures should be avoided and reliance should be placed more on the history and progress of your patient (*e.g.*, avoiding frequent sigmoidoscopies in a child with ulcerative colitis).

Drug Therapy. The disease determines the medicine; relatively few drugs are used in pediatric gastroenterology, but advances in understanding intestinal mechanisms are leading to the introduction of newer drugs.

In most cases, drug therapy can be minimal when a child has confidence in his doctor (Table 13-3). This principle applies to simple drugs such as Pro-Banthine (for irritable bowel syndrome) as well as for potent drugs such as steroids and immunosuppressive agents for inflammatory bowel disease.

CONSTIPATION (FECAL RETENTION WITH OR WITHOUT SOILING)

Definition

It is useful to understand constipation as "a problem of elimination of feces with or without fecal soiling."

Pathophysiology

With normal anatomy, the basic mechanisms of an inability to eliminate feces are not well understood. Feces that remain longer in the large intestine undergo more water reabsorption, become inspissated, and are harder to pass rectally. This is the usual mechanism of simple constipation. However, many children who retain large amounts of feces but soil may fail to properly defecate for 3 to 4 months. Despite this, their feces can remain soft and even difficult to palpate abdominally. In place of passage of stools, fecal liquid material may leak out and cause anal soiling. This frequently leads to a mistaken diagnosis of diarrhea, which may be treated with agents to retard colonic activity. The result is further retention of bowel contents.

Emotional stimuli can indirectly affect intestinal function. Many children become temporarily unable to defecate for several days in a new environment such as school or summer camp. Others who become anxious and are emotionally immature may involuntarily withhold feces for many weeks or months at a time.

In abnormal anatomy, difficulty with bowel movements is usually self-explanatory. Conditions such as painful anal fissures, malrotation, imperforate anus or Hirschsprung's disease can be responsible.

The process of defecation is complicated. First, a colonic signal must be recognized, then, in addition to a massive propulsive colonic contraction, there must be closure of the glottis associated with Valsalva's maneuver, increased intra-abdominal pressure, reflex relaxation of the internal anal sphincter, and relaxation of the external anal sphincter and puborectalis sling. There is elevation of the pelvic floor as the bowel

TABLE 13-3. Commonly Used Drugs

Drugs	Dose	Disease
Pro-Banthine	7.5–15 mg/dose	Irritable bowel syndrome
Lomotil	2.5–15 mg/day	Loose stools with abdominal pain
Azulfidine (sulphasalazine)	3–5 g/day initially 2 g/day maintenance	Inflammatory bowel disease
Corticosteroids (prednisolone)	2 mg/kg/day initially 5–10 mg/day maintenance	Inflammatory bowel disease
Azathioprine (Imuran)	2 mg/kg per day	Inflammatory bowel disease
Antibiotics	Appropriate dose	Infections
Antacids	Titrated by symptomatic relief	Ulcer disease, Esophagitis

movement passes through the anus. If any one of these mechanisms is impaired (*e.g.*, congenital absence or weak abdominal musculature), defecation becomes difficult.

Another mechanism involves incoordination of these maneuvers which is unrecognized by the patient; there may be contraction of the external anal sphincter during defecation that prevents easy passage of the bowel movement. This often persists for 45 seconds or longer until the colonic propulsive contraction ceases. Other patients develop a very high threshold of recognition of colonic propulsive activity (usually acquired) so that normal propulsive activity goes unrecognized and associated defecation maneuvers are not brought into play (*e.g.*, the busy executive dealing with multiple daily crises or the busy child engrossed in play). Once acquired, this threshold allows more feces to accumulate and when large enough, normal rectal contraction and expulsion of the large stool becomes impossible. Soiling frequently occurs as a safety valve under these circumstances.

It is commonly believed that the primary mechanism (all too often the only one considered by many physicians in dealing with a toddler age group), is related to a painful event such as fissure formation in the anus. This mechanism is represented schematically in Figure 13–1.

This form of constipation should respond quickly to simple remedies such as lubricants or stool softeners, but, unfortunately, anal manipulations are frequently used to relieve the pain and crying of young children. These manipulations may become frequent without the physician or family realizing it. The result is the turning of a self-limited process into a prolonged problem. As seen in Figure 13–1, the emotional factors are reinforced, and a severe family emotional disturbance with ensuing behavioral abnormalities can develop in a child's formative years of emotional growth.

In summary, the known mechanisms for constipation in the absence of organic disease are as follows:

1. Simple constipation is a temporary event of inspissated feces without soiling, usually self-limited or responding to simple treatment.

2. Voluntary incoordination of the defecation process is usually acquired, for example, following a painful event like fissure formation or by conscious suppression of colonic propulsive defecation signals and consequent development of high colonic thresholds (usually in older children and adults). In general, these are short-term problems.

3. With involuntary incoordination of the defecation process, usually the stools are soft and bulky and paradoxical external anal sphincter squeeze may occur during defecation, always unrecognized by the patient and usually present in varying severity from birth.

This group emerges clearly through objective studies after 5 to 6 years of age, by which time the normal child should have developed full control of defecation. This problem can be falsely interpreted as withholding on an emotional basis and mistakenly treated psychiatrically after traditional simple methods of treatment fail. These patients respond poorly to psychotherapy, and in the past have been long-term problems persisting with symptoms into the late teens and early 20s. Categories 2 and 3 are a large group, accounting for 60% of the patients who do not fall into category 1.

4. Coordinated processes of defecation by objective criteria, yet retention of feces with persistent soiling is usually associated with deep-seated emotional disturbances and requires full psychotherapeutic measures. Again, this group only emerges clearly when objective studies can be made at 5 to 6 years of age. Invariably, long-term therapy is required. They account for approximately 30% of the patients who do not fit into category 1.

Organic Disease. Many disease states can have associated constipation on a temporary or long-term basis, depending on the type of disease. Frequently when the disease is appropriately treated, the constipation will cease.

Techniques of Study

A careful history and physical examination should be done (Table 13-4).

Plain Film of the Abdomen. Feces can frequently be seen by radiograph. They

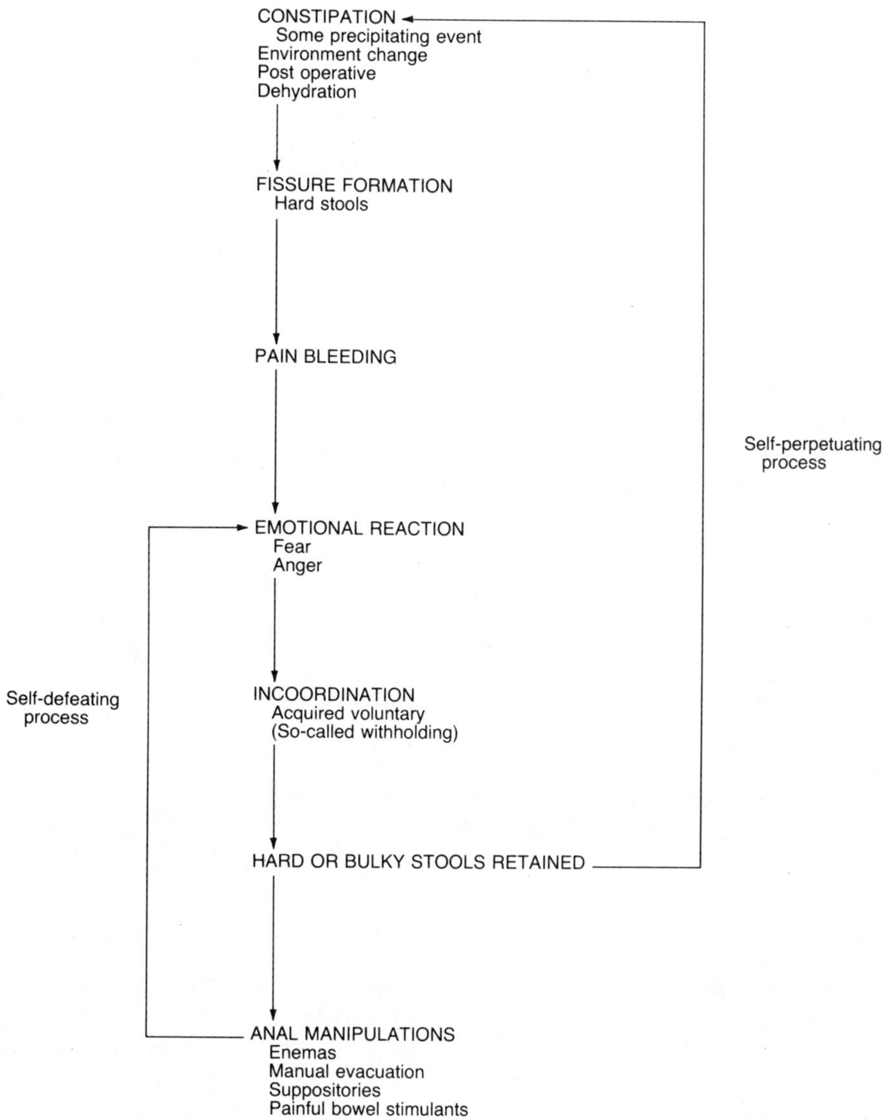

Fig.13-1. A common series of events leading to chronic constipation.

TABLE 13-4. Constipation: Differential Diagnosis and Symptoms

Disease Mechanism	Symptoms	Signs	Soiling	Barium Enema	Sigmoidoscopy	Anal Tonometry
Functional						
Simple (any age)	Cannot defecate, pain	Hard feces in sigmoid (pellets)	None	Normal colon, pellet stools, normal post-evacuation film	Pellet stool, normal rectum	Normal
Voluntary incoordination	Cannot defecate, pain	Firm or soft feces in colon, fissures	Usually none	Large colon, inadequate evacuation	Hard or soft feces, dilated rectum	High colonic threshold, normal sphincter function
Involuntary incoordination	Cannot defecate, pain	Soft feces, whole colon	Present	Large colon, inadequate evacuation	Soft homogenous feces not adherent to mucosa, dilated rectum, fluid feces at periphery	High colonic threshold, external sphincter squeeze during defecation
Coordinated	Cannot defecate, usually no pain	Soft feces, present whole colon: severe emotional disturbance	Present	Large colon, inadequate evacuation	"	Normal colonic threshold, normal external sphincter function, normal internal sphincter function

Other	Age Group	Cause
	Newborn	Anatomic obstruction Hirschsprung's disease Meconium plug Abdominal muscles (weak or absent) Anorectal stenosis
	Infancy and Childhood	Normal variations Insufficient milk, sugar or water 1. Vomiting, pyloric stenosis, esophageal reflux, toxemia 2. Metabolic conditions associated with polyuria, hypercalcemia, adrenocortical hyperplasia, renal acidosis, diabetes insipidus Hypothyroidism Congenital spinal palsy Hypotonia Lead poisoning

may take the form of pellets or balls as in simple constipation, or may have a diffuse granular appearance throughout a large part of the colon, even as far as the cecum. This is frequently seen in fecal retention with soiling.

Abnormal gas shadows of various types can be seen, and it is possible to diagnose obstruction, malrotation, a narrow rectum or short-segment Hirschsprung's disease, and many other conditions.

Barium Enema. In problems of elimination, it is important to perform the barium study without the usual bowel preparations most radiology departments do routinely. We are interested in a problem of elimination, the nature of the colon, the nature of the feces, and the propulsive capabilities of the colon, rectum, and sphincter under the circumstances of the illness. Very frequently when the bowel is cleaned out by preparation, much of this information is lost. The most important film of the barium enema is the film showing the postevacuation capability of the colon and the presence or absence of retained feces.

Limited pictures can be taken, perhaps showing one overhead film outlining the whole colon to the cecum, anteroposterior and lateral views of the rectum, and a postevacuation film. It is important to avoid inserting a balloon-tipped catheter as this obscures information required about the rectum. The barium should be run in under gravity through an open-tipped catheter so that it is not too painful for the patient.

Intravenous Pyelogram and Urinalysis. A urinalysis is an important study. Some children—particularly girls—who have fecal retention with soiling may have chronic urinary tract infection.

Occasionally, the fecal material occupying the pelvis may cause compression of the ureters and may lead to dilatation of the renal pelvis and ureters. If this is the case, management must be aimed vigorously at removing the fecal material to avoid hydronephrosis.

Sigmoidoscopy. Sigmoidoscopy provides useful information not easily determined by finger rectal examination. It is possible to see an internal anal fissure. The mucosa should be normal since feces usually do not adhere to the mucosal wall. The nature of the stool is important. In the child with simple constipation, the stool is pellet or ball-shaped or lies free in a dilated rectum as a column, which does not usually extend beyond 15 cm. In fecal retention with soiling, the feces are soft and the instrument can be passed readily into it. Frequently, such material will be present well beyond 15 cm. Spontaneous relaxation of the internal sphincter can be observed occasionally on insufflation of air into the rectum during sigmoidoscopy.

Anal Tonometry. The anal tonometer is a pressure-recording device consisting of three air-filled balloons supported on a thin metal introducer. Two of the balloons are placed in the anal canal, one at the level of the internal sphincter and one at the level of the external sphincter. These two are filled with a fixed volume of air while the third balloon, which is placed higher in the rectum or sigmoid, can be filled with varying amounts of air, producing differing degrees of colonic stimulation (Fig. 13-2).

Variations in pressures recorded in the sphincter balloons reveal autonomic and voluntary sphincter responses to colonic distention. Normally, the resting tone maintained in both sphincters is such that they close the anal orifice and must be opened for the passage of a bowel movement. The internal sphincter has only smooth muscle controlled by the autonomic nervous system. The external sphincter is capable of both reflex and voluntary responses.

Normally when the rectum or sigmoid is stretched by the proximal balloon, there is a spontaneous relaxation of the internal sphincter and momentary constriction of the external sphincter (Fig. 13-3).

During normal defecation, the internal sphincter relaxes and the external sphincter is not actively contracted. As a result, the instrument is pushed outward through the anal canal and the pressure falls on the external sphincter balloon (Fig. 13-4). The increase in pressure recorded by the internal balloon is transmitted by intra-abdominal pressure from the Valsalva movement during defecation. These normal responses may be altered in various disease states (*e.g.*,

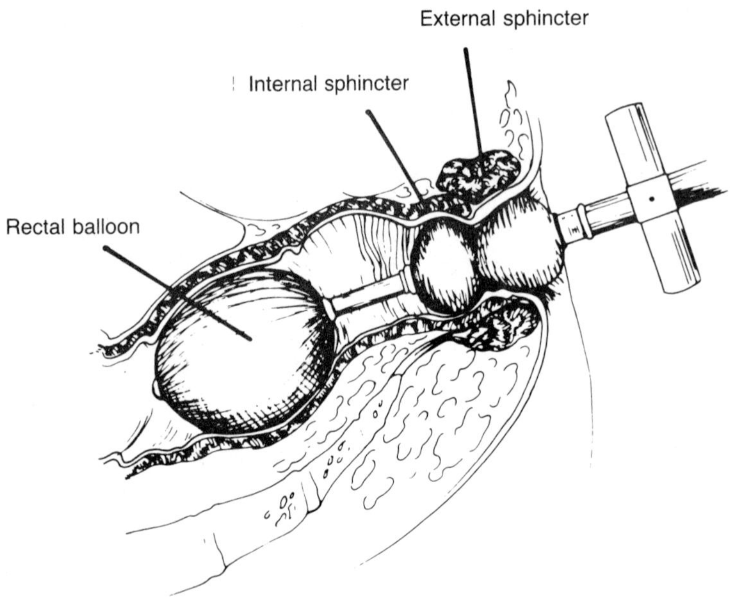

Fig. 13-2. The anal tonometer.

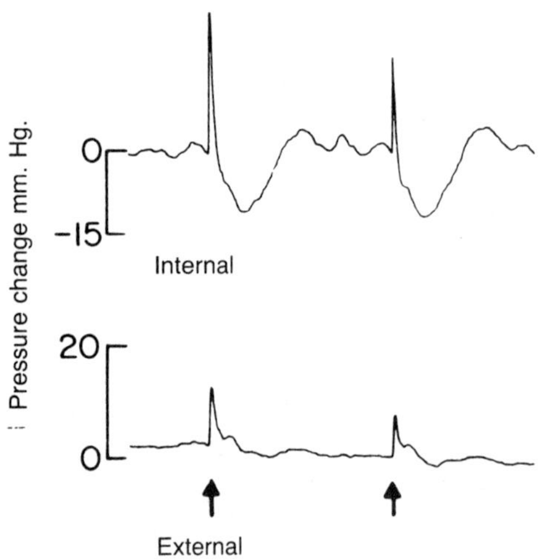

Fig. 13-3. Sphincteric responses to transient rectal distension. (Arrows indicate balloon distention.)

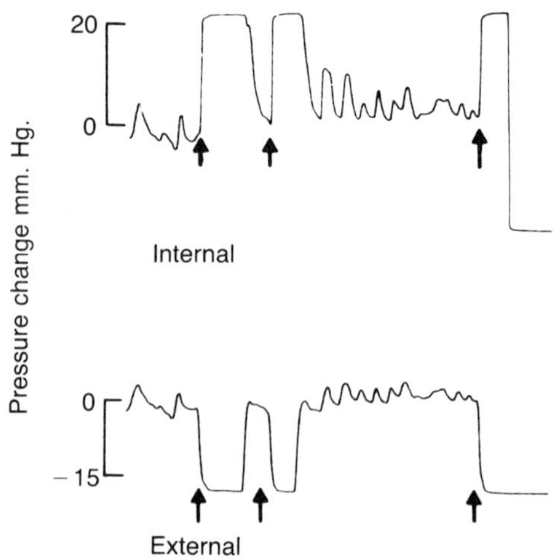

Fig. 13-4. Sphincter pressure reponses during normal defecation. (Arrows indicate voluntary attempts to defecate.)

Hirschsprung's disease in which the internal sphincter will fail to relax normally).

Evaluation of Emotional Growth and Development. An essential part of any study of a patient with a problem of elimination and should go hand-in-hand with evaluation of the physical state.

Blood Tests. A number of disease states with alteration in chemical values in the blood may have associated constipation. Examples are: hypothyroidism, hypopituitarism, lead poisoning, or hypercalcemia.

Management of Common Causes of Elimination: General Principles

Evaluation of Emotional Growth and Development. Problems of elimination tend to be chronic and associated either primarily or secondarily with internal conflicts for the child and disturbed family relationships.

A psychological examination is often indicated and appropriate supportive action begun. Evaluation of the child's scholastic performance may be important, and previously unrecognized problems must be faced. Emotional immaturity relating to self-image and peer relationships can be prominent difficulties. Differing opinions of siblings and parents in dealing with the problem increase the child's internal conflicts and further distort the normal process of defecation.

A child who has been manipulated by his family may discover that he can turn the tables and manipulate them by failing to defecate normally. This can be an unconscious phenomenon and its unraveling may require psychotherapy if it has existed for many years. Emotional factors may become self-perpetuating and purely medical approaches will fail.

Management of Organic Causes. The underlying organic problem should be dealt with directly, if possible. Normal defecation will resume, provided intrinsic mechanisms of intestinal function, abdominal musculature, and sphincter control are intact.

Anal Manipulations. Repetitive anal manipulations should be avoided; they produce temporary relief at best and may set up serious emotional reactions in the older child. The infant who has frequent enemas, suppositories, or finger dilations of the rectum may come to believe these are *necessary* for defecation and may not learn the normal process. It must be remembered that the entire process of defecation is *not* reflex and that some aspects (such as sphincter control and colonic signal recognition) have to be learned.

Dilatation of the anal sphincter in a constipated infant is not indicated. After stretching, a normal sphincter will rapidly return to its previous resting state, and only if fibers are torn will it return to a weaker resting tone. This may lead to involuntary soiling.

Impacted masses do occasionally require manual evacuation; if a fecal mass is compressing a ureter, it must be vigorously evacuated and prevented from reaccumulating.

Laxatives, Lubricants, and Stool Softeners. Laxatives (such as milk of magnesia) may be useful in managing simple constipation but should be used sparingly. If the problem becomes chronic, investigation is needed to determine the mechanism.

Stimulant cathartics (cascara, senna, bisacodyl) are best avoided because they may cause frightening and severe abdominal cramps. Prolonged use (many years) may permanently damage the normal propulsive power of the colon.

Stool softeners (which act by inhibiting colonic reabsorption of water) can be effective in a young child who has hard stools. They may be given for long periods without harm until a regular pattern of defecation is established.

Lubricants (such as mineral oil) are most effective in patients who are attempting defecation when a pattern of fear has developed. Such children who have normal mechanisms of defecation may lose this fear when lubricants allow a less painful bowel movement. They are not habit-forming and are nonstimulating; used in reasonable doses they do not lead to vitamin deficiency. Lipoid pneumonia will not occur unless the child is forced to swallow the lubricant.

Biofeedback. When the anal tonometer is used in diagnosis, there is usually a printed expression of pressure changes. If a child of 5 to 6 years of age or older is shown this, he can readily learn to control his anal sphincter in response to colonic distention. He can be taught to respond to progressively lower colonic stimuli by external anal sphincter squeeze and thus prevent soiling. If he has inappropriate external sphincter squeeze during defecation, he can see this on paper, associate it with physiologic sensation, and be rapidly taught to reverse the phenomenon.

As with lubricants, softeners, and psychotherapy, biofeedback can be a useful adjunct in management. However, the correct diagnosis must be established first.

Supportive Counseling. Abdominal pain should involve an understanding of the child and family. Supportive counseling should be used by the primary physician in every case of chronic constipation. The principles depend upon: (1) the child being motivated to help himself with his problem and being actively involved in the process, and (2) the parents and siblings believing that their child or sibling is capable of normal function. They should show their confidence by their behavior and verbal and nonverbal communication. Disparaging the child should be avoided. Psychotherapy, if it is needed, should be directed toward these two main objectives.

Remember that children seldom grow into adulthood with fecal retention and soiling. Most learn to control bowel movement when their internal motivations have been developed and skills of bodily awareness are appropriately applied to restore normal function. The physician can be a helpful catalyst in achieving this.

RECTAL BLEEDING (MELENA)

Pathophysiology

The adage that children are not little adults applies particularly to the diagnosis and management of the child with gastrointestinal hemorrhage. Causes of rectal bleeding vary from a simple anal fissure to failure to define any cause in a high proportion of cases, especially in patients with transient bleeding. Previously unrecognized causes of gastrointestinal hemorrhage in the child may be revealed as modern instrumentation in skilled hands widens the scope of diagnosis. In general, melena indicates disease from the duodenum and distally but does not exclude bleeding from a higher source: the stomach, nose, pharynx, or even the chest.

The age of the patient may help in diagnosis; for example, most diseases occur in any age group, but melena from swallowed maternal blood is confined to the newborn while melena from inflammatory bowel disease tends to occur most commonly in the older child.

The quantity of melena may indicate a possible source of bleeding. Profuse melena stool with shock, nausea, or pallor more often suggests higher small intestinal bleeding or extensive inflammatory disease of the colon. Bright blood of smaller amounts in an otherwise well child is more suggestive of a rectal polyp or anal fissure.

The tarry stool color so often helpful in indicating a higher source of bleeding in adults is not as useful in the child. This is because intraluminal bleeding increases intestinal motility and speeds the rate of passage of the contents so that bleeding from the duodenum may produce bright red melena.

The location of the blood in relation to the stool is important. Blood on the outside of the stool suggests a lesion low in the sigmoid or rectum. Similar low sources of bleeding with anal fissures are commonly associated with several drops of blood following passage of hard or soft stools.

Pain and abdominal cramps with melena suggest a partial or complete obstructive lesion such as an intussusception, volvulus, or pedunculated polyp.

A question that should always be asked is: is it blood? Food colorings, beets, Kool-Aid, gelatin desserts, ampicillin, and lincomycin can all simulate rectal bleeding. The simplest test for blood is the hematest for hemoglobin.

Techniques of Study

A careful history and physical examination should be made and the bowel movement observed for appearance and odor. Do not rely entirely on the observation of others.

Rectal Examination. Observation of the anus for pigmentation, scars, fissures, polyps, skin tags, worms, hemorrhoids, asymmetric folds and other local lesions is helpful. In children, examination with the finger for causes of bleeding will yield little information except for the nature and position of stool or a pelvic mass. Palpable rectal mucosal lesions causing bleeding (like cancer of the rectum in adults) are extremely rare in childhood. Occasionally, a polyp may be felt. A rectal examination should always be done and bimanual palpation included.

Sigmoidoscopy. Appropriately sized instruments are required, for sigmoidoscopy. The procedure should be done without general anesthesia; in only a few instances is sedation necessary. The older child should have each step of the procedure explained, and the infant must be properly held by trained assistants. The procedure should be considered early in the diagnosis of melena and it should be done the first time without colon cleaning procedures. Enemas and other preparations are holdovers from dealing with adults. These preparations may severely exacerbate disease (*e.g.,* ulcerative colitis) and frequently cause terror in the patient who may refuse to cooperate for the subsequent sigmoidoscopy, leading to unnecessary general anesthesia and its potential complications. If the rectum is full, it is better to wait until the child has his next bowel movement and repeat the study immediately afterward. When distal inflammatory bowel disease has been excluded by sigmoidoscopy, careful preparation of the colon is necessary before barium films are taken.

Colon Biopsy. If abnormal mucosa is seen during sigmoidoscopy, a suction colon biopsy should be taken from the abnormal area. This can be carried out safely with an all-purpose Rubin suction biopsy tube.

Plain Film of the Abdomen. Plain films may show abnormal thickening, distention, position of bowel shadows, soft-tissue masses, or a foreign body.

Barium Enema. When inflammatory bowel disease is not suspected, thorough colon preparation is required because small polyps may be missed if small amounts of feces are present.

Upper Gastrointestinal and Small Bowel Radiographic Series. Because high intestinal lesions may cause melena, upper gastrointestinal and small bowel radiographic series are important. If colonic inflammatory bowel disease is present, the antegrade study followed through the colon is not likely to produce toxic megacolon as does a barium enema. Sufficient information about the colon can often be obtained in this way.

Technetium Scan. Technetium scan is a radioactive study in which the injected material sometimes localizes in the ecotopic gastric mucosa of a Meckel's diverticulum and aids diagnosis.

Selective Angiography. If severe bleeding persists and no obvious cause is found, selective arteriography helps the surgeon localize a bleeding point in the gastrointestinal tract. This may avoid blind procedures of intestinal resection in an effort to stop catastrophic bleeding.

Upper Gastrointestinal Endoscopy. Fiberoptic instruments with excellent visibility, suitable for use in small infants, are available. Lesions not easily seen by radiographs (*e.g.*, a Mallory-Weiss tear) and the cause of hematemesis and unexplained rectal bledding can be detected.

Blood Tests. Abnormal bleeding tendencies or blood dyscrasias occasionally present as gastrointestinal hemorrhage. Liver disease with associated esophageal varices should always be looked for.

Chest Film. Chest x-ray study should be done to exclude causes of hemoptysis in the young child who cannot spit up sputum and may swallow blood.

Diagnosis

Because high intestinal lesions may cause melena, the differential diagnosis should include causes of gastrointestinal hemorrhage.

Causes of Gastrointestinal Bleeding. The causes of gastrointestinal bleeding in children cover the same range as for adults, with certain differences. The more important causes of gastrointestinal bleeding in children are enumerated below. The causes of melena include all those of hematemesis, with the emphasis changing according to the age group (Tables 13-5, 13-6).

Principles of Management

Management for a first bleeding episode should begin conservatively unless bleeding is catastrophic and the hemoglobin drops to 6 g or less in a shocked patient, or unless there is a complicating condition such as leukemia or congestive heart failure. As many as half of all episodes of gastrointestinal bleeding in children resolve spontaneously and a specific cause may never be found, even after laparotomy. Furthermore, there may never be another episode.

The pediatric patient should *never* be sent to an adult intensive care unit. The patient should not be put into the pediatric intensive care unit if it can be avoided (in most cases of an initial bleeding episode this is possible). The atmosphere of strange noises, rapid movement, comings and goings, physician anxiety and concern, other sick patients and their care, and the general hubbub will not help the patient and generally will make things worse. In particular, the sight of a half-naked elderly adult lying exposed and semiconscious with many tubes attached, is terrifying for children of all ages.

Family visits should not be restricted, no matter what one's opinion of the parents or the relatives may be. A much sounder approach is enlisting the support of the family in the management of their child in a caring fashion.

Use of a nasogastric tube in the stomach for hematemesis is not recommended

TABLE 13-5. Differential Diagnosis and Symptoms of Melena

Age	Disease	Other Major Symptoms	Other Signs
Newborn	Acute colitis (infective or inflammatory bowel disease)	Diarrhea	Frequent stools, blood, mucus in stools
	Disseminated intravascular coagulation	Overwhelming illness	Many bleeding sites
Infants	Anal fissure (any age)	Painful defecation	Fissure at anus, retained feces
	Infectious diarrhea	Vomiting, diarrhea, loss of appetite	Fever, weight loss
	Cow's milk allergy	May be none	Eczema
	Malrotation	Abdominal pain, vomiting	Abdominal distention
Preschool	Juvenile polyps	Painless, usually	Polyp may appear at anus
	Meckel's diverticulum	Abdominal pain	Tender abdomen, severe bleeding
	Intussusception	Abdominal pain	Sausage-shaped palpable mass, mucus mixed with blood
	Rectal prolapse	Frequent bulky stools	Prolapsed bowel seen
School age	Inflammatory bowel disease	Pain, anorexia, diarrhea	Poor growth, weight loss
	Peptic ulcer	Pain relieved by food	Epigastric tenderness
	Esophageal varices	Those of the primary disease	
	Esophagitis	Heartburn	May be none
	Malignancy	Multiple symptoms	Weight loss, fever

TABLE 13-6. Differential Diagnosis and Symptoms of Hematemesis

Age	Disease	Other Major Symptoms	Other Signs
Intrauterine	Intestinal perforation	Postnatal vomiting	Tender, distended abdomen
	Peptic ulceration	Postnatal vomiting	
Newborn	Swallowed maternal blood	Placental or vaginal bleeding	Hematemesis
	Swallowed hemoptysis	Respiratory distress	Abnormal air entry, pulmonary signs
	Iatrogenic (*e.g.*, aspirin for fever)	Related to need for aspirin	Fever
	Hemorrhagic disease	Respiratory distress	Bruises, bloody urine, signs of CNS hemorrhage
	Congenital thrombocytopenic purpura	Depend on bleeding site	Purpura
	Hemorrhagic gastritis	Abdominal pain	Signs of infection or septicemia
	Pyloric outlet obstruction (stenosis, webs)	Avid hunger, projectile vomiting	Severe weight loss, visible gastric peristalsis
	Stress ulcer	Associated disease	Tender epigastrium, anemia
	Necrotizing enterocolitis	Pallor, weak suck reflex	Distended abdomen, shock
	Chalasia (severe)	Regurgitation of feeds	Aspiration pneumonia
	Hiatus hernia with esophagitis	Vomiting feeds	Failure to grow
	Esophageal, gastrogenic cysts	May be none	May be none
Any age group	Iatrogenic (*e.g.*, aspirin)	Related to need for aspirin	Fever
	Esophageal varices	Cough (cystic fibrosis)	Malabsorption
		Poor appetite (cirrhosis liver)	Enlarged spleen, hard liver, xanthomata
	Peptic ulcer (Zollinger-Ellison syndrome)	Abdominal pain	Anemia, tender epigastrium
	Telangiectasia	May be none	Skin telangiectasias
	Hemangiomatosis	Dependent on site	Consumption
			Coagulopathy
	Foreign body	Pain, dysphagia	Local or none

unless the patient is unconscious or there is a depressed cough reflex that makes aspiration a hazard. This procedure is not necessary for diagnosis or assessment of continued bleeding because a child may vomit blood from as high as the nose or as low down as the jejunum. A thorough physical examination and history-taking will serve the clinician just as well for diagnosis. Furthermore, placement of a nasogastric tube is extremely repugnant to most children; sometimes they will fight and pull out the tube, thus compounding the bleeding. The danger of a Mallory-Weiss lesion (tear of the esophageal mucosa) should preclude the placement of a nasogastric tube.

There should be no dietary restrictions for conscious patients unless the diagnosis indicates an acute surgical condition of the abdomen, esophageal varices, or Mallory-Weiss lesion. The diet should not be restricted because of infrequent vomiting episodes. It is appropriate to ask the family what the child's favorite foods are, and, if possible, provide them in accordance with a dietitian's advice.

It is prudent to avoid the insertion of an intravenous line; it is better for the child to be free to move and be held by relatives or nurses and go to the toilet normally. Frequently repeated venipunctures or fingersticks should be avoided, and all the specimens necessary for diagnosis should be obtained during the first venipuncture. In addition, it is very important not to order *routine* repeated fingersticks (*e.g.*, hemoglobin and hematocrit determinations two, three, or four times a day). These tests should be done only when vital signs, history, and physical examination indicate a further loss of blood. Children in certain age groups can be reduced rapidly to bundles of fear and apprehension, or can become violent fighters, by frequent, routine sticking.

It is not advisable to give blood in the face of a stable condition unless the hemoglobin is 6 g or less, or unless the patient has a special need for increased oxygen (*e.g.*, cyanotic congenital heart disease, pulmonary insufficiency, or severe infections). Most children are resilient, and will manage with a hemoglobin of 6 g without difficulty. Because of the risk of hepatitis or other disorders, blood transfusion can be more dangerous to the patient than a gastrointestinal bleed that has stopped at 5 or 6 g and does not recur.

All too often the pediatric patient in a busy setting is physically restrained by having an arm or leg tied for an intravenous line, or because he wishes to move about. A child will govern his own movements depending on how he feels. The arm or leg should be tied down only if it is absolutely necessary to maintain a life-saving blood infusion.

Further Steps in Management

Vital signs such as pulse rate, respiration, and blood pressure are recorded every half-hour. A gradual increase in pulse rate is the best indicator of continued bleeding. The blood pressure will fall if the patient has decompensated and is in shock, and it is not usually necessary to disturb a sleeping child to take frequent blood pressure recordings if the pulse rate remains steady.

The initial essential blood tests include determinations of hemoglobin, hematocrit, white blood cell count, differential, and sedimentation rate. Always incorporate a coagulation profile, ascertain the child's blood group, cross-match, and hold blood ready for transfusion. Other blood tests depend on the tentative clinical diagnosis.

Whole blood is best for replacing blood loss. Packed red blood cells should be used in long-standing chronic anemia or congestive heart failure. The amount of blood necessary can be based on 15 ml/kg of whole blood. The rate of infusion depends on the urgency of the patient's need.

Discussion

Without doubt, it is true that children are different. They will reward the clinician with resilience, response, and recovery after confident, considerate management. It is important to gain the child's confidence by talking with him on his own level. The nurses should be familiar with children and their specific needs, as well as being firm and sympathetic. All too often in adult units unaccustomed to children there is an overindulgence by adult patients and staff alike; this can be detrimental to a child's overall growth and development.

Schooling, play, peer interaction, and the presence of parents and siblings are of importance to a child. These needs should be given due consideration with any child with gastrointestinal bleeding, no matter how severe. The presence of familiar things will help the child to recover rapidly, and will reduce the apprehension that can only increase the risk of continued hemorrhage. It is not uncommon, after many transfusions, to see bleeding stop when the intravenous line is removed and a child is provided the right environment. When a child is restricted, venipunctured, frightened, and transfused too often to increase the hemoglobin, he may continue to bleed; these patients may undergo laparotomy unnecessarily.

BIBLIOGRAPHY

Anderson CM, Burke V (eds): Pediatric Gastroenterology. London, Blackwell, 1975

Davidson M (ed): Clinics in Gastroenterology—Pediatric Gastroenterology. Philadelphia, WB Saunders, 1977

A concise monograph, limited in scope, but which deals well with important common problems.

Galler JR, Neustein S, Walker WA: Clinical aspects of recurrent abdominal pain in children. Adv Pediatr 27:31 1980

A review of causes, treatment, and outcome of chronic abdominal pain in childhood.

Gryboski J: Gastrointestinal Problems in the Infant. Philadelphia, WB Saunders, 1975.

Roy CC, Silverman A, Cozetto FJ: Pediatric Clinical Gastroenterology. St. Louis, CV Mosby, 1975

These are good general tests of pediatric gastroenterology which focus on clinical aspects of of diagnosis and treatment.

Vomiting

14

James A. Hallock

Vomiting is one of the most common signs and symptoms in infancy and childhood. It may occur with any acute infection or emotional stress and is a sign of abnormality in either the gastrointestinal tract, urinary tract, or nervous system. It is important to know the main etiologic factors and their variation in different age groups.

PATHOPHYSIOLOGY

The mechanisms responsible for vomiting depend upon stimulation of brain centers. The vomiting center is located in the medulla, near the tractus solitarius at the level of the dorsal motor nucleus of the vagus. The center receives stimuli from the visceral organs by the vagus or sympathetic afferent nerves. These stimuli may arise in any abdominal organ but the strongest stimuli arise from the stomach and duodenum. Following stimulation of the vomiting center, the act of emesis is transmitted through motor impulses by cranial nerves V, VII, IX, X, XII. This mechanism is responsible for the vomiting seen with gastrointestinal and renal disease. Vomiting with increased intracranial pressure also results from stimulation of this center.

Another mechanism involves stimulation of the chemoreceptor trigger zone (CTZ), which is located in the floor of the fourth ventricle above the area postrema. This area is sensitive to toxins and drugs such as apomorphine. The vomiting associated with infection is thought to be mediated by this mechanism.

The stimulus for vomiting in motion sickness arises from labyrinthine receptors. Impulses produced are transmitted either directly to the cerebellum or by way of the vestibular nuclei to the CTZ, with emesis the result.

The chemical mediators involved with these mechanisms are unknown at this time.

Metabolic Changes Following Vomiting

Vomiting is followed by disturbances in fluid and electrolyte balance since there is loss of water, hydrochloric acid, and electrolytes. As a result of these losses, clinical dehydration becomes evident with contraction of extracellular fluid volume and development of hypochloremic metabolic alkalosis.

The potential for dehydration should be considered in all cases of vomiting, especially in infants and small children. Documentation of fluid loss and ability to ingest fluids is a critical step in the evaluation of all children with vomiting.

CHARACTER OF VOMITUS

The appearance of the vomited material is helpful in determining the significance of the vomiting and the level of involvement of the gastrointestinal tract (Table 14-1).

Undigested or unchanged food suggests that the lesion is in the esophagus or stomach (*e.g.*, esophageal atresia or stenosis). Digested food which is not bile-stained suggests a lesion proximal to the ampulla of Vater (*e.g.*, pyloric stenosis). Bilious vomiting is suggestive of obstruction distal to the ampulla (*e.g.*, small bowel obstruction). Fecal vomitus is an emergency suggesting distal gastrointestinal obstruction or peritonitis. Hematemesis is always pathologic and must be investigated thoroughly (see Neonatal Period).

PATTERN OF VOMITING

The pattern of vomiting may be a clue to the diagnosis. Although each of the following patterns is suggestive, none is pathognomonic of a specific diagnosis (Table 14-2). Vomiting with nausea is a common sign of acute illness such as infection or ingestion of toxic material. Vomiting without nausea may be a sign of increased intracranial pressure and should be rapidly evaluated. Projectile vomiting also requires prompt evaluation and usually indicates the presence of gastrointestinal obstruction or increased intracranial pressure.

APPROACH TO DIAGNOSIS

The etiology of vomiting is usually considered in relation to the age of the child. The three age periods are: (1) neonatal period, (2) infancy through 2 years, and (3) childhood (after 2 years). In assessing a symptom such as vomiting, the history and physical examination are important keys to diagnosis. The vomiting should be categorized as acute or chronic, since the approach varies depending on the duration of the vomiting.

Attention must be paid to the child's development. When growth and development are "normal" for his age and vomiting is chronic, a psychosomatic cause is likely, and an extensive laboratory and radiologic evaluation is unnecessary. If there is retardation of either growth or development, a search should be made for one of the causes of chronic vomiting listed for each age period below.

TABLE 14-1. Character of Vomitus

Character of Vomitus	Probable Level of Involvement	Example Lesion
Undigested food	Esophagus	Esophageal atresia
Digested food, no bile	Proximal to ampulla of Vater	Pyloric stenosis
Bile-containing material*	Distal to ampulla of Vater	Jejunal atresia
Fecal vomiting*	Distal gastrointestinal tract	Peritonitis
Blood*	Upper gastrointestinal tract	Ulcer

*Should be initially approached as an emergency situation.

TABLE 14-2. Types of Vomiting

Type	Significance	Etiology
Projectile vomiting	Pathologic and requires evaluation	Upper gastrointestinal tract Increased intracranial pressure
Vomiting without nausea	Pathologic and requires evaluation	Increased intracranial pressure
Vomiting with nausea	Common	Infection Toxicity

In each of the following discussions, an attempt will be made to demonstrate the probable diagnosis and to present guidelines for evaluation.

Neonatal Vomiting

Vomiting is common (50%) in normal full-term newborns and is related to either swallowed amniotic fluid, swallowed blood, or faulty feeding techniques. If the baby is feeding well, gaining weight, and physical examination reveals no abnormalities, then no evaluation should be performed unless the vomiting is persistent. The evaluation of a vomiting neonate who appears ill is critical. This is a symptom of a potentially rapidly fatal process and one which quickly leads to difficulty with fluid and electrolyte balance.

The signs and symptoms listed below are the ones associated with pathologic causes of vomiting in the newborn. Certain findings including dehydration, hematemesis, bilious vomiting, projectile vomiting, and abdominal mass, demand immediate evaluation since they indicate an emergency situation, surgical or medical. Maternal polyhydramnios, increased gastric contents (more than 25 ml) at initial aspiration, abdominal distention, lack of meconium stools, decrease in feeding, lethargy, and irritability are signs or symptoms which demand close observation but not necessarily immediate evaluation. The appearance and physical examination of the baby should be the major factor in evaluation. When indicated, this evaluation must be as rapid, thorough, and atraumatic as possible.

Signs and Symptoms of Disease Associated with Neonatal Vomiting

Dehydration—loss of 5%–10% of birth weight
Hematemesis: This could be the presentation of upper GI bleeding or swallowed maternal blood. (An APT* test with 10% NaOH should be performed to differentiate adult from fetal hemoglobin.)
History of maternal polyhydramnios in this pregnancy
Increased gastric contents (>25 ml) at initial aspiration after birth
Progressive abdominal distention
Lack of meconium stools
Bilious vomiting
Decrease in feeding
Lethargy
Irritability
Projectile vomiting
Abdominal mass

* APT test: Reaction of the specimen with NaOH. Reduction as indicated by a change in color to yellow or brown, signifies adult hemoglobin. No change indicates fetal origin.

Differential Diagnosis of Vomiting in the Neonate

Gastrointestinal lesions (usually represent acute surgical emergencies in the neonate)
- Esophageal atresia—tracheoesophageal fistula
- Duodenal, jejeunal, or ileal atresia
- Annular pancreas

- Congenital bands
- Intestinal malrotation with volvulus
- Imperforate anus
- Toxic megacolon (Hirschsprung's disease)
- Meconium ileus (cystic fibrosis)
- Meconium plug syndrome
- Trauma to upper GI or respiratory tracts

Infections (medical emergencies)
- Generalized sepsis
- Meningitis
- Urinary tract infection
- Pneumonia

Central nervous system
- Subdural hematoma
- Intracranial hemorrhage

Renal disorders
- Renal tubular acidosis

Metabolic (inborn errors)
- Galactosemia
- PKU
- Congenital adrenal hyperplasia
- Hypercalcemia
- Aminoacidurias
  - Maple syrup urine disease
  - Hyperglycinemia
  - Citrullinemia
  - Hypervalinemia
  - Hyperammonemia
  - Argininosuccinicaciduria

To rule out a surgical lesion such as intestinal obstruction, plain radiographs of the abdomen or radiographs using air as the initial contrast medium should be taken. Further radiologic evaluation may include contrast enema and upper gastrointestinal films. If a surgical lesion is diagnosed, prompt stabilization and hydration should be accomplished prior to operation. These lesions are usually upper intestinal and include esophageal atresia with or without tracheoesophageal fistula, and duodenal obstruction secondary to atresia, annular pancreas, or congenital bands.

If no surgical lesion is demonstrated, infection is the next major category to be considered. A blood culture, urine culture (suprapubic aspiration), lumbar puncture and other cultures must be performed if the baby appears ill with no obvious cause for vomiting. In this situation, antibiotic therapy is frequently initiated prior to culture results.

Further evaluation should be performed as indicated by the patient's status. The differential diagnosis is listed and can serve as a guide to most likely possibilities and studies needed. This is the presentation for many of the metabolic disorders listed.

Infancy

Most acute vomiting during infancy is in conjunction with infectious diseases. Although any of the listed causes of chronic vomiting may start acutely, these are not thought of in the initial patient encounter unless some other factor is present. Infant regurgitation causes much maternal anxiety. Therefore, when you are presented with an infant 1 to 2 months of age, certain facts must be elicited. Probably all normal infants bring up some milk after feeding but the pattern is very important in deciding whether it is necessary or desirable to investigate for organic disease.

Since the child can give no history of nausea or abdominal pain, the physical examination frequently provides the answer. Each of the causes listed below must be considered and the likely ones ruled out by physical examination or appropriate laboratory study (*e.g.,* urine culture for suspected urinary tract infection). Also, during physical examination strict attention must be paid to fluid balance to ensure no problem with dehydration. Persistent or chronic vomiting associated with any of the following requires a more thorough investigation: projectile vomiting, decreased feeding, failure to grow or develop properly, bilious vomiting, hematemesis, abdominal mass, distention, bloody diarrhea, and episodes of apnea.

Causes of Vomiting During Infancy

Gastrointestinal lesions
- Pyloric stenosis (2–12 weeks)
- Intussusception*
- Malrotation with volvulus*
- Achalasia of esophagus
- Chalasia
- Hiatal hernia
- Duodenal bands
- Gastroesophageal reflux

Infectious problems
- Gastroenteritis*
- Urinary tract infections
- Meningitis*
- Pneumonia*
- Otitis media*
- Pertussis*
- Sepsis*
- Any URI*

Central nervous system
- Subdural hematoma

Hydrocephalus

Renal disease
- Nephrotic syndrome
- Renal tubular acidosis
- Polycystic kidneys
- Nephrogenic diabetes insipidus
- Uremia

Metabolic (inborn errors)
- Diabetes mellitus*
- Galactosemia
- Fructosemia
- Congenital adrenal hyperplasia*
- Aminoacidurias (as in neonate)

* A cause of acute as well as chronic vomiting in this age group (see text).

The two most important nonorganic causes of chronic vomiting are regurgitation and rumination. (1) *Regurgitation* or spitting-up represents the nonforceful expulsion of small amounts of food shortly after feeding. It may be related to faulty feeding techniques or social/environmental factors. One- to three-month-old babies experience this, and it disappears when the baby begins to walk. These children have "normal" growth and development; this, together with a "normal" physical examination, supports the diagnosis. (2) *Rumination* is a rare but serious form of chronic vomiting with its onset during the latter half of the first year. The child deliberately causes himself to vomit food which has recently been ingested. The problem is psychogenic in origin due either to maternal deprivation or maternal inadequacy. There is usually associated failure to thrive. If the child can be seen gagging himself, the diagnosis can be readily made. However, this is difficult to observe and document, and is a difficult diagnosis to confirm.

Gastroesophageal Reflux. Decreased pressure in the lower esophageal sphincter, may lead to regurgitation and vomiting, particularly when the infant is prone. It can cause failure to thrive, neurologic abnormalities, or apnea. Diagnosis may require X-ray motility studies, pressure measurements of the distal esophagus, or evidence of regurgitated acid (*e.g.*, Tuttle test). The child may benefit from being kept upright and given small frequent feedings, and calcium-containing antacids. In refractory situations, plication of the fundus of the stomach should be considered.

Childhood Vomiting

As in the case with infants, this is not a variant of "normal" in children over the age of 2 years; therefore, all children with vomiting must be evaluated. The type of evaluation depends on whether the symptom is acute or long-standing.

Chronic Vomiting. The most common etiology for chronic vomiting in childhood is functional vomiting. When this complaint is made, the major thrust of evaluation should be a physical examination that includes blood pressure, and ocular fundi and visual field examinations. When evaluating this symptom, do not attempt a "full workup." The following are helpful indicators and should lead to a search for a specific diagnosis: deterioration in health, weight loss, disturbance in growth pattern, urinary symptoms, neurologic symptoms, pallor, and unilateral abdominal pain. If the above are absent and physical examination is "normal," you are justified in following the child and observing the pattern.

Functional Vomiting. Usually the diagnosis of functional vomiting is made as a diagnosis of exclusion. However, an attempt must be made to gather historical data sufficient to support this diagnosis (*e.g.*, evaluate school phobias or stresses in the child's environment).

Acute Vomiting. As with younger children, the most common association is with infections; these should be evaluated. In addition, ingestion of unusual substances gains in importance and must always be considered in any child with vomiting. Note the following list of some of the causes for acute vomiting in this age group.

Appendicitis. Special mention is made of this condition since in many reported series, more than half the children less than 6 years of age operated on for appendicitis have suffered a ruptured appendix. In order to prevent this, the diagnosis must be considered and made earlier.

SUMMARY

In any age group, the keys to proper evaluation are the history and physical examination. These should point to the diagnosis or provide the information needed to decide whether further studies are necessary. In addition, the history and physical examination should give a clear picture of the child's growth and development and how they are affected by the complaint of vomiting.

Vomiting in Childhood

Acute infection
- Any infection may present with vomiting but it is most commonly seen with:
  - Gastroenteritis*
  - Urinary tract infections (see below)*
  - Pharyngitis*
  - Pneumonia*
  - Viral exanthems*
  - Otitis media*
  - Hepatitis*

Gastrointestinal
- Appendicitis*
- Small bowel obstruction*
- Meckel's diverticulum*
- Hiatal hernia
- Peptic ulcer
- Pancreatitis (rare)*

Renal
- UTI*
- Acute glomerulonephritis*
- Nephrosis
- Hypertension*
- Uremia

Intracranial disease
- Increased intracranial pressure
  - Brain tumor
  - Pseudotumor cerebri
  - Hydrocephalus
  - Others
- Migraine headaches
- Meningitis*
- Seizure disorders

Poisoning (drug ingestion)
- Lead*
- Salicylates*
- Most medications or drugs*
- Any toxin

Metabolic diseases
- Diabetes mellitus*
- Hypertension*
- Hyperlipidemia

* Acute or chronic vomiting in this age group. (See text.)

BIBLIOGRAPHY

Batzdorf U: The management of cerebral edema in pediatric practice. Pediatrics 58:78, 1966

This article deals with the management of cerebral edema, but also points out the recognition of vomiting as a manifestation of increased intracranial pressure and the evaluation of a patient for intracranial pressure.

Euler AR, Ament ME: Detection of gastroesophageal reflex in the pediatric age group. Pediatrics 60:65, 1977

This article discusses the use of esophageal pH to confirm diagnosis of gastroesophageal reflex.

Sheinbein M: Treatment for hospitalized infantile ruminator. Clin Pediatr 14:719, 1975

An approach to recognition and management of rumination.

Talbert JL, Felman AH, DeBush FL: Gastrointestinal surgical emergencies in the newborn infant. J Pediatr 76:783, 1970

This is an excellent summary of all the findings present in newborns with intestinal obstruction and surgical emergencies and outlines the diagnostic approach in evaluation of signs and symptoms.

Taneja OP, Taneja S, Lal A: Intestinal obstruction in infancy and childhood. Arch Surg 97:544, 1968

This gives the statistical review of the causes of intestinal obstruction and an evaluation of children with intestinal obstruction.

Vulliamy DG: Recurrent abdominal pain and vomiting in childhood. Br Med J 1:1113, 1965

This article is an approach to nonorganic causes of vomiting in childhood and offers a good perspective on evaluating vomiting as a symptom in helping to decide whether the problem is organic or inorganic.

Diarrheal Diseases

15

John I. Malone

Diarrhea is not a disease but a symptom of a number of other disease processes that involve various organ systems including the gastrointestinal tract.

The term "diarrhea" is not precise. Thus it is important to have the patient or parent describe in other terms what they mean when using the word diarrhea. The medical definition is "an abnormally frequent discharge of *fluid* and *fecal material*." The exact meaning of "abnormally frequent" and its implication regarding the total amount of material lost continues to be vague and subjective, particularly at younger ages. Infants vary considerably in the number and consistency of normal stools passed per day. Four to six in a day may be normal for one infant, while one in two or even three days may be normal for another. Therefore, the definition of diarrhea must be modified to an increase in the frequency and looseness of stools beyond that which is common for a particular individual.

As the child grows older and the intestinal tract matures, the normal consistency and frequency of stooling becomes less variable. There is less response to variation in the components of the diet, (*e.g.*, sugar, fat, protein) as the mechanisms of absorption mature, thus the "normal" stooling pattern of a person becomes more predictable with increasing age.

Acute diarrhea is commonly a self-limited minor problem or inconvenience for older children, adolescents, and adults. This must be contrasted, however, with the life-threatening potential of acute diarrhea during the first year of life. Acute diarrhea during infancy has a much greater potential for massive fluid loss and resultant cardiovascular collapse than in older children.

Chronic diarrhea (more than 2 weeks' duration), an even more life-threatening situation for an infant, also has significant morbidity and mortality for older children. This is due largely to the resultant malnutrition.

Diarrhea is a frequent and important problem in pediatrics. An understanding of the mechanisms that cause diarrhea may make its treatment more rational.

MECHANISMS OF DIARRHEA

Damaged Intestinal Brush Border Membrane

Damage to intestinal brush border membrane is caused either by toxins or mechanical trauma. It results in impaired transport of water, electrolytes, and products of digestion in and out of the intestinal lumen.

Increased Intraluminal Unabsorbed Osmotically Active Substances

In turn damaged intestinal brush border membrane may be the cause of increased intraluminal unabsorbed osmotically active substances. Drinking water that contains increased amounts of soluble sulfates is an example. The brush border membrane is unaffected, but the unabsorbed sulfate osmotically pulls extra water into the intestinal tract. Hereditary deficiency of intestinal enzymes (*e.g.*, lactase, lipase, amylase) which break down ingested food to absorbable particles, results in increased intraluminal osmotically active substances. Certain antibiotics are believed to inhibit enzymes important for the absorption of digested food. Acquired enzyme deficiencies may occur secondary to certain antibiotics (ampicillin, tetracycline, erythromycin) or to mechanical or toxic injury to the intestinal mucosa of diarrhea.

Intestinal Microorganisms

Intestinal microorganisms may cause diarrhea by damaging the intestinal brush border by released enterotoxin or by direct invasion of the epithelial lining of the mucosa. Another way that intestinal microorganisms cause diarrhea is by biotransformation of bile acids and saturated long chain fatty acids to substances that impair fat absorption and cause steatorrhea.

Bile Acids

Bile acids are normally absorbed in the ileum. Surgical resection of the ileum or pathologic processes such as inflammation which prevent their absorption results in increased amounts of bile acids in the colon. Bile acids in the colon interfere with the absorption of water and electrolytes and induce the colon to secrete and increase the stool volume.

Diarrhea Due to Hydroxy-Fatty Acids

Deficient absorption of long chain fatty acids allows biotransformation by colon flora of these substances to hydroxy-fatty acids which are well-known cathartics.

Abnormal Intestinal Motility

Altered intestinal motility produces disturbances in digestion and absorption. Increased motility is the result of an excess of smooth muscle active substances such as prostaglandins and serotonin. It has been reported that the interaction of the pituitary polypeptide coherin with serotonin in mucosal receptors alters intestinal motor activity.

Decreased intestinal motility may occur in diabetes and scleroderma. This allows increased bacterial colonization which plays a role in the malabsorption and diarrhea observed in these patients.

Hypersecretory State

A hypersecretory state is an exudative enteropathy. This category varies from gastrin-induced gastric hypersecretion and hypersecretory states provoked by the chronic inflammation of ulcerative colitis and regional enteritis to intestinal lymphangectasia involving the loss of lymph and protein through the colon.

Unknown Mechanisms

The mechanisms responsible for the diarrhea of immune disorders, acrodermatitis enteropathica, and food intolerances, *are speculative at present.*

DISEASES CAUSING ACUTE DIARRHEA

Improper Feeding

The most common cause of acute diarrhea of infancy is improper feeding. Infants vary widely in their tolerance to both the quantity and the quality of food. A quantity of formula that is tolerated by one infant may cause diarrhea in another. The commonly used infant formulas differ in the amount and types of protein, fat, and carbohydrate. Each of these components may affect the stool volume in variable ways. Stool volume and water content seem to vary directly with the fat and sugar content of the formula. Thus, babies on a formula high in polyunsaturated fats (Similac) have looser stools than those on a formula containing a greater percentage of saturated fats (SMA). Switching from one formula to another for nonspecific problems such as colic may result in a stool pattern interpreted as diarrhea. In a similar fashion, if the sugar content in a formula is much greater than 7.2% weight per volume (W/V), the stools tend to become soft and watery. Some family feeding practices allow for the addition of honey to the proprietary formula to "enrich the formula." This usually loosens the stools. This type of intolerance decreases as the gastrointestinal tract matures and is, therefore, less apparent with increasing age.

Infections

Infections are the most common causes of diarrhea during infancy and childhood. Table 15-1 shows the clinical features useful in identifying the infectious diarrheas.

Infections outside the intestinal tract are frequently associated with diarrhea in younger children. This is called "parenteral" diarrhea. In such patients, cessation or persistence of the diarrhea parallels the clearing or continuation of the primary infection. This suggests that parenteral diarrhea is associated with the response of the immature colon to nongastrointestinal disease. This is supported by the observation that young infants are more sensitive than adults to the development of parenteral diarrhea. Diarrhea that results from the use of antibiotics, moreover, is much more common in children than adults and may have the same mechanism.

Protozoal infections cause both acute and chronic diarrhea. The onset is not likely to be sudden. The stools lack the odor and appearance of an infectious diarrhea. The mucus is white or yellowish, and the odor suggests an autolytic rather than a suppurative process. The children may have a variety of complaints that can be traced to the intestinal tract and appear to have a malabsorption syndrome such as celiac disease prior to the onset of diarrhea. The diagnosis requires reliable microscopic laboratory examination of several small quantities of stool.

Food Poisoning

Food poisoning as a cause should also be considered. This type of diarrhea is of acute onset and usually occurs in a large group of people within 4 to 6 hours of ingesting a specific food item. One type of food poisoning is called botulism and is caused by a toxin released by the *Clostridium botulinum,* an anaerobic spore-forming organism. The source of the organism is chiefly home-canned foods, especially underprocessed nonacid meat, fish, and vegetables. Some patients have acute nausea, vomiting, and abdominal pain. Central nervous system symptoms develop in 12 to 48 hours and are due to a curarelike action of the toxin on the motor end plate.

Some strains of staphylococci and

TABLE 15-1. Typical Clinical Features of Infectious Diarrheas

					Shigella			
	Cholera	Enterotoxigenic E. coli*	Enteroinvasive E. coli*	Entero-pathogenic E. coli	Diarrheic Form	Dysenteric Form	Salmonella	Reoviruslike Organism
Site of action	Small bowel	Small bowel	Large bowel	Small bowel?	Small bowel	Large bowel	Small and large bowels	Small bowel
Mechanism of action	Toxin	Toxin	Invasion	?	?	Invasion	?	?
Age	Any	Any?	Any?	<1 yr	>2 yr	Any	Any	<7 yr
Diarrhea in household	+ +	+	+	0	+ +	+ +	+	+
Season	Epidemic	Any	Any	Fall	Fall	Fall	Any	Winter
Character of onset	Abrupt	Abrupt	Abrupt	Gradual	Abrupt	Gradual	Gradual	Abrupt
Vomiting	+ (Late)	+ +	0	+	+ +	+	+	+ +
Cramps	+ +	+ +	—	?	0	+ +	+	?
Tenesmus	0	0	?	?	0	+ +	+	?
Fever >102° F	0	0	+ +	0	+ +	+	0	0
Convulsions	0	0	0	0	+ +	0	0	0
Anal sphincter tone	Normal	Normal	Normal	Normal	Lax	Lax	Normal	Normal
Stool volume	Large	Large	Small	Moderate	Large	Small	Moderate	Large
Stool consistency	Watery	Water	Slimy	Slimy	Watery	Viscous	Slimy	Watery
Stool odor	Odorless	Oderless	Foul	Musty	Odorless	Odorless	Foul	Odorless
Stool blood	0	0	+ +	+	0	+ +	0	0
Stool mucus shreds	+ +	+ +	+	0	+ +	0	0	0
Stool pus	0	0	+ +	+	0	+ +	+	0
Stool color	Colorless	Colorless	?	Green	Colorless	Bloody	Green/brown	Colorless/brown
Stool leukocytes	0	+	+ +	+	+	+ +	+ +	0
Granulocytosis	?	+	+	+	+ +	+ +	0	0
Duration (untreated)	3–6 days	5–10 days	?	7–14 days	2–3 days	7–14 days	3–7 days	5–7 days

*Based on observations in adults.
Key: ?, Insufficient data available; 0, usually absent; +, sometimes present; + +, commonly present.
(Adapted from Nelson JD, Hieber JP. From Krugmun S, Ward R, Katz S: Infectious Diseases of Children. St. Louis, C. V. Mosby, 1977).

TABLE 15-2. Clinical Features of Acute Diarrhea (Nonbacterial)

Clinical Feature	Overfeeding	Parenteral	Protozoal	Food Poisoning
Age	0–2 years	Any	Any	Any
Well-being	Normal	ill	ill	Severely ill
Weight	Normal	Stable	Loss	Loss
Diarrhea in household	No	No	Variable	Yes
Vomiting	Variable	No	Occasionally	Yes
Fever	No	Variable	Occasionally	No
Abdominal discomfort	No	No	Variable	Yes
CNS signs	No	Variable	No	Yes
Stools				
Consistency	Loose	Loose	Watery	Watery
Odor	Normal	Normal	Variable	Variable
Blood	No	No	Yes	Variable

streptococci produce an exotoxin that causes nausea, vomiting, abdominal pain, and acute prostration in addition to diarrhea, within 1 to 6 hours of ingesting contaminated food. Foods commonly infected are pastries, salads, chicken, ham, beef in hash, whipped cream, and custards.

Table 15-2 lists some of the clinical features that are helpful in differentiating the noninfectious causes of diarrhea.

CHRONIC DIARRHEA

In infants and children, chronic diarrhea is often a diagnostic and therapeutic challenge. The clinical spectrum ranges from benign normal physiologic responses misinterpreted as problems to disorders which are life-threatening and frequently associated with severe nutritional deficiencies (Table 15-3).

Although novel techniques have been applied to the diagnosis of chronic diarrhea, a well-taken history (*e.g.*, feeding history, stool description, general health) offers important clues which channel and identify priorities in the workup of such a patient. The age of the patient should direct one's thinking (Fig. 15-1). The physical exam must include an evaluation of the patient's growth and physical development. Normal growth and development are not likely to be associated with a process of a severe nature. Examination of the diarrheal stool is part of the complete physical examination of such a patient. The presence or absence of excessive mucus and water and their characteristics are very useful information. Purulent mucus suggests an infectious process; bloody mucus, an ulcerative process. Disaccharidase deficiency results in the excretion of large quantities of watery stool. In the absence of free water in the stool, a disaccharidase deficiency is unlikely. The indirect tests used to make this diagnosis are the findings of an acid stool pH and the presence of unabsorbed sugar in the stool. In the absence of the intestinal disaccharide that hydrolyzes the sugar, it acts as an osmotically active substance which increases stool water. This same sugar is in turn metabolized by the enteric flora to produce lactic acid which lowers the pH of the stool water below pH 5. To test for reducing substance in the stool, on part liquid stool is mixed with two parts water. Fifteen drops of this mixture are then added to a test tube and a fresh clinitest tablet is

TABLE 15-3. Causes and Features of Chronic Diarrhea

Disease	Vomit	Stool					Abd. dist.	Hereditary	Acquired	Other
		H_2O	Mucus	pH	Red sub	Fat				
Deficiciency disaccharidase	N	+	N	<5	+	+	+	±	+	Renal calculi
Glucose-galactose intol.	N	+	N	<5	+	N	N	+	N	—
Cystic fibrosis	N	N	N	6.5–7.5	N	+	±	+	N	Pulmonary disease
Pancreatic insufficiency	N	N	N	6.5–7.5	±	+	±	+	N	Cyclic neutropenia
Giardiasis	N	+	N	6.5–7.5	N	+	±	N	+	Immune deficiency
Blind loop syndrome	+	+	+	<5	N	+	+	N	+	—
A-beta lipoproteinemia	N	N	N	6.5–7.5	N	+	N	+	N	Acanthocytosis, retinitis pigmentosia
Liver failure	N	N	N	6.5–7.5	N	N	+	N	+	—
Ileal resection	N	N	N	6.5–7.5	N	+	+	N	+	—
Proteolytic enzyme deficiency	+	N	+	6.5–7.5	–	–	+	+	+	Hypoproteinemia
Intestinal lymphangiectasis	N	N	+	6.5–7.5	N	+	+	–	–	Chylous ascites—hypoproteinemia
Protein intolerance	+	N	+	6.5–7.5	N	N	++	±	±	Abdominal pain—eosinophilia
Cow's milk protein intol.	+	+	+ Bloody	<5	+	+	+	N	+	Edema hypoproteinemia
Gluten-sensitive enteropathy	N	+	+	6.5–7.5	+	+	+	+	+	Villous dystrophy
Familial protein intol.	N	+	N	6.5–7.5	±	+	+	+	N	Hepatosplenomegaly, rickets, hyperammonemia
Ulcerative colitis	N	N	+	6.5–7.5	±	+	N	N	+	Skin, joint, and liver disease
Regional enteritis	N	N	Bloody	6.5–7.5	±	+	N	N	+	Fever, arthritis erythema nodosum
Ileal disease	N	±	+	6.5–7.5	±	+	N	N	+	B_{12} deficiency
Tumors catecholamines	N	±	N	6.5–7.5	+	+	+	N	+	Urinary VMA, cystathionine
Antibody deficiency	N	±	N	6.5–7.5	+	+	+	+	±	Recurrent infections
Hirschsprung's disease	N	±	N	6.5–7.5	–	–	+	N	+	Delayed passage of first stool
Congenital chloride diarrhea	N	+	N	<5	N	N	–	±	–	Metabolic alkalosis
Irritable colon	N	+	N	6.5–7.5	N	N	N	±	±	Pos. family history, self-limited Ends 3–4 years

N = Negative + = Postive

Note: All these disorders are associated with failure to thrive. The relationship of the etiology to the age of the patient is seen in Figure Table 15-1.

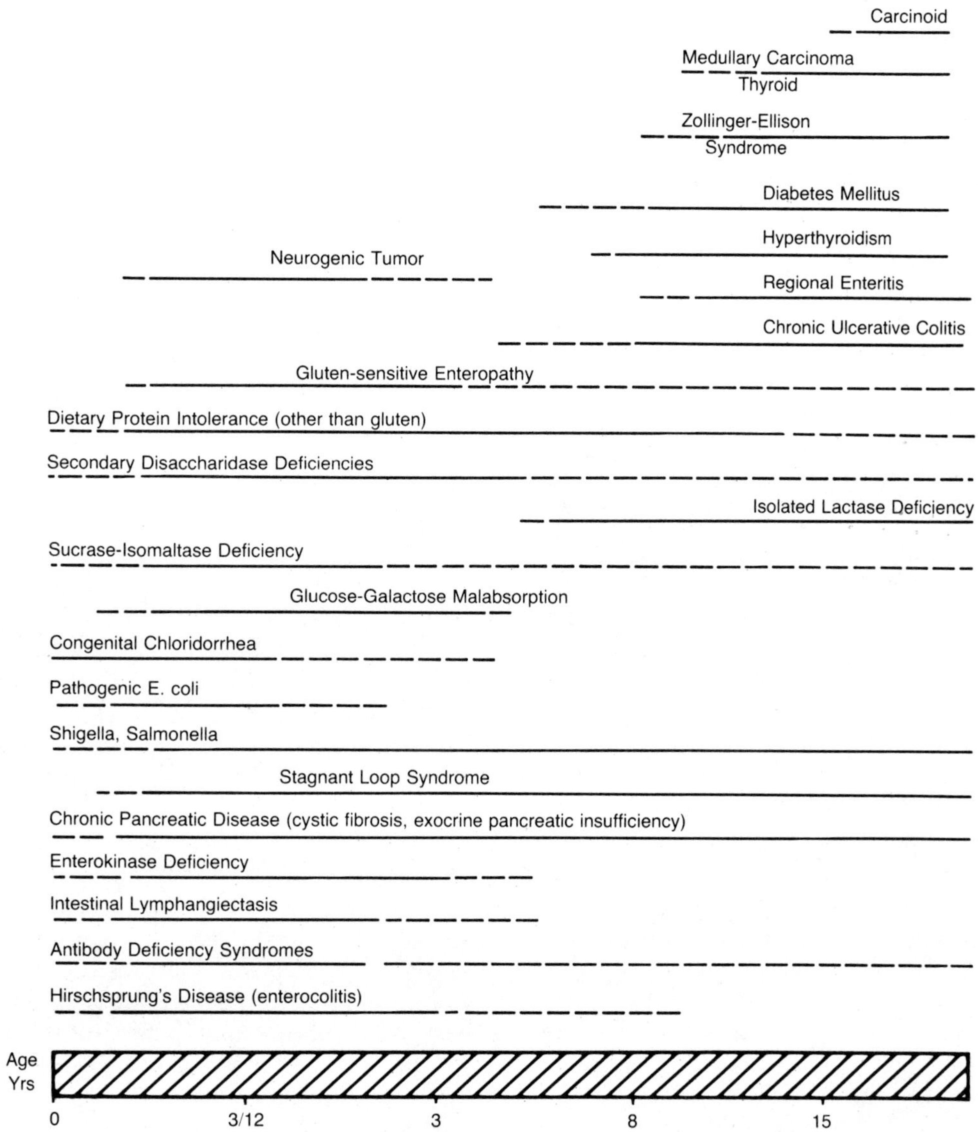

Fig. 15-1. Relation of etiology to age of patient in chronic diarrhea in children. Solid lines: estimated greatest frequency of occurrence or diagnosis. Broken lines: possible occurrence or establishment of diagnosis at a younger or older age. (From Poley JR: Chronic diarrhea in infants and children, Part I. South Med J, *66*:1050, 1973.)

added to the tube. The color chart for sugar in the urine (5-drop method) is employed. A reading of 0.5% or greater is considered positive. If the stool water is missed and these substances are looked for in water in which the stool particles were emulsified, many false-negatives will occur.

While following the course of a patient with chronic diarrhea, daily weights must be noted. This is particularly important in untrained infants who may pass large quantities of fluid into the diaper with no solid material left as evidence. This can result in a significant fluid and weight loss during a time interval when the nursing observations indicate that the diarrhea has stopped.

The evaluation of poor fat absorption (steatorrhea) characteristically involves the measurement of the 24-hour excretion of fat in the stool. If consuming a diet of at least 50 g of fat, a stool fat greater than 7 g in 24 hours measured for 3 consecutive days, is considered abnormal. An easier indirect measurement of fat absorption is the level of the fat-soluble vitamins (A, D, E, K) in the serum.

Chronic nonspecific diarrhea is the most common cause of prolonged diarrhea in children less than 5 years of age not associated with failure to thrive. It is characterized by diarrhea of at least 3 weeks' duration, a normal pattern of growth and development, and no evidence of malabsorption or enteric infections. The stool frequency is usually lower than for other causes of chronic diarrhea, but the stool consistency is no different. The stools contain no blood, but mucus is a prominent feature. Most affected children consume diets low in fat content (less than 27% of total calories) with either adequate or low caloric content for their age. A few (about 20%) have diet histories with apparently normal caloric and fat content. All these children respond within 2 weeks of increasing the fat content of the diet (minimum of 4 g/kg of body wt/day) with a decrease in stool frequency and improved stool consistency.

TREATMENT

The initial therapeutic approach to diarrhea is to make sure the patient is not in impending shock. If the patient is in shock, proper fluids and electrolytes must be administered immediately. Following that determination, the patient's diarrhea is then categorized as either mild, moderate, or severe. When making a decision about the seriousness of diarrhea, it is very helpful to know the daily weights of the patient. Therefore, a weight must be recorded on each visit of such a patient and may be the only objective evidence available during the clinical observations of a specific patient to determine the severity of the diarrhea (Table 15-4).

Mild diarrhea is treated effectively by a modified fast that includes sweetened tea or apple juice offered only at the usual feeding times. This is continued for 12 to 24 hours depending on the response. The basic plan is to put the intestinal tract at rest. If this stops the diarrhea, the patient is gradually titrated back to a normal diet after 12 hours.

Moderate diarrhea differs from mild by having some degree of dehydration. Oral therapy may be successful, but close observation is required to be sure that intravenous fluids are not required to correct the dehydration. Vomiting is frequently associated with more severe diarrheal conditions. This would preclude the use of oral fluids in the initial management.

Severe diarrhea merits hospitalization and intravenous fluid therapy. Then the patient should be maintained on appropriate intravenous fluids for 24 hours after the diarrhea stops while receiving no oral feedings. After 24 hours, clear liquids should be offered by the method previously described and the intravenous fluids discontinued when the oral feedings seem to be tolerated (Table 15-5).

TABLE 15-4. Severity of Diarrhea Based on Weight Loss

Onset	Mild	Moderate	Severe
Acute*	3%	3–6%	> 6%
Chronic†	10%	10–20%	>20%

*Weight loss/24 hr
†Weight loss/2 wk

TABLE 15-5. Treatment of Nonspecific Diarrhea

Therapy	Mild (hours)	Moderate (hours)	Severe (hours)
Correction of dehydration and acidosis with IV therapy	0	0–24	24–48 hr
↓	↓	↓	↓
Trial of oral clear liquids	12–24	12–24	24 hrs
↓	↓	↓	↓
¼ strength milk (full liquids for older children)	0	0–12	24 hrs
↓	↓	↓	↓
½ strength milk (soft diet for older children)	12–24	12–24	24 hrs
↓	↓	↓	↓
Full strength milk (full diet for older children)	As desired		

Note: If diarrhea recurs, return to preceding step or step 2 and advance more slowly.

TABLE 15-6. Etiologies of Treatment Failure

Problem	Mechanism	Solution
Damaged brush border membrane plus increased unabsorbed osmotically active substance	Damaged intestinal brush border membrane, increased intraluminal unabsorbed osmotically active substance	Dilute formula
Acquired lactase deficiency	Increased intraluminal unabsorbed osmotically active substance	Change from formula containing lactose to one with a different sugar
Steatorrhea	Intestinal microorganisms, diarrhea due to hydroxy-fatty acids, hypersecretory state	Use formula with medium chain triglycerides
Cow's milk protein intolerance	Unknown mechanisms	Change to milk providing soy protein
Chronic idiopathic diarrhea	Unknown mechanisms	Hyperalimentation

This routine is generally successful. However, diarrhea may again commence with realimentation. If this is so, possible mechanisms and solutions are suggested in Table 15-6.

BIBLIOGRAPHY

Hodes HL: Gastroenteritis with special reference to rotavirus. Adv Pediatr 27:195, 1980

Nelson JD, Haltalin KC: Accuracy of diagnosis of bacterial diarrheal disease by clinical features. J Pediatr 78:519, 1971

A discussion of clinical features useful for differentiating bacterial from nonbacterial diarrhea.

Poley RJ: Chronic diarrhea in infants and children: Part I. South Med I 66:1035, 1973

Poley RJ: Chronic diarrhea in infants and children: Part II. South Med I 66:1133, 1973

A review of the diseases responsible for most chronic diarrheal syndromes with special emphasis on pathophysiology.

Dehydration and Fluid Replacement

16

John S. Curran

Few entities in clinical pediatrics demand greater attention to detail than the management of infants with dehydration. Application of principles of rational fluid management tempered with a knowledge of fluid and electrolyte depletion states enable the physician to evaluate logically, investigate, and assemble a mode of therapy tailored to the individual patient. No single "cook book" approach to the dehydrated patient exists; however, sufficient latitude exists because of intrinsic lung, renal, and endocrine homeostatic mechanisms that mean values may be given as empiric guides to therapy.

Dehydration may perhaps be defined best as a net loss of body water and salts engendered by a pathologic or environmental state. Dehydration is never a primary disorder in itself. Salt loss is not only restricted to the major cations (sodium and potassium) but includes other cations such as calcium and magnesium in addition to anions such as chloride. Since most disease states leading to dehydration as a primary or secondary disorder produce their effect first on extracellular water and then upon intracellular fluid, greatest emphasis must be placed on three elements of dehydration—water, sodium, and potassium.

Pathologic states which frequently result in dehydration are listed in Table 16-1 along with the relative contribution of the three basic mechanisms.

EFFECTS AND TYPES OF DEHYDRATION

The effects of dehydration upon the patient and correlation with his chemical state can perhaps be appreciated by a consideration of the disturbances in the so-called internal environment. Basically, the disturbances are of five types, which are found in the following list; the primary contribution is from the first two.

Disturbances in Dehydration

1. ↓ Circulating blood volume → ↓ output → diminished perfusion-effects on multiple organ systems esp. CNS, renal, pulmonary, cardiac.
2. Acute Δ body fluid osmolality → altered CNS function via either cerebral edema or intracellular dehydration; impaired cellular integrity end function.
3. ↑ (H^+) via intracellular − extracellular (H^+) shifts → systemic acidemia and metabolic acidosis → altered CNS regulation of respiration, altered renal regulation of (H^+), altered cellular and enzymatic function in all body systems.
4. Loss of intracellular ions − (K^+), (Mg^{++}) → altered cardiac and neuromuscular contractility.
5. Interchange of extracellular fluid ions ⇄ skeletal pool (predominantly Ca^{++}).

The major disturbances that require therapeutic assistance from the clinical practitioner are restricted to changes of volume and osmolality. Given correction of these

TABLE 16-1. Pathologic States Producing Dehydration

Disorder	Pathogenetic Mechanisms ↑ Loss H_2O	↑ Loss salts	↓ Intake
Diarrhea	+	+	±
Anorexia	0	0	+
Vomiting	+	+	+
Fever	+	+	±
Hyperventilation	+	0	0
Excess renal solute load	+	±	±
Diabetes mellitus	+	+	±
Diabetes insipidus	+	+	− ↑
Adrenocortical insufficiency	±	+	±
Burns	+	+	+
Salt-losing renal diseases			
Postobstructive	+ +	+	0
Medullary cystic diseases	+	+	0
Iatrogenica Pediatrica	+	+	+
Hyperosmolal contrast media	+	+	±
Hypertonic bicarbonate, mannitol	+	±	0
Emetics	+	+	0
Induced hyperglycemia	+	+	±
Radiant warmers in neonate	+	0	±
Prematurity	+	0	+
Diuretic overutilization	+	+	±

+—positive effect
±—variable
0—no definite effect

disturbances, body homeostatic mechanisms usually readjust the latter three except in pathologic states with lung, renal, or endocrine disease. Clinically, the disturbances in osmolality have given rise to three classic types of dehydration disorders (Table 16-2).

Fundamental to understanding the occurrence of dehydration is the principle that dehydration will only occur if intake (fluid + electrolyte) < output + insensible losses, that is:

intake = output + insensible loss → normal state of hydration

Diarrhea, Anorexia, Vomiting } intake < output + insensible loss → dehydration

intake > output + insensible loss → overhydration

Assessment of dehydration *per se* requires scrupulous attention to details of the antecedent history, physical findings, and objective measurements. Expertise is manifest by prompt recognition of the primary disorder causing dehydration, magnitude, and judgment as to the type of dehydration from details of the history and physical examination. In this way prompt institution of an appropriate fluid and electrolyte therapy may be begun in the emergency room environment without undue dependence upon laboratory studies and results.

Basically, the three types of dehydration may be divided into two major groups which can be differentiated clinically prior to knowing electrolytes or osmolality values. Specific details are enumerated in Table 16-3.

Table 16-3 can be summarized by emphasizing that the signs of hypertonic de-

TABLE 16-2. Clinical Class of Dehydration

Disorder	Ratio salt/water (relative to plasma)	Osmolality	Serum (Na +)
1. Isotonic	Loss salt/water - equal	270–285 mOsm/l	131–144 mEq/l
2. Hypotonic	Loss salt>water	↓	<130 mEq/l
3. Hypertonic	Loss water>salt	↑	>145 mEq/l

hydration are different from those of hypotonic or isotonic dehydration because of the relative preservation of circulating blood volume in the presence of hyperosmolarity. Since sodium is primarily an extracellular cation, water is drawn into the interstitial and intravascular space to maintain circulating volume at the expense of cellular desiccation, particularly of the brain and skin. This provides perfusion and prevents the occurence of many of the signs associated with the hypotension seen in the other types of dehydration. Nevertheless, children with hypertonic dehydration rapidly pass into hypovolemic shock when body compensatory mechanisms have been exhausted.

With hypernatremia (hyperosmolar syndrome), circulation is not affected until late in the disease. Often there are neurologic symptoms, and hypocalcemic tetany can occur frequently with treatment. Renal tubular necrosis also may occur. If sodium is greater than 150 mEq/l in 50% of patients, there may be hyperglycemia. Most patients have moderately severe metabolic acidosis if enteric disease is present. Metabolic acidemia (release of H^+ from desiccated cells) is frequent.

The clinical estimation of the magnitude of dehydration can, of course, be easily assessed if a recent weight of the patient is known:

$$\frac{PRW - pw}{PW} \times 100 = \%\ \text{dehydration}$$

Rarely is there such objective evidence so one must rely on the following clinical approximations for determining the severity of *acute* dehydration:

1. Extracellular fluid loss
   Mild—Early minimal signs (? dehydration): positive history, intake less than output and insensible loss and a less than 5% decrease in body weight.
2. Extracellular fluid loss + intravascular fluid loss
   Moderate—Early circulatory impairment: classic signs (See Table 16-3) as well as a 10% decrease in body weight.
3. Extracellular fluid loss + intravascular fluid loss + Cardiovascular signs and shock
   Severe—Circulatory collapse: moribund and a 10%–15% decrease in body weight.

TREATMENT

Successful therapy of dehydration mandates consideration of the etiologic process(es) causing dehydration as outlined in Table 16-1. Dehydration is a secondary process preceded by one or more pathologic states. Correction of dehydration requires thorough understanding of normal daily fluid, electrolyte, and glucose requirements, estimation of deficits, and estimation of con-

TABLE 16-3. Comparison of Clinical Findings

Symptoms & Signs	Hypotonic (hypoosmolar)	Isotonic (isoosmolar)	Hypertonic (hyperosmolar)
History			
Fever	±	±	+ +
↓ intake	+	+	+
↓ urine output	+	+	+
Weight loss	+	+	+
Improper formula	Too dilute	−	Salt added or too little water
Physical examination			
Pulse*	↑	↑	± ↑ to normal
Respiration (if acidemic)	↑	↑	↑
Blood pressure*	↓ ↓	↓	Normal to ↓ late
Neurologic status*	Coma, lethargic	Lethargic	Irritable, restless
Seizures	May occur rarely	Uncommon	Usually occur late
Stiff neck	−	−	Common
Fontanelle	Sunken, soft	Sunken, soft	Not sunken till late
Skin*			
Color	Pallor	Pallor	May be flushed
Temperature	Cold	Cold	May be warm
Turgor	Creases, tenting	Tenting	"Doughy"
Mucous membranes	Slightly moist	Dry	Parched

+ = Present ↑ = Increased
± = Variable ↓ = Decreased
− = Absent

*Indicates major differential points between hyperosmolar dehydration and others

tinuing losses. This can be exemplified by the therapeutic equation:

fluid + electrolyte required =
maintenance + ongoing losses + replacement

Calculation of fluid requirements can be done in a number of different ways: per kilogram (varies with weight), per meter^2 (surface area), and by water requirements for each 100 kcalories metabolized. Each method has its advantages and disadvantages but the methods utilizing surface area and weight are more simple (Table 16-4).

Deficits of water and electrolytes may be estimated from Tables 16-5 and 16-6. In addition, the assessment of ongoing losses may necessitate consideration of the electrolyte content of various body fluids.

Therapeutic management of dehydration demands attention to three phases of correction: emergency, repletion, and recovery. Figure 16-1 is an example of the approach to the dehydrated patient in the emergency phase.

Reassessment and Repletion

Hypernatremic Dehydration. After urine output has been reestablished for two to four hours, start K^+, 40 mEq/l. To determine the total fluid loss, calculate: deficit + ongoing loss + 2–3 days maintenance. Plan the total correction in 48–72 hours (if $Na^+ > 160$ mEq/l correct over 72 hours or more) and administer fluids evenly throughout the entire 48–72 hours. These fluids should consist of Na^+ 40–75 mEq/l, usually as NaCl. [Rarely, in association with

TABLE 16-4. Maintenance Requirements

		H_2O (ml)		Na^+(mEq)		K^+(mEq)		Glucose (g)	
Wt in kg	SA (m)^2	Per kg	Per m^2	Per kg	Per m^2	Per kg	Per m^2	Per kg	Per m^2
3	0.20	100	1500	3	60	2	50	6–10	150
5	0.27	90	1500	3	60	2	50	6–10	150
10	0.45	75	1500	3	60	2	50	6–10	150
15	0.64	65	1500	–	60	–	50	—	150
30	1.10	55	1500	–	60	–	50	—	150
50	1.50	45	1500	–	60	–	50	—	150
70	1.73	40	1500	–	60	–	50	—	150

* Surface area may be approximated if a nomogram is not available by the equation SA (m)^2 = $0.1 + \frac{\text{wt in lbs}}{60}$ for children.

TABLE 16-5. Deficits of Water and Electrolytes: Moderate Dehydration (Assumed 10% Dehydration)

		Per kg body weight		
Disorder	H_2O (ml)	Na^+ (mEq)	K^+ (mEq)	Cl^- (mEq)
Fasting and thirsting	100–120	5–7	1–2	4–6
Diarrhea				
Isotonic	100–120	8–10	8–10	8–10
Hypotonic	100–120	10–12	8–10	10–12
Hypertonic	100–120	2–4	0–4	−2 to −6
Pyloric stenosis	100–120	8–10	10–12	10–12
Diabetic acidosis	100–120	8–10	5–7	6–8

TABLE 16-6. Electrolyte Content of Body Fluids

Source	Na^+ (mEq/l)	K^+ (mEq/l)	Cl^- (mEq/l)
Gastric juice	20–80	5–20	100–150
Pancreatic	120–140	5–15	90–120
Small intestine	100–140	5–15	90–130
Bile	120–140	5–15	80–120
Ileostomy	45–135	3–15	20–115
Diarrhea	10–90	10–80	10–110
Sweat			
Normal	10–30	3–10	10–35
Cystic fibrosis	50–130	5–25	50–110
Burns	140	5	110

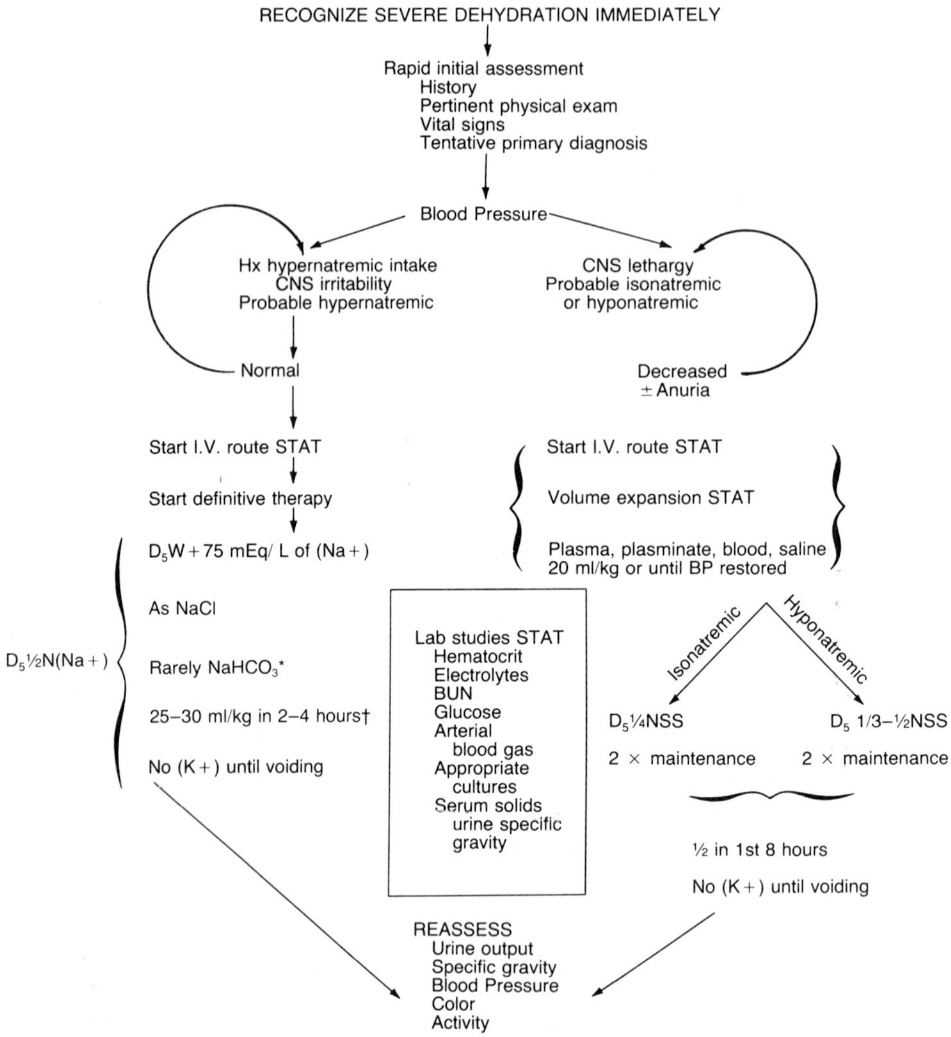

D_5¼NSS = 40 mEq Na+/L with 5% glucose/water

D_5 1/3NSS = 50 mEq Na+/L with 5% glucose/water

D_5½NSS = 75 mEq Na+/L with 5% glucose/water

Fig. 16-1. An approach to the dehydrated patient in the emergency phase. *See text, p. 169. †See p. 166 for subsequent therapy.

severe acidosis ($< pH7.1$), the administration of $NaHCO_3$ up to one-fourth of total (Na^+) solute may be considered, recognizing that its use may be associated with paradoxical CNS and other tissue acidosis.] Severe hypernatremia > 180mEq/l mandate Na^+ solute density up to 120mEq/l. Optimally, the decrease in plasma Na should not exceed 0.5 mEq/l/h. Check calcium and if it has decreased, you may use 10% calcium gluconate, 1 ml/kg, slowly while the heart is monitored.

Isonatremic Dehydration. After the initial reestablishment of perfusion, give one-half the first day's fluid + electrolyte within eight hours. The total should equal two times the maintenance for the first day as D5¼NSS. Potassium should be added only after voiding; give one-and-one-half to two times maintenance and do not exceed 40 mEq/l.

On the second day, give one-and-one-half times the maintenance volume of fluid. Usually this is given as D5¼NSS (40 mEq Na^+/l). Follow closely the electrolytes, urine output, and urine-specific gravity.

Plan on total rehydration within 2 to 3 days. Usually oral realimentation can begin on the second day. Deduct 50% oral intake from the day's IV orders if the fluids are given combined IV and PO.

Hyponatremic Dehydration. After the initial stabilization of perfusion, continue with two times the maintenance volume, one-half in the first eight hours of D5 ⅓–½NSS (deduct the volume of plasma expander used from the total day's fluids). Add K^+, one-and-one-half to two times the maintenance volume. This should be added to fluids after voiding has been established. Follow the parameters listed under isonatremic dehydration so that total hydration will be established over 2 to 3 days. If seizures occur early in the disorder, use 3% NaCl, 1 ml/min intravenously up to a maximum of 12 ml/kg, until seizures stop.

Fluid and Electrolyte Calculation

As an example, take the case of a hypotensive, 10 kg infant with moderate to severe isonatremic dehydration:

Maintenance fluid/day =
$0.45 \times 1500 \text{ ml/m}^2 = 675$ ml
Deficit 10% depleted =
1000 ml, repair 2 days
Deficit Na^+ 80 mEq (10 kg × 8 mEq/kg)
K^+ 80 mEq (10 kg × 8 mEq/kg)
Maintenance Na^+ = 27 ($0.45 \times 60 \text{ mEq/m}^2$)
K^+ = 23 ($0.45 \times 50 \text{ mEq/m}^2$)
Plasma to expand 20 ml/kg × 10 kg = 200 ml
First day fluid total 675 + 500 ml = 1175 ml
Less 200 ml plasma −200 ml
975 ml

Give one-half this solution in the first 8 hours; this equals 61 ml/hr × 8 hours for a total of 488 ml. The second half is administered during the next 16 hours. This equals 31 (30.5) ml/hr × 16 hours for a total of 488 ml. The total for the 24 hours is 1176 ml.

The electrolyte content is determined by:

Maintenance Na^+ = 27 mEq
+ ½ deficit Na^+ = 40 mEq
67 mEq/1176 ml
= 57 mEq Na/L

Maintenance K^+ 23 mEq
+ ½ deficit K^+ 40 mEq
63 mEq/1176 ml
= 53 mEq K^+/L

But K^+ *cannot* exceed 40 mEq/l

Thus, the IV orders will read: 1000 ml D_5W + 57 mEgNaCl mEq NaCl + 40 mEq KCl to run at 61 ml/hr × 8 hours, then 31 ml/hr × 16 hours.

Much of the above cumbersome calculation can be avoided by simply figuring two times the maintenance fluid + electrolyte as D_5¼NSS (40 mEq/l) during the first 24 hours in isonatremic dehydration. Thus the calculation becomes:

$0.45 \times 1500\ ml/m^2 = 675\ ml$
$2 \times$ maintenance $= 1350\ ml$
Less $= -200\ ml$ plasma
$1150\ ml$

One-half in first 8 hours $= \frac{575\ ml}{8\ hours} = 72\ ml/hr \times 8$ hours

Second 16 hours $= \frac{575\ ml}{16\ hours} = 36\ ml/hr \times 16$ hours

Thus, the IV fluid is: 1000 ml D_5W + 40 mEq NaCl + 34 mEq KCl. The infusion rates are as above.

Principles to Remember

Certain principles should be followed if dehydration is to be treated successfully:

1. Treat hypotension aggressively.
2. Never give solute-free fluid.
3. Never give fluids rapidly to a patient with hypernatremic dehydration unless hypotension is present.
4. Fluid and electrolyte administration to the dehydrated patient serves to restore body homeostatic mechanisms. Calculations are necessarily imprecise and follow more the "art" than the "science" of medicine.
5. Never give potassium before the patient voids, because serious arrythmia may result.
6. Never forget to reassess the patient frequently with a physical examination hourly, or more frequently if need be.
7. Never base all treatment solely upon laboratory results but rather correlate them with clinical assessment of the patient.

There are a number of special fluid and electrolyte problems which do not fall into the framework previously outlined. These will be discussed. For brevity, they are presented in outline form.

A. Newborn infants (maintenance)
   1. Premature infant > 1500 g
      a. Maintenance fluid: 80–100 ml/kg/day
         Usually sodium and potassium not needed first day; 2nd and 3rd days, add 20 mEq Na^+/l; 4th day and thereafter 40 mEq/l. Begin maintenance K^+ (2 mEq/kg/day) 2nd day and thereafter.
      b. Fluid may be D_5W or $D_{10}W$. If $D_{10}W$ is used, monitor for glycosuria or hyperglycemia, particularly in sick infants.
      c. Increase fluids 1 ml/kg/hr for infants under radiant heaters.
      d. In infants receiving phototherapy and weighing > 1500 g add 1.4 ml/kg/hr
   2. Premature infants < 1500 g
      a. Maintenance fluid—start with 90 ml/kg/day. Salt administration as previously noted above, but may need major increase if critical.
      b. Always start D_5W, monitor as above and increase caloric content stepwise to $D_{10}W$ as per blood sugars and absence of glycosuria.
      c. Infants under radiant warmers:

         maintenance fluid

         <1,000 g add up to 50%
         1000–1500 g add 25%
      d. Phototherapy

         <1500 g add 1–2 ml/kg/hr
      e. Attempt to establish urine flow ~ 2ml/kg/hr, urine SG ~ 1.005 –1.010
   3. Term infants
      a. Fluid D_5W or $D_{10}W$ with salts as above

b. 70 ml/kg — Day #1
80 ml/kg — Day #2
90 ml/kg — Day #3
100 ml/kg — Day #4

B. Dehydrated newborns—treat as previously outlined
C. Vomiting
   1. Volume and composition as previously outlined
   2. Replace volume of vomitus or nasogastric drainage as equivalent to pysiologic saline as per Table 16-6.
D. Heat exhaustion
   1. Give fluids as D_5W glucose with 50–80 mEq Na^+/l. Volume as per dehydration.
E. Anuria
   1. Give 5%–10% DW at 400 ml/m^2 plus urinary losses.
   2. May be necessary to give fluid challenge prior to confirmation of diagnosis of anuria.
   3. Watch for hyperkalemia or hyponatremia. Appropriate therapy if present.
F. Inappropriate secretion of antidiuretic hormone—postoperative, with CNS disease, or trauma
   1. Establish diagnosis—hypo-osmolality with high urinary osmolality or specific gravity. Edema and overhydration may be present clinically.
   2. Treat with fluid restriction.
G. Cardiac disease with failure
   1. Clinical assessment (serial) with pharmacologic therapy and fluid restriction to less than maintenance until stabilized.
H. Fever: add 10% volume for each degree temperature elevation $>101°$.
I. CNS disease (head trauma, meningitis)
   1. High risk of syndrome of inappropriate antidiuretic hormone secretion.
   2. Restrict fluids in advance to $\frac{2}{3}$–$\frac{3}{4}$ maintenance, urine SG—1.010 to 1.015.

SUMMARY

The preceding presentation has demonstrated multiple facets of fluid balance in disease states. Intrinsic to the outlined therapy is the maintenance of an adequate intravascular fluid administration route for acute management of fluid and electrolyte deviations. One must never forget that an intravenous route places the patient in potential jeopardy if there are errors in medications, volumes, compositions, or rates of administration. Several axioms of intravenous maintenance must always be remembered:

1. Always establish a *secure* intravascular route in hypotensive patients.
2. Always interpose a pediatric administration set between a large volume of fluid and the patient to prevent accidental, rapid administration of large volumes.
3. Always limit the maximum amount of fluid directly connected to a patient to an 8-hour supply.
4. Always write IV orders clearly, legibly, and include all desired components.
5. Number IVs consecutively.
6. Treat IV sites as areas of potential infection and prepare accordingly before venipuncture; sterile technique should be maintained.
7. Rotate IV sites to minimize phlebitis.
8. Scalp needles are preferred to intravascular catheters since there is less risk of infection.
9. Never mix sodium bicarbonate and calcium in IV fluid.
10. Check for drug incompatibilities before mixing in infusate.

These recommendations should be regarded merely as guidelines. The repeated clinical assessment of the individual patient may dictate deviation from these suggestions.

BIBLIOGRAPHY

Barness LA, Young LN: A simplified view of fluid therapy. Pediatr Clin North Am 11:1091, 1964

Older but excellent brief overview of fluid therapy.

Clarke TA, *et al:* Hypernatremic dehydration resulting from inadequate breast-feeding. Pediatrics 63:931, 1979

Describes a new association with hypernatremia.

Finberg L: Hypernatremic (hypertonic) dehydration in infants. New Engl J Med 289:196, 1973

Review of hypernatremic dehydration.

Finberg L: The role of oral electrolyte-glucose solutions in hydration for children—international and domestic aspects. J Pediatr 96:51, 1980

Editorial review of practical information on oral hydration solutions.

Fortin J, Parent MA: Dehydration scoring system for infants. J Trop Pediatr 24:110, 1978

Practical scoring system for dehydration.

Kahn A, Brachet E, Blum D: Controlled fall in natremia and risk of seizures in hypertonic dehydration. Intensive Care Med 5:27, 1979

Prospective study to define rates of infusion and sodium decrement.

Kingston NE: Biochemical disturbances in breast-fed infants with gastroenteritis and dehydration. J Pediatr 82:1073, 1973

Large series studying special problems of dehydration in breast-fed infants.

Robson AM: Parenteral fluid therapy. In Vaughn VC, McKay RJ, Nelson WE (eds): Textbook of Pediatrics, pp. 250–270. Philadelphia, WB Saunders, 1975

Excellent overview of dehydration with valuable tables.

Rosenfeld W, de Romana GL, Kleinman Q, Finberg L: Improving the clinical management of hypernatremic dehydration. Clin Pediatr 16:411, 1977

Observations retrospectively from management of 67 infants.

Abnormalities of Urine

17

Edward R. Root
Lewis A. Barness

The routine urinalysis is a test ordered for many conditions and is part of the complete pediatric physical examination. When abnormal findings in the urine are approached systematically, the routine urinalysis is a most useful aid in differential diagnosis.

Early in their careers students should develop a standard method of examining urine. Some prefer no centrifugation while others prefer spun urines. The advantage of learning to look at unspun urine is that the variance of centrifugation need not affect one's standard.

Elements of a Routine Urinalysis

Specific gravity
Protein
pH
Sugar-reducing substance
Acetone
Red cells (test for blood optional)
White cells
Casts
Ferric chloride
Color
Odor

ELEMENTS OF A ROUTINE URINALYSIS

Specific Gravity

Specific gravity in children ranges normally between 1.000 and 1.036 on random specimens; therefore, a specific gravity in an isolated specimen is never abnormal. Specific gravity of 1.007 corresponds to an isotonic state or osmolality of 280 mOsm per liter (isosthenuria). Suspect a concentrating defect if the child has hypotonic urine in the first morning void, if he has a history of arising several times each night to drink or, if he always has large volumes of urine in the absence of glycosuria. (Low specific gravity is normal for infants less than 4 months of age.)

Osmolality, which measures osmotic work done by the kidneys, is preferable to specific gravity which is influenced by weight of solutes.

Among the causes of low specific gravity (hyposthenuria) are:

1. Dilutional states, *e.g.*, water intoxication and psychological polydipsia. The latter often resolves with counseling.

2. Pituitary (or central) diabetes insipidus—partial or complete lack of antidiuretic hormone (ADH). This may signify a brain tumor or hypothalamic injury. Differentiating central from psychogenic polydipsia, often difficult, is best evaluated by water deprivation, then by challenging patients with vasopressin. Central diabetes insipidus is treated by injecting or sniffing ADH or by taking oral chlorpropamide. The vasopressin analogue 1-deamino 8-D-arginine vasopressin (DDAVP) requires intranasal use only twice daily.
3. Nephrogenic diabetes insipidus—also related to ADH. Distal renal tubules respond to neither endogenous nor a trial of exogenous ADH (vasopressin). Low-sodium diet and diuretic may be used to diminish urine volume.
4. Sickle-cell disease and sickle-cell trait. When discovered early, the defect is reversible by transfusions of normal blood, but later, due to medullary infarcts, there is permanent loss of concentrating ability.
5. Other renal tubular defects. Obstructive nephropathy, polycystic kidney disease, renal amyloidosis and chronic pyelonephritis are renal structural causes of a concentrating defect. Electrolyte problems such as chronic hypokalemia (*e.g.*, in cystinosis, renal tubular acidosis, or Bartter's syndrome) or hypercalcemia (*e.g.*, in prolonged immobilization, vitamin D intoxication, or neoplasms) may lead to moderate, usually reversible, concentrating defects. Advanced chronic renal failure usually demonstrates polyuria and inability to maximally concentrate the urine. Thus, patients with chronic renal failure may develop dehydration if not allowed free access to water.
6. Diarrhea in infants. This is perhaps a failure of secretion of ADH. In spite of dehydration, the patient excretes dilute urine.

High urinary specific gravities are appropriate in instances of hypovolemia. Burn patients and those with dehydration exhibit elevated urinary specific gravity. Inappropriately high urinary concentration is seen with plasma hypotonicity in the syndrome of inappropriate ADH secretion, which occasionally accompanies pulmonary or CNS disorders. Elevated urinary osmolalities are also seen in patients with glycosuria and proteinuria, and in patients who have received radiocontrast materials.

*p*H of Urine

*p*H varies normally from about 4.5 to 7.5, so that any isolated urinary *p*H is normal. Urine *p*H assumes significance in several clinical situations, the most important of which is obtaining a *p*H of 6.5 or higher when the *p*H of the blood is less than 7.2. This occurs when the kidney is unable to establish an adequate hydrogen ion gradient in the distal tubule, leading to deficient hydrogen ion excretion—distal or classic renal tubular acidosis. In proximal renal tubular acidosis, urinary acidification to maximal levels is possible since the defect is a low bicarbonate threshold in the proximal tubule. However, this does not affect the ability of the distal tubule to establish an adequate hydrogen ion gradient.

The proximal tubule is concerned with the reabsorption of isotonic saline, glucose, amino acids, and phosphorus. Both proximal and distal tubules regulate *p*H by exchanging hydrogen ion for sodium in the tubule lumen, and by converting secreted ammonia to ammonium. It is helpful to know the distinctions between proximal and distal acidosis (see Table 17-1).

Another clinically important use of urinary *p*H determination occurs in those children, particularly newborn or young infants, whose urinary *p*H persists at approximately 4.5 with a serum *p*H less than 7.2. It is normal for infants fed human milk or milk with less than 1.5 g protein/dl to have a urine *p*H of 6.5 or higher. If particularly low *p*H is found, it may be considered that the child has a metabolic error.

Lactic acid is a normal metabolic product in the glycolytic pathway. It accumulates in exercise but may become excessive, especially in states of anoxemia, or with decreases in perfusion, especially in shock. Hyperosmotic states, such as diabetic ketoacidosis, also produce lactic acidemia. Attention should be directed to the cause; treatment of lactic acidemia with sodium bicarbonate may increase hyperosmolality and worsen the patient's condition. Because CO_2 (as carbonic acid) rapidly traverses the cerebrospinal fluid while HCO_3 enters more slowly, addition of bicarbonate in the presence of lactic acidosis causes a rise in serum *p*H but a fall in CSF *p*H and may be responsible for central nervous system deterioration during such treatment.

Other causes of resistant acidosis include: methylmalonic acidemia, propionic acidemia, maple syrup urine disease, lactic-pyruvic acidemia, isovaleric acidemia, and others.

Since all of these may be amenable to treatment, specific diagnosis should be reached rapidly by identifying the acids in the urine or serum. Some patients with methylmalonic acidemia respond to vitamin B_{12}, some with propionic acid to biotin, and some with maple syrup urine disease or branched-chain amino aciduria respond to dietary management. Other patients with lactic-pyruvic acidemia may respond to thiamin, while those with isovaleric acidemia may respond to dietary management. Acidosis of metabolic cause should be accompanied by acid urine.

Urine *p*H can be either alkaline or acid in patients with metabolic alkalosis, usually accompanied by hypokalemia due to renal potassium losses. Two categories of metabolic alkalosis have different etiologies. A sodium chloride deficient type is seen with vomiting, diarrhea, diuretic therapy, or cystic fibrosis. A mineralocorticord excess type is caused by hyperaldosteronism, Cushing's syndrome, or Bartter's syndrome. Clinically, the two categories can be distinguished by

TABLE 17-1. Proximal and Distal Renal Tubular Acidosis

	Proximal	Distal
Presenting complaint	Failure to thrive Hyperchloremic acidosis Vomiting, constipation, diarrhea	Failure to thrive Hyperchloremic acidosis Vomiting, constipation, diarrhea Urolithiasis Nephrocalcinosis Osteomalacia
Urine *p*H	As low as 4.5–5.0	Never below 6.0
Causes	Idiopathic Cystinosis Lowe's syndrome Wilson's disease Galactosemia Fructose intolerance Tyrosinemia Lightwood's syndrome Poisons	Idiopathic Malnutrition Hyperparathyroidism Vitamin D intoxication Fabry's disease Hyperthyroidism Renal tubular necrosis Medullary sponge kidney Poisons
Inheritance of idiopathic	Mainly males	Autosomal dominant
Age of onset	0–2 years	2 years +
Bicarbonate requirement	>6 mEq/kg/day	<2 mEq/kg/day
Prognosis of idiopathic	Reversible	Permanent

a spot urine chloride determination (except when diuretics have been administered within 36 hr). Less than 10 mEq/1 indicates sodium chloride depletion and greater than 20 mEq/1 indicates mineralocorticord excess. Postprandial urine *p*H may be elevated temporarily due to the alkaline tide. Very high urinary *p*H may indicate presence of urea-splitting bacteria such as proteus and calls for urine culture.

Protein

Beyond the neonatal period, children normally excrete 60 mg/m²/24 hr. Teenagers excrete up to 300 mg protein per 24 hours, but by adulthood the normal excretion is less than 60 mg/m²/24 hr. Abnormally high total 24-hour urinary protein excretion (obtained at bedrest) suggests renal disease. There is a general but unreliable correlation between size of the urinary protein molecule and degree of glomerular damage, for example, if the protein is mainly albumin, a relatively small molecule, the glomerular damage is generally less than that which produces globulinuria. The following must be considered:

Nephritis. (Refer to section on *Hematuria* if hematuria is prominent or if hypertension, renal insufficiency, or red cell casts are present.) Most nephritides develop varying degrees of proteinuria: patients with Berger's IgA nephropathy may have normal protein excretion, whereas patients with severe nephritides with guarded prognosis, such as membranoproliferative glomerulonephritis, may present as nephritic nephrotics, exhibiting full-blown nephrotic syndrome.

Nephritides may present with *only* proteinuria and no nephrotic syndrome. These include lupus nephritis, focal segmental glomerulosclerosis, membranoproliferative and tubulo-interstitial nephritis. Significant urinary protein excretion may be an indication for renal biopsy.

Nephrotic syndrome and nephrosis. (Refer to Chapter 19, "Edema and Hypertension" if proteinuria is severe enough to cause edema or serum changes such as hypoalbuminemia and hyperlipidemia.) Some other causes of the nephrotic syndrome are listed below. The prognosis for these is related to the prognosis for the underlying disease.

Congenital Nephrosis. Apparently inherited as an autosomal recessive disease congenital nephrosis manifests proteinuria and edema in the first few weeks of life. Treatment is ineffective.

Renal Vascular Occlusion. Children with sepsis or kidney trauma, and in particular, infants born of diabetic mothers may develop proteinuria and the nephrotic syndrome. Usually an enlarged kidney can be felt. Renal arteriograms, umbilical aortogram, and intravenous pyelogram aid in diagnosis. Some resolve spontaneously, though removal of the kidney may be necessary. Some children with sickle-cell disease may develop the nephrotic syndrome probably secondary to renal vascular occlusion.

Polycystic Disease and Renal Dysplastic Disease. Anatomic kidney abnormalities, including varying degrees of renal agenesis, may present only with proteinuria. As the child gets older, serum proteins decrease and the nephrotic syndrome ensues.

Collagen-Vascular Diseases. (See Hematuria.) Children with collagen-vascular diseases may present with proteinuria and the nephrotic syndrome, but the urinary abnormality first noted is usually hematuria.

Obstructive Uropathy. Children with obstructive uropathy and hydronephrosis may develop proteinuria and abdominal masses. Frequently, a renal tumor is suspected but pyelograms lead to correct diagnosis. When infection or the nephrotic syndrome supervenes, the diagnosis is usually more obvious. Occasionally, pyelonephritis alone may present as the nephrotic syndrome.

Metabolic Disease. Some children with diabetes develop severe renal disease (Kimmelstiel-Wilson syndrome) with the nephrotic syndrome.

Poisons. Multiple poisons, particularly heavy metals, cause tubular damage, protein loss, and the development of the nephrotic syndrome.

Structural Anomalies of the Kidneys. Structural anomalies may be present with no urinary abnormalities and are detected only when signs of renal failure ensue. When other causes of proteinuria are not discovered, structural anomalies should be sought. These include polycystic disease, hydronephrosis, renal tumors, and obstructive disease.

Renal Tubular Disease. (See *p*H of the Urine.) Proteinuria is found in renal tubular acidosis and renal tubular necrosis.

Toxins. A variety of toxins cause tubular disease and result in proteinuria. This occurs in ingestion of heavy metals, papillary necrosis, and metabolic diseases, especially aminoacidurias and galactosemia.

Orthostatic Disease. Some children, particularly those with lordosis, develop proteinuria on standing, presumably because of renal venous congestion. The child should be tested after lying down and after exercise. Many otherwise normal children excrete protein after vigorous exercise. These children do not have renal disease.

Fever. Infants and children with fever and no renal disease may have 2 to 3+ proteinuria.

Heart Failure. Proteinuria in children with heart failure is apparently also due to renal venous congestion.

Hematuria. In the presence of hematuria, protein from the red cells results in a positive test for protein. Centrifuging the urine and testing the supernate gives a truer test for protein. Proteinuria without hematuria is much more likely to be benign than that associated with hematuria. Even more striking for prognosis, hematuria alone is more frequently a reversible finding than hematuria associated with proteinuria.

Summary. If the proteinuria is of short duration, the child should be tested for orthostatic proteinuria and observed for the possibility of febrile proteinuria. If the patient's condition is inconsistent with these, the diagnosis should be pursued. Most frequently the patient has an acute poststreptococcal glomerulonephritis with other urinary and physical findings that are consistent with this diagnosis: edema, hypertension, elevated antistreptolysin titer, hematuria, red cell casts.

If these are not present, intravenous pyelogram and renal biopsy may be helpful. The type of protein in the urine may help in the prognosis of some diseases; for example, if the protein is mainly albumin, a relatively small molecule, the tubular damage is generally less than that which produces globulinuria. Tests for type of protein require electrophoresis.

Reducing Substance

In pediatrics, any reducing substance in the urine is important. The testing papers containing glucose oxidase identify only glucose. Therefore, if a paper is used to determine pH, protein, acetone, sugar, and blood, the urine must be tested at least once to measure for reducing substances with clinitest or similar agents.

Glucose is the most common reducing substance. Excessive glucose ingestion may cause elevated blood sugar. When glucosuria is present, blood sugar should be determined. Glucosuria is found in the following conditions:

Diabetes Mellitus. Generally, a glucose tolerance test should be abnormal before making a diagnosis of diabetes mellitus.

Poisons, Particularly Heavy Metals. History, specific tests for heavy metals and other urinary abnormalities should be sought. Glucosuria from metal poisoning, like proteinuria, is due to tubular damage. Some poisons have specific antidotes; for example, copper can be chelated with penicillamine or lead with EDTA. Other poisonings can be reversed by removing the poison.

Increased Intracranial Pressure. The mechanism by which increased intracranial pressure causes glycosuria is poorly understood. It is usually associated with hyperglycemia.

Adrenal Cortical Excess, Cushing's Syndrome. Cortisol is gluconeogenic and causes hyperglycemia.

Low Renal Threshold. Usually renal tubules can reabsorb sugar when the blood sugar does not exceed 180-200 mg/dl. For unknown causes, in some children, maximal tubular reabsorption of glucose is decreased and glucosuria occurs at lower levels of blood sugar. Such children are usually normal otherwise, though some may fail to thrive due to caloric loss.

Renal Tubular Disease, Fanconi's Syndrome. Any renal tubular disease may cause glycosuria. In the autosomal recessive disease cystinosis (Fanconi's syndrome), cystine crystals are stored in the lysosomes of all tissues; in addition to glycosuria, infants develop polyuria, aminoaciduria, rickets, and renal tubular acidosis. The condition is seen in adolescents as a milder disease and in adults with few symptoms. Cystine crystals appear in the corneas.

Reducing substances other than glucose include the following: *galactose,* which may be the first sign of galactosemia. The presence of *lactose* usually is due to excessive ingestion. The presence of *pentose* occurs as a recessively inherited condition with no known disease. The presence of *ascorbic acid* is due to excessive ingestion. Reducing *amino acids* such as in alcaptonuria may be present. *Fructose* in the urine may occur in children with fructose intolerance, but usually this is due to excessive ingestion.

Whenever reducing substances are found, they must be identified and quantitated. Diabetes mellitus, of all the causes, must be considered first.

Ketonuria

Ketonuria is easily tested with nitroprusside-containing papers. This condition occurs whenever a considerable proportion of the child's energy needs are obtained from fat rather than from sugar. Likely causes of ketonuria are: diabetes with insulinopenia, persistent vomiting, starvation, reducing diet, heavy exercise, fever, lead poisoning, glycogen-storage disease, and hyperinsulinism with hypoglycemia. Sometimes in the very young, any of these causes may be present without ketonuria. The mechanism of the lack of ketonuria is obscure.

Aspirin poisoning may produce vomiting, dehydration, and ketonuria. In addition, the breakdown products of salicylates may alter the color of the nitroprusside. If so, urine may be boiled first, removing the acetone. It is better to test for salicylates with ferric chloride.

Hematuria

Normally 0-1 red cell may be present in the urine in a high-power field. If the fresh urine occult blood test is positive but there are few intact red cells in the sediment, consider hemoglobinuria or myoglobinuria. Blood in the urine of pubertal females may be of menstrual origin.

Sources of hematuria are most often either renal or urologic:

Glomerulonephritis (Renal). Acute postinfections glomerulonephritis may occur following many types of infections including staphylococcus, leptospirosis, scarlet fever, mononucleosis, mycoplasma pneumonia, and viral infections. However, the most common nephritis in childhood and the most common of the postinfectious nephritides is that which follows a streptococcal infection.

Acute Poststreptococcal Glomerulonephritis. About 7 to 14 days after a streptococcal infection of the throat or skin, a child 2 or more years old may develop headache and hematuria. Edema, vomiting, fever, and abdominal pain may occur. In addition to hematuria, proteinuria is found. White cells may be present early. Most children develop hypertension. Oliguria and renal failure may occur. At the onset, BUN, creatinine, erythrocyte sedimentation rate (ESR), and streptococcal enzymes are elevated and C-3 complement is decreased. ANA should be checked to rule out systemic lupus erythematosus, the modern "great masquerader."

The complications of the acute period of hematuria may be severe and are the same as for acute renal failure—hypertension secondary to fluid overload and hyperkalemia. Usually salt and water restriction and aggressive use of antihypertensives are indicated. However, occasionally in a child dehydrated from previous vomiting, oliguria and hypertension may be corrected by judiciously replacing the calculated deficit. If the child is edematous or weighs more than his usual weight, this should not be attempted since he is already overloaded with fluid.

Penicillin is usually prescribed if there is evidence of ongoing streptococcal infection.

ASO titer elevation, ESR elevation, and hematuria persist several months but do not indicate an unfavorable prognosis.

If C-3 does not return to normal by 4 to 6 weeks from onset, membranoproliferative or lupus nephritis must be considered. Restriction of activity is generally not necessary unless the patient is very edematous; increases in hematuria with activity do not alter the prognosis and are reflections of the disease rather than contributors to the nephritis. Almost all these children recover. However, if anuria or severe renal insufficiency (GRF less than 15%) occurs, or if the patient does not improve 10 to 14 days after onset of the illness, another diagnosis should be sought, preferably by renal biopsy.

Membranoproliferative Glomerulonephritis. The pathologic entity of membranoproliferative glomerulonephritis may start clinically like poststreptococcal glomerulonephritis or may present as nephrotic syndrome, especially in older children, or as isolated proteinuria noted on a routine urinalysis. Hematuria is usually present. The disease is generally progressive over months or a few years with gradual loss of renal function, perhaps accompanied by nephrotic syndrome and hypertension. Some patients experience intervals of disease quiescence. C-3 is either constantly or intermittently depressed in certain of these patients. C-3 nephritic factor and partial lipodystrophy are associated with one type of this disease.

Rapidly Progressive Glomerulonephritis. Clinical presentation of rapidly progressive glomerulonephritis may be as a severe acute poststreptococcal glomerulonephritis with hypertension and severely compromised renal function; indeed, one form of the disease is like acute poststreptococcal glomerulonephritis pathologically but with crescents surrounding more than 60% of the glomeruli. Occasionally, the disease presents with severe hypertension or even late in the course as vomiting associated with uremia.

Treatment is supportive. Pulses of methyl prednisolone, if instituted early enough, reverse the disease to a great extent.

Hereditary Nephritis. Most often manifested as Alport's syndrome, hereditary nephritis usually presents in males in their second decade, with gross hematuria, mild or moderate renal failure, and perhaps hypertension. There is usually a history of deafness in the patient or his male relatives. Audiometry confirms the presence of high-tone sensorineural hearing loss. Also suggestive is a finding of microscopic hematuria in female relatives.

Inheritance appears to be autosomal dominant with preferential segregation of the somatic gene with the X-chromosome. Thus, more females have the disease but for unknown reasons they are usually much less severely affected. Males develop progressive renal failure eventually requiring dialysis or transplantation. There is no known treatment for the disease itself, which appears to involve defective basement membrane synthesis.

Pyelonephritis, Cystitis, Vaginitis, Urethritis. In both pyelonephritis and cystitis, pyuria is more common than hematuria. Hematuria occurs, particularly with tuberculous infections of the kidney, coliform or viral infections of the bladder. Bubble baths and infection with pinworms, particularly in females, may cause vaginitis or cystitis. Look for foreign bodies, especially in the uretha, which should be observed for prolapse.

Neoplasms, Polyps, Bladder Tumors. Tumors anywhere in the urinary tract may cause hematuria. First consider more common causes such as glomerulonephritis or pyelonephritis before diagnostic studies are used. These studies, such as cystoscopy, may hurt the child.

Trauma. Trauma to any part of the urinary tract causes hematuria. Trauma may occur following a blow to the kidney or bladder area, or after introduction of foreign bodies. Children who have been battered may present with hematuria. If battering is suspected, the child should be admitted to the hospital and protective services notified. Investigation and treatment of the hematuria should be instituted, including a bone survey for fractures or other evidence of battering or neglect.

A psychosocial history should be obtained to determine methods of discipline, parent-child and parent-parent relationships, and parents' ability to escape temporarily from the child's needs. Psychiatric consultation should be obtained early. The battered child needs more frequent follow-up than most children, and the physician should participate in the decisions regarding disposition and care of the child before discharge. Placement of the child may be necessary.

Trauma to the kidney can result in rupture with extravasation or intrarenal bleeding. Bladder or urethral rupture can result in intra- or extraperitoneal bleeding. In addition to hematuria, there may be pain or palpable masses. Radiograms, including urograms, reveal the extent of injury or possible pelvic fracture.

Calculi. Calculi and disease in which crystals are formed can cause hematuria. Certain toxic substances including drugs such as sulfonamides cause crystal formation. In children with fever and dehydration, hematuria may occur that is possibly due to crystal formation by urates, phosphates, or oxalates.

Collagen-Vascular Disease. The collagen-vascular diseases are multisystemic; children develop joint pains, skin rashes, arthritis, and gastrointestinal and kidney involvement. Hematuria as part of the presentation may occur in children with any of these diseases.

In children with rheumatoid arthritis, fever and arthritis of one joint or of many joints may be the initial complaint. A fleeting salmon-colored skin rash and painful subcutaneous skin nodules may occur. Some children develop iridocyclitis or pericarditis. Positive laboratory findings include elevated ESR and other acute phase reactants as well as the presence of histocompatibility antigen HLA B27. Antinuclear antibodies and rheumatoid factor may be present.

Treatment should be directed to maintaining and avoiding deformities. Aspirin, 60–130 mg/kg/day, usually controls symptoms although prednisone or other anti-inflammatory agents may be necessary.

Systemic lupus erythematosus. SLE is one of the causes of glomerulonephritis in childhood. Patients with severe renal involvement may mimic acute poststreptococcal glomerulonephritis, but the typical presentation is in a teenage girl with a vague history of a month or more of nonspecific malaise, tiredness or joint aches and pains. The "butterfly" malar rash may be present in a minority of patients. Other presentations for lupus include purpura, vomiting, headache, edema, gross hematuria, sinusitis, otitis media, abdominal pain, chorea, catatonia, and psychiatric illness. ANA and Sm-antibody are positive. C-3 and C-4 depression may reflect the degree of renal involvement. Occult renal involvement and progression with time can be detected by biopsy.

Mild cases of lupus without severe renal involvement can be treated symptomatically. More severe cases should be treated with prednisone 2 mg/kg/day up to 80 mg every morning from 4 to 8 weeks. Thereafter, withdraw the steroid gradually, always watching for relapses. Cyclophosphamide may help some patients who do poorly. Pulses of methylprednisolone may achieve control. Plasmapheresis appears to have a role in the early treatment of florid cases of lupus with rapidly deteriorating renal function.

In children with other collagen-vascular diseases such as dermatomyositis, polyarteritis, and scleroderma, renal involvement with hematuria can also occur.

Henoch-Schönlein Purpura (HSP). HSP or anaphylactoid purpura may present initially as nephritis, mimicking acute poststreptococcal glomerulonephritis, with hematuria, renal insufficiency, and hypertension. Usually this disease presents with lower extremity purpura, abdominal pain, or melena and joint swelling. Children who develop significant renal disease do so within two months of onset.

C-3 levels are invariably normal. IgA levels may be elevated, and on the basis of biopsy of involved tissues including kidney and skin, the disease appears to be a systemic IgA-related small artery vasculitis.

A short course of steroid usually alleviates the abdominal pain, but the role of high-dose steroids, including pulses of methylprednisolone, is less well defined.

Recent evidence suggests that *Berger's IgA nephropathy* is a mild form of HSP nephritis without the typical rash. This nephropathy is clinically distinct because gross hematuria occurs at the time of an intercurrent infection. Occasionally there is temporary renal insufficiency; proteinuria is slight.

Hemolytic Uremic Syndrome (HUS). HUS presents a day or two after gastroenteritis in children 1 to 4 years of age, with oliguria, pallor, gross hematuria, and edema. Fibrin strands deposited in the kidneys cause not only renal insufficiency but microangiopathic hemolytic anemia. The patients experience acute renal failure, hypertension, anemia, and thrombocytopenia. BUN and creatinine are elevated in spite of fluid overload, and the peripheral blood smear shows fragmented red blood cells.

Disseminated intravascular coagulation (DIC) is not present in children with HUS, and those treated with peritoneal dialysis do better than those treated with heparin. Dialysis is begun for hyperkalemia, hyponatremia, fluid overload prior to or after blood transfusion, severe metabolic acidosis, prolonged malnutrition, and hypocalcemia.

Plasma infusions to replace a deficient PGI_2 inhibitor have yet to be proven successful.

Two other forms of the syndrome appear without prodrome: (1) recurrent HUS in older children and (2) hereditary HUS in siblings in whom the disease occurs months or years apart. The recurrent form may be prevented by daily low-dose salicylate.

Chronic Renal Failure. The causes of chronic renal failure in children are not always found, although frequently it is assumed that a preceding acute or chronic nephritis had occurred. Biopsy, if indicated, often shows only a sclerotic end-stage kidney.

Kidney function may be reduced for a long time before any abnormalities, including those in the urine, are noted. Eventually, the child develops an inability to concentrate urine which is followed by oliguria.

As the child develops progressive renal insufficiency and becomes more uremic, he may also develop hypertension, headache, anorexia, pallor, anemia, acidosis, renal rickets, and bone pain.

When the glomerular filtration rate is 10% of normal, the child should be observed closely. Blood pressure should be maintained as near normal as possible, and the child should be investigated and treated for infections. As renal function further decreases, the polyuric child will no longer require large salt and fluid intake. Phosphate binders are administered orally for elevated phosphate or parathyroid hormone levels. Phosphate must be lowered toward normal before the hypocalcemia of renal rickets is treated with calcitriol (1,25-dihydroxy-cholecalciferol). The danger of metastatic calcification is avoided if the calcium-phosphorus product is kept below 60. Severe metabolic acidosis may be treated orally with citrate (Shohl's solution) or bicarbonate. For nutritional reasons, protein should not be restricted; instead, the patient should be placed on maintenance dialysis or provided with a kidney transplant.

Acute Renal Failure (ARF). ARF presents with oliguria (less than 0.5 ml/kg/hr) and a rising BUN and creatinine. Hematuria and proteinuria are usually mild. The cause should be sought and treated. Prerenal causes include dehydration due to vomiting, diarrhea, shock, or hypovolemia of any etiology. Congestive heart failure can also cause acute renal failure. The kidneys continue to function to reabsorb salt and water. Therefore, urine sodium is less than 20 mEg/l and urine creatinine is concentrated (urine creatinine/plasma creatinine greater than 40).

Renal causes of ARF include hemolytic uremic syndrome, acute glomerulonephritis, poisons, ischemia, shock, and myoglobinuria secondary to viral rhabdomyolysis or crush injury. Acute tubular necrosis (ATN) is a pathologic diagnosis often assumed to be the cause of ARF except when the renal failure is glomerular in origin. Renal disease is evidenced by urine sodium above 20 mEq/l and isosthenuric urine with U/P creatinine ratio less than 20.

If treatment of the underlying condition does not reestablish urine formation or if diuresis does not occur following one trial of mannitol (0.5 to 1 g/kg IV) or furosemide (2 mg/kg IV) fluid is restricted to insensible losses plus urine output. Sodium and potassium are restricted. Electrolytes are carefully monitored, especially for the development of hyponatremia and hyperkalemia.

Dialysis should be instituted. Nutritional intake can be supplemented with Aminade which is low in sodium but high in carbohydrate and protein.

Wilms' Tumor. Wilms' tumor, the most common childhood renal tumor, usually presents as an abdominal mass. Ultrasonogram or pyelogram may be helpful.

Benign Recurrent Hematuria. Benign hematuria is microscopic or gross hematuria without known cause that is not associated with any other evidence of renal disease such as significant proteinuria, hypertension, or renal insufficiency. This is a diagnosis of exclusion. Isolated hematuria rarely develops into a significant disease. However, if significant proteinuria, hypertension, or renal failure are present or subsequently appear, the child should be evaluated for glomerulonephritis.

Bleeding Diseases. Hematuria can occur in children with any bleeding diathesis.

Infectious Diseases. Certain infections, particularly leptospirosis, scarlet fever, and occasionally infectious mononucleosis, are likely to be associated with hematuria. Children with subacute bacterial endocarditis almost always have hematuria, while other acute infections can produce hematuria. Prognosis is related to the successful treatment of the infection.

Sickle-Cell Anemia. Children with sickle-cell anemia or sickle-cell trait frequently develop microscopic hematuria, perhaps due to microthrombi or anoxia.

In diseases with hematuria with over 150 mg protein per dl, consider upper urinary tract disease first; when the concentration of protein is less, consider cystitis of urethritis first.

The cause of hematuria must be found. If other signs of acute glomerulonephritis exist (headache, hypertension, proteinuria, edema, or typical chest film) wait for the state to resolve. If this diagnosis seems unlikely, proceed with urine culture, intravenous pyelogram, voiding cystourethrogram, retrograde studies, and renal biopsy.

If hematuria is found, the urine should then be centrifuged and the supernatant retested for protein. In this way, the amount of protein directly related to the red cells will not distort the estimation of protein. If available, also test for blood. This not only confirms the presence of red cells, but if the test for blood is much more positive than expected from the number of red cells, this is an indirect indication of hemolysis, either systemic or localized in the urinary tract.

White Cells (Pyuria)

Normally, 0-2 white blood cells may be seen in urine per high-power field but it is also possible to have urinary tract infection without pyuria. Therefore, either significant pyuria or the presence of symptoms of urinary tract infection (fever, dysuria, gross hematuria, chills, flank pain, and so on) demands examination of unspun urine for bacteria and culture of clean voided or suprapubic aspirate urine.

Other causes of pyuria include early poststreptococcal glomerulonephritis (check blood pressure, renal function), tubulo-interstitial nephritis (eosinophils on Wright's stain of urine sediment) and, rarely, advanced renal tuberculosis.

Casts

Urinary casts originate in the upper urinary tract. Most casts are normal—hyaline, granular, or waxy. White cell casts indicate pyelonephritis, early poststreptococcal glomerulonephritis, or possibly interstitial nephritis; specific for the latter is presence of eosinophiles detected by Wright's stain of the urine sediment.

Red cell casts are abnormal and indicate significant renal disease, usually nephritis. They may be distinguished from red cell clumps or hyaline casts with adherent red cells by the presence of cast matrix with red cells embedded within, not merely adherent to the cast surface.

Crystals

Many urines, particularly concentrated ones, contain crystals. Most commonly, these are phosphates and disappear when the urine is rewarmed. Some crystals may be indicative of disease.

Cystinuria is a cause of renal stones. Patients may also excrete lysine. High urine volume, alkalinization, and penicillamine therapy prevent stone formation. The urine gives a positive test with nitroprusside-ferricyanide.

Oxalate crystals occur in oxaluria, which involves two enzymic errors. Pyridoxine may be helpful.

Calcium crystals following hypercalciuria are usually excreted with oxalate.

Urate crystals occur in children with hyperuricemia (*e.g.,* Lesch-Nyhan syndrome). In this syndrome, the patients are self-mutilating and hyperirritable; antihistamines may be beneficial. Gout occurs in older patients and may respond to xanthine oxidase inhibitors.

Also, crystals of administered medicines may appear.

Ferric Chloride

One of the important urinary screening tests is with ferric chloride. This reagent is stable on paper and in liquid as a 10% solution. The urine should be tested fresh, and poisonings or inborn errors of metabolism may be suggested by the change in color.

Among the causes of color change are: drugs or poisons (especially salicylates or phenothiazines), aminoacidurias, autosomal recessive diseases, such as phenylketonuria, tyrosinemia, histidinemia, oasthouse urine disease, maple syrup urine disease, alcaptonuria, and pyridoxine disorders. Tumors (*e.g.,* melanin) may cause color changes, as may severe acidosis and other organic acids. When the test with ferric chloride is positive, exact identification of the substance is necessary.

Color

Urine is normally light yellow. Dark yellow or brown coloring of the urine suggests the presence of bile. This is usually due to excessive conjugated bilirubin, hemoglobin (especially in acute hemolytic states), myoglobin (as occurs with muscle breakdown), and dehydration due to concentration of pigment.

Red urine occurs in children with hematuria, hemoglobinuria, and porphyria; it can be due to congenital porphyria or poisonings with excessive porphyrin production. Beeturia occurs in iron-deficient anemic children when they eat beets. Dyes and *Serratia marcescens* in the diaper of the newborn also cause color changes. Blue urine may be seen in infants with disorders of tryptophan metabolism, and black urine is an indication of alcaptonuria or melanuria.

Odor

Urine frequently mimics body odor. For example, in diphtheria or phenylketonuria, urine smells "musty." Urine smells like fish in some patients with disorders of sulfur amino acid metabolism, and smells like maple syrup in children with disorders of branched-chain amino acids.

It should be remembered that almost no urine test is diagnostic. Urine tests are screening tests and indicate the direction for proceeding in further diagnostic work-up.

BIBLIOGRAPHY

Arneil G: Management of the nephrotic syndrome in the child. In Lieberman E (ed): Clinical Pediatric Nephrology, Philadelphia, JB Lippincott, 1976

Practical review of causes, diagnosis, and treatment of various forms of childhood nephrotic syndrome.

Leake R: Perinatal nephrobiology: a developmental perspective. Clin Perinatol 4: 321, 1977

Comprehensive review of the subject including clinical and therapeutic implications.

West C, McAdams AJ: The chronic glomerulonephritides of childhood. Parts I and II. J Pediatr 93: 1, 167, 1978

Thorough discussion of both primary and secondary nephritides of childhood and their therapy.

Enuresis

18

Walter W. Tunnessen, Jr.

Enuresis is the involuntary passage of urine, usually at night or during sleep. Enuresis is a symptom, not a disease. The involuntary passage of urine may be "normal" or it may be associated with serious underlying anatomic abnormalities or other problems, depending on the age of the child. In the majority of children with enuresis, a clear-cut pathologic disorder cannot be demonstrated, and there is considerable controversy regarding the etiology of this common symptom.

Before discussing enuresis, a few terms should be defined.

Diurnal enuresis—the involuntary passage of urine both during the day and night
Primary enuresis—the persistence of enuresis from infancy without interruption by prolonged dry periods
Secondary enuresis—the recurrence of enuresis after a dry period of at least 3 to 6 months
Essential enuresis—the presence of involuntary wetting without identifiable cause

PREVALENCE OF ENURESIS

Enuresis is not a disorder of modern society. Reference to enuresis as a problem dates back as far as 1500 BC. Enuresis may be normal expected behavior. Obviously, the young infant involuntarily passes urine, while the 15-year-old is expected to have gained control. Somewhere in between these two ages, control of bladder emptying should have been achieved. Most investigators who have attempted to study the symptom of enuresis identify it as a problem in children over 5 or 6 years of age. This definition, however, may ignore younger children whose enuresis may be pathologic rather than essential.

By 3 years of age, 80% of children are able to maintain daytime dryness and 50% night-time dryness (see Oppel). By 5 years of age, approximately 90% of children remain dry during the day and 70% remain dry through the night. When children reach age 10 years, more than 95% are dry during the day, but only 85% remain dry without relapse during sleep. By age 12, all but 1% to 2% of children maintain daytime control, but as many as 8% have occasional relapses of nocturnal enuresis (Fig. 18-1). Males are more frequently enuretic than females, but both sexes show a gradual decline in the numbers of children reported to have had enuretic episodes with advancing age.

The symptom of enuresis, though common, does not mean that the physician should deal with it casually. Simply stating that the child will outgrow the problem is inappropriate. In a small number of cases, this symptom may be indicative of significant underlying disease. But, even if we are not able to define the cause of enuresis in the

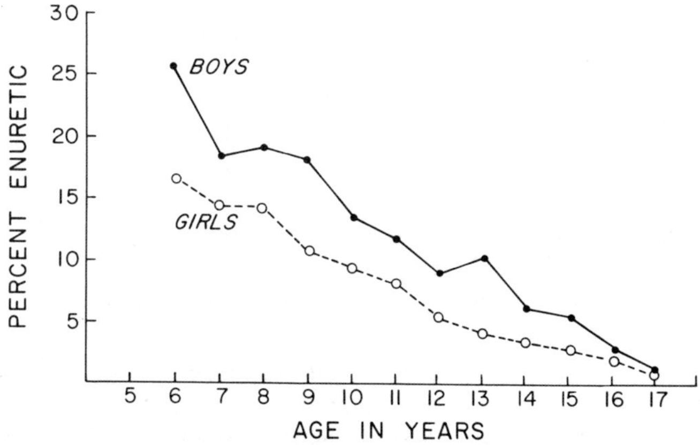

Fig. 18-1. National Health Survey 1963–1970. Percent of children reported to have wet the bed during the past 12 months. Vital and Health Statistics, Series II No. 137 Table B p.7.

majority of cases, the symptom is important, because it is embarrassing and perplexing to the child and his family, and it may promote family stress and discord.

DIFFERENTIAL DIAGNOSIS OF ENURESIS

With few exceptions, most of the disorders associated with enuresis may be diagnosed by a careful history and physical examination and a few simple laboratory tests (see list). Children with essential enuresis appear well and their growth is normal. They have a good urinary stream, no evidence of anatomic or neurologic abnormalities, and no polyuria or genitourinary tract infections.

Etiologic Classification of Enuresis

I. Essential
II. Psychogenic-environmental
    A. Toilet-training difficulties
    B. Environmental stress
    C. Psychologic disturbances
III. Organic-anatomic abnormalities
    A. Obstructive lesions
        1. Urethral valves
        2. Ectopic ureters
        3. Diverticulum of the anterior urethra
        4. Urethral stricture
        5. Meatal stenosis
        6. Contraction of the bladder neck
        7. Bladder diverticuli
        8. Prostatic tumor or abscess
        9. Hydrocolpos-hematocolpos
        10. Labial atresia
        11. Marked phimosis
    B. Neurogenic
        1. Myelomeningocele
        2. Sacral agenesis
        3. Occult neuropathic bladder
        4. Seizures
        5. Spinal cord injuries
        6. Spinal cord tumors
        7. Diastematomyelia
    C. Infections
        1. Urinary tract infections
        2. Osteomyelitis of a vertebral body
        3. Spinal epidural abscess
    D. Disorders associated with Polyuria-polydipsia
        1. Diabetes mellitus
        2. Sickle cell anemia
        3. Renal disorders
IV. Miscellaneous
    A. Allergies
    B. Global retardation

Psychogenic or environmental causes of enuresis are usually easily uncovered. An example of environmental stress resulting in enuresis is the birth of a new sibling, whereupon the previously toilet-trained child under 5 years of age may suddenly begin wetting the bed at night or his clothing during the day. Hospitalization or family disruption may also promote regression in bladder control. Psychological disturbances associated with enuresis are usually obvious because of the presence of other behavioral manifestations. A few decades ago emotional disorders were purported to be the major cause of essential enuresis. Although some psychologists and psychiatrists still attribute this symptom to causes such as an unresolved Oedipal complex, substitution for masturbation, or the result of faulty toilet training, most physicians today consider emotional disturbances to be a rare cause of enuresis.

Obstructive lesions resulting in enuresis can be suggested by a history of dribbling, poor urinary stream, difficulty in initiating or stopping urination, recurrent urinary tract infection, failure to empty the bladder completely, or poor growth. Prospective, controlled studies have failed to document structural abnormalities as a cause of enuresis without the suggestive signs and symptoms mentioned above (see Committee on Radiology, biblio.). Still, many physicians continue to subject their patients with essential enuresis to radiographic procedures. Structural abnormalities may be a cause of enuresis, but "silent" defects are not the explanation of essential enuresis.

Neurogenic causes of enuresis are usually detected by history, inspection, and neurologic examination. Although children with seizures may have urinary incontinence during convulsive episodes, essential enuresis is not a manifestation of an unsuspected seizure disorder.

The child with a urinary tract infection may present with the sudden onset of enuretic episdoes, but asymptomatic infections are a rare cause of long-standing enuresis. A urine culture should be performed.

The child with polyuria may have enuresis. A urinalysis with specific gravity, tests for glucose, protein and blood, and a microscopic examination of the spun sediment will uncover many of these disorders. Children with sickle-cell anemia have hyposthenuria and polyuria and, occasionally, enuresis may be a presenting symptom. Although children with essential enuresis may have increased urinary frequency, they do not have an increased urinary output.

Children with severe mental retardation may have delayed control of bladder function or never attain it. Occasionally children with hidden food allergies have enuresis. These children usually have allergic stigmata such as allergic shiners, Dennies' lines (transverse creases on the lower eyelid), an allergic salute, and perennial rhinitis. Additional nonspecific symptoms of the so-called allergic tension—fatigue syndrome secondary to hidden food allergy—include recurrent headaches, abdominal pain, leg aches, lethargy, and irritability. It is likely that food allergy plays only a minor role in the etiology of essential enuresis.

ESSENTIAL ENURESIS

Children with essential enuresis are expected to have gained bladder control, but are still wetting involuntarily. Although many urologists feel enuresis is a structural problem and many psychiatrists support an emotional basis, most pediatricians adhere to the concept that essential enuresis is usually a manifestation of delayed maturational control of bladder function. In support of this hypothesis are a number of well-known associations.

1. Genetic Influence. One of the most strikingly consistent bits of evidence for a maturational delay of bladder control is the incidence of enuresis in families. Table 18-1 contains information on the familial

TABLE 18-1. Family Incidence of Enuresis

Concordance of enuresis in family members	Percent
Monozygotic twin: co-twin	67.9
Both parents: child	77.3
Father: child	42.5
Mother: child	43.5
Dizygotic twin: co-twin	35.7
Neither parent enuretic: child	15.2

(After Bakwin H, Bakwin RM: Behavior Disorders in Children, 4th ed, pp. 432–446. Philadelphia, WB Saunders, 1972)

association of enuresis generated by the Bakwins (see biblio.). If one monozygotic twin is enuretic, the other twin will be enuretic in two out of three pairs. Dizygotic twins, however, are concordant for enuresis in only one-third of cases. If both parents were enuretic, their children have a 75% chance of being enuretic. If only one parent was enuretic, the chances are about 4 in 10 that each offspring will have a similar problem.

The familial incidence of enuresis has been supported in many studies. In a report of children in kibbutzim in Israel, where the children are raised in child care centers and the influences of family customs are eliminated, enuresis was present in 11% of children between the ages of 3½ and 12 years, a rate similar to children in Israel not raised in kibbutzim. In addition, when sibling pairs were raised by different nurses in these situations, if one child was enuretic, over 40% of their siblings were also enuretic (see biblio. Committee on Radiology).

2. Bladder Capacity. The amount of urine passed per 24 hours does not differ between enuretics and dry controls. What is apparent is that enuretic children have a smaller functional bladder capacity than their dry peers. Manometric studies of the urinary bladder have documented that children with enuresis demonstrate bladder irritability and involuntary contractions with smaller amounts of bladder filling than control children.

The typical enuretic child needs to urinate more frequently during the day, and if he senses the need to void he must do so almost immediately. Long car trips must often be interrupted for "bladder relief."

3. Spontaneous "Cures". Another significant fact that supports the developmental delay hypothesis is the yearly rate of spontaneous resolution of enuresis. There is an annual attrition rate of enuresis of approximately 15% *without intervention.* One would not expect enuresis secondary to structural abnormalities to diminish with time to such a degree.

A popular notion prior to the advent of sleep research was that enuretics were heavier sleepers than nonenuretics. Parents of bed wetters often state that their children are difficult to arouse from sleep. Enuresis may occur during any stage of sleep, and is not limited to nonrapid eye movement periods.

One of the more difficult bits of information to incorporate into the developmental delay hypothesis is the frequency of secondary enuresis. Two-thirds of children with essential enuresis have primary enuresis, never having been free of this symptom. The other third of essential enuretics has secondary enuresis, referring to the presence of a dry period of at least 3 to 6 months prior to the recurrence of the problem. Some physicians advocate more extensive investigation of people with secondary enuresis looking for anatomic or organic disorders.

APPROACH TO THE CHILD WITH ENURESIS

The most important contribution a physician can make to the enuretic child and his family is one of care and concern. If the physician does not set aside ample time to discuss the problem and show interest in its resolution, he should avoid an intervention because it could create more harmful than helpful effects.

Many families are reluctant and embarrassed to discuss the problem. During a routine office visit, it is incumbent upon the physician to *ask directly* about the presence of enuresis rather than to rely on the child or his family to raise the issue. A careful history must be obtained to differentiate between children with essential enuresis and those in whom this symptom indicates another disorder.

History

The age of the child is important. Are the parents unrealistic about when they expect their child to develop bladder control? However, the possibility that a 3- to 5-year-old may have an underlying structural or other pathologic problem should not be overlooked.

Has the enuresis been continuous since infancy, or is it of recent onset? Does it occur daily, nightly or both, a few times a week, or once a month? Have the parents observed the urinary stream? The child should be able to voluntarily initiate voiding without straining. The urinary stream should be full and not splayed. The presence of dribbling of urine between enuretic episodes should be ascertained.

If the enuresis is secondary, have there been any associated symptoms? Does the child experience dysuria? If he urinates, does he feel that the bladder is empty, or will he have to urinate again within a short period of time? Are there systemic symptoms such as fever, failure to gain weight or grow, abdominal or back pain? Does the child also have encopresis, the involuntary passage of stool? Ten to fifteen percent of enuretics are also encopretic.

A careful family history should be obtained. Are there other family members with enuresis? The parents may be reluctant to acknowledge that they have had enuresis, or one parent may not know that the other had the problem. The parents may have repressed the fact that they were "bed-wetters." Grandparents may offer assistance in the history.

The pregnancy, labor, and birth histories may indicate significant perinatal insults that could affect bladder control. Social and environmental information might prove important. Did the enuresis develop after the birth of a sibling, a family move, hospitalization, or family stress such as separation, divorce, or death?

It is helpful to gather information about the family's response to the enuresis. What is their understanding of the problem? Is their approach one of ridicule, embarrassment, or punishment? Are the parents in agreement and consistent in their approach? If possible, discuss the bedwetting separately with the child to evaluate his perception of the problem. Do the parents limit fluid intake, wake the child during the night, give him all responsibility for changing and washing clothing and bedding? Simple questions such as the accessibility of the bathroom in the home are often neglected. The child may be limited in his social life by this symptom. Is he allowed to sleep at grandmother's or friends' houses? Is he allowed to go to camp, or is he too embarrassed to go if allowed? Have other forms of therapy such as drugs, diet, alarm systems and the like been tried?

Physical Examination

The child's behavior during the history taking and physical examination should be noted. Inappropriate responses to the examination might indicate a need for further psychologic evaluation or may indicate a difficult home environment.

The child's height and weight should be plotted on standard growth charts. Growth failure may occur in a number of disorders. Similarly, the blood pressure must be obtained, since hypertension may reflect renal disease.

The abdomen should be carefully palpated for masses, particularly bladder and kidney enlargement. If possible, palpate the child's abdomen before and after voiding to determine whether the bladder empties completely. The external genitalia are examined for abnormalities, particularly meatal stenosis and hypospadias in the male. Cryptorchidism might suggest structural genitourinary defects. The female genitalia should also be inspected for abnormalities such as labial adhesions, imperforate hymen, or an ectopic urethral meatus.

The child's back should be carefully palpated searching for vertebral defects. A rectal examination will give some indication of anal sphincter tone and will also reveal chronic constipation that could be playing a role. Perineal sensation should be checked by pinprick. The lower extremities are examined for muscle tone, strength, deep tendon reflexes, and sensory changes.

The physician should watch the child void. The character of the child's urinary stream as well as his ability to start and stop may offer helpful clues that need further laboratory evaluation.

Laboratory Investigation

All children with enuresis should have a clean catch urine screened for specific gravity, protein, sugar, blood, and ketones. The spun sediment should be examined for cellular elements. A urine culture or screening culture (available for office use in simple inexpensive packages) is also suggested. Although radiographic studies were commonly performed in the past, the current recommendations are that these studies (intravenous pyelograms, voiding cystourethrograms, and others) are not indicated unless other signs or symptoms suggest underlying disorders. These studies are not only expensive, but they subject the child to unnecessary radiation and the inherent stresses of urologic examination as well.

Management of Essential Enuresis

Although the etiology of essential enuresis is unknown, the physician must not assume that his duties end with the separation of essential enuresis from structural, metabolic, emotional, or other causes of this symptom. The physician is a teacher and should educate the child and his family about this symptom. Often a frank discussion, optimistic reassurance, and a few helpful suggestions may diminish or end the problem. Enuresis is not managed by one office visit. The physician must show his concern and interest by a willingness to work with the child and his family.

The spontaneous "cure" rate for enuresis is approximately 15% per year. A number of studies have demonstrated an additional significant response in children even after one visit to the physician. The factors involved in this response may include improvement in the child's self-esteem and changes in family attitudes.

In the 5- to 7- or 8-year-old group, a simple behavior modification approach might be tried. A calendar of wet and dry nights (or days) is kept, and dry nights are rewarded by a gold star. Small rewards, such as movie privileges or other "special treats" may be offered for significant improvements. The calendar system also serves the purpose of giving the physician an indication of the frequency of the enuresis and allows him to evaluate the response to other therapeutic recommendations in the future.

Bladder-stretching Exercises

A successful response in one-third to two-thirds of children with enuresis has been reported with a technique called bladder stretching (see Starfield). The impetus behind this approach was the recognition that children with enuresis have a smaller bladder capacity than their dry, age-matched peers. Studies have shown that by increasing bladder capacity, control of enuresis may be attained. The child is encouraged to restrain from voiding for as long as possible during a regular daytime period, perhaps after school. The volume of urine passed is then carefully measured and recorded on a calendar along with "dry and wet" notations. The child is then encouraged to increase the volume by holding the urine longer each day. As the urine volume increases, enuresis may be abolished. This method is the only one in current use that actually offers the youngster a sense of control over and responsibility for his problem. Naturally, this method is not useful for all children or families, but the cooperative and motivated child as young as 7 or 8 may comply.

Drugs

Significant improvement in enuresis has been reported in children treated with a tricyclic antidepressant, imipramine hydrochloride. The exact mechanism by which this drug exerts its effect is not known, but it seems to be its anticholinergic rather than its antidepressant effect. Some children treated with imipramine hydrochloride are affected by unpleasant side-effects such as dry mouth, irritability, sleep disturbances, constipation, and others. A more serious problem is the potential for ingestion by the child or a younger sibling. There have been numerous warnings of significant toxicity, reporting cardiac arrhythmias and convulsions, or death in children who have ingested excessive amounts of imipramine hydrochloride. Its margin of safety is not great. Prescribing imipramine hydrochloride promotes the impression that a drug must be used for every symptom or illness, creating a generation of children who will rely on drugs in years to come.

Forty to ninety percent of children treated with imipramine are expected to improve. A starting dose of 25 mg in the evening is recommended for children under 10 years of age with an additional 25 mg added if there is no response in two weeks. Children under 7 years of age generally are not considered candidates for drug therapy. The relapse rate after stopping this drug is high.

Conditioning

Another method of therapy is the alarm mattress. A number of different alarm systems are available that use the electrolyte content of urine to trigger a battery-operated alarm. When the child urinates in his sleep, the alarm sounds, waking the child. Reported success rates with this method have also ranged from 50% to 90%. The alarms must be used for 3 to 4 months and, as with other methods of therapy, the relapse rate is high. The alarm systems may be rented, but the cost is high. Occasional reports of skin ulcers secondary to the mattresses are of minor severity.

Miscellaneous Therapies

Numerous other treatment methods for enuresis have been employed by parents and physicians, including urethral dilatation. The withholding of fluids after supper is rarely effective and serves more as a punitive than a therapeutic measure. Some parents use alarms to wake their child at intervals during the night to have him void. This method is disruptive to the child as well as the family and rarely proves helpful.

Occasionally, children may respond to the elimination of certain foods from their diet. Milk, chocolate, and eggs are the most frequently reported offenders. A 2- to 3-week elimination diet may be tried in selected children, particularly those with other allergic manifestations.

Counseling by a psychiatrist or psychologist is not necessary unless the child is emotionally disturbed. Counseling by the primary physician, however, is a cornerstone of rational therapy.

As is typical of disorders of uncertain etiology, hundreds of therapies have been suggested for the treatment of enuresis. None has been shown to be uniformly effective; however, bladder-stretching exercises, treatment with imipramine hydrochloride, and use of alarm mattresses have been popular and relatively successful therapies. Education and support of the child and his family are the most important aspects of medical care of this problem, with therapeutic interventions tailored to meet the needs of the specific situation.

SUMMARY

Enuresis, the involuntary passage of urine, is a common symptom in children. A small minority of children have enuresis as a result of underlying anatomic, metabolic, infectious, or other recognizable disorders. The majority have essential enuresis, a disorder of uncertain etiology, possibly related to delayed functional maturation of bladder control.

There is a high familial incidence of enuresis. Children with enuresis have been demonstrated to have a decreased functional capacity of their bladders. Smaller amounts of urine in the bladder will result in involuntary bladder contractions in enuretics than is seen in dry controls. This diminished functional capacity seems to improve with age without specific therapy, since there is an annual attrition rate of 15% in enuretic children.

BIBLIOGRAPHY

Bakwin H, Bakwin RM: Behavior Disorders in Children, 4th ed, pp 432–446. Philadelphia, WB Saunders, 1972.

A superb, objective, and clearly written discussion of enuresis by two experienced and highly regarded child psychiatrists.

Committee on Radiology: Excretory urography for evaluation of enuresis. Pediatrics 65:644, 1980

An expert panel opinion regarding the controversial topic of the radiologic evaluation of children with enuresis.

Oppel WC, Harper PA, Rider RV: The age of attaining bladder control. Pediatrics 42:614, 1968

Data are presented on the age of attaining bladder control for waking and sleeping hours from a 12-year prospective study of 859 children.

Starfield B: Enuresis: its pathogenesis and management. Clin Pediatr 2: 343, 1972.

A well-written overview of enuresis coupled with data collected from the author's own investigations. A practical approach to bladder-training exercises that may be presented to enuretics and their families is included.

Edema and Hypertension

19

Lewis A. Barness
Edward R. Root

Interstitial fluid, whether present in normal or excessive amounts, is an ultrafiltrate of plasma and the milieu, or "primordial sea," in which the cells are bathed. An abnormal accumulation of interstitial fluid is edema and in most instances results from excessive salt and water retention caused by the kidney's response to an underlying pathologic state such as massive proteinuria, starvation, cirrhosis, congestive heart failure, or inappropriate antidiuretic hormone. In addition, renal failure itself can cause excessive salt and water retention.

DETECTING EDEMA

Pressure over a part of the body which is larger than normal results in indentation, pitting edema. Measurement of the part, for example, the leg, compared with the normal part indicates an increase in circumference due to an increase in volume. Similarly, measuring the circumference of the the abdomen may indicate the progress of abdominal fluid, ascites. Nevertheless, the best method presently available for the detection of and the following of the progress of edema in the child is determining the daily weight of the child and noting weight changes. Even in the newborn, lack of physiologic weight loss in the first week of life may be the earliest evidence of abnormal water accumulation.

Edema usually accumulates in dependent parts and in easily distensible tissue. Thus, generalized edema may be distributed over the entire body but detected only in the face or over the eyes in the morning (periorbital edema), and then disappear as the child becomes upright and the fluid shifts to the scrotum and lower legs and feet in the afternoon. This is shifting edema and occurs in all cases, but is more marked in those with lesser amounts of edema fluid. Anasarca is generalized massive edema and includes leg and sacral edema and ascites. Localized edema and nonpitting edema may have special causes. These are discussed below.

Mechanism of Edema Formation

Edema is formed when those factors holding water in the intravascular space are less than those allowing fluid loss out of this space (Starling's law). The two main forces causing loss of fluid to the interstitium are increased capillary hydrostatic pressure and decreased capillary colloid oncotic pressure.

1. *Hydrostatic pressure changes.* Increased intravascular pressure changes drive water and solutes into the extracellular spaces. For example, cardiac output decreases, leading to increased hydrostatic pressure; vascular constriction causes local increase in hydrostatic pressure; or, venous obstruction

causes an increase in hydrostatic pressure distal to the obstruction.

2. *Osmotic pressure,* regulated by osmoreceptors, located in the nucleus supraopticus and in the portal circulation: These regulate the release of ADH and perspiration. This is regulated by hepatic protein synthesis; nutrition, depending on protein and calorie intake; losses, especially through kidney (*e.g.*, nephrosis); hypermetabolic states. Osmotic pressure can be caused by electrolytes, the concentration of which are regulated by intake; mineralocorticoids which control sodium and chloride retention (any state resulting in increased aldosterone secretion results in an increase in tubular reabsorption of sodium), changes in excretion, as in renal disease, with decreased filtration (increased osmotic pressure) or decreased reabsorption (decreased osmotic pressure), as well as in heart failure, with secondary decreased renal perfusion, and excess losses, (*e.g.*, sweating, cystic fibrosis of pancreas). Nonelectrolytes, (*e.g.*, urea, glucose) also cause osmotic pressure. (Fig. 19-1)

In most situations, formation of edema is related to a decrease in plasma oncotic pressure caused by decreased albumin. As the serum protein level falls, two related events occur. First, intravascular fluid is lost to the interstitial space and intravascular volume decreases. Intravascular volume is 50 ml/kg, and therefore a partial loss of this volume due to decreased oncotic pressure can account for only a small portion of the massive edema. The second event leads to accumulation of edema and is due to a similar mechanism seen in other hypovolemic states such as dehydration: the kidney avidly retains water and sodium. A vicious cycle is established since reabsorbed salt and water cannot be held in the intravascular space. Thus, patients with nephrotic edema have increased total body sodium and water in the face of decreased intravascular volume. This is a practical consideration in sodium restricting a nephrotic; intravascular volume is determined not so much by sodium and water ingested but by the level of serum protein.

Diseases Associated with Edema Formation

Edema occurs in children with heart failure, volume overload, kidney disease, diseases of the capillaries, improper fluid therapy, severe anemia or polycythemia, carcinoid, or any illness associated with low-serum proteins.

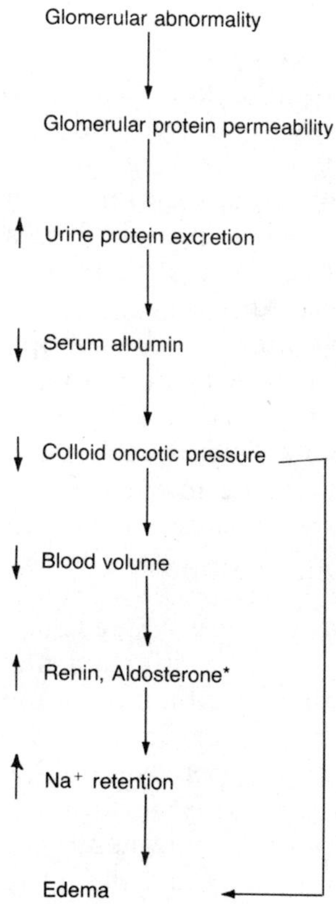

Fig. 19-1. Mechanism of edema formation in nephrotic syndrome.* Recent evidence indicates that the renin-angiotensin system does not play the major role in renal sodium and water retention in nephrotic syndrome; proximal tubular factors may play a role.

Decreased blood volume on the arterial side occurs with left-sided failure; increased systemic venous pressure is termed backward failure. With heart failure edema fluid is a transudate, an ultrafiltrate of plasma. Protein content is less than 3% and specific gravity less than 1.015. Exudates, as in infections, contain more than 3% protein and specific gravity is greater than 1.018.

Kidney Disease. Kidney diseases associated with decreased filtration, increased tubular reabsorption of electrolytes, or albumin loss include those diseases described in the proteinuria section.

Diseases Associated with Decreased Oncotic Pressure. Diseases that are due to decreased production or increased losses of proteins, particularly albumin, include: nephrosis and nephrotic syndrome (see Proteinuria) and malabsorption syndromes. Any malabsorption syndrome may cause such severe protein losses that hypoproteinemia occurs. These syndromes include: celiac disease, sprue, cystic fibrosis, the dysenteries, abetalipoproteinemia (though the carrier protein for fat is absent, protein is also lost), colitis (particularly ulcerative colitis), ileitis, and protein-losing enteropathy, which may be associated with anatomic or vascular anomalies of the intestinal tract.

Liver Disease. (see Chap. 12) Children with cirrhosis in particular do not produce sufficient albumin. Some children with storage diseases or with Wilson's disease in which the copper in the liver is high, or with cystic fibrosis develop this type of cirrhosis. Some chronic hemolytic anemias cause hemosiderosis and defective albumin production.

Hypothyroidism. Albumin production may be decreased or excessive albumin metabolized in hypothyroidism.

EVALUATION OF EDEMA PATIENTS

In evaluating the child with edema, first make certain he does not have congestive heart failure, not because this is the most common cause of edema, but because failure to recognize this cause early may lead to catastrophe. Look for a history of heart disease, history of fatigue, history of streptococcal infection, history of rheumatic fever, and history of tuberculosis (? constrictive pericarditis). Also, look for these physical signs: tachycardia, tachypnea, orthopnea cardiomegaly (scratch percussion), hepatomegaly, rales, murmurs, cyanosis, hypertension, low pulse pressure, and clubbing. Take a chest film to see whether the heart is enlarged, or small, or whether there is decreased cardiac motion. Take an EKG and measure hemoglobin levels and determine whether hematocrit is high or low. Finally, get an echocardiogram.

If heart disease is not present, eliminate kidney disease next as a cause of edema. Look for a history of previous infection (nephritis), familial kidney disease, deafness (Alport's syndrome), oliguria, polyuria, polydipsia, history of hypertension, hematuria, headache, and exposure to poisons. The physical signs to check are mass in abdomen, costovertebral angle, or bladder tenderness and hypertension.

A urinalysis will measure protein, specific gravity, hematuria (casts), reducing substance, white cells (casts), heavy metals, bacteria, and culture. Check the blood for anemia, urea nitrogen (creatinine), serum proteins, antistreptococcal antibodies, ANA and hepatitis-associated antigen.

Most children between the ages of 1 and 6 who have nephrotic syndrome (idiopathic nephrotic syndrome of childhood) need not undergo a percutaneous renal biopsy; it can be assumed that they have minimal change (nil) disease unless one or more atypical signs or symptoms are present: arthralgias, malar or purpuric rashes or abdominal pain, hematuria, severe hypertension, significant renal failure or depressed C3. These atypical findings suggest that the patient is a nephritic nephrotic. Another atypical feature eventually becomes evident—poor response to steroid. These atypical patients usually require renal biopsy to differentiate, for therapeutic and prognostic reasons, lupus nephritis, Henoch-Schönlein purpura nephritis, membranoproliferative glomerulonephritis, focal-segmental glomerulosclerosis and others, all of which can present as nephrotic syndrome. (See discussion on Hematuria, Chap. 17.)

Over the age of 6, minimal change disease is less common. Teenagers, especially females, who are nephrotic with low-serum albumin and elevated serum cholesterol, usually have either lupus nephritis or membranoproliferative glomerulonephritis. Renal biopsies are often indicated in nephrotics over 6 years old. However, teenagers with long-standing diabetes mellitus who become nephrotic can be assumed to have Kimmelstiel-Wilson syndrome.

When the nephrotic child is under 1 year old, the common causes of nephrotic syndrome just listed are to be considered, as well as Finnish-type hereditary congenital nephrotic syndrome and nephrotic syndrome secondary to syphilis or topoplasmosis, rubella, cytomegalovirus, herpes virus (TORCH) infections. Open renal biopsy is usually necessary.

Nephritic edema is also common in children, for example, in acute poststreptococcal glomerulonephritis or in nephritides that present similarly. (See Hematuria, Chap. 17.)

If the patient does not have heart failure or kidney disease but has generalized edema, suspect low serum proteins, particularly albumin. If this is found, be sure to obtain a dietary history, social history, and history of jaundice, liver disease, and chronic infection.

Physical examination may indicate only a large, tender, or hard liver. Then obtain liver enzymes (*e.g.*, SGOT), bilirubin, serum proteins (electrophoresis), and blood ammonia, urea (urea frequently decreased and ammonia elevated).

If liver tests are positive, test for specific liver causes, although cirrhosis may have no other abnormalities.

If dietary history is poor, first try the child on an adequate diet before doing extensive tests and making bizarre diagnoses. As his diet improves, the child may not gain weight for as long as 6 weeks, though serum proteins will increase and edema will decrease.

If diarrhea is a problem, do a careful rectal examination looking for signs of megacolon. Then obtain stool cultures, stool ova, and parasites, stool blood, stool pH (pH below 5 suggests intestinal enzyme deficiency), stools for fat, sugar, and protein, sweat test for cystic fibrosis, and tuberculin test, and look at a blood smear for acanthocytes.

If these are not diagnostic, proceed with a GI series including barium enema and sigmoidoscopy. Specific malabsorption syndromes may be detected. If history suggests chronic infection, the sources of infection must be sought. These include cultures of blood, urine, stools, and perhaps ears, cerebrospinal fluid, and radiographs of sinuses.

If the source of edema is neither heart, liver, or kidney disease, or low serum proteins, look for diseases or states causing increased capillary permeability. Capillary permeability is probably the most common cause of localized edema and may be associated with generalized or localized edema. Diseases or states causing increased capillary permeability include: anaphylaxis or shock, allergies—angioneurotic edema, insect bites, measles, gonadal dysgenesis, hypothyroidism (get T4, T3, and TSH), scurvy, beriberi, rickets, poisons, position (*e.g.*, facial edema in morning, obstruction to flow by crossing legs) and lymphatic obstruction (*e.g.*, filariasis). Do not make a diagnosis of allergic or angioneurotic edema without examining the patient thoroughly (particularly for heart disease) and performing a urinalysis.

PRINCIPLES OF MANAGEMENT

In general, salt intake should be monitored or decreased in all patients retaining fluid. This is probably not as important in children with the nephrotic syndrome with normal blood pressure. More important for this group of children is *that* they eat rather than *what* they eat.

For children with heart failure, digitalis and diuretics are the basis of treatment. If anoxia is present, oxygen is helpful. For those with myocarditis, corticosteroids should be tried.

Usually, renal disease causing edema is acute poststreptococcal glomerulonephritis. Penicillin therapy for several months usually suffices. If hypertension is present, salt should be restricted, the patient should be kept at rest, and antihypertensives such as phenobarbital, reserpine, and hydralazine should be used.

If the diagnosis is nephrosis or the nephrotic syndrome, corticosteroids should be used for at least 4 weeks. For some of the poisonings, specific antidotes are available. Some children have surgically correctable kidney lesions; these should be corrected.

In children with hypoalbuminemia, suitable diets should be tried first. If these do not help, intravenous albumin may be necessary. Generally for those with allergy, antihistamines help.

HYPERTENSION

Hypertension results from increased salt retention, either from diet or excessive mineralo-corticoids and aldosterone, or from the renin-angiotensin mechanism following renal stimulation of the juxtaglomerular apparatus. Other renal substances may also cause hypertension.

Most hypertension in children is due to unknown causes or to renal disease. Normal blood pressure is best obtained with a proper cuff size (see Chap. 1). Some children have elevated blood pressures only occasionally (labile hypertension); the relation of labile hypertension to true hypertension is unknown. Exercise and excitement cause sporadic hypertension and may be precursors of fixed hypertension. The most common cause of acute onset of hypertension in children is acute glomerulonephritis. Signs of hypertension include headache, vomiting, and bradycardia. It is also common for both acute and chronic hypertension to be symptom-free. Signs of hypertensive encephalopathy include papilledema, irritability, seizures, and (rarely) retinal hemorrhages. Chronic hypertension, other than exhibiting typical funduscopic changes, is often asymptomatic until target organ damage occurs: blindness, seizures, stroke, congestive heart failure, or renal failure.

Evaluation

If there is a familial history of hypertension, renal or adrenal disease, direct the workup to similar systems in the child. A history of excess ingestion of licorice which contains an aldosteronelike compound, or a history of heavy metal exposure or of other drug ingestion may be obtained. Physical examination may reveal coarctation of the aorta. Hypertension will be found in upper extremities, hypotension in lower extremities, and femoral pulses will be diminished. Abdominal or flank bruit may be heard.

In the absence of a leading history or physical finding, study the child's genitourinary system. Careful urinalysis may reveal abnormalities. Intravenous rapid sequence urogram may indicate intrinsic or destructive renal disease and is helpful in determining unilateral renal disease. Aortography and renal arteriography with differential renal vein renin levels, as well as renal scan, help delineate vascular or unilateral disease. Renal biopsy may also be helpful.

If all studies are negative, catecholamine-producing lesions such as neuroblastoma, pheochromocytoma, or carcinoid should be suspected. Urinary catecholamines, VMA, and cystathionine help distinguish these. Removal of a pheochromocytoma is complicated by paroxysms of hypertension and hypotension. Phentolamine should be given preoperatively and levarterenol should be available at operation for decreased blood pressure.

In the absence of specific cause of hypertension, a diagnosis of essential hypertension may be made. Organic cause of hypertension is much more common in children than in adults.

Hyperthyroidism. Enlarged thyroid, tachycardia, hyperhidrosis, and tremor may be present.

Increased Intracranial Pressure. Many children with signs of meningitis, encephalitis, or brain tumor develop hypertension, usually with bradycardia. Sometimes it is difficult to distinguish signs of primary encephalopathy with hypertension from encephalopathy due to hypertension.

Obesity. Obese children may have hypertension. Often it is difficult to get an accurate blood pressure measurement in obese children.

Riley-Day Syndrome. Signs of familial dysautonomia such as absence of tears, decreased pain sensation, vomiting, and failure to thrive may indicate Riley-Day syndrome.

Treatment

Hypertensive emergencies, such as hypertensive encephalopathy or a diastolic pressure reading greater than 120, should be treated at once with either hydralazine 0.5 mg/kg intravenously to be repeated every 2 hours as needed (up to a total dose as high as 6 mg/kg/day) or diazoxide (Hyperstat) 5 mg/kg (up to 300 mg per dose) rapid IV push, which may be repeated once 30 minutes after.

To achieve control of ongoing acute hypertension or to maintain control in chronic hypertension, it would be best to combine, if needed, a peripheral dilator, adrenergic inhibitor, and a diuretic. However, in practice whatever combination works should be used, especially if once daily medications can be used. Once control is achieved, it may be possible to taper off previously added medications. One cause of poor blood pressure control is taking different medications at irregular intervals throughout the day; the best combined effect is achieved by taking the medications at the same time at regular intervals (See list and Table 19–1).

General Guidelines in Management of Pediatric Hypertension

1. For children with mild hypertension or significant hypertension risk factors reduce dietary sodium and achieve weight control.
2. For children with blood pressure determinations repeatedly above the 95th percentile for their age or 140/90, despite the above dietary prophylactic measures, initiate pharmacologic therapy. Select an agent from *one* category; diuretics or beta-blockers or neurologically active agents. Particularly in cases

TABLE 19-1. Antihypertensive Medications

Medication	Dose	Route	Advantages	Disadvantages
Diuretics				
Hydrochlorothiazide (Hydrodiuril)	0.5-1 mg/kg/dose	oral		hypokalemia
Chlorthalidone (Hygroton)	0.5-1 mg/kg/dose	oral	once a day	hypokalemia
Furosemide (Lasix)	3-6 mg/kg/dose	oral, IV	rapid onset	hypokalemia
Spironolactone (Aldactone)	2-3 mg/kg/dose	oral	K+ sparing	slow onset (days)
Triamterene (Dyrenium)	1-4 mg/kg/day	oral	K+ sparing	
Beta-Blockers				
Metoprolol (Lopressor)	1-7 mg/kg/dose	oral	renin inhibition specific beta-1 inhibitor	bradycardia (rare)
Propranolol (Inderal)	1-10 mg/kg/day	oral	renin inhibition	bradycardia (rare) fatigue
Agents Acting on Nervous System				
Methyldopa (Aldomet)	5-10 mg/kg/day	oral		rare liver disorders, drowsiness, rarely effective
Clonidine hydrochloride (Catapres)	0.05-0.80 mg total per day	oral	renin inhibition	drowsiness, dry mouth
Guanethidine (Ismelin)	5-20 mg total per day	oral	usually effective before puberty; once a day	postural hypotension
Resperine	0.005-0.015 mg/kg/ day (0.5 mg max)	oral		nasal stuffiness, depression
	0.02 mg/kg q 4 hr	IM		
Vasodilators				
Hydralazine (Apresoline)	1-6 mg/kg/day	oral,IM,IV		
Prazosin hydrochloride (Minpress)	0.5-20 mg total per day	oral		initial syncope
Diazoxide (Hyperstat)	5-10 mg/kg/dose	IV push	rapid onset	hypotension
Nitroprusside (Nipride)	2-8μg/kg/min	IV drip	rapid onset	
Minoxidil (Loniten)	0.2-1.0 mg/kg/day	oral	usually effective	hirsutism, fluid overload, blocker & diuretic required

Prepared by Bonita Falkner, MD

of secondary hypertension, a drug should be selected which will interact with the underlying pathology (*e.g.*, diuretics would be a first choice in Cushing's disease but of little value in hyperthyroidism or anuric renal failure). Begin at low dosage and titrate until satisfactory blood pressure control is achieved.

3. If blood pressure control is unsatisfactory or there are side-effects, a second drug should be added. The second drug is selected from another category. If a diuretic is not given as first drug it should be given as second drug (exception: anuric renal failure).
4. If blood pressure control is unsatisfactory with two agents, a third should be added. Oral vasodilators are generally given as the third drug in therapy.
5. In cases of acute hypertension with CNS symptoms,

the blood pressure should be rapidly reduced. The drugs of choice in hypertensive emergencies are vasodilators administered parenterally (diazoxide, nitroprusside, or hydralazine).

* Prepared by Bonita Falkner, MD

BIBLIOGRAPHY

Ganer OH, Henry JP, Behn C: The regulation of extracellular fluid volume. Ann Rev Physiol 32:547, 1970

A discussion of the physiologic mechanisms involved in the regulation of body fluids.

Winters RW (ed): The Body Fluids in Pediatrics. Boston, Little, brown, 1973

A thorough discussion of body fluids and their regulation, and a discussion of the diagnosis and treatment of errors in fluid balance.

Richard GA, Garin EH, Fennell RS: A pathophysiologic basis for the diagnosis and treatment of the renal hypertensions. Adv Pediatr 24:339, 1977

A clear concise description of the steps necessary for the diagnosis and treatment of hypertension in children.

Disturbances of Growth

20

Allen W. Root
Edward O. Reiter

RETARDATION OF LINEAR GROWTH

Determinants of Growth

The most important factor that determines the linear growth of a person is the genetic potential for growth which he inherits from his ancestors. Genetic influences govern the rate of cell division and increase in cell size which are reflected ultimately as the patient's height. The genetic growth potential may be directly related to the growth of one or both parents or may reflect an inherited influence of more distant progenitors (grandparents, great grandparents, and so on). Superimposed upon the familial genetic potential for growth are internal and external factors which determine whether the person will realize his or her genetic growth potential.

Nutritional deprivation *in utero* may result in permanent retardation of growth. Fetal malnutrition due either to severe maternal malnutrition or more frequently to placental dysfunction of many sorts may permanently imprint a pattern of retarded growth upon the developing fetus by restricting cell division and cell size.

Causes of Small-for-Gestational-Age Births

- Placental insufficiency
  - Maternal toxemia, cardiac disease, hypertension, ulcerative colitis
  - Placental malformations, infarctions
  - Twinning
- Intrauterine infections
  - Rubella
  - Cytomegalic inclusion disease
- Intrauterine drugs
  - Narcotics
  - Aminopterin
  - Alcohol
- Chromosomal anomalies
  - Autosomal
    - Trisomies 21, 15, 18
  - Sex chromosomal
    - XO, XXXXY
  - Chromosomal breakage
    - Fanconi's anemia (pancytopenia, absent radius)
    - Bloom's syndrome (telangiectasies, broad thumbs)
- Endocrine abnormalities
  - Hypothyroidism (rare)
  - Growth hormone insensitivity
  - Human chorionic somatomammotropin deficiency (?)
- Primordial
  - Russel-Silver
  - Conradi
  - Virchow
  - Multiple congenital anomalies

A similar effect is observed if there is significant nutritional deprivation at puberty. In the latter instance, sex hormone secretion in the nutritionally deprived state is associated with epiphyseal maturation and fusion without corresponding increase in chondrogenesis and linear growth. Malnutrition at other times of childhood probably does not permanently impair linear growth potential. "Catch-up" growth may ensue after many years of malnutrition if nutrition is improved. Specific dietary deficiencies of vitamins (A, D), trace elements (zinc, copper), and other dietary components may also impair growth.

Human pituitary growth hormone acting in part through induction of hepatic, renal, and skeletal muscle synthesis of a group of proteins, the "somatomedins," which stimulate growth in diverse tissues (*e.g.*, cartilage, fibroblasts, erythroblasts), plays a key role in cell division. Insulin is a fundamental growth hormone exerting effects not only upon carbohydrate metabolism but also stimulating amino acid transport, protein synthesis, and cell division in a manner identical with that of the somatomedins. Thyroid hormone influences the rate of cell division and growth of cell size. Androgens increase the rate of cartilage cell division but accelerate epiphyseal maturation (calcification) to an even greater extent. Estrogens also stimulate chondrogenesis but advance epiphyseal maturation at an even faster rate. Glucocorticoids inhibit cell division in part by diverting amino acids from protein synthesis into gluconeogenic pathways. Other hormones such as glucagon, the enterohormones (gastrin, secretin, cholecystokinin-pancreozymin), parathyroid hormone, and calcitonin also influence growth directly or indirectly by affecting the rates of cell growth and division.

Major diseases may temporarily or permanently impair the rates of cell division and cell growth. In the majority of instances termination of the disease state is followed by accelerated linear (catch-up) growth which is maintained until the premorbid growth channel is again achieved. The molecular and hormonal mechanisms of the accelerated growth following the termination of starvation or illness are poorly understood; thyrotropin and thyroid hormones are necessary for the recovery process.

Evaluation

An aberration of linear growth should be considered when the child's height falls more than three standard deviations below the mean height for his age, when the patient's growth channel shifts from a higher to a lower position, or when a patient is inappropriately small for family size. A decline in the linear growth velocity is the earliest sign of an abnormal growth pattern.

A precise history of the patient's growth pattern together with accurate past measurements of height (and weight) are needed. Past measurements may be obtained from parental baby books, school, and summer camp physical examinations, or physician's records. The linear growth of a child is not steady. In order to define the child's growth velocity, measurements should be obtained no less than 6 months apart and preferably yearly. There may be a seasonable variation in growth acceleration observed during the spring and summer months.

One should determine when the decline in growth occurred and what symptoms and signs preceded, accompanied, and followed the alteration in growth pattern. Maternal exposure to potential teratogens (drugs, alcohol) or complicating diseases (diabetes mellitus, infectious processes) at the time of conception and during gestation, the conditions of labor (analgesia, anesthesia, duration, fetal position), delivery (head position, umbilical cord position), and the early postnatal period (resuscitative measures) should be noted. Thereafter, the child's growth pattern, health, and associated disease states, symptoms and signs up until the interview are recorded in a chronologic manner. Historical data relative to the health and growth patterns of the parents, siblings, grandparents, and other relatives are accumulated.

Measurements of height, weight, limb length, and head circumference are recorded in a uniform manner. Blood pressure and other vital signs are recorded. Thereafter, physical examination of the integumentary, musculoskeletal, cardiorespiratory, central nervous system, and other systems is performed and the appropriate positive and negative findings recorded. Often the physical examination alone will provide diagnostic clues (*e.g.*, of rickets, chondrodystrophy, hypothyroidism, congenital heart disease).

After completion of the historical review and physical examination, height measurements are plotted; growth velocity should be calculated and plotted:

$$GV\left(\frac{cm}{yr}\right) = \frac{Ht_2 - Ht_1(cm)}{Time\ (yr)}$$

The height age (HA) is the chronologic age corresponding to the 50th percentile for the patient's height. The number of standard deviations that the patient's height falls below the mean height for age can be determined (Table 20-1).

Linear growth potential may be assessed by determining the skeletal maturation or bone age (BA) of a person through roentgenograms of the epiphyseal centers appropriate to bracket both the patient's chronologic age (CA) and HA.

Assuming that the historical review and physical examination do not provide significant diagnostic probabilities, it is possible to classify the patient into one of three groups of patients with growth retardation (see outline).

Causes of Linear Growth Retardation

Genetic short stature
- Familial
- Intrauterine growth retardation (see outline)
- Chromosomal anomalies
  - Trisomies 21, 15, 18
  - Gonadal dysgenesis—XO, XO/XX, XX pi . . .

TABLE 20-1. Means and Standard Deviations of Height (centimeters)

	Males				Females			
	White		Black		White		Black	
Age (years)	Mean	SD	Mean	SD	Mean	SD	Mean	SD
1	76.0	2.68	75.7	2.53	74.4	2.60	74.5	2.62
2	86.9	3.11	86.6	3.12	85.5	3.10	86.0	3.28
3	95.2	3.67	95.6	3.59	94.0	3.56	95.0	3.98
4	102.6	4.14	103.8	4.07	101.7	4.00	103.0	4.48
5	109.5	4.41	110.8	4.40	108.6	4.32	110.4	4.59
6	115.9	4.80	117.3	4.93	115.1	4.72	116.9	5.43
7	122.3	5.22	123.2	5.10	121.2	5.03	123.4	5.96
8	128.1	5.74	129.3	5.25	127.2	5.49	129.2	6.20
9	133.9	5.96	135.1	5.44	132.8	5.76	134.9	6.20
10	140.3		139.6		140.8		141.8	
11	145.7		145.7		147.3		149.2	
12	152.3	8.40	152.1	6.87	155.0	7.43	156.5	6.59
13	159.9	9.11	159.7	9.29	158.7	7.02	159.0	6.55
14	166.9	8.70	165.7	8.62	161.4	6.25	161.5	5.69
15	171.6	7.23	170.4	7.81	162.4	6.98	161.7	6.16
16	174.4	6.94	174.0	6.80	162.8	6.41	161.9	6.51
17	175.7	6.99	174.5	7.01	163.0	6.32	162.7	6.61

(Adapted from: Ages 1–9: Wingerd J, *et al:* Pediatrics *52*:555, 1973. Ages 10–11: Hamill PVV, *et al:* National Health Survey, Series 11, 1970. Ages 12–17: Hamill PVV, *et al:* National Health Survey, Series 11, 1973. National Center for Health Statistics, Public Health Service)

Chondrodystrophies
Mucopolysaccharidoses
Primordial
Russel-Silver dwarf
Bird-headed dwarf of Seckel
Cockayne's syndrome with advanced bone age

Constitutional delay in growth and development

Malnutrition

Emotional deprivation (psychogenic)

Systemic disease
Cardiorespiratory
Congenital cardiac malformation
Asthma
Gastrointestinal
Malabsorption syndromes
Gluten-induced enteropathy
Cystic fibrosis
Regional enteritis
Genitourinary
Renal tubular acidosis
Chronic renal insufficiency
Nephrogenic diabetes insipidus
Hematologic
Chronic anemia
Endocrinologic
Growth hormone deficiency
Hypothyroidism
Hypoadrenocorticism
Hyperadrenocorticism
Diabetes mellitus, poorly controlled

Genetic Short Stature. (HA<BA = CA). The most common form of genetic short stature is familial. However, certain disease states are also characterized by genetic short stature, such as chondrodystrophies, chromosomal anomalies (Down's syndrome [trisomy 21], gonadal dysgenesis [XO and other aberrations of sex chromosome complement], trisomy 15-18), eponymic entities (Cockayne's syndrome, leprechaunism, Seckel's bird-headed dwarfism), intrauterine insults (rubella, placental insufficiency, maternal alcoholism, other drug use), storage diseases (mucopolysaccharidosis), central nervous system abnormalities, and others (see Causes of Small-for-Gestational-Age Births).

Constitutional Delay in Growth and Adolescent Maturation and Malnutrition. (HA = BA < CA). The growth pattern of children with constitutional delay represents a normal variation in the timing of linear growth and sexual maturation. Growth velocity is normal; HA and BA are usually similar and equally retarded behind (but more than 75% of) CA.

Frequently this growth pattern is familial, the mother or father having been delayed in growth and sexual development. Suboptimal nutrition may also delay growth and sexual maturation, but these effects are potentially reversible with restoration of adequate caloric intake prior to the onset of puberty. Frequently, the suboptimal nutritional state reflects decreased appetite of the patient; this can be related to emotional problems, trace element deficiency or unknown factors involved in the regulation of appetite.

Chemical or radiographic studies do not positively identify the child with constitutional delay in growth and sexual development. This diagnosis is based upon the characteristic patterns of linear growth and skeletal maturation, family history, absence of detectable diseases and the maintenance of the anticipated growth pattern during prolonged observation.

***Emotional Deprivation* (Psychogenic).** A wide variety of intrafamilial psychological abnormalities may lead to diminished growth. Clinical appearance may reflect "functional" panhypopituitarism, simple malnourishment, or psychologic aberrations. Relationship of HA and BA to CA is variable. Removal of the child from the offending environment often enhances the growth velocity and may be necessary to confirm the diagnosis.

Systemic and Endocrine Diseases. Many systemic diseases and endocrinologic abnormalities may interfere with a child's linear growth, causing the patient's growth velocity to be abnormally slow. HA or BA are often less than 75% of the CA.

Careful historical review and physical examination may provide the clues necessary to pursue the correct diagnostic pathways, for example, skeletal deformities—rickets, chondrodystrophy, mucopolysaccharidosis; heart murmur or cyanosis—congenital or acquired abnormality of the cardiorespiratory system; hypothyroidism; frequent foul-smelling, greasy stools with ravenous appetite—malabsorption syndrome, and so on. However, disorders of renal (renal tubular acidosis, chronic renal insufficiency), gastrointestinal (regional enteritis), and pituitary (hyposomatotropism) function may be occult.

It is necessary, therefore, to screen patients with suspected systemic or endocrine abnormalities. However, most of the children screened do not have an identifiable disease process and represent more extreme examples of constitutional delay in growth and development than those identified by the criteria previously listed.

In the authors' clinic the following screening studies are carried out on selected children: skull films, complete blood count, sedimentation rate, urinalysis (including pH and specific gravity), serum sodium, potassium, chloride, bicarbonate and calcium concentrations, thyroxine and triiodothyronine resin uptake, a screening test for growth hormone secretion, such as a brief exercise tolerance test and a plasma somatomedin-C determination. A buccal smear is obtained on all short girls, and chromosomal karyotype is performed when there is clinical suspicion of gonadal dysgenesis. If any study is abnormal, appropriate diagnostic steps are pursued. If studies are normal, the patient is observed with periodic (6-month) measurements of height. Observation is continued as long as growth velocity is constant and additional signs and symptoms do not appear. With further deviation of growth pattern, additional investigative efforts are mandatory, including radiographic survey of the gastrointestinal tract and other measures appropriate to the situation.

Management

Management of the child with linear growth retardation depends upon accurate identification of the etiology of the growth pattern. The patient with familial genetic short stature cannot realize a height greater than the genetically determined growth potential. The rate of growth may be accelerated in such children by androgen administration, but this therapy is only used in specific instances. These children and their parents require explanation, reassurance, and reeducation of attitudes concerning the importance of height. Every effort should be made to emphasize the other talents and traits of the child that do not rely upon height.

In children with defined disease processes, appropriate therapy should be undertaken. If the disease state can be identified and treated, the illness-induced impediment to growth can often be overcome and linear growth resumed. Patients undergoing treatment for hypothyroidism with thyroid hormone experience accelerated linear growth velocity, but skeletal maturation often advances still more rapidly. Human growth hormone administered to a patient with hyposomatotropism accelerates linear growth velocity to a greater extent than that of skeletal maturation. Appropriate treatment of the child with malabsorption syndrome or regional enteritis is followed by increased linear growth velocity. However, prolonged exposure to glucocorticoids, either therapeutically or, rarely, as a consequence of a glucocorticoid-secreting tumor, may permanently impair linear growth.

In the nutritionally deprived child, increased caloric intake, often extremely difficult to effect, accelerates growth (see below). A group of children with growth retardation attributed to psychogenic and nutritional factors are members of disturbed families characterized by discord, alcoholism, or infidelity. These children have bizarre behavioral and eating patterns (eating from garbage cans, wolfing loaves of bread and jars of mayonnaise, drinking from toilet bowls). There is decreased secretion of growth hormone and ACTH; after the child is removed from the home these levels return to normal and rapid growth resumes. The abnormal growth and endocrine patterns have been attributed to psychogenic factors, but recent observations suggest that the basic abnormality may be severe nutritional deprivation.

Management of the boy with constitutional delay in growth and development requires reassurance and careful explanation of the normal variability of growth patterns. Prediction of adult height (range) may be helpful. The boy should be observed periodically to be certain that the anticipated patterns of growth and sexual maturation ensue. Occasionally these children are disturbed by the difference between their body image and that of their peers. Verbal reassurance may be insufficient and attempts to accelerate the rates of growth and development may be indicated. Testosterone (by intramuscular depot administration as the propionate or enanthate, or sublingually as methyltestosterone) or a synthetic derivative (fluoxymesterone or oxandrolone) may be administered for brief periods. In view of the potential hazards of androgen therapy, such a rapid acceleration of skeletal maturation and hepatocellular carcinoma, these drugs should be administered only under the supervision of experienced physicians.

In girls with constitutional delay in growth and development, therapy with androgens and estrogens is usually withheld unless there is an extreme degree of growth retardation and parental or patient concern. The decision to employ hormonal therapy in such children should be considered on an individual basis.

FAILURE TO GAIN WEIGHT

Etiology

Frequently a mother complains that her child fails to gain weight, but evaluation of this complaint is warranted only if weight gain is documented to be inadequate or weight loss is actually noted. The causes of failure of weight gain are listed below. In most instances, inadequate weight gain reflects inadequate calorie intake. However, with the exception of underdeveloped countries, unavailability of food seldom accounts for decreased food intake. Inadequate calorie intake in the infant often reflects disturbance in the mother-infant relationship which may be of a complex nature. Although generous quantities of foodstuffs are offered, the feeding period may be shortened because the mother is busy with other children, or there may be (unrecognized) conflict between the mother and child during mealtime. In children with genetic short stature and a fragile bony structure, a small appetite seems appropriate for body size. Frequently, however, slow growth velocity and poor weight gain are due to a small appetite; in such patients a cause for the decreased appetite is usually not identified.

Infrequently, low body levels of zinc may be associated with decreased sensations of taste and smell, leading to anorexia. Zinc supplementation may reverse these abnormalities and improve appetite in selected patients. The diencephalic syndrome secondary to a tumor in or near the third cerebral ventricle is characterized by anorexia and disproportionate happiness with inappropriate affect. Children with this syndrome may grow linearly but are emaciated; surgical or radiation therapy of the tumor may temporarily reverse these findings.

Patients with anorexia nervosa are frequently females whose weight loss began with a self-imposed diet initiated because of actual or suspected overweight. Dieting continues to the point where appetite is lost and the thought, sight, and smell of food become revolting. Frequently there is deep psychopathology, although vigorous interruption of the weight loss before it has progressed to the point of debility may reverse the process. Many disease processes (such as congenital heart disease, chronic renal insufficiency and diabetes insipidus) may be associated with anorexia; thus, children with these illnesses fail to grow, in part, because of decreased calorie intake. Electrolyte disturbances, particularly hypercalcemia, may be associated with anorexia.

Causes of Failure to Gain Weight

- Caloric deprivation
  - Inadequate nutrition (economic deprivation, protein-calorie malnutrition)
    - Marasmus
    - Kwashiorkor
    - Marasmic-kwashiorkor
    - Breast-feeding
    - Zinc deficiency
    - Hypothyroidism
    - Hypercalcemia (subcutaneous fat necrosis, idiopathic hyperparathyroidism, vitamin A or D intoxication)
  - Maternal deprivation
    - Psychosocial deprivation
    - Emotional deprivation
  - Anorexia nervosa
- Organic diseases
  - Congenital anomalies
    - Cleft palate
    - Glossoptosis
    - Megacolon
    - Congenital cardiac anomalies
    - Biliary atresia
    - Obstruction of gastrointestinal tract
  - Malabsorption syndromes
    - Cystic fibrosis
    - Disaccharide intolerance
    - Monosaccharide intolerance
    - Celiac disease
    - Parasitic infestation
    - Hypocalcemia
- Excessive utilization of calories
  - Hyperthyroidism—congenital or acquired
  - Narcotic addiction (maternal)
  - Infections
    - Urinary tract
    - Septicemia
  - Diencephalic syndrome
  - Neoplasia
- Failure to utilize calories
  - Renal insufficiency
  - Renal tubular acidosis (cystinosis)
  - Hypothyroidism
  - Hypopituitarism—hyposomatotropism
  - Hypoadrenalism
  - Galactosemia
  - Glycogen storage disease
  - Diabetes mellitus, poorly controlled
  - Acrodynia
  - CNS insult
  - Diabetes insipidus, central or renal

Gastrointestinal malabsorption characterized by diarrhea and steatorrhea prevents normal absorption of food. Patients with malabsorption usually have large calorie intakes but poor linear growth and weight gain. Stools may be frequent, loose, foul-smelling, or greasy. Certain foods may provoke these symptoms, particularly if the malabsorption syndrome is due to a specific intestinal enzyme deficiency. Hypermetabolic states such as hyperthyroidism, narcotic intoxication, diabetes mellitus, and neoplasia may also be associated with weight loss or failure to gain weight despite excessive calorie intake.

Evaluation

Evaluation of the child who fails to gain weight normally begins with a thorough history and physical examination. A detailed dietary history may distinguish between the quantity of food offered and the amount actually ingested and retained, excluding food remaining on the plate, chair, floor, ceiling, or bib. A description of the frequency, quantity, and type of stool and an extensive systemic review searching for clues to associated illness should be obtained. An attempt to define the mother-child relationship should be undertaken. The interaction between mother and child during the examination and subsequent evaluation should be observed. In most children with inanition, the height is within the low normal range but the weight is below average for the height. Evidence of systemic illness is sought during the physical examination. Most frequently, both the historical review and physical examination are uninformative.

If the child with failure to thrive is hospitalized, the child's calorie intake should be measured. Every effort should be made to ensure sufficient calories for normal growth (in infancy, 120 calories/kg). If observation reveals that the child fails to grow or gain weight despite adequate calorie intake, then, depending upon the clinical findings, a more extensive evaluation should be undertaken. Diseases of the cardiovascular, central nervous, gastrointestinal, genitourinary, and endocrine systems should be eliminated. Studies should include the determination of skeletal maturation, radiographs of the skull, blood glucose, urea nitrogen, serum electrolytes, creatinine, calcium, *p*H, blood count, urinalysis, and examination of stool for ova and parasites, *p*H, reducing substances, and fat content.

Management

If a specific systemic disorder is identified, appropriate and rational therapy should be undertaken. Management of the child with failure to gain weight is difficult after treatable diseases or nutritional deficiencies have been eliminated as possible causes. Close supervision of the child in addition to frequent visits to the physician's office and frequent visits to the home by a visiting nurse, social worker, or physician may reinforce the mother-child relationship and permit more adequate nutrition of the child. Nevertheless, follow-up reports of infants in whom failure to thrive was clearly demonstrated to be due to decreased calorie intake indicate that at older ages these children are still considerably underweight for height. No appetite-stimulating medications are effective. Generally it is recommended that the child be offered substantial calories, but that no confrontation between child and parent over his food intake be permitted, since this is often a self-defeating action. The child should be encouraged to eat more, but not threatened. A reward for weight gained and maintained may be considered in certain instances. Behavior modification of the child with anorexia nervosa is often quite rewarding; he is rewarded only for specific weight gain and must be made to earn even the most limited privilege by weight gain.

OBESITY

Etiology

Most frequently the obese child (weight more than 2.5 standard deviation above the mean or increased skin-fold thickness) presents a subject in whom calorie intake far exceeds calorie expenditure. Patients with exogenous (regulatory) obesity eat large meals (some state they miss breakfast), between meals, and bedtime snacks. They eat frequently, even without hunger, and experience no feeling of satiety; this is a chronic pattern frequently beginning in early infancy and present for several years. It sometimes occurs in previously thin children following tonsillectomy. In addition to the large calorie intake, these children enjoy sedentary activities such as reading, watching television, knitting, or model building. They sit stoically and immobile, conserving every possible calorie. The obese child is often a member of a family with obese parents and siblings. The *pickwickian syndrome* is characterized by excessive and inappropriate somnolence secondary to hypercapnia, hypoxemia, and right heart decompensation due to alveolar hypoventilation, a consequence of the relative immobility of the obese thorax.

Causes of Obesity

Excessive calorie intake
- Exogenous
- Emotional disorder

Organic diseases
- Hyperadrenocorticism
- Hypothyroidism
- Lawrence-Moon-Bordet-Biedl syndrome
- Pseudohypoparathyroidism
- Prader-Willi syndrome
- CNS injury
- Polycystic ovary syndrome

It is rare for an obese child to have a serious underlying disorder. The obesity may reflect an emotional problem. Although the majority of obese children seem perfectly happy and content, this appearance often belies fundamental concern with body image, family strife, or school performance. The possibility of a central nervous system hypothalamic lesion should be considered in children whose obesity begins after meningitis, encephalitis, or head injury.

Rarely is a patient with hypothyroidism confused with the obese subject. In general, the child with *hypothyroidism* presents with severe growth retardation. Occasionally, however, the hypothyroid child may be seen shortly after onset of the hypothyroid state; he is distinguished by the clinical symptoms (lethargy, fatigue, cold intolerance, constipation), physical signs (myxedema, delayed relaxation of deep tendon reflexes, bradycardia, low pulse pressure), and laboratory findings (low thyroxine, and so on) of hypothyroidism. The child with *hypopituitarism* may be slightly obese but is markedly short.

Although exogenously obese children often secrete excessive amounts of glucocorticoids, these levels are appropriate for the increased surface area. The child with *Cushing's syndrome* has a centripetal distribution of fat, violaceous striae, low-set hair line, increased eyebrow hair, and is usually short in stature. In early adolescent females with polycystic ovarian disease, obesity may be accompanied by hirsutism and irregular menses. Children with the *Prader-Willi syndrome* are characterized by severe hypotonia in the neonatal and early infancy periods, which gradually improves thereafter; there is an initially difficult feeding pattern with poor weight gain followed at approximately 1 year of age by excessive weight gain and obesity along with hypogenitalism and hypomentia. The incidence of diabetes mellitus in these children is high. Patients with pseudohypoparathyroidism are characterized by classic phenotype (round facies, modest obesity, short stature, brachymetacarpals, brachymetatarsals, submentation) and biochemical abnormalities (hypocalcemia, hyperphosphatemia). Patients with the *Lawrence-Moon-Bordet-Biedl* syndrome are obese, short, and dull, with hypogonadism, polydactyly and retinitis pigmentosa.

Diagnosis

The diagnosis of exogenous obesity is established by historical and physical findings. The majority of children with regulatory obesity are excessively tall (HA>CA) with weight exceeding height (WA>HA); the bone age is advanced over chronologic age (BA>CA). Additional laboratory studies are not indicated unless other findings suggest the possibility of an underlying disease process.

Management

Management of the obese child is difficult. In the younger child whose diet is controlled by the family, decreased calorie intake may be possible, particularly if one eliminates from the household all foods inappropriate for the child (and usually the rest of the family). If continued rapid weight gain is prevented, the child's future growth will permit redistribution of mass and ultimate loss of obesity without actual weight reduction.

In older children who have achieved adult stature, weight reduction is most difficult to achieve. Dietary restrictions are successful only if the child is an active and willing participant in the prolonged therapeutic process. This requires a mature, thoughtful subject who believes that the long-term rewards of weight reduction are greater than the immediate gains of oral gratification and who is able to withstand the self-inflicted discomfort of decreased calorie intake. Stringent dieting may be accompanied by hyperuricemia which should be specifically monitored. The use of anorexigenic agents is usually without benefit, although these drugs occasionally may reinforce the will to forego immediate gratification for the future rewards of weight reduction. A protein-sparing modified fast may accelerate initial weight loss and enhance compliance through ketosis-induced anorexia. Older children benefit greatly by association with a peer group with similar problems, such as in professional weight reduction groups (Weight-Watchers). In patients with the pickwickian syndrome, immediate weight reduction is mandatory, because this is a life-threatening complication of obesity.

Recent attempts at behavior modification by requiring strict recording of all dietary intake, prolonged and thorough mastication of food, and increased duration of meal time seem promising but will require more prolonged evaluation before their ultimate and long-lasting effects are known. Psychiatric counseling is occasionally of benefit. In extreme instances, a bowel bypass operation has been recommended as a last resort.

GIGANTISM

Etiology

The mean adult height of males and females in America is increasing gradually due to improved nutrition and the absence of serious diseases during the periods of growth in infancy and childhood. Excessively tall stature is most frequently a consequence of genetic inheritance; tall children are often the offspring of tall parents. This is usually of no consequence to the male, but the excessively tall preteenage girl (and her mother) is often concerned about ultimate height. Modestly tall stature is also observed at diagnosis in children with obesity, hyperthyroidism, and diabetes mellitus. *Marfan's syndrome* is an autosomal dominant disorder of mesodermal tissues, characterized by tall stature, long thin fingers and toes (arachnodactyly), subluxation of the lenses, and aortic aneurysm. A similar phenotype occurs in patients with homocystinuria. *Cerebral gigantism* is a sporadic disorder characterized by excessive height and weight, macrocrania, high arched palate, large extremities, and mental retardation. Normal sexual development occurs at the appropriate chronologic age. Bone age may be commensurate with chronologic or height age. Infants with *Wiedemann-Beckwith's syndrome* are large at birth and also have visceromegaly, omphalocele, and hypoglycemia. Rarely does excessive secretion of the pituitary growth hormone, usually associated with a pituitary tumor, cause gigantism and acromegaly characterized by excessive growth (increased deposition of membrane bone in the skull with coarse facial features, enlargement of hands and feet, cardiomegaly, visceromegaly, and so on). Patients with gigantism are often sexually infantile.

Causes of Tall Stature

Genetic tall stature
- Familial

Obesity
Hyperthyroidism
Diabetes mellitus

Disorders associated with excessive stature
- Marfan's syndrome
- Homocystinuria
- Wiedemann-Beckwith's syndrome
- Cerebral gigantism
- Growth hormone excess
- Primary hypogonadism (late)
- Sexual precocity

In children with sexual precocity (see Chap. 21), there is excessive linear growth, but bones mature more rapidly than height increases. Ultimately these children become short adults unless the process of sexual precocity is terminated. Some patients with primary hypogonadism (Klinefelter's syndrome) display long extremities (eunuchoid habitus) and are of tall stature.

Diagnosis

The cause of tall stature is frequently apparent after review of history and physical examination. In the genetically tall subject, growth velocity is normal, physical examination is appropriate for age, and bone age is equal to chronologic age. In patients with disorders cited previously, the clinical findings are usually sufficiently obvious to alert the examiner. The diagnosis of cerebral gigantism is established on the basis of clinical observations (prognathism, antimongoloid slant to the eyes, depressed nasal bridge, dolicocephaly), absence of a definable pituitary tumor, and normal secretion of growth hormone. In patients with acromegalic gigantism, the sella turcica is enlarged and serum concentrations of growth hormone are elevated and often not suppressed by hyperglycemia. The diagnosis of Marfan's syndrome depends upon a positive family history and the presence of typical clinical characteristics. In patients with isosexual precocity, the bone age is markedly advanced and the urinary and plasma levels of gonadotropins and gonadal sex steroids may be elevated.

Management

Males with familial genetic tall stature are reassured as to their basic good health. Attempts to foreshorten excessively tall females by estrogen administration have been advocated. Estrogens accelerate the rate of bone age maturation to a greater extent than the attendant increase in linear growth velocity and height age. The efficacy of this therapy is questionable. In the authors' clinic, the use of estrogens in such females is restricted to those whose predicted adult height is 6 feet or above. For greatest efficacy these medications should be initiated between 8 and 10 years of age and continued until the bone age has reached 14 to 15 years. The attendant hazards of such therapy (excessive vaginal bleeding and potential injury to the delicate hypothalamic-pituitary-ovarian axis) must be appreciated.

There is no specific treatment for patients with cerebral gigantism or Marfan's syndrome. Although neurosurgical removal of the growth hormone-secreting pituitary tumor has been advocated in patients with acromegalic gigantism, the recent identification of hypothalamic growth hormone-release inhibiting factor (somatostatin) suggests that medical therapy for this abnormality may become feasible. Bromocriptine, a dopamine agonist has also been useful in the treatment of this disease. Management of the child with sexual precocity or hypergonadism is discussed in Chapter 21.

BIBLIOGRAPHY

Brasel JA, Blizzard RM: The influence of the endocrine glands upon growth and development. *In* Williams RH (ed): Textbook of Endocrinology, 5th ed, pp 1030–1058. Philadelphia, WB Saunders, 1974

The authors present a comprehensive discussion of the influence of the endocrine system upon normal growth and illustrate the aberrations of growth which may occur in patients with varied endocrinopathies.

Falkner F, Tanner JM (eds): Human Growth: 1. principles and prenatal growth; 2. postnatal growth; 3. neurobiology and nutrition. New York, Plenum Press, 1978

Green M: Pediatric Diagnosis, 3rd ed, pp 369–381. Philadelphia, WB Saunders, 1980

This reference lists causes of aberrations of growth and the evaluation and management of these abnormalities with little descriptive text.

Root AW, Bongiovanni AM, Eberlein WR: Diagnosis and management of growth retardation with special reference to the problem of hypopituitarism. J Pediatr *78:737*, 1971

This article discusses the problem of retardation of linear growth and presents clinical and laboratory data on patients with hypopituitarism.

Supported by National Foundation—March of Dimes Grants 1-323, C-199, and Basil O'Connor Starter Grant 5-71.

Normal and Abnormal Sexual Development

21

Mary L. Voorhess

Sexual development in the human represents a continuum which begins with differentiation of the embryonic gonad and gonaducts, includes development of the hypothalamic-pituitary gonadotropic-gonad system in the fetus and young infant, and extends through sexual maturation at puberty and the attainment of fertility. Intricate control mechanisms govern each stage of differentiation and maturation. This chapter provides the reader with a review of the primary events in normal sexual development and a description of the common abnormalities.

EMBRYONIC SEXUAL DIFFERENTIATION

The human embryo is bipotential and sexual differentiation involves (1) differentiation of the primordial gonads into testes or ovaries, (2) differentiation and development of Wolffian duct structures in the male with inhibition of Müllerian anlage or differentiation of Müllerian duct structures in the female with disappearance of Wolffian anlage, and (3) formation of the external genitalia from common primordia—the urogenital tubercle, the urogenital swellings, and the urogenital folds.

Male Differentiation

The testes develop at approximately the 7th week of gestation by a complex process which appears to be under control of H-Y antigen, a cell surface molecule which is the product of a male determining gene located on the short arm of the Y-chromosome. A regulatory gene on the X-chromosome activates the H-Y gene on the Y-chromosome. H-Y antigen causes the cells of the undifferentiated embryonic gonad to develop into a testis. The Leydig cells of the fetal testis then secrete testosterone, which stimulates development of the Wolffian ducts into the vas deferens, seminal vesicle, and epididymis, and the Sertoli cells of the testis secrete an anti-Müllerian duct factor which specifically inhibits the Müllerian anlage. In specific target areas, testosterone is converted by 5 α reductase enzyme to dihydrotestosterone, which forms an androgen-receptor complex in the cell and induces differentiation of male external genitalia. The urogenital sinus gives rise to the prostate and the prostatic urethra. The genital tubercle develops into the glans penis, the genital folds into the shaft of the penis, and the genital swellings into the scrotum. Fusion of the genital swellings and folds takes place before the 12th week of fetal life, and phallic enlargement occurs throughout intrauterine life under the influence of androgenic hormones. Fetal pituitary gonadotropins are essential for normal growth and development of the testes and external genitalia.

Female Differentiation

In the absence of H-Y antigen, the primordial gonad becomes an ovary. Development begins at the 13th week of gestation and the first follicles appear after the 16th week. The 46,XX-chromosome complement is necessary for differentiation and maintenance of normal ovarian tissue. Fetal pituitary gonadotropins also are essential for development of the ovary. Females with a 45,X-karyotype have only streak gonads containing connective tissue at birth.

Differentiation of the female phenotype, however, does not depend on the presence of a functioning fetal gonad. It results, regardless of chromosomal sex, when fetal testicular hormones are absent. The Müllerian duct structures differentiate into the fallopian tubes, the uterus and the upper one-third of the vagina. The Wolffian anlage regresses, and female differentiation of the external genitalia takes place. The urogenital sinus gives rise to the urethra and lower portion of the vagina. The genital tubercle develops into the clitoris, and the genital folds and swelling differentiate into the labia minora and labia majora. The female fetus may develop varying degrees of masculinization of the external genitalia if exposed to andro-

TABLE 21-1. Disorders of Sexual Differentiation

Classification	Karyotype	External Genitalia and Other Features
Undervirilization of male infant (Male Pseudohermaphrodism)	XY	
1. Defects in both cortisol and testosterone synthesis		
a. 3-β hydroxysteroid dehydrogenase deficiency		Incomplete male, salt loss
b. 17-α hydroxylase deficiency		Female, hypertension
2. Defects in sex steroid synthesis		
a. 17–20 desmolase deficiency		Incomplete male
b. 17-β hydroxysteroid reductase deficiency		Incomplete male
3. Syndromes of androgen resistance		
a. 5-α-reductase deficiency		Ambiguous, with virilization at puberty
b. syndrome of testicular feminization		Female
4. Embryologic defects in testes or penis		Incomplete male
Virilization of female infant (Female Pseudohermaphrodism)	XX	
1. Congenital virilizing adrenal hyperplasia		
a. 3-β hydroxysteroid dehydrogenase deficiency		Ambiguous, salt loss
b. 21-hydroxylase deficiency		Ambiguous, with or without salt loss
c. 11-β-hydroxylase deficiency		Ambiguous, hypertension in late childhood
2. Transplacental maternal androgen		Ambiguous
3. Associated anomalies of genitourinary and gastrointestinal tracts		Ambiguous or incomplete female
Gonadal Disorders		
1. True hermaphrodite	XX, XY or XX/XY	Ambiguous, with ovary and testis or ovotestes
2. Syndrome of gonadal dysgenesis	45 X, 45 X/XX 45 X/XY, etc.	Female
3. Seminiferous tubular dysgenesis (Klinefelter syndrome)	XXY or XXYY	Male, with small testes and occasional gynecomastia

genic substances during critical periods of embryonic development but these compounds have no effect on differentiation of the Müllerian duct structures.

Abnormalities in Sexual Differentiation

Abnormalities in sexual differentiation result from a variety of factors which interfere with one of the stages in embryonic development. These factors include: (1) sex chromosome abnormalities which affect gonadogenesis, (2) defects in testosterone and dihydrotestosterone biosynthesis and end-organ resistance to testosterone, which cause varying degrees of undervirilization of the male fetus, (3) defects in fetal glucocorticoid biosynthesis and prenatal exposure to maternal androgens which cause virilization of the female fetus, and (4) embryologic defects of unknown cause (Table 21-1).

■ SEX CHROMOSOME ABNORMALITIES

Gonadal Dysgenesis (Turner's Syndrome)

Clinical Findings. In 1938, Dr. Henry Turner wrote the first description of gonadal dysgenesis. His report included seven short, sexually infantile girls with similar congenital anomalies including webbed neck and cubitus valgus deformity. Since then, a host of abnormalities (see list) has been described in affected persons. The clinical features are so distinctive in most girls with monosomy X that diagnosis is suspected before confirmation by chromosomal analysis (Fig. 21-1). This is particularly true in the neonatal period when lymphedema of hands and feet and extra skin folds in the neck are hallmarks of the syndrome of gonadal dysgenesis.

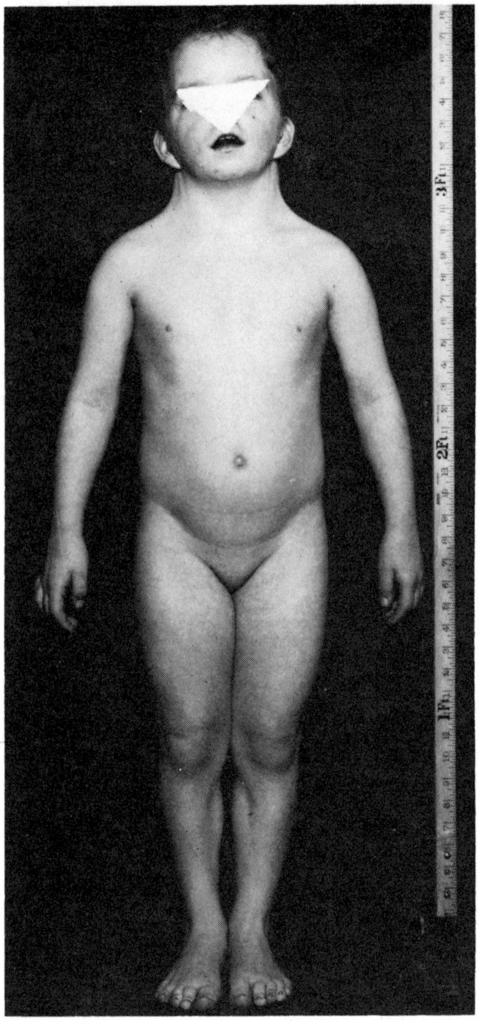

Fig. 21-1. Nine-year-old girl with an XO sex chromosomal pattern and gonadal dysgenesis including coarctation of the aorta. (Neu RL, Gardner LI: Abnormalities of the sex chromosomes. In Gardner LI (ed): Endocrine and Genetic Diseases of Childhood and Adolescence, 2nd ed. Philadelphia, WB Saunders, 1975)

Features of Gonadal Dysgenesis

Short stature—height, <3rd percentile	100%
Low-set and malformed ears	80%

Hypoplastic mandible—high arched palate	70%–80%
Low posterior hairline and short neck	80%
Webbed neck	50%
Shield chest and widely spaced nipples	80%
Congenital heart disease—coarctation of aorta most common	20%
Renal anomalies, especially horseshoe kidney	50%–60%
Increased carrying angle—arms	
Brachymetacarpelia	
Lymphedema of hands and feet	80%
Deeply set fingernails and toenails	70%–80%
Hypoplastic nails	
Multiple nevi	
Sexual infantilism due to ovarian dysgenesis	100%
Mental retardation	10%–15%

Typically, affected persons have a short, stocky build with broad shoulders and a short neck. Pubic and axillary hair usually appear at puberty but there is lack of breast development and no menarche because the ovaries have been replaced by fibrous streaks. The external genitalia are normal but infantile in appearance. Multiple nevi are present over the trunk and upper extremities. The fingernails and toenails are deeply set and hypoplastic.

The phenotypic expression of the disorder is varied, however, and some girls have few somatic abnormalities (Fig. 21-2). A modest degree of breast enlargement may occur but menarche seldom occurs. Regular, cyclic menses are rare. Patients with a mosaic sex chromosome pattern, *i.e.,* monosomy X in a portion of the cells and an XX pattern in the remainder, or those with only a part of one X missing, generally have less severe malformations.

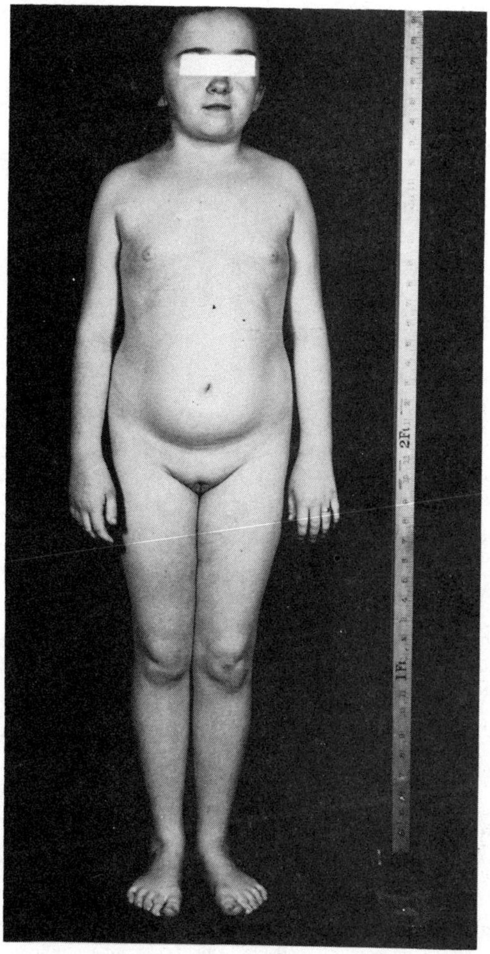

Fig. 21-2. Twelve-year-old girl with the syndrome of gonadal dysgenesis and XX/XO mosaicism. Buccal smear contained 14% chromatin positive cells.

Diagnosis. The sex chromatin pattern is negative, and chromosomal analysis reveals a total count of 45 with a single X in many affected persons. Others have sex chromosomal mosaicism with XX/X, X-isochromosome X, X-deleted X or X/XY patterns. A sex chromatin mass may be present in 7% to 15% of cells when monosomy X occurs in a portion of the cells while persons with XX have 20% to 35% chromatin-positive cells. An X/XY pattern often is associated with virilization of the external genitalia as well as the stigmata described above. Before age 11 to 12 years, bone age is compatible with chronologic age or slightly retarded but it is almost always delayed in older girls. At the age of adolescence, pituitary gonadotropins rise to high levels due to end-organ (ovarian) failure. Estrogen levels are low and adrenal steroid excretion is normal. Plasma growth hormone levels usually are normal.

Females with the somatic appearance of Turner's syndrome who have a positive sex chromatin pattern, a 46,XX-karyotype, and normal ovarian function (Noonan's syndrome) have been described. Congenital heart disease with atrial septal defect or pulmonic stenosis is common in this disorder.

Treatment. Treatment includes correction of the anomalies and use of cyclic estrogen and progesterone beginning at the age of puberty. Sometimes intermittent courses of anabolic steroids also are prescribed to enhance linear growth. Mean adult height of affected girls is only 55 to 56 inches.

Psychological support is an important component of therapy. Most girls are stressed because there is no effective treatment for their short stature. In late childhood, they should be told that hormone therapy probably will be required to induce breast development and menses because the ovaries are incompletely developed. Their need to adopt children also should be discussed.

Patients whose karyotype contains a Y-chromosome require surgical excision of their streak gonads because of the high incidence of gonadoblastoma in these cases.

Seminiferous Tubule Dysgenesis (Klinefelter's Syndrome)

In 1942, Klinefelter, Reifenstein, and Albright described a syndrome in males which is characterized by small, firm testes, hyalinization of the seminferous tubules with absent spermatogenesis but normal Leydig cells, increased secretion of follicle-stimulating hormone, and gynecomastia. Affected persons tend to be taller than average during childhood and to have a eunuchoid build at puberty. Arms and legs are long so the upper segment/lower segment ratio is lower than that found in normal boys and span usually exceeds height. Sexual hair and penile growth appear at puberty but the testes remain small because seminiferous tubule structures account for most of the size of the mature testes. Gynecomastia may be severe. There is a high incidence of emotional disturbance and some boys are mentally retarded.

Diagnosis. The presence of gynecomastia, fairly normal secondary sexual maturation (except small testes) in a tall, pubertal boy strongly suggests Klinefelter's syndrome. Approximately 75% of patients have a positive sex chromatin pattern and a total chromosome count of 47 with an XXY sex chromosome pattern. Others with less severe physical findings and more normal gonadal function may have sex chromosomal mosaicism with XY/XXY patterns.

It is rare that a male with the phenotypic appearance of Klinefelter's syndrome without tall stature and abnormal body proportions is found to have a chromatin-positive buccal smear and a 46,XX-karyotype. These XX males are H-Y antigen-positive, so it is possible there is translocated Y-chromosomal material present somewhere.

Treatment. When there is deficient virilization at adolescence, treatment with androgens is helpful. Cosmetic surgery may be necessary to correct severe gynecomastia and to improve body image. Psychosocial counseling of patients and parents is an important part of medical care.

Undervirilization of the Male (Male Pseudohermaphrodism)

Affected males have gonads identified histologically as testes and varying abnormalities of the gonaduct system and external genitalia. Their sex chromatin pattern is negative, and their sex chromosomal constitution includes a Y-chromosome. There may be unilateral or bilateral cryptorchidism, hypospadias, and hypoplastic scrotum and penis; or, the external genitalia may have a female appearance while the internal duct structures are male (Fig. 21-3). The testes may be located in the pelvis, in the inguinal area or in the labioscrotal folds. There may be such marked alteration in anatomic structures that sex assignment at birth is difficult. The various abnormalities are due to defects in testosterone synthesis, impaired end-organ response to fetal androgens (androgen resistance), or failure of the fetal testes to produce appropriate Müllerian duct inhibiting factor.

Deficient Androgen Formation. Enzyme deficiencies common to both cortisol and testosterone pathways or defects limited to sex steroid synthesis cause decreased androgen formation and incomplete male development. Table 21-1 lists the various deficiency syndromes. Those defects which occur early in the biosynthetic pathway of cortisol are associated with severe salt wasting in addition to ambiguity of the genitalia. Males with 17-α hydroxylase deficiency have hypertension due to accumulation of 11-deoxycorticosterone and corticosterone and female external genitalia.

Rare disorders associated with Leydig cell agenesis or other embryologic defects in the fetal testis also cause deficient androgen formation.

Diagnosis. When a neonate with an XY-karyotype has marked ambiguity of the external genitalia due to undervirilization and salt-wasting syndrome, detailed biochemical studies are required to define the error in steroid hormone synthesis and metabolism. When there is no biochemical defect, injection of x-ray contrast media into the urogenital sinus and a pelvic laparotomy usually are necessary to define the gonads and gonaduct structures.

Some patients will be found to have dysgenetic gonads and a 46,XY, 45,X-karyotype.

Treatment. Cortisol and salt-retaining hormone are necessary for infants

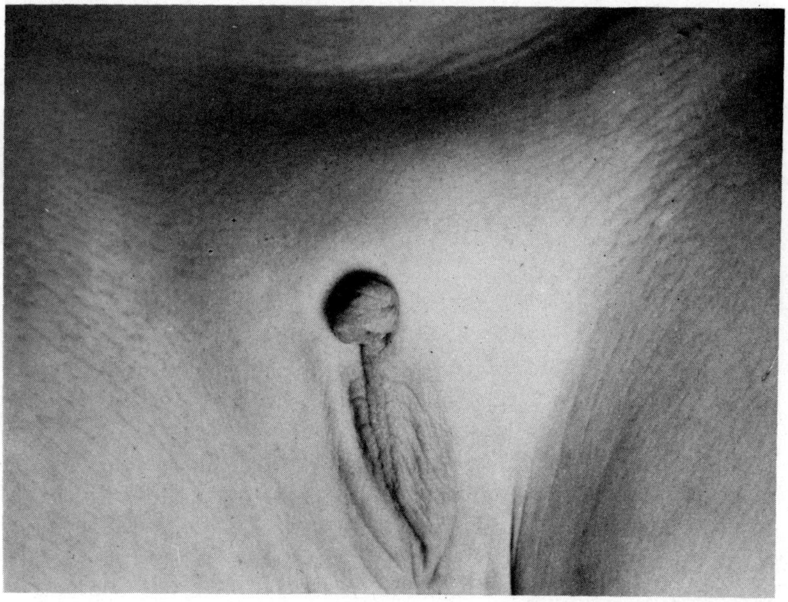

Fig. 21-3. Incomplete masculinization of the external genitalia in a 4½-year-old boy. The phallus and gonads are markedly hypoplastic.

with 20-22 desmolase or 3-β hydroxysteroid dehydrogenase deficiency. The sex of rearing is determined by the functional capacity of the external genitalia. Reconstructive surgery is performed appropriate to the sex assignment and dysgenetic gonads are removed because of their malignant potential. Testosterone or other androgen therapy is prescribed as necessary to enhance masculine development. Whenever severe genital abnormalities are present, extensive psychosocial counseling of parents and patient is an essential part of therapy from the onset. The obstetrician, pediatrician, surgeon, endocrinologist, and psychological counselor should work closely as a team in providing for the needs of the patient and his family.

Impaired End-Organ Response to Fetal Androgen. In impaired end-organ response, testosterone synthesis and Müllerian duct regression are normal but there is an abnormality in androgen action. In the pathway of androgen action, free circulating testosterone enters a cell where it may or may not be converted to dihydrotestosterone by 5-α reductase enzyme, depending on the cell type. The two hormones then bind to the same androgen receptor protein in the cytosol, enter the nucleus, and interact with acceptor sites before affecting a biologic response. When abnormalities are present at a step in this pathway, androgen resistance occurs with varying degrees of defective virilization of the affected male.

5-α Reductase Deficiency. Males with 5-α reductase deficiency have a 46,XY-karyotype, external female phenotype at birth, testes, and normal Wolffian duct structures (epididymis, vas deferens, seminal vesicle, and ejaculatory duct) that terminate in the vagina. At puberty, there is variable virilization of the external genitalia and normal axillary and pubic hair development because testosterone production increases normally.

Deficiency of 5-α reductase is believed to represent the homozygous state of an autosomal recessive disorder that causes abnormal sexual development only in the male.

Testicular Feminization. Testicular feminization is thought to be the most common form of male pseudohermaphrodism. Affected males usually are not identified at birth. They have a female phenotypic appearance and are given a female sex assignment. Diagnosis is made later in life when testicular tissue is discovered in a hernial sac or when an XY sex chromosome pattern is discovered during evaluation of primary amenorrhea.

Clinical Findings. In the complete form of testicular feminization, the external genitalia are unambiguously female, and there is no clitoromegaly. The vagina characteristically ends as a blind pouch. Occasionally, testes are palpable in the labia majora or the inguinal area. Müllerian structures are absent. At the expected time of puberty, enhanced production of 17-β-estradiol by the testes causes feminization of the body habitus, breast development, and estrinization of the vaginal mucosa, but menarche does not occur. Pubic and axillary hair are sparse or absent.

Incomplete or partial variants of testicular feminization have been described. Varying degrees of clitoromegaly and posterior fusion of the labioscrotal folds are present in these cases. The vagina is short and blind-ending. Some virilization as well as feminization may occur at puberty.

There frequently is a family history of the disorder. It is thought to be an X-linked recessive defect or a sex-limited autosomal dominant. When family history is negative, a new mutation may have occurred.

Diagnosis. The combination of a female phenotype, 46,XY-karyotype and gonads which are testes provides strong evidence for the syndrome of testicular feminization. The androgen resistance is due to abnormalities of the androgen receptor. Testosterone synthesis is normal. Therefore, most patients have plasma testosterone levels in the normal range for males. Estrogen production may be in the high normal range for males or in the female range. Since the hypothalamic feedback mechanism also is unresponsive to androgen, luteinizing-hormone (LH) levels are high but follicle-stimulating hormone (FSH) concentration usually is normal. Vaginogram demonstrates a blind-ending vagina without evidence of a cervix. No Müllerian structures can be found on pelvic sonography.

In the prepubertal patient, a normal rise in plasma testosterone following stimulation with human chorionic gonadotropin (HCG) indicates the absence of a defect in testosterone biosynthesis.

Treatment. Malignant degeneration may occur in the gonads of patients with testicular feminization. Incidence increases with advancing age, so most physicians recommend gonadectomy after the second decade of life. Prior to that age, there is no general agreement regarding whether surgical removal of the gonads should be done at the time of diagnosis or after breast development has occurred at puberty. Patients with the partial form should have their testes removed before puberty to prevent unwanted virilization.

Estrogen therapy is prescribed to induce or maintain breast development. Treatment with surgery or dilators may be required to enhance vaginal depth before sexual intercourse. Psychosexual counseling is an important facet of medical care.

Virilization of the Female Fetus (Female Pseudohermaphrodism)

Persons with female pseudohermaphrodism have normal ovaries and normal Müllerian duct differentiation (normal fallopian tubes, uterus, and upper vagina). The abnormality in sexual differentiation is limited to the distal vagina and external genitalia when varying degrees of labioscrotal fusion or clitoral enlargement are found. In almost all cases, the disorder results from exposure of the female fetus to androgenic hormones, the degree of masculinization depending on the potency of the androgen and the stage of fetal development during which exposure occurs. Labioscrotal fusion indicates that there was excessive androgenic stimulation prior to 12 to 13 fetal weeks; by this time, female differentiation of the external genitalia is completed. Often, this fusion extends anteriorly with enclosure of the urogenital sulcus so that there is a single perineal opening and the urethral and vaginal orifices are obscured. Clitoral hypertrophy results from androgen stimulation at any stage of intrauterine development or after birth.

Because congenital virilizing adrenal hyperplasia is the most common cause of female pseudohermaphrodism, it is appropriate clinically to group the disorders into adrenal and nonadrenal causes. Nonadrenal causes include (1) fetal virilization caused by transplacental passage of androgen from the mother, (2) ambiguity of the genitalia associated with abnormalities of the genitourinary and gastrointestinal tracts, and (3) unknown causes.

Congenital Virilizing Adrenal Hyperplasia. A biochemical error in adrenocortical biosynthesis results in cortisol deficiency, an increase in ACTH production, adrenal cortical hyperplasia, and overproduction of intermediary steroid metabolites and androgens. The most common form of the disorder is due to a deficiency of 21-hydroxylase enzyme with or without salt loss; a less common defect is deficiency of 11-hydroxylase enzyme. When the female fetus is exposed to excessive adrenal androgen before the 12th fetal week, there are varying degrees of masculinization of the external genitalia manifested by labioscrotal fusion, a urogenital sinus, and clitoral hypertrophy. The vaginal orifice and urinary meatus usually are found within the perineal opening of the urogenital sinus. Since Müllerian duct development is not influenced by adrenal androgen, the fallopian tubes, uterus, and upper vagina are normal, as well as the ovaries.

Clinical Findings. The appearance of ambiguous genitalia at birth usually leads to prompt identification of females with congenital virilizing adrenal hyperplasia. In severely affected females, virilization of the genitalia may be so marked that the newborn girls are mistakenly thought to be males with bilateral cryptorchidism with or without hypospadias. The enlarged phallus is similar to a penis and is bound down in chordee; the urogenital sinus resembles a perineal hypospadias, and the empty labioscrotal folds have the appearance of bifid scrotum with cryptorchidism (Fig. 21-4). A complete phallic urethra is rarely present.

Because their genitalia are normal at birth, males with nonsalt-losing congenital virilizing adrenal hyperplasia often are not suspected of having the disorder until they are several years old. By then, the excessive production of androgenic steroids has caused acceleration in the rate of somatic growth and progressive virilization with growth of sexual hair, enlargement of the penis, acne, and deepening of the voice. The testes, however, usually remain small.

Both male and female neonates with the salt-losing form of the disorder have difficulties early in life. Weight gain is poor. Vomiting and severe dehydration develop shortly after birth, and sudden death may occur unless prompt treatment is given. The symptoms resemble an addisonian crisis.

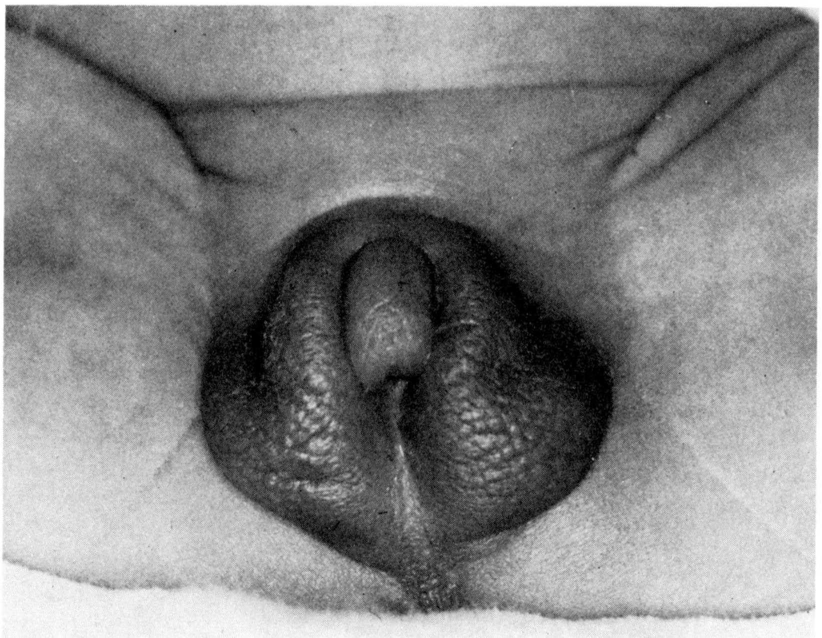

Fig. 21-4. External genitalia of a newborn girl with salt/losing congenital virilizing adrenal hyperplasia (Schlegel RJ, Gardner LI: Ambiguous and abnormal genitalia in infants. In Gardner LI (ed): Endocrine and Genetic Diseases of Childhood and Adolescence, 2nd ed. Philadelphia, WB Saunders, 1975)

Patients with the C-11 hydroxylase enzyme defect also have virilization, and they develop hypertension due to production of excessive amounts of desoxycorticosterone.

Diagnosis. Neonates born with ambiguous genitalia but without palpable gonads should be considered females with a virilizing syndrome (most likely congenital virilizing adrenal hyperplasia) until proven otherwise. Immediate steps should be taken to establish a diagnosis to avoid the danger of an unrecognized salt-losing disorder. No less urgent is the need to determine the appropriate sex assignment.

Genitography, with introduction of radiopaque material into the perineal opening, usually demonstrates a vagina and cervix in females with virilized external genitalia. Pelvic sonography is helpful in identifying the presence of a uterus. Chromosomal analysis should be performed to confirm a 46,XX-karyotype.

Persons with congenital virilizing adrenal hyperplasia and a 21-hydroxylase deficiency have high plasma concentrations of 17-hydroxyprogesterone and their urine contains abnormally large amounts of 17-ketosteroids. Urinary pregnanetriol excretion also is elevated, particularly if treatment is delayed a few days after birth. Measurement of plasma 17-hydroxyprogesterone is a particularly helpful diagnostic test in identifying affected neonates because the analysis can be done rapidly without a 24-hour delay for urine collection. Patients with the salt-losing form of 21-hydroxylase deficiency develop low serum sodium and high serum potassium concentrations by 5 to 7 days of age. In the hypertensive form of the disease, associated with 11-β hydroxylase deficiency, excessive quantities of tetrahydro- compounds derived from 11-desoxycortisol appear in the urine.

Female neonates with nonadrenal causes for virilization of their external genitalia have normal plasma 17-hydroxyprogesterone levels and normal urinary excretion of adrenocorticosteroids and their metabolites.

Treatment. The principle of therapy in congenital virilizing adrenal hyperplasia is to provide physiologic doses of cortisol for the patient. This inhibits ACTH overproduction because of the negative feedback mechanism and prevents accumulation of steroid metabolites with androgenic and hypertensive properties. Patients with the salt-losing form of the disorder also must receive desoxycorticosterone to correct their electrolyte disturbance. Following treatment, the pattern of urinary adrenal steroid excretion becomes normal. Progressive virilization ceases and the child grows normally.

In addition to steroid therapy, most affected girls need perineoplasty to correct the abnormalities of their external genitalia. Usually, a clitoral recession procedure is done during the first year of life, together with exteriorization of the urinary meatus and vaginal orifice. Vaginal reconstruction may be necessary during adolescence or early adulthood. Because congenital, virilizing adrenal hyperplasia is an autosomal recessive disorder, appropriate genetic counseling of the family is an important part of therapy.

Maternal Androgen and Progestogen as Nonadrenal Cause of Fetal Virilization

Sometimes progestational steroids with androgenic activity are given to mothers during pregnancy to conserve the products of conception after threatened abortion or habitual abortion. Placental transfer of the androgenic compounds occurs, and varying degrees of masculinization of the external genitalia of the female fetus may take place, the severity depending on the dose of medication, duration of therapy, and stage of pregnancy. If the drug is administered prior to the 13th week of fetal life, varying degrees of labioscrotal fusion occur. Clitoral enlargement may result from androgenic stimulation at any time during gestation. Steroids such as 17 α-ethynyl-19 nortestosterone (Norlutin), norethindrone with mestranol (Ortho-Novum), norethynodrel (Enovid), and testosterone have been implicated. It is rare for a virilizing ovarian tumor in a pregnant woman to cause a similar picture.

When female pseudohermaphrodism is caused by maternal androgen, urinary steroid excretion of the infant is normal, and progressive virilization does not occur since the baby is separated at birth from the source of androgen. Surgical correction of the genital abnormalities may be necessary in selected cases.

Congenital Abnormalities of Unknown Cause

Some female neonates have ambiguous genitalia and varying congenital abnormalities of the genitourinary or gastrointestinal tract such as absent fallopian tubes, rudimentary uterus, rectovaginal fistula, and absent distal vagina. Their sex chromosome pattern is XX and adrenocorticosteroid excretion is normal. Pelvic laparotomy may be required to evaluate the gonads and the Müllerian duct derivatives.

True Hermaphrodism

Persons with true hermaphrodism have both an ovary and a testis or, more commonly, two ovotestes. Most have an ambiguous phallus with hypospadias or nearly normal-appearing male genitalia. Completely normal female external genitalia rarely are found. Breast development and menstrual periods may occur at puberty.

About two-thirds of true hermaphrodites are sex chromatin-positive, and one-third are sex chromatin-negative even though an XX sex chromosomal pattern in peripheral leukocytes is much more common than an XY constitution. Occasionally, a mosaic sex chromosome pattern is found.

After the sex of rearing has been selected, an effort should be made to preserve the appropriate gonad and remove the inappropriate one. The external genitalia should be reconstructed, as necessary, consistent with the sex assignment.

GUIDELINES TO DIAGNOSIS OF ABNORMALITIES OF SEXUAL DIFFERENTIATION

It is important that any abnormality of sexual differentiation be recognized and correctly diagnosed as soon after birth as possible so that the proper sex of rearing can be assigned and appropriate treatment initiated. The etiology of an abnormality cannot be determined from history and physical findings alone. Diagnostic studies should be performed. Some disorders such as the syndrome of testicular feminization and Klinefelter's syndrome often are not suspected until the adolescent years when normal pubertal development fails to take place.

An abnormality of sexual development should be suspected when the following are present: (1) ambiguous external genitalia, (2) phenotypic male with bilateral cryptorchidism, (3) phenotypic female with masses in groin or labia, (4) congenital edema of hands and feet and extra skin folds in neck of a newborn female, (5) primary amenorrhea in an adolescent female with breast development and decreased or absent sexual hair, (6) small testes in an adolescent male with or without gynecomastia, (7) phenotypic females with short stature and other stigmata of gonadal dysgenesis, and (8) sibling with a disorder of sexual differentiation.

Figure 21-5 outlines a plan for evaluating infants with abnormal external geni-

History	Other affected family members Neonatal deaths Maternal hormone ingestion Maternal health
Physical Examination	Size of phallus—position of urethral meatus Appearance of labioscrotal folds Perineal openings Source of urinary stream Masses in inguinal region or labioscrotal folds Rectal examination (pelvic structures)

Bucccal Smear for Sex Chromatin Pattern and Chromosomal Analysis

Gonads Palpable		Gonads Not Palpable	
Chromatin Negative	**Chromatin Positive**	**Chromatin Negative**	**Chromatin Positive**
1. Defect in testosterone synthesis or metabolism 2. Congenital non virilizing adrenal hyperplasia 3. Androgen resistance syndrome 4. True hermaphroditism 5. Anatomic defect	1. True hermaphrodite 2. Sex chromosomal abnormality	1. Syndrome of gonadal dysgenesis 2. Androgen resistance syndrome 3. True hermaphroditism	1. Female with virilizing adrenal hyperplasia 2. Extra fetal androgens (maternal) 3. True hermaphroditism 4. Anatomic defect

Fig. 21-5. Evaluation of ambiguous genitalia.

talia. Syndromes of marked undervirilization of the genitalia and salt-wasting in male infants are rare disorders.

A careful history from the parents and the obstetrician is an important aid in diagnosis. Since virilizing adrenal hyperplasia is an autosomal recessive disorder, the history may reveal that a sibling died early in infancy with dehydration and collapse (a possible salt-losing crisis), that siblings were born with abnormal genitalia, or that siblings had progressive virilization during childhood. Information about medications taken by the mother during pregnancy may suggest that virilization of the neonate is related to maternal hormone ingestion. It is rare for mssculinization of a female offspring to be due to transplacental passage of androgen from a maternal tumor.

Systematic inspection and palpation of the external genitalia including a rectal examination are an integral part of the evaluation. Masses in the inguinal area or labioscrotal folds usually are testes or ovotestes and suggest a diagnosis of male pseudohermaphrodism or true hermaphrodism. Neonates with phallic enlargement, fusion of the labioscrotal folds, a single perineal opening, and no palpable gonads most likely are female pseudohermaphrodites. Thus, the presence or absence of gonads can be used by the examiner as a guide in approaching the evaluation of an infant with abnormal genitalia.

When no gonadal structures are palpable but the external genitalia are virilized, it is important to look for Müllerian duct structures. The combination of genitography and pelvic sonography are helpful diagnostic aids in identifying a vagina, cervix, and uterus. A chromatin-positive buccal smear also supports the presence of female pseudohermaphrodism (although XX neonates can have a chromatin-negative pattern). Since most females with ambiguous genitalia have congenital adrenal hyperplasia due to 21-hydroxylase deficiency, these studies and measurement of plasma 17-hydroxyprogesterone will lead to diagnosis and permit assignment of sex of rearing within 24 hours of birth. Additional studies including karyotype, urinary steroid analyses, and measurement of serum sodium and potassium also are required to complete the evaluation. Female infants with masculinization of their external genitalia from maternal androgens or from unknown causes will have Müllerian duct structures, XX-sex chromosome pattern and normal levels of adrenal hormones and metabolites.

Patients with palpable gonads and ambiguous genitalia are male infants with undervirilization of the external genitalia or true hermaphrodites. The buccal smear usually is chromatin-negative. Male pseudohermaphrodites have a Y-chromosome or are H-Y antigen-positive while infants whose gonads contain both ovarian and testicular tissues may be 46,XX or 46,XY. Many infants require laparotomy to ascertain the pelvic contents and gonadal biopsy. Biochemical studies including measurement of gonadotropins, adrenal, and testicular hormones and an HCG stimulation test often are necessary.

Male neonates with microgenitalia and hypoglycemia should be suspected of having congenital hypopituitarism. Some infants may have a micropenis and normal scrotum and testes. The cause of this abnormality is unknown.

General Management

Usually, chromosomal sex, gonadal sex, sex hormones, the gonaducts, and the external genitalia are consistent with each other and sex assignment at birth is easy. When abnormalities are present, the physician has the responsibility to evaluate the problem carefully, make a diagnosis as soon as possible, and be sure that the patient is assigned an appropriate sex of rearing. Then, serious psychosocial problems will be obviated for the patient and the parents.

Female pseudohermaphrodites should be reared as females, and the genital defects should be corrected, if necessary by surgery during infancy. Patients with congenital adrenal hyperplasia need adrenal steroid therapy as well.

Male pseudohermaphrodites should be assigned a sex of rearing appropriate to the functional capacity of the external genitalia. If the phallus is markedly hypoplastic or the external genitalia resemble female anatomy making reconstruction of male structures impossible, the person should be reared as a female. The genitalia should be made to conform to the assigned sex as early in life as possible. If the gonads are not consistent with the expected secondary development at puberty, surgical excision will be necessary.

Psychosexual orientation is not due to chromosomal sex, gonadal sex, or sex hormones but is the result of the gender role and life experiences of a person. If the child is raised in the gender role for which he is best suited and there is no uncertainty in the mind of the parents and the physician about the sex assignment, there need be no psychosexual problems or abnormal sexual behavior.

PUBERTAL SEXUAL MATURATION

Puberty is that stage of development between childhood and adulthood which is characterized by acceleration of somatic growth, appearance of secondary sexual characteristics, and attainment of reproductive capacity. It represents the terminal phase of a process of neuroendocrine maturation which begins during fetal life after differentiation of the embryonic gonad into testes and ovaries.

Maturation of Hypothalamic-Pituitary-Gonadal Axis

Gonadotropin-releasing hormone (GnRH) secreted by the fetal hypothalamus activates release of luteinizing-hormone (LH) and follicle-stimulating hormone (FSH) from the fetal pituitary by 10 to 12 weeks gestation; these pituitary gonadotropins, in turn, stimulate gonadal growth and sex steroid production. After 21 fetal weeks, GnRH release is inhibited by the development of negative feedback and increasing sensitivity of the hypothalamic-pituitary gonadotropin axis to sex steroids. There also appears to be an intrinsic central nervous system control mechanism which suppresses GnRH.

After birth, the gonadotropins and sex steroids rise for a few months and then gradually decline and remain suppressed during childhood. At 7 to 8 years of age, maturation of the androgenic zone of the adrenal cortex (adrenarche) begins. Then, CNS inhibition decreases, sensitivity of the GnRH negative feedback threshold changes, and there is pulsatile increase in the secretion of LH and FSH. Subsequently, secretion of sex steroids by the ovary or testis occurs. Prolactin levels rise and the adrenal cortex matures completely.

As the quantity of gonadal steroids increases, pubertal development ensues. Finally, the gonadal hormones themselves are capable of further stimulating the hypothalamic-pituitary axis to secrete gonadotropins (positive feedback). This positive feedback control is particularly important in the female for menarche and ovulation.

Female Changes of Puberty

As puberty approaches, the levels of estrogens increase and bring about development of the nipples and mammary ducts, stimulate growth of the uterus and vagina, and enhance linear growth and skeletal maturation. Production of adrenal androgens increases, and these compounds stimulate growth of pubic and axillary hair, contribute to oily skin and seborrhea and also accelerate the rate of linear growth and skeletal maturation. The mechanism that leads to increased secretion of adrenal androgen is not precisely known; however, it is probably mediated through the anterior pituitary because it is absent in children with hypopituitarism.

Menarche occurs when sufficient estrogen has been produced to cause proliferation of the uterine mucosa. The cyclic vaginal bleeding which occurs during the reproductive years is related to a cyclic pattern of gonadotropin and ovarian steroid production. Besides the negative or inhibitory feedback mechanism by which the changes in the concentrations of circulating sex steroids cause reciprocal changes in secretion of gonadotropin-releasing hormones and gonadotropins, there is a positive or stimulating feedback mechanism in which a critical level of circulating estrogen results in synchronous release of LH and FSH. The negative feedback mechanism is functional in prepubertal children and adults, but the positive feedback mechanism does not appear until late puberty and continues during adulthood. It is this positive feedback that causes the LH surge which leads to ovulation.

There is considerable individual variation in the age of onset of secondary sexual characteristics, in the rate of progression of the changes of puberty, and in the temporal relation of one event to another. The majority of healthy American girls begin sexual maturation between 8 and 13 years. Standards for normal breast and pubic hair development have been described by Marshall and Tanner (Tables 21-2, 21-3) and are used to provide an objective measure of progress in development. Breast enlargement is usually the initial finding but pubic hair appears first in some healthy girls. The average time of transition from Tanner stages 2 to 5 is about 4 years, although some girls may complete their development in 1½ years. On the average, menarche occurs at 12.5 years in America. Peak height velocity usually is reached early in the course of puberty, and significant deceleration in linear growth takes place after menarche. The relation between the events of puberty is more meaningful than the chronologic age of occurrence, however.

Primary amenorrhea in an 18-year-old girl who has stopped growing and has reached stage 5 breast development 3 years previously warrants investigation. Primary amenorrhea in an 18-year-old girl who had onset of breast budding and appearance of pubic hair at age 14 to 15 years and who has shown progressive evidence of growth and development probably represents simple delayed adolescence.

Male Changes of Puberty

At puberty, pituitary gonadotropin secretion increases and stimulates testicular maturation. LH acts on Leydig cells causing them to secrete testosterone and estrogen while FSH acts on the seminiferous tubules to induce and maintain spermatogenesis. A negative feedback mechanism exists between testosterone and LH levels, while a nonsteroidal product of the Sertoli cells called inhibin probably is the inhibitory factor of FSH secretion.

Testosterone and adrenal androgens stimulate (1) growth of the penis and scrotum, (2) growth of facial and body hair, (3) recession of scalp hair, (4) lowering of the voice, (5) increase in muscle mass, and (6) acceleration in the rate of linear growth and

TABLE 21-2. Stages of Breast Development

Tanner Stage	Mean Age + SD in Years at Achievement of Stage
1. Preadolescent; elevation of papilla only	Prepubertal
2. Breast bud stage: elevation of breast and papilla as a small mound, enlargement of areola diameter	11.15 ± 1.10
3. Further enlargement of breast and areola, with no separation of contours	12.15 ± 1.09
4. Projection of areola and papilla to form a secondary mound above level of the breast	13.11 ± 1.15
5. Mature stage; projection of papilla only, due to recession of the areola to the general contour of the breast.	15.33 ± 1.74

(Adapted from Marshall WA, Tanner JM: Variations in the pattern of pubertal changes in girls. Arch Dis Childhood *44*:291, 1969)

TABLE 21-3. Stages of Pubic Hair Growth in Girls

Tanner Stage	Mean Age + SD in Years at Achievement of Stage
1. Preadolescent; no pubic hair	Prepubertal
2. Sparse growth of long, slightly pigmented, downy hair, straight or slightly curled, appearing chiefly along labia	11.69 ± 1.21*
3. Considerably darker, coarser, and more curled. Hair spreads sparsely over junction of the pubes.	12.36 ± 1.10
4. Hair adult in type but area covered is smaller than in adults. No spread to thighs	12.95 ± 1.06
5. Adult hair distributed as an inverse triangle. Spread to medial surface of thighs	14.41 ± 1.12

(Adapted from Marshall WA, Tanner JM: Variations in the pattern of pubertal changes in girls. Arch Dis Childhood *44*:291, 1969)
* Probably occurs earlier. See original article.

skeletal maturation. Testosterone is necessary for full maturation of the seminiferous tubules and for growth of the prostate and seminal vesicles.

Marshall and Tanner have described the variations in the physical changes of puberty in boys and have classified pubic hair and genital growth into five stages of development as noted in Tables 21-4 and 21-5. The initial physical sign of puberty in most boys is testicular enlargement. Prepubertal testes are less than 2 cm in greatest length so the presence of gonads which are more than 2.5 cm in length indicates early pubertal development. By stage 3, the stretched penis is usually more than 6 to 7 cm in length. On the average, the genitalia reach the adult stage within 3 years. Facial hair growth is not abundant until after genital stage 5.

Figure 21-6 diagrams the sequence of events at puberty in relation to age in years for the average boy and girl. Girls begin their pubertal growth spurt early in the course of development of their secondary sexual characteristics, while it is unusual for boys to reach their peak height velocity until their genitalia are quite well developed. Most girls have completed their linear growth at the age when boys attain their maximum adolescent spurt.

Disorders of Sexual Maturation

It is convenient, clinically, to consider disorders of sexual maturation on the basis of (1) overproduction, (2) underproduction, and (3) normal production of the hormones involved in the various stages of development. There also may be increased or decreased tissue responses to the hormones. The higher centers in the cerebral hemispheres, the hypothalamus, the anterior pituitary, the gonads, and the adrenals may play primary or secondary roles in the disturbance. Intrinsic factors of genetic, neural, infectious, metabolic, or neoplastic origin and extrinsic factors such as environment and drugs may interfere with normal physiologic processes, leading to overproduction or underproduction of hormones. The patient, in turn, may exhibit precocious, delayed, or absent secondary sexual development.

Sexual Precocity. When secondary sexual characteristics develop at an ear-

TABLE 21-4. Stages of Pubic Hair Growth in Boys

Tanner Stage	Mean Age + SD in Years at Achievement of Stage
1. Preadolescent. No pubic hair	Prepubertal
2. Sparse growth of long, slightly pigmented downy hair, straight or slightly curled, chiefly at base of penis	13.44 ± 1.09*
3. Considerably darker, coarser, and more curled. Hair spreads sparsely over junction of the pubes.	13.9 ± 1.04
4. Hair adult in type but area covered is still small. No spread to medial surface of thighs	14.36 ± 1.08
5. Adult in quantity and type. Inverse triangle. Spread to medial thighs but not up linea alba.	15.18 ± 1.07

(Adapted from Marshall WA, Tanner JM: Variations in the pattern of pubertal changes in boys. Arch Dis Childhood 45:13, 1970)
* Probably occurs earlier. See original article.

lier age than normal, the child has the syndrome of *precocious puberty. Isosexual precocity* refers to sexual development consistent with the phenotype of the child, whereas, *heterosexual precocity* implies that development of sexual characteristics deviate from the phenotype of the person. In *true (complete) precocious puberty*, normal hypothalamic-pituitary-gonadal function is activated at an abnormally early age, whereas, in *pseudoprecocious puberty*, secondary sexual characteristics develop because of abnormal production of estrogens or androgens without maturation of the gonads. True precocious puberty arises from dysfunction of the central nervous system and is characterized by an adult pattern of sexual function, *i.e.,* menstruation in girls and testicular maturation and spermatogenesis in boys. Girls with incomplete precocious puberty do not have ovulatory cycles, and spermatogenesis does not occur in affected boys because the disorder occurs without pituitary gonadotropic stimulation.

Complete precocious puberty is five to six times more common than pseudoprecocious puberty and occurs much more often in girls than in boys. About 80% of prematurely developed girls have no demonstrable lesion of the hypothalamic-pituitary-gonadal axis or other identifiable etiology for their precocious development and are said to have "constitutional" or "idiopathic" sexual precocity. In contrast, more than 60% of boys with precocious development have serious organic disease.

When breast development occurs in girls prior to age 8 years without other evidence of precocious sexual maturation, it is called *premature thelarche.* The isolated appearance of axillary or pubic hair before age 8 years in girls and age 10 years in boys is called *premature adrenarche.* Both of these disorders are benign. The physician should always be alert to the possibility that these findings are the first evidence of what later will be complete sexual precocity.

Etiology. Even though no etiology can be identified for the precocity in most girls and in some boys, a thorough study of each child is required. A diagnosis of idiopathic or constitutional precocity should be made only after organic causes have been ruled out.

Heterosexual precocity in girls is caused by abnormalities which result in excessive circulating androgens such as arrhenoblastoma of the ovary, tumor, or biochemical defect in steroid hormone synthesis of the adrenal or ingestion of androgens. Heterosexual precocity in boys is rare and may

TABLE 21-5. Stages of Genital Growth in Boys

Tanner Stage	Mean Age + SD in Years at Achievement of Stage
1. Preadolescent. Testes, scrotum, and penis are same size and proportion as in early childhood.	Prepubertal
2. Scrotum and testes have enlarged and there is some reddening and change in texture of scrotal skin.	11.64 ± 1.07
3. Growth of penis has occurred, at first mainly in length but with some increase in breadth. Further growth of testes and scrotum	12.85 ± 1.04
4. Penis further enlarged in length and breadth with development of glans. Testes and scrotum further enlarged.	13.77 ± 1.02
5. Genitalia adult in size and shape	14.92 ± 1.10

(Adapted from Marshall WA, Tanner JM: Variations in the pattern of pubertal changes in boys. Arch Dis Childhood *45*:13, 1970)

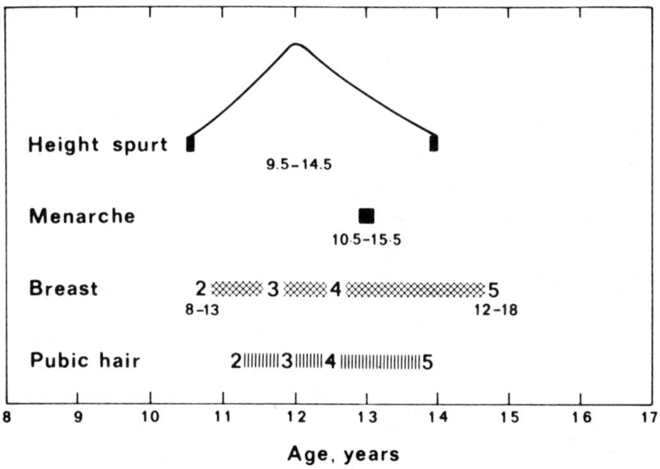

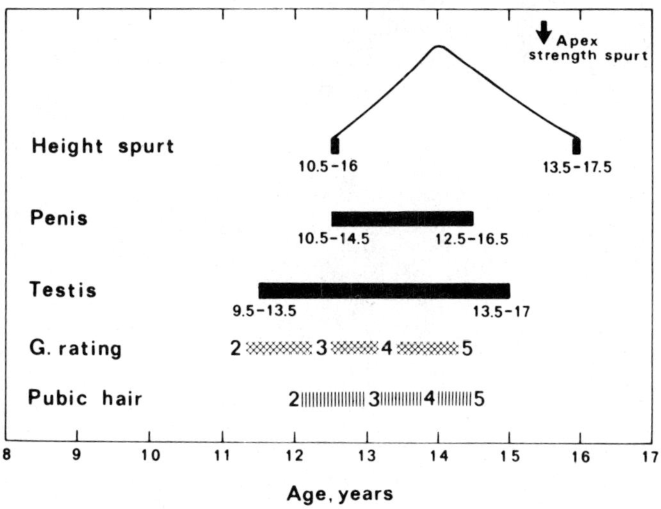

Fig. 21-6. Diagram of sequence of events at adolescence in girls and boys. An average girl and boy is represented; the range of ages within which each event charted may begin and end is given by the figures placed directly below its start and finish. (Tanner JM: Growth and endocrinology of the adolescent. In Gardner LI (ed): Endocrine and Genetic Diseases of Childhood and Adolescence, 2nd ed. Philadelphia, WB Saunders, 1975)

be caused by excessive estrogen produced by a feminizing tumor of the adrenal or other estrogen-producing neoplasms as well as ingestion of estrogen.

Clinical Evaluation of the Patient. A carefully taken history is an important part of the initial evaluation of sexual precocity. The physician should document the chronology of the sexual development and chart any growth data. The various stages of pubertal development may follow the usual sequence or occur in random fashion; sometimes vaginal bleeding is the first sign of precocity in girls. Acceleration of the linear growth rate usually starts at the onset of precocious development. Inquiry should be made about ingestion of drugs and vitamins as well as application of hormone-containing ointments. Signs and symptoms that can be referred to the central nervous system (visual disturbances, convulsions, behavior changes, polydipsia and polyuria, trauma, and infection) are particularly important. A history of precocious development in relatives may be helpful in identifying familial precocity or congenital adrenal hyperplasia.

Accurate measurements of head circumference, length or height, arm span, lower segment, weight, and blood pressure are essential. A young child with a large head may have hydrocephalus, a congenital cyst, or another expanding intracranial lesion. Hypertension may occur in association with CNS lesions or adrenal disorders. The physical examination should include careful inspection for *café au lait* spots and asymmetric growth which occur in the McCune-Albright syndrome and in neurofibromatosis. Abdominal examination may reveal a mass in the renal, hepatic, or ovarian region.

Facial acne, a muscular habitus, sexual hair growth, and penile enlargement in the male or clitoromegaly in the female suggest excessive androgen production. Breast development, sexual hair, and appearance of genitalia should be rated according to the criteria of Tanner. It is desirable to record breast size, stretched penile length, and testicular dimensions so a reference will be available to judge the subsequent rate of progression of the precocity. Bilateral testicular enlargement indicates gonadotropin stimulation while unilateral increase in size occurs in the presence of tumor, adrenal rest cells, or other localized pathology. Estrogen production in girls not only causes breast development but also results in a white vaginal discharge or vaginal bleeding which is apparent on examination of the introitus. Rectal examination is necessary to delineate adnexal anatomy and to check uterine size in girls. The uterus enlarges in response to estrogen but remains age-appropriate in size in the presence of androgens. Enlargement of the prostate may be found in males with precocity.

A detailed neurologic examination including perimetry is essential. Visual field defects may occur before other signs of an intracranial lesion when a tumor impinges on the optic tracts or chiasm.

Diagnostic Studies. In most cases, a careful review of the history and physical findings provide clues which indicate the appropriate direction to pursue in the diagnostic evaluation. It is best to draw up a protocol at the outset which lists the tests to be performed during each day of investigation to avoid needless delays.

For instance, x-ray contrast material which is excreted by the kidneys may interfere with analyses of certain urinary hormonal metabolites; therefore, 24-hour urine specimens should not be collected while radiologic studies are in progress. Furthermore, urine samples may be inadvertently lost, particularly from young patients, during x-ray procedures.

Radiologic Studies. Androgens and estrogens accelerate osseous maturation, so the bone age of children with progressive sexual precocity will be advanced except in the rare cases of hypothyroidism and isosexual precocity in which osseous maturation usually is delayed. Skeletal maturation is usually assessed by comparing x-rays of the hand and wrist with an atlas of bone age radiographs.

Skull radiographs may reveal an abnormality of the sella turcica, intracranial calcifications, or increased intracranial pressure. Patients with McCune-Albright syndrome often have sclerosis at the base of the skull as well as osteolytic lesions of polyostotic fibrous dysplasia.

A skeletal survey should be done when asymmetry of the extremities or cutaneous abnormalities suggest a bone dysplasia.

When an intracranial lesion is suspected, computerized axial tomography of the head usually is indicated. Brain scan, arteriography, or pneumoencephalography are required in selected cases only.

Computerized axial tomography and ultrasonography are important noninvasive diagnostic aids when a mass in an adrenal, ovary, or some other site in the abdomen or pelvis is suspected. Intravenous pyelography will assist in detection of suprarenal lesions. Venography and arteriography may be necessary to define specific lesions.

Laboratory Studies. Children with isosexual precocity of cerebral origin have levels of urinary 17-ketosteroids (17-KS) and dihydroepiandrosterone (DHA) which are appropriate for their maturational ages. Urinary pregnanetriol and plasma 17-OH progesterone levels are normal. Plasma estradiol and testosterone concentrations are compatible with the stage of sexual maturation. Cytologic examination of a vaginal smear or of urinary sediment cells in girls indicate the presence of ovarian sex steroids. A single plasma follicle-stimulating hormone (FSH) and luteinizing-hormone (LH) measurement may be low or in the pubertal range because of the pulsatile release of gonadotropins from the pituitary. Thus, it is preferable to obtain a timed overnight or a 24-hour uine collection for analysis of gonadotropins. These measurements are diagnostic only in situations in which elevation of gonadotropins from extra pituitary sources, such as a trophoblastic neoplasm, are suspected. Marked elevation of human chorionic gonadotropins (which cross-react in the LH assay) is found in patients with chorionic gonadotropin-secreting tumors. Gonadotropin levels which are minimally elevated, normal, or low for age do not provide other diagnostic information.

Plasma and urinary estradiol levels usually are markedly elevated in girls with granulosa cell tumors of the ovary. Urinary pregnanediol, the metabolite of progesterone, is elevated in thecomas as well as in cycling precocious girls during the luteal phase. Some ovarian tumors secrete androgens as well as estrogens.

Urinary 17-ketosteroid, dihydroepiandrosterone (DHA), and pregnanetriol excretion is increased in children with congenital virilizing adrenal hyperplasia due to 21-OH deficiency, and the levels fall to normal following dexamethasone suppression. The concentration of plasma 17-OH progesterone follows a similar pattern. In patients with adrenal tumors, steroid production is autonomous and not under ACTH control, and 17-ketosteroid and DHA levels cannot be suppressed by dexamethasone. 17-OH progesterone levels are normal. Leydig cell tumors of the testis in boys also are androgen-producing neoplasms which function autonomously.

Treatment. Surgical removal of hormone-secretory tumors of the ovary, adrenal gland, or testis obviously is necessary. Unfortunately, tumors of the central nervous system rarely are amenable to curative surgery. Radiation therapy and chemotherapy may be helpful in selected cases.

The course of idiopathic isosexual precocity in girls is variable, sometimes remaining stationary, sometimes progressing slowly, and sometimes moving rapidly to complete sexual maturation. Thus, it is necessary to observe the patient carefully for as long as one year after initial evaluation to determine the course of the sexual development. There is no satisfactory treatment to stop the process. Medroxyprogesterone therapy may be used to depress levels of gonadotropins and cause cessation of menses and regression of breast development. However, it usually has little effect on rate of linear growth or skeletal maturation.

Boys with nonfamilial isosexual precocity of undetermined etiology must be followed very carefully because a central nervous system lesion can remain undetected for years.

Particular attention must be given to the psychological management of children with sexual precocity. Affected children appear much older than their chronologic age because of their physical maturity, yet they have psychosexual development consistent with their chronologic age.

Gynecomastia. Enlargement of mammary tissue in the male is called *gynecomastia.* It is common in the neonate due to transplacental passage of maternal estrogen; it usually disappears within a few weeks and is rare during childhood years. Seventy percent or more of boys have gynecomastia during adolescence, however. It may consist of a 3 to 4 cm button of tissue beneath the areolae or it may be severe enough to result in pendulous breast development. The enlargement is usually bilateral but occasionally is limited to one breast. The growth of mammary tissue is thought to result from a decrease in the testosterone-estradiol ratio during rapid pubertal maturation. Mastectomy may be required when the hyperplasia is marked or causes profound psychological problems.

Testicular and adrenal tumors rarely cause gynecomastia. It may occur in Klinefelter syndrome or be associated with drug therapy, use of marijuana, and liver disease.

Delayed Sexual Maturation. Delayed adolescence may result from hypothalamic-pituitary dysfunction leading to gonadotropin deficiency (hypogonadotropic hypogonadism) or from gonadal disease (hypergonadotropic hypogonadism). Causes of delayed adolescence are listed below.

Causes of Delayed Adolescence

- Normal Variation
  - Constitutional delay—more common in boys
- Abnormal
  - *Hypothalamic-Pituitary Axis* (hypogonadotropic hypogonadism)
    - Congenital anomalies—absence of releasing hormones
    - Inflammatory disorder—encephalitis, sarcoidosis
    - Tumors—craniopharyngioma, hamartoma, glioma
    - Trauma—basilar skull fracture
    - Suppression by exogenous hormone
  - *Gonads* (hypergonadotropic hypogonadism)
    - Ovary
      - Chromosomal abnormality—syndrome of gonadal dysgenesis
      - Tumors requiring oophorectomy
      - Trauma—bilateral torsion of pedicle, radiation therapy
    - Testis
      - Chromosomal abnormality—Klinefelter's syndrome
      - Inflammation—mumps orchitis
      - Tumor
      - Trauma—torsion, atrophy following orchidopexy
  - *Others*
    - Chronic systemic illness
    - Congenital absence of uterus or vagina or both
    - Anorexia nervosa

Constitutional Delay (Normal). When delay in sexual maturation merely represents retardation in activation of the hypothalamic-pituitary-gonadal axis at the time of puberty, it is called constitutional delay or idiopathic delay in growth and development. These children have a normal growth rate at or near the third percentile until age 11 to 12 years when deceleration occurs. Skeletal maturation is delayed and usually consistent with height age and stage of puberty development. Often there is a history of late adolescent development in other family members. It may be difficult to differentiate severe constitutional delay from permanent hypogonadotropic hypogonadism in certain people for many years.

Hypogonadotropic Hypogonadism. Hypogonadotropic hypogonadism is due to a permanent deficiency of hypothalamic gonadotropin-releasing hormone or pituitary gonadotropins. Congenital abnormalities, inflammatory disorders, trauma, or tumors may be causative factors. Sometimes there is familial occurrence of hyposmia or anosmia as well as other defects such as cleft lip and palate in association with hypogonadotropism.

Hypergonadotropic Hypogonadism. Elevations of FSH and LH are found during early adolescence because there is deficient gonadal steroid hormone production. The most common primary gonadal disorder in girls is the syndrome of gonadal dysgenesis which is usually associated with a sex chromosome abnormality. Primary testicular dysgenesis is found in males with Klinefelter's syndrome. Other boys may have congenital hypoplasia or agenesis of the testes with or without associated somatic abnormalities. Occasionally, Leydig cell function is preserved so that virilization occurs, but the patients are sterile. In both cases, the gonads may lose function subsequent to trauma or inflammation.

Other Causes. Chronic diseases as well as malnutrition or significant weight loss from dieting often cause varying degrees of delayed sexual maturation. Primary amenorrhea rarely is caused by an imperforate hymen leading to hematocolpos or by absence of the uterus or vagina.

Clinical Evaluation of Patient with Delayed Sexual Maturation. A historical review beginning with the obstetrical data is essential. Inappropriate birth weight and length for gestational age may indicate intrauterine growth failure. Babies who sustain cerebral anoxia during a difficult delivery and resuscitation sometimes grow poorly from birth as do those who have significant illness during the neonatal period.

Malnutrition, chronic illness, and endocrine disorders in childhood can cause deceleration in the rate of growth, delayed osseous maturation, and delayed sexual development. Information about school achievement, psychosocial relations, and family constellation provides clues to growth retardation due to emotional deprivation.

Review of the family history may show that other members have had delayed growth and sexual maturation. All past measurements should be plotted on growth charts so that the pattern can be evaluated. Deceleration in the rate of linear growth usually indicates organic disease and requires thorough diagnostic evaluation, while children with constitutional short stature and delayed adolescence grow at a constant rate through the years to the age of puberty.

When partial sexual maturation has taken place, it is important to determine the exact chronology of the stages of pubertal development. A healthy 14-year-old boy who is prepubertal in development may have simple delayed adolescence, whereas a boy of similar age who has had Tanner stage 4 genital development for 2 to 3 years except for small, prepubertal sized testes needs detailed evaluation.

General inspection of the patient at the outset of the physical examination provides useful clues. There may be no evidence of secondary sexual characteristics, or partial development may be present. A girl with gonadal dysgenesis may have pubic and axillary hair but no breast development. Boys with Klinefelter's syndrome may have gynecomastia, sexual hair, and pubertal enlargement of the penis but small testes. The physician should look for associated somatic abnormalities (see Gonadal Dysgenesis). Accurate measurements of head circumference, height and weight, arm span, and lower segment are made. Boys with a eunuchoid habitus and hypogonadism have a long arm span and a decreased ratio of upper/lower body segments. On the other hand, the ratio is increased in hypothyroidism and patients with hypopituitarism usually have normal body proportions.

Examination for evidence of systemic disease is essential in patients with delayed maturation. A careful neurologic evaluation including perimetry should be done. Since some patients with hypogonadism have anosmia, olfactory sensation should be checked.

Careful inspection of the genitalia in girls permits visualization of the hymen, and the uterine cervix can be palpated on rectal examination. In boys, particular attention should be directed toward the location of each testis and its size and consistency. The stage of sexual maturation of all patients should be assessed by the criteria of Tanner.

Diagnostic Studies. After the history, physical examination, and review of all available growth data, the physician must decide the appropriate diagnostic approach.

Most often, particularly in boys, lack of secondary sexual characteristics is due to constitutional delay. Skeletal maturation of the patient is determined by x-ray examination of the hand and wrist and comparison of the film with plates in an atlas of standards for bone age. Height age and bone age usually are equally delayed.

Serum and urine gonadotropin levels and concentrations of gonadal hormones are appropriate for the degree of sexual maturation of the patient. As time progresses, there is increase in the gonadotropins, particularly at night, and then physical signs of sexual maturation appear.

Pubertal girls with gonadal dysgenesis or with ovarian agenesis and boys with Klinefelter's syndrome or other types of testicular dysgenesis have high plasma and urinary gonadotropin levels because of hypogonadism and lack of a normal negative feedback mechanism. Their gonadal steroid hormone concentrations typically are low. As discussed previously, females with gonadal dysgenesis and males with Klinefelter's syndrome have sex chromosome abnormalities. The culdoscope may be used to visualize the ovaries and other pelvic structures in selected girls when ovarian agenesis is suspected. Boys with anorchia do not increase plasma levels of testosterone after human chorionic gonadotropin (HCG) stimulation in contrast to males with cryptorchidism whose testosterone levels rise significantly.

When linear growth rate has not been constant through the years, when there is interruption in the usual sequence of secondary sexual development, or when subjects with suspected constitutional delay do not mature as expected, further evaluation is necessary. After nonendocrine systemic disease and chromosomal abnormalities have been ruled out, each component of the hypothalamic-pituitary-gonadal axis should be investigated in an orderly sequence.

Skull radiographs are obtained and visual field examination is done. When there is evidence of tumor or other expanding lesion, computerized axial tomography of the head is indicated. Electroencephalography, brain scan, and cerebral angiography may be helpful in defining a lesion in specific cases.

When hypogonadism is the result of a hypothalamic-pituitary abnormality, serum and urinary gonadotropin levels are low. After administration of synthetic gonadotropin-releasing hormone, the secretion of FSH and LH increases to the normal range when there is hypothalamic dysfunction but remains abnormally low in hypopituitarism.

Children whose delayed growth and development is on the basis of panhypopituitarism also have low levels of growth hormone following provocative stimulation by agents such as insulin and arginine. Thyrotropin secretion can be evaluated by measurement of serum TSH and T4 levels. Function of the hypothalamic-pituitary-adrenal axis is assessed by determining plasma cortisol response to insulin-induced hypoglycemia and by using the metyrapone test. ACTH can be measured by radioimmunoassay but the test is not performed in most clinical laboratories.

Treatment. Patients with constitutional delay in growth and sexual maturation should be followed regularly to be certain that pubertal development occurs and to reassure the patient and the parents. Boys, particularly, are subject to teasing by their peers and may develop behavioral and school problems. All persons with uncomplicated constitutional delay eventually will have normal secondary sexual characteristics without treatment. Occasionally, when profound psychological problems arise, it is appropriate to give boys a short course of androgen or HCG therapy to enhance development. It is usually not necessary to treat girls who have constitutional delay.

Males with hypogonadotropic hypogonadism or primary gonadal failure are given testosterone to promote virilization, and females are given estrogen and progesterone therapy to induce feminization. When fertility is desired, gonadotropins can be prescribed for selected patients with hypothalamic-pituitary dysfunction. Patients with deficiency of other pituitary hormones also may require treatment with growth hormone, thyroid hormone, and hydrocortisone.

BIBLIOGRAPHY

Grumbach MM: The neuroendocrinology of puberty. In Kreiger DT, Hughes JC (eds): Neuroendocrinology. The Interrelationships of the Body's Two Major Integrative Systems in Normal Physiology and Clinical Disease, pp 249–258. MA Sunderland, Sinauer Associates, 1980

A current review of the endocrine events of puberty beginning with sexual differentiation in the fetus. Excellent diagrams.

Imperato-McGinley J, Peterson RE: Male pseudohermaphroditism: the complexities of male phenotypic development. Am J Med 61:251, 1976

A comprehensive description of the basic steps in human sexual differentiation, especially in the male.

Kaplan SA: Diseases of the adrenal cortex II. Congenital adrenal hyperplasia. Pediatr Clin North Am 26:77, 1979

A review of the pathophysiology, clinical presentation, and treatment of congenital adrenal hyperplasia.

Lemli L, Smith DW: The XO syndrome: a study of the differentiated phenotype in 25 patients. J Pediatr 63:577, 1963

A clinical description of the findings in the 45 X syndrome.

Marshall WA, Tanner JM: Variation in the pattern of pubertal changes in girls. Arch Dis Child 44:291, 1969

Marshall WA, Tanner JM: Variations in the pattern of pubertal changes in boys. Arch Dis Child 45:13, 1970

The Marshall and Tanner texts are classic descriptions of normal pubertal development in girls and boys.

Nora JJ, Nora AH, Sinha AK, Spangler RD, Lubs HA: The Ullrich-Noonan syndrome (Turner phenotype). Am J Dis Child 127:48, 1974

Sizonenko PC: Endocrinology in preadolescents and adolescents. I. Hormonal changes during normal puberty. Am J Dis Child 132:704, 1978

Sizonenko PC: Preadolescent and adolescent endocrinology: physiology and physiopathology. II. Hormonal changes during abnormal pubertal development. Am J Dis Child 132:797, 1978

Styne DM, Kaplan SL: Normal and abnormal puberty in the female. Pediatr Clin North Am 26:123, 1979

A comprehensive review of the subject with excellent tables and figures as well as numerous references.

Juvenile Diabetes: Insulin-Dependent Diabetes

22

Robert Kaye

The onset of diabetes in children is usually accompanied by the classic symptoms of polyuria and polydipsia. Untreated, the disease progresses with weight loss, ketoacidosis, dehydration, coma, peripheral circulatory failure, and death. The fully developed manifestations are the consequences of an essentially complete deficiency of insulin production by the pancreas compounded by a relative excess of glucagon.

PREVALENCE

Estimates of the prevalence of diabetes in children under the age of 15 years range from 1 in 600 to 1 in 1200, or approximately 85,000 children with diabetes in the United States. It is the most common childhood endocrine disorder. A recent survey reports the female-to-male ratio as 5:3. The average age of onset is 10 to 11 years, although the disease has appeared as early as 11 days of life.

Diabetes in children has been characterized as juvenile diabetes, growth-onset diabetes, ketosis-prone diabetes, and insulin-dependent or type I diabetes. These designations have served to emphasize certain differences between the disease (Table 22-1) as it occurs in the child and as it occurs in the adult (maturity-onset, insulin-independent or type II diabetes).

Childhood diabetes does not always occur abruptly. Children with impaired glucose tolerance are being identified prior to the exhibition of frank diabetic symptoms—especially asymptomatic siblings of diabetic children, approximately 20% of whom exhibit impairment in glucose toler-

TABLE 22-1. Differential Features of Juvenile and Adult Onset Diabetes

	Juvenile Diabetes	Adult Diabetes
Exogenous insulin	Required for long-term management	Usually not
Ketosis	Prone	Resistant
Obesity	Not characteristic	80%
Response to caloric restriction alone	Poor, leads to cachexia	Often restores glucose tolerance to normal
Oral hypoglycemic agents	Effective only in partial remission	Usually effective
Insulin response to glucose	Decreased or lacking	Delayed, may be increased
Life expectancy reduction	Approximately 30%	Less with advancing age
Quality of control	Labile	Stable
Brittleness or hyperlability	Common	Rare
Insulin sensitivity	Marked	Reduced
Major complications	Microangiopathy	Macroangiopathy

ance without apparent symptoms of diabetes (chemical diabetes). Five to ten percent of siblings of insulin-dependent diabetics develop the disease, often within one year. The risk for offspring is about 2% to 5%. Chemical diabetes will also be detected in glucose tolerance testing of some children studied because of symptoms suggestive of reactive hypoglycemia. Fasting glucose concentrations are usually normal, but 1- and 2-hour values are elevated with a rapid fall to low normal or hypoglycemic levels between the 3rd and 5th hours.

Genetic Considerations

Predisposition to diabetes is genetically determined. There is an increased frequency in some families compared with the general population and in monozygotic compared with dizygotic twins. Some believe that genetic data best fit a multifactorial inheritance pattern—a number of genes on separate loci which contribute equal and additive effects to the development of the characteristic. Others consider a recessive pattern with incomplete penetrance to be operative. No single genetic mechanism is compatible with all observations. Pyke has observed that among identical twins almost all twin pairs are concordant for diabetes when the onset occurred over age 40, and only 50% when the index case appeared earlier. Such observations suggest the presence of environmental in addition to genetic factors as causes of diabetes. Heterogeneity in the clinical and genetic aspects of diabetes in young people is apparent in the group of diabetics studied by Tattersall and Fajans. These subjects exhibited a mild diabetic state characterized as "maturity onset diabetes in the young" (MODY). In these cases, approximately 85% of the parents were diabetic in contrast to only 11% of parents of patients with typical juvenile onset diabetes, observations compatible with a dominant mode of inheritance. Of further genetic interest is the association of juvenile diabetes with histocompatibility loci, DW3, DW4, DR3, DR4, B8, B15, and B18. B7 and DR2 may be protective.

Environmental Factors

Two diabetic parents do not always produce diabetic offspring and identical twins are not necessarily concordant for diabetes, suggesting a role of nongenetic factors in the etiology of diabetes. Viral infection is a possibility; antibody to Coxsackie B virus has been implicated in some studies. Diabetes occurs in children affected by the intrauterine rubella syndrome; outbreaks of mumps have been followed by an increase in the incidence of diabetes in children. Several viruses are capable of producing inflammation in the pancreas of experimental animals resulting in diabetes. An interplay of genetic factors is suggested by species specificity in susceptibility to virus-induced diabetes.

Immunologic elements in some cases of diabetes are suggested by the finding of a 30-fold increase in the frequency of antibodies against thyroid, adrenal, and gastric antigens in diabetic compared with normal children. In addition, antibodies against pancreatic islets have been detected in the sera of juvenile diabetics. These observations suggest that prevention of some cases of diabetes may be achieved by the use of vaccines or antiviral drugs.

PATHOPHYSIOLOGY

Insulin Biosynthesis and Secretion

The insulin molecule is made up of two polypeptide chains, A and B, joined by a pair of disulfide bridges. A single-chain polypeptide precursor, proinsulin, has been identified which includes in its structure both the A and B chains of insulin. Proinsulin is transformed into insulin by enzymic cleavage of the connecting peptide, C-peptide. C-peptide measured in blood or urine serves as a marker for insulin secretion. Greatly reduced insulin responses to glucose occur in juvenile diabetes. Because of a decrease in the number of insulin receptors on the cell surface, obese subjects show an increase in fasting- and glucose-stimulated insulin levels indicative of insulin resistance. The obese adult diabetic, while exhibiting higher basal and glucose-stimulated insulin levels than the nonobese, nondiabetic adult, responds with a lower insulin output than the obese nondiabetic control.

Glucose is the most potent stimulus for release of insulin. Others include proteins and amino acids, medium and short chain fatty acids and ketones, glucagon, fructose ACTH, beta adrenergic agents, gastrointestinal hormones, and some sulfonylureas.

Metabolic Effects of Insulin

Insulin plays a major role in regulating the glucose concentration of blood and extracellular fluid. It is the only hormone which suppresses glucose influx from the liver and facilitates glucose outflow into insulin-responsive tissues. Its action permits conservation of excess nutrient energy absorbed with meals.

The target sites and metabolic actions of insulin are summarized in Table 22-2.

During fasting, when exogenous nutrients are unavailable, suppression of insulin release is appropriate. Low levels of insulin facilitate lipolysis and provide free fatty acids for energy needs at a rate that does not result in accumulation of excess ketone bodies. Fasting levels of insulin do not stimulate glucose uptake by muscle. Glucose is then available to meet the obligatory requirements of the brain, kidney, adrenal, and formed elements of the blood. Suppression of insulin secretion during fasting further ensures an adequate supply of glucose to the brain by increasing the availability of gluconeogenic substrates (amino acids and glycerol) with the mediation of glucagon, cortisol, and catecholamines. Concomitantly, there is increased glycogenolysis and hepatic glucose output, facilitated by glucagon and catecholamines.

The metabolic sequence set in motion by insulin deficiency (diabetes mellitus) can be regarded as an exaggeration of the physiologic suppression of insulin release during fasting. The primary effects of insulin deficiency are (1) decreased peripheral uptake of glucose, (2) increased gluconeogenesis and hepatic output of glucose, and (3)

TABLE 22-2. Target Sites and Metabolic Actions of Insulin

Metabolic Fuels	Liver	Adipose Cell	Muscle
Carbohydrate	↑ Glucokinase ↑ Glycogen synthetase ↓ Phosphorylase ↓ Gluconeogenesis	↑ Glucose transport ↑ Glycerol synthesis	↑ Glucose transport ↑ Glycolysis ↑ Glycogen synthesis
Fat	↑ Lipogenesis	↑ Triglycerides ↑ Fatty acid synthesis ↓ Lipolysis	—
Protein	↓ Proteolysis	—	↑ Amino acid uptake ↑ Protein synthesis

uncontrolled lipolysis leading to ketosis. These metabolic changes are the key features in the pathogenesis of diabetic ketoacidosis and are illustrated in Figure 22-1.

Polyuria and polydipsia are the result of hyperglycemia and consequent glycosuria. As the concentrating ability of the kidney is exceeded, marked glycosuria obligates an increase in renal excretion of water compensated by an increase in intake. Uncontrolled lipolysis leads to accumulation of the strong acids, beta-hydroxybutyric and acetoacetic, which augment the body's hydrogen ion pool and overwhelm the bicarbonate buffering mechanism. In health, ketone bodies are oxidized by means of the Krebs cycle to yield carbon dioxide and water.

The solute diuresis accompanying hyperglycemia augments the acidosis as dehydration decreases renal perfusion, and compromises renal excretion of hydrogen ions derived from fatty acid and protein catabolism. Solute diuresis also contributes to dehydration by decreasing renal reabsorp-

PATHOGENESIS OF DIABETIC ACIDOSIS

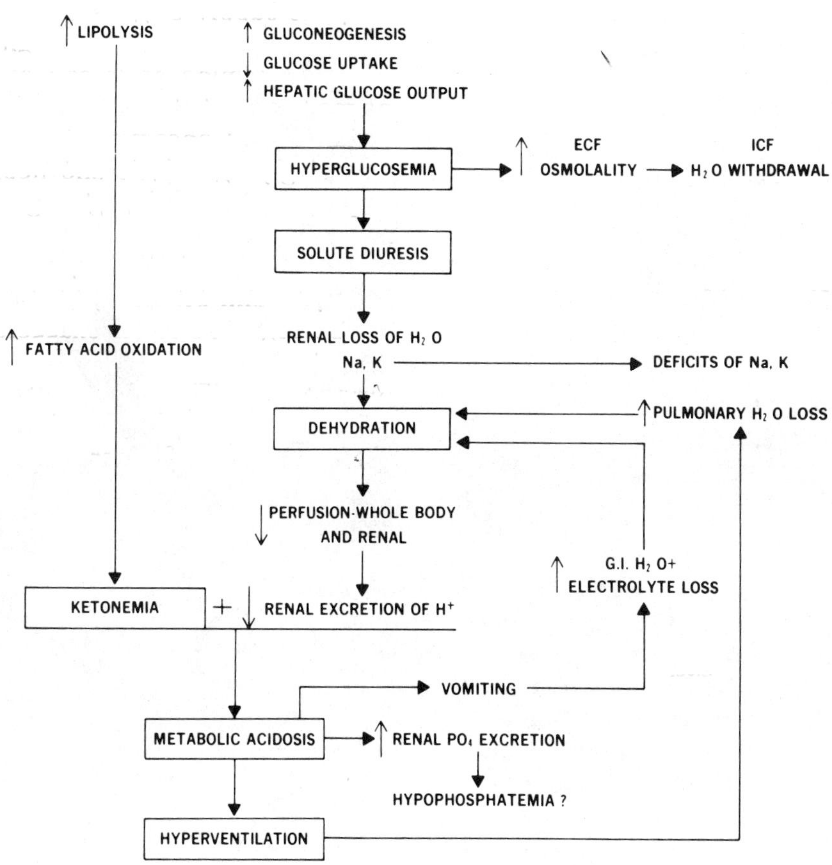

Fig. 22-1. Pathogenesis of diabetic acidosis. (Kaye R: Juvenile diabetes. In Sherkey HC (ed): Pediatric Therapy, 6th ed. St. Louis, C. V. Mosby, 1980)

tion of sodium and potassium. Compensatory hyperventilation initiated by metabolic acidosis increases the deficit of body water. As acidosis and ketonemia progress, nausea and vomiting occur and reduce water and electrolyte intake; the development of acidosis, dehydration, and hypovolemic shock are accelerated.

Hyperglycemia causes the extracellular fluid to become hypertonic and osmotic shifts of water from the intra- to the extracellular compartment take place. The intracellular deficit of potassium is increased by its movement to the extracellular fluid consequent to metabolic acidosis. Potassium returns intracellularly with appropriate treatment with insulin, water, electrolytes, and glucose.

DIAGNOSIS

Diabetes as the cause of polyuria and polydipsia is usually considered prior to the development of profound ketoacidosis. A positive test of urine for glucose leads to determination of blood glucose concentration which in symptomatic children usually exceeds 250 mg/dl and is diagnostic of diabetes mellitus.

In preverbal or non-toilet-trained infants, increased thirst and urine output may not be noticed and diabetes may progress to ketoacidosis. The child with brain damage may fail to sense the need for increased water intake to compensate for polyuria; extremely high blood glucose concentrations and dehydration may lead to the development of hyperglycemic, hyperosmolar nonketotic diabetic coma.

Other symptoms suggesting diabetes mellitus are weight loss, enuresis in a child previously toilet-trained, monilial vulvitis, and abrupt disturbances of visual acuity.

If glycosuria is observed and the random blood glucose concentration is normal or borderline, a glucose tolerance test should be performed to rule out renal glycosuria and to establish the diagnosis of diabetes. Oral glucose tolerance testing is more sensitive than intravenous. See outline for dosage and diagnostic values for glucose tolerance in normal children, children with impaired glucose tolerance (chemical diabetes), and normals.

Diabetes Mellitus in Children

Either of the following are considered diagnostic of diabetes:

A. Presence of the classic symptoms of diabetes, such as polyuria, polydipsia, ketonuria, and rapid weight loss, together with a random plasma glucose >200 mg/dl.
B. In asymptomatic individuals, *both* an elevated fasting glucose concentration and a sustained elevated glucose concentration during the OGTT on more than one occasion. Both the 2-h sample *and* some other sample taken between administration of the glucose dose (1.75 g/kg ideal body weight, up to a maximum of 75 g) and 2 h later must meet the criteria below.

Fasting value:

venous plasma ≥ 140 mg/dl (7.8 mmol/dl)
venous whole blood ≥ 120 mg/dl (6.7 mmol/dl)
capillary whole blood ≥ 120 mg/dl (6.7 mmol/dl)

2-h OGTT value and an intervening value:

venous plasma ≥ 200 mg/dl (11.1 mmol/L)
venous whole blood ≥ 180 mg/dl (10.0 mmol/L)
capillary whole blood ≥ 200 mg/dl (11.1 mmol/L)

Impaired Glucose Tolerance (IGT) in Children

Two criteria must be met: the fasting glucose concentration must be below the value that is diagnostic of diabetes, and the glucose concentration 2 h after an oral glucose challenge must be elevated.

Fasting value:

venous plasma < 140 mg/dl (7.8 mmol/L)
venous whole blood < 120 mg/dl (6.7 mmol/L)
capillary whole blood < 120 mg/dl (6.7 mmol/L)

2-h OGTT value:

venous plasma > 140 mg/dl (7.8 mmol/L)
venous whole blood > 120 mg/dl (6.7 mmol/L)
capillary whole blood > 120 mg/dl (6.7 mmol/L)

Normal Glucose Levels in Children

Fasting value:

venous plasma < 130 mg/dl (7.2 mmol/L)
venous whole blood < 115 mg/dl (6.4 mmol/L)
capillary whole blood < 115 mg/dl (6.4 mmol/L)

2-h OGTT value:

venous plasma < 140 mg/dl (7.8 mmol/L)
venous whole blood < 120 mg/dl (6.7 mmol/L)
capillary whole blood < 140 mg/dl (7.8 mmol/L)

National Diabetes Data Group: Classification and diagnosis of diabetes mellitus and other categories of glucose intolerance. Diabetes 28:1049, 1979. Reproduced with permission from the American Diabetes Association, Inc.

Situations in which nondiabetic hyperglycemia may be encountered include (1) carbohydrate deprivation followed by glucose loading, (2) stress (physical, emotional, or infection), (3) drugs (epinephrinelike compounds, thiazide diuretics, oral contraceptive agents, phenytoin), or (4) excessive production of anti-insulin hormones (growth hormone, catecholamines, [neuroblastoma], pheochromocytoma, adrenal glucocorticoids, ACTH, thyroid, aldosterone).

Starvation is accompanied by an appropriate suppression of insulin secretion which serves to protect against hypoglycemia. Patients with head injury or intracranial infection may develop hyperglycemia secondary to central stimulation of adrenergic neurons inhibitory to insulin secretion. Insulin-antagonistic hormonal concomitants of stress—growth hormone, cortisol, and catecholamines—may also be involved.

TREATMENT

Hospitalization

Hospitalization of the newly diagnosed diabetic child may be indicated so that the family can assimilate the considerable body of new information requisite for the supervision of their child's illness. If the patient is hospitalized, it is especially important that this instruction is not turned over to routine nursing personnel, who may be too busy and may not have sufficient experience to provide this important educational exposure. However, the essentials of diabetic management, insulin administration, meal planning, and home glucose monitoring (urine or blood) can easily be managed and effectively taught to the family with the patient as an outpatient.

Educational objectives are the functions of insulin, especially the type being used by the child, the role of diet, recognition and treatment of hypoglycemia, recognition of ketosis, management of vomiting episodes, and the use of home glucose monitoring.*

Diet

Opinion varies concerning the relative merits of "unmeasured" in contrast to "prescribed" diets in management of diabetic

---

* Autolet, Ulster Scientific Inc., Highland, N.Y. This device makes use of a sharp, spring-activated lancet, to make a controlled skin puncture yielding a drop of blood which is applied to a reagent-strip calibrated to approximate glucose concentrations over the range of 20 to 800 mg/dl. Chemstrip b.g., Bio-Dynamics, Indianapolis, Ind. More accurate blood glucose estimations can be made using reagent strips and reflectance meters.

children. Proponents of both recommend a diet conforming to acceptable nutritional practices for all children with appropriate response if the diet proves to be excessive or fails to lead to satiety and satisfactory weight gain. If a free diet is used, parents are helped by initial prescription of the quantity and composition of the diet, with the explanation that it is an estimate that may be modified according to their child's individual requirements. It is physiologically sound to permit some flexibility in the daily calorie intake. It should be assumed that the nonobese diabetic child possesses the normal homeostatic mechanisms which balance calorie intake and expenditure. Increased physical activity requires an increase in calorie intake, and hunger is often a manifestation of hypoglycemia.

Insulin

Symptomatic diabetes mellitus in children always requires insulin therapy in the initial and later phases of treatment. A small group (perhaps 5%) experience a period of weeks or months of improved carbohydrate tolerance in which blood glucose levels remain in the normal range without the administration of exogenous insulin. It is important to explain that the remission or "honeymoon period" will be temporary and that insulin therapy will again be required.

Fundamental to an understanding of the difficulties encountered in the treatment of the diabetic child is the fact that juvenile diabetes is associated with a reduced or almost absent endogenous secretion of insulin. Current methods of insulin treatment sustain life and well-being for long periods but are not adequate replacements for the rapidly responding homeostatic system involving insulin and its counterregulatory hormones operative in the normal subject. In health, insulin release is stimulated in seconds by increments of blood glucose (about 10 mg) and falls to basal values when the glucose level is restored to normal. In the diabetic patient, insulin is administered peripherally rather than intraportally in anticipation of, rather than in response to, nutrient ingestion. The metabolic lability of the juvenile diabetic, though primarily due to inadequate endogenous insulin, is compounded by variations in nutrient intake, physical activity, growth and maturation, and in some instances emotional arousal. These considerations should temper the degree of metabolic control demanded of a partially unphysiologic system inherently lacking in the rapid and precise adjustments characteristic of the metabolic-homeostatic hormone complex in the normal subject.

Numerous types of insulin are available and grouped conveniently on the basis of rapidity and duration of action (Table 22-3). A mixture of regular and NPH insulins is used for the treatment of most of our patients. Rapid-acting regular insulin facilitates utilization of the breakfast calories and also quickly reverses the inhibition of insulin action present in the fasting state when free fatty acid levels are elevated. In about 25% of patients, the combined use of NPH insulin permits utilization of calories ingested during the balance of the day.

The lente insulins have the theoretical advantage of being free of the foreign protein, protamine, present in NPH and protamine zinc insulins. Ultralente insulin is sometimes useful in limiting excessive overnight glycosuria when intermediate-acting insulins fail to do so. In many instances, ultralente does not accomplish this purpose. Therefore, approximately 75% of children require a second injection of an intermediate-acting insulin that is approximately 20% of their morning dose.

More highly purified insulin preparations have been introduced for general use and contain only small amounts of noninsulin

TABLE 22-3. Some Properties of Currently Used Insulins

Type of Insulin	Onset (hr)	Peak (hr)	Duration (hr)	Intensity of peak
Rapid-acting				
Crystalline zinc (insulin injection, USP) ("regular" insulin)	½	2–4	6–8	Marked
Semi-lente (prompt) insulin zinc suspension, USP)	½	2–4	10–12	Marked
Intermediate-acting				
Globin (globin zinc insulin injection, USP)	2	6–10	12–18	Moderate
NPH (isophane insulin suspension, USP)	2	8–10	18–24	Moderate
Lente (insulin zinc suspension, USP)	2	8–12	20–26	Moderate
Prolonged-acting				
Ultralente (extended insulin zinc suspension, USP)	6	18–24	36+	Mild
Protamine zinc (PZI) (protamine zinc insulin suspension, USP)	6	14–20	24–36	Mild

(Kaye R: Juvenile diabetes. *In* Shirkey HC (ed): Pediatric Therapy, 6th ed. St. Louis, CV Mosby, 1980.)

proteins. They are available only in a concentration of 100 units/ml (U100) as regular, NPH, semilente, lente, and ultralente. There are indications that these preparations produce less subcutaneous atrophy than the previously available products and often correct insulin lipoatrophy when injected directly into affected sites.

The details of insulin treatment are beyond the scope of this chapter. Patients who are not significantly acidotic are treated initially with regular insulin four times daily. After 5 to 6 days of such treatment, a decrease in insulin requirement occurs as shown by diminishing blood and urinary glucose concentrations, indicative of a partial remission. At this time, treatment with a mixture of a rapid-acting and intermediate-acting insulin given in one or two injections per day is begun.

For patients with dehydration and acidosis, intravenous fluids and more frequent administration of insulin are required. Equally effective are low-dose constant intravenous insulin infusions, low-dose intramuscular, high-dose intravenous bolus, and initial intravenous with repeated subcutaneous injections. Treatment is directed at restoring water and electrolyte deficiencies and reversing the metabolic alterations of insulin deficiency described above.

The development of simple and relatively painless techniques of obtaining and estimating glucose concentrations in capillary blood makes it feasible for patients to use blood rather than urinary glucose determination as the basis for adjustment of insulin dosage.

A number of investigations have documented improved metabolic control by the use of a battery-driven pump which delivers insulin by continuous subcutaneous infusion with bolus injections before meals. Low concentrations of insulin must be made available to the liver in order for it to function appropriately in glucose homeostasis, by the release of glucose when concentrations are low and by uptake when glucose levels are elevated. In the absence of basal levels of insulin, glucose may be released by the liver in spite of hyperglycemia. There is some evidence that multiple injections of rapid-acting insulin combined with a prolonged-acting insulin may be equally effective.

PATHOGENESIS OF LATE COMPLICATIONS

The consensus of studies designed to gain an understanding of the late complications of diabetes has tended to implicate hyperglycemia in the pathogenesis of lesions of the peripheral nervous system, the lens of the eye, and capillaries throughout the body. Increased activity of the polyol pathway consequent to hyperglycemia may play a role in the development of diabetic cataracts, neuropathy, and lesions of major arteries. *Polyols* are organic alcohols derived from sugars by reduction of the terminal aldehyde or ketone group.

Sorbitol is the polyol derived from glucose. The reaction is catalyzed by aldose reductase; the rate of the reaction varying directly with increasing glucose concentration permitting sorbitol to accumulate in tissues in hyperglycemic states. Sorbitol accumulation has been demonstrated in lenses of human diabetics where its osmotic activity can result in increased water content as well as interference with the sodium and potassium "pumps" regulating the intracellular concentration of these ions. Similar mechanisms may be of pathogenic significance in the metabolism of Schwann's cell contributing to the development of diabetic neuropathy and in the wall of the aorta in which edema may interfere with the diffusion of O_2 and other nutrients to the deeper portions of the blood vessel wall.

Hemoglobin and other proteins may be nonenzymatically glycosylated to an extent proportional to the average glucose concentration to which they are exposed. Measurement of glycosylated hemoglobin (hemoglobin A_{1C}) is now widely used as a measure of the quality of diabetic control.

The microangiopathic lesions of diabetes involve thickening of the basement membrane which surrounds the capillaries of all tissues. In the kidney, both the glomerular capillary loops and mesangial regions are affected, leading to an impairment in the function of the glomerulus as a selective filter. Similar changes have been shown in the capillaries of the retina, skin, nerves, and muscle. These changes may result from alterations in chemical composition of glycoproteins of the basement membrane secondary to hyperglycemia.

The prevalence and magnitude of thickening of the basement membrane of muscle capillaries increase with the duration of the disease.

Pathology

Hyalinization of the Langerhans islets is characteristic of the findings in the pancreas of the older diabetic patient. Gepts has described autopsy findings in subjects developing diabetes under the age of 21 years. In 22 diabetics who died less than 6 months after onset, the number of beta cells was found to be reduced to less than 10% of normal. Lymphocytic inflammatory infiltrates in or around the islets were prominent and fibrosis was evident. The inflammatory changes noted are compatible with an infectious, toxic, or autoimmune mechanism.

COMPLICATIONS AND PROGNOSIS

Ketoacidosis as a cause of death in diabetic children is relatively infrequent. Sepsis is no longer a significant threat to the survival of the young diabetic.

Vascular injury remains the most important cause of late morbidity and mortality in juvenile-onset diabetes. White has reported that large vessel calcifications occur between the ages of 10 and 19 in about 6.5% of juvenile diabetics. These changes lead to significant impairment of health. Among 30-year survivors of childhood diabetes, 4% experienced cerebral vascular accidents and 19% suffered myocardial infarctions. Retinopathy is the earliest of the microangiopathic lesions to occur. These have been classified into exudative, angiopathic, and proliferative types. Angiopathy includes dilated venules, microcapillary aneurysms, hemorrhages, and neovascular formation. Retinal lesions that threatened vision occurred in 3% of patients after 15 years of diabetes; this figure rose to 30% by 40 years, at which time 8% of patients were blind.

Nephropathy, though second in frequency of microangiopathy, is first as a cause of morbidity and mortality. It is present in 18% of patients by 15 years and 44% by 30 years of disease. The prognosis of diabetic renal disease correlates best with elevation of blood urea nitrogen. Sustained elevation to 25 mg/dl is associated with an average life expectancy of 6 years. Duration of life is adversely affected by the occurrence of diabetes in childhood. A youngster becoming diabetic at age 15 has a life expectancy of 56 years in contrast to 73 years for his nondiabetic peers. It is hoped that more effective methods of insulin delivery or pancreas transplantation will improve the present unsatisfactory prognosis.

BIBLIOGRAPHY

Committee on Professional Education of the American Diabetes Association: Diabetes Mellitus, 5th ed. 1980

This volume provides an up-to-date summary of the major topics of pathophysiology and treatment of diabetes. It is issued periodically by the Committee on Professional Education of the American Diabetes Association, Inc, 600 Fifth Avenue, New York, NY 10020

Ganda OP, Soeldner SS: Genetic, acquired, and related factors in the etiology of diabetes mellitus. Arch Intern Med 137:461, 1977

An excellent review of genetic, viral, and autoimmune factors in diabetic etiology.

Kaye R: Diabetes. In Shirkey HC (ed): Pediatric Therapy, 6th ed. St Louis, CV Mosby, 1980

A detailed discussion of the treatment of juvenile diabetes.

Marble A, White P, Bradley RF, Krall LP: Joslin's Diabetes Mellitus, 11th ed. Philadelphia, Lea & Febiger, 1971

An excellent reference book dealing comprehensively with physiologic and clinical aspects of diabetes.

Tamborlane WV, Sherwin RD, Genel M, Felig P: Outpatient treatment of juvenile-onset diabetes with a preprogrammed portable subcutaneous insulin infusion system. Am J Med 68:190, 1980

A description of the technique and results of pump therapy.

Tattersall R, Gall E: Patient self-monitoring of blood glucose and refinements of conventional insulin treatment. Am J Med 70:177, 1981

An excellent discussion of the advantages of self-monitoring of blood glucose and the effectiveness of a three times daily insulin injection regimen.

23

Respiratory Signs and Symptoms

Douglas S. Holsclaw

The diagnosis, assessment, and management of pediatric pulmonary diseases require an understanding of the normal structure and an appreciation of the major presenting signs and symptoms of deviations from the normal. The history and physical examination are of primary importance; laboratory studies of lung functions are less important. Most of the pulmonary function tests used for adults are difficult for younger children to perform, and few of the available tests are critical for the diagnosis of the majority of clinical conditions in pediatrics.

Rather than dwell on a detailed review of respiratory physiology, an approach has been chosen to integrate structure of the respiratory tract with function and to introduce some of the terms and symbols used in the assessment of respiratory physiology. Since deranged pulmonary function is expressed in the child by certain symptoms which are usually the reason for the patient being brought to the physician's attention, consideration of the major presenting signs and symptoms and their implications for certain disease processes follow.

Principles of clinical evaluation applicable to a broad spectrum of lung diseases conclude the chapter.

PULMONARY STRUCTURE AND FUNCTION

The main function of the lung is to enable air to come into close proximity to the red blood cells flowing through the pulmonary capillaries. In this way oxygen (O_2) can diffuse into the blood and carbon dioxide (CO_2) can diffuse out.

Several structural adaptations are needed to produce this functional relationship. Included are the development of the right ventricle and the pulmonary vascular system, by means of which all blood returning to the heart is pumped through a vast array of thin sheets infolded into a relatively small space, and an airway system that can deliver a large volume of air at almost zero velocity when it comes into contact with these sheets of blood. The large internal surface area of the adult human lung—approximately 1 m^2/kg body weight at 75% of total lung capacity (TLC)—is not related to the act of distributing air into the lung (ventilation, V). Instead, it fulfills the need to distribute a large quantity of blood (perfusion, Q), into a very fine film so that

1. The capillary transit time, during which gas exchange occurs, is long enough to permit equilibration
2. The tissue phase of gas diffusion is minimized
3. The resistance to flow in the pulmonary vascular bed remains low

The structures that allow this to take place are discussed with particular reference to the function of each segment involved.

AIRWAYS

There are about 25 generations or branches of airways that can be classified longitudinally into three groups: the cartilaginous airways (trachea and bronchi) generations 0 to 7, the membranous airways (bronchioles) generations 8 to 22, and the gas exchange airways (respiratory bronchioles and alveolar ducts) generations 23 to 25.

Cartilaginous Airways

Structure. Cartilaginous airways include the trachea and all its branchings down to the small bronchi (approximately 0.1–0.3 cm in diameter when the lung is fully inflated). The main structural supports for the bronchi are C-shaped cartilaginous rings and plates supporting their anterior and lateral walls connected by a strong fibrous layer. The cartilaginous plates become smaller and fewer in number with each successive branching of the bronchial tree. Within this framework is a layer of circularly arranged smooth muscle whose motor innervation is the parasympathetic branch of the autonomic nervous system (vagus nerve). This smooth muscle is also capable of being contracted, thus narrowing the airway by direct stimulation.

The mucous membrane is pseudostratified, ciliated epithelium. Interspersed between the ciliated cells are mucus-secreting goblet cells in, roughly, a 1-to-5 ratio. A distinctive feature of the large cartilaginous bronchi is the presence of bronchial glands situated deep within the submucosa connecting to the surface through ducts. These glands contain both mucus and serous-secreting elements and may be stimulated to secrete by the vagus nerve. The bronchial glands are particularly dense in the medium-sized bronchi, decreasing in number and size distally, finally disappearing altogether near the transition from cartilaginous bronchi to membranous bronchioles.

The mucosal surface of the cells is covered by a thin blanket formed by continuous serous and mucus secretion of the airway epithelium and glands. In a normal adult, the mucous membrane of the tracheobronchial tree secretes about a half liter of fluid in a 24-hour period. This blanket is propelled continuously upward through the airways to the pharynx (mucociliary escalator), pushed along by the constantly beating cilia (1000 strokes/minute). Two hundred cilia are on each ciliated cell, each cilium being 4–6 μm long).

The sensory innervation of the large airways is by vagal nerve fibers whose receptor endings appear to be adjacent to the surface epithelial layer. These fibers are sensitive to irritation and appear to be identical with cough receptors that are particularly abundant in the trachea and largest bronchi.

Blood is supplied to the bronchi by way of the bronchial circulation arising from the aorta (systemic circulation).

Function. The cartilaginous airways are the conduits through which gas enters and leaves the respiratory gas exchange areas of the lung. Since these airways do not allow gas exchange across their walls, they contribute to that portion of the freshly inspired breath that does not undergo gas exchange—the dead space. Indeed, the cartilaginous airways, together with the nose and throat, account for almost all the anatomic dead space volume. In addition, because of the air flow through this system of branching and narrowing tubes, the cartilaginous airways contribute to a large portion of the total resistance to breathing. Resistance to gas flow in the bronchi can be increased by reflex or local stimulation of the smooth muscles, which causes narrowing of the airways. Both inert particles impinging on the airway surface and chemically active agents may stimulate the irritant constrictor mechanism.

The cartilaginous airways also aid in

the warming and humidification of incoming air, particularly during mouth breathing when the nasal mechanism is bypassed.

Inhaled particles in the size range between 2 and 10 μm usually settle or impact onto the mucociliary surface layer during inspiration and are transported out of the airways to the pharynx where they are swallowed. This remarkable mechanism, which propels particles at a rate of 1.0 cm/min in the upper airway, is dependent on stable temperature and humidity and can be temporarily inactivated by noxious substances such as cigarette smoke. Highly soluble gaseous materials (sulfur dioxide) are very efficiently scrubbed out of the inspired air; none reaches the distal delicate gas exchange surfaces.

Chronic irritant stimuli appear to cause hypertrophy of the mucus-secreting elements and glands of the upper airway with a parallel increase in the production and secretion of the airway mucus.

Membranous Airways

Structure. The bronchioles, direct continuations of the airways, end in the terminal bronchioles which are approximately 0.4 mm in diameter. The chief difference between them and the bronchi is the absence of both the fibrocartilage framework and the secretory glands. The patency of the bronchioles is greatly influenced by the negative intrapleural pressure.

Structural support of the bronchioles comes from their being directly embedded into the connective-tissue framework of the lung. They contain a continuous circular layer of smooth muscle whose innervation is believed to be similar to that of the bronchi.

The mucosa is continuous with that of the bronchi. The epithelial layer consists of low ciliated columnar cells which gradually become more cuboidal as the terminal bronchiole is approached. Interspersed with the ciliated cells is a decreasing number of goblet cells which normally disappear completely at the terminal bronchiole.

Blood supply to the bronchioles is also from the bronchial artery. Sensory innervation consists mainly of undifferentiated fibers in the subepithelial portion of the mucosa.

Function. The functional difference between small bronchi and large bronchioles is not as sharp as the anatomic description suggests; there is a gradual transition. Although the bronchioles contribute to the dead space and airflow resistance, this contribution is normally considerably less than that of the bronchi. The bronchioles are affected by lung volume since these airways are embedded in the lung tissue and are passively dilated during lung inflation and, conversely, narrowed in lung deflation (expiration).

Edema of the bronchiolar mucosa, mucus accumulation, or active contraction of the circular smooth muscle by reflex or by local irritation can greatly increase the resistance to airflow through these very small tubes.

The mucociliary blanket in the terminal bronchioles is mainly a watery fluid, but it gradually accumulates mucus as it moves up the airways. With chronic irritant stimulation, the mucus-secreting goblet cell population in the bronchioles may markedly increase.

Gas Exchange Airways

Structure. The respiratory bronchioles and alveolar ducts are the final branchings of the airways. They are continuous with the terminal bronchioles. Chief distinguishing feature of these gas exchange airways is the presence of alveoli, an estimated 300,000,000 in number, in whose walls the pulmonary capillaries are distributed and where the O_2 and CO_2 exchange occurs.

All the gas exchange airways are approximately the same diameter (0.05 cm) and, like the bronchioles, receive their structural support from the connective-tissue framework of lung tissue. There is an interrupted circular layer of smooth muscle whose motor innervation is probably similar to that of the bronchioles; however, this is not clearly defined. The mucosa of the respiratory bronchiole is a single layer of low cuboidal epithelial cells some of which contain cilia. The Clara cell, recently discovered and believed to secrete a surfactantlike material, is interspersed. There are no goblet cells. Sensory nerves in the mucosal layer are the undifferentiated type, similar to those seen in the bronchioles, but much less numerous.

Blood is supplied to the gas exchange airways by means of the pulmonary circulation, not the bronchial circulation.

Function. The gas exchange airways serve to distribute the inspired gas by bulk flow within the terminal respiratory units. Because of their blood supply via the pulmonary circulation, the smooth muscle of these units (particularly the respiratory bronchioles) may be selectively influenced by agents present in the pulmonary blood. These airways dilate and narrow with changes in lung volume. They account for approximately one-third of the total alveolar gas exchange volume.

PULMONARY CIRCULATION

Structure. The quantity of blood flowing through the lungs is equal to that flowing through the systemic circulation. The muscle wall of the right ventricle is only one-third as thick as that of the left ventricle, yet the right ventricle pumps as much blood as the left at much lower pressure. The entire output of the right ventricle enters the pulmonary artery and is distributed to the lungs through the pulmonary arteries. These branch out with the airways down to the respiratory bronchioles. Thus, at all levels the pulmonary arteries are adjacent to the airways. The branches of the pulmonary artery are all very short and accommodate very small quantities of blood in comparison with the relatively large amounts that can be stored in the systemic arterial system. The average blood pressure in the pulmonary artery reaches 22 mm Hg during systole and falls to 8 mm Hg during diastole with a mean pressure of about 13 mm Hg. If it were not for the extreme distensibility of the thin pulmonary arteries, the pulmonary arterial pulse pressure would have to be greater than it is. Larger pulmonary arteries are elastic, whereas the smaller ones that accompany the terminal bronchioles are described as muscular. The pulmonary arteries are richly innervated from the sympathetic branch of the autonomic system.

Pulmonary microcirculation consists of an extensive capillary network which some investigators believe behaves more as a sheet of blood than as individual channels. The pulmonary capillaries are somewhat larger than systemic capillaries. The capillary network originates in short precapillary vessels branching at right angles from the small arteries. Each capillary network is continuous over several alveoli before condensing into the pulmonary venous system.

The pulmonary venous system is not closely related to the airways and, in fact, lies as far from the airways as anatomically feasible. The pulmonary veins drain into the left atrium. The venous system contains smooth muscle and is well innervated, presumably by the sympathetic branch of the autonomic nervous system.

Function. The pulmonary vascular bed is highly distensible and has a low resistance to blood flow. All the right ventricular output passes through the pulmonary vascular bed at a driving pressure that is about one-seventh that of the systemic circulation. Pressure in the pulmonary capillaries is about 5 mm Hg when measured by catheterization. Blood passes through the pulmonary capillaries in about 0.8 of a second. This allows time for the red cells to remain in contact with the gas phase and is sufficient for O_2 and CO_2 equilibration under all except the most severe conditions, such as heavy exercise while breathing low oxygen tensions.

With a normal increase in cardiac output into the pulmonary circuit, this transit time remains at about 0.8 of a second. The increased blood flow is accomplished by a reserve of capillaries which normally remain collapsed, but which open up to accommodate increased blood flow.

Since the pulmonary circulation is a flow-through system, there is no dead space comparable to that in the airways. Because all venous blood passes through the pulmonary microvascular bed before entering the systemic circulation, the pulmonary capillaries act as a filter for removal of embolic material and as a site of inactivation of certain chemical substances in blood.

Because the pulmonary arteries are adjacent to the airways, inflammatory airway disease may cause scar tissue to encompass the adjacent pulmonary artery, thereby affecting the distribution of blood flow to the distal segment.

The smooth muscle of the pulmonary microvascular bed, particularly the small muscular pulmonary arteries, is sensitive to the partial pressure of oxygen in the surrounding airspaces (PaO_2). Breathing low oxygen concentrations (which results in hypoxia) stimulates the smooth muscle to constrict.

The endothelium of the pulmonary microvascular bed forms a substantial component of the tissue structure of the alveolar walls (approximately 30% by volume). There are data that suggest that the endothelial cells are more sensitive to damage by toxic substances than other cells such as high levels of oxygen and endotoxins.

THE TERMINAL RESPIRATORY UNITS

Structure. Beyond the last membranous airway (terminal bronchiole), the airways contain alveoli, in whose walls the pulmonary capillaries course and where the exchange of O_2 and CO_2 occurs. The respiratory bronchiole, the alveolar duct and the alveolar sacs constitute the terminal respiratory unit (TRU). The basic functional structure of the lung is that of a very large number (100,000 in man) of TRUs arranged in parallel fashion. Each of these units receives ventilation through a terminal bronchiole and perfusion through a pulmonary arteriole.

At the end of a normal expiration, the total volume of gas in all the TRUs is the functional residual capacity (FRC) of the lung. In the normal adult, the FRC is approximately one-third of the maximal possible volume that all the TRUs can hold (total lung capacity—TLC).

The principal cellular structures of the alveolar epithelium are the broad pavement cells that cover 95% of the alveolar surface (type I cells), granular pneumonocytes, which are smaller, more numerous, and more active-appearing cells (type II cells), and alveolar macrophages. Type II cells contain peculiar, dense granules thought to be the precursors of alveolar surfactant. Found in varying numbers, alveolar macrophages are migratory phagocytic cells submerged in the extracellular lining of the alveolar surface. There is general agreement that alveolar macrophages originate from stem cell precursors in the bone marrow and reach the lung through the bloodstream, presumably as circulating monocytes. Alveolar macrophages are of considerable interest because they constitute the chief mechanism for clearance of bacteria and particles deposited in the terminal respiratory units. Deficiencies in their function undoubtedly contribute to the pathogenesis of pulmonary infections.

As mentioned in the section on pulmonary circulation, the capillary endothelium accounts for about 30% of the non-blood portion of the alveolar walls, making it a large tissue in its own right.

On the surface of the alveolar epithelium, separating the gas phase from the epithelial cells, is a thin film of fluid on whose surface is distributed a monomolecular phospholipid film (alveolar surfactant). Surfactant is believed to be actively secreted by type II alveolar cells.

The respiratory membrane is between 1 and 4 μm in thickness, and is composed of three layers: the endothelial cells of the capillary wall, the epithelial cells of the respiratory epithelium, and the interstitial layer. The capillaries are about 8 μm in diameter; therefore, the red blood cells, which are a little over 7 μm, actually squeeze through the pulmonary capillaries. The surface membrane of the red blood cell contacts the walls of the capillaries, and oxygen traverses very little plasma before it enters the red blood cells. These narrow clearances facilitate rapid oxygen uptake by the red blood cells.

To recognize the magnitude of the blood-air interface at the respiratory membrane and the capability for rapid, thorough exchange of gases, imagine a wall 20 ft high and 30 ft long, 85% to 95% of which is covered with pulmonary capillaries. In the normal adult, about 60 to 100 ml of blood occupy the pulmonary capillaries at one time. A third of a billion red blood cells are exposed over a 600 ft^2 respiratory membrane surface at any instant. This area of surface contact is 40 times greater than that of the body's external skin. Within 0.8 of a second the alveolar gases and pulmonary capillary blood of a normal man are in close equilibrium.

An addition to having an important but passive role in gas and liquid exchange, the capillary endothelium is thought to be the site of active biochemical events, such as the inactivation of polypeptides, prostaglandins and amines that have important physiologic functions.

Function. Current evidence indicates that the entire TRU expands and contracts proportionately with breathing, but over the range of the lung volume from FRC to TLC the alveoli remain inflated.

In breathing, the gas exchange airways receive the bulk of fresh air flow coming down the airways, whereas the alveoli receive the air that was in the gas exchange airways and dead space at the end of the previous expiration. Aerosol particles, in the size range from 0.3 to 2 μm in diameter, do not impact or settle in the conducting airways and, therefore, reach the respiratory bronchioles and alveolar ducts by bulk flow. Gases and particles less than 0.3 μm in diameter diffuse from the gas exchange airways into the alveoli themselves and are generally exhaled with a subsequent breath.

The phospholipid monolayer at the alveolar air-liquid interface has the special property of varying surface tension with TRU volume. Its most important attribute is to decrease surface tension to nearly zero because TRU volume decreases during expiration, and thus avoids the collapse of the alveoli.

The surfactant film is critical to normal breathing. It decreases the work of breathing, permits alveoli to remain inflated at low distending pressures, and reduces the net forces causing tissue fluid accumulation (pulmonary edema). Changes in alveolar surface area with breathing causes movement in the surface film with loss of some surfactant material and replacement by new molecules. Movements of the alveoli cause the surface film to flow over alveolar walls to the central airway (first-order respiratory bronchiole) of the TRU. Alveolar clearance of surfactant and entrapped particles is predominately by macrophage ingestion or, alternatively, by penetration through the alveolar epithelium and clearance through the interstitium by way of the lymphatics.

Fresh air ventilation of the TRU is only useful if it is matched by a proportionate blood flow through the pulmonary capillaries of that unit. The relationship of alveolar ventilation (V) to blood flow (Q) for each TRU is called the *ventilation/perfusion ratio* (V/Q). The ventilation/perfusion ratio averaged from all the TRUs of the lung is the overall ventilation-to-perfusion ratio of the lung and determines the arterial O_2 and CO_2 pressures by which the efficiency of the gas exchange process is judged. Within limits, each TRU can regulate V/Q through changes in respiratory bronchiole and pulmonary artery smooth muscle tone. The earliest manifestation of uneven V/Q is a fall in PaO_2, while $PaCO_2$ is essentially normal if overall V is normal.

The extremes of V/Q unevenness are zero (blood flow without ventilation) and infinity (ventilation without blood flow). The former is an anatomic or physiologic shunt; the latter is wasted ventilation, also known as physiologic dead space. The process by which oxygen penetrates from the gas phase of the TRU into the red blood cells in the capillaries is called *diffusion.* Ordinarily, there is rapid diffusion of O_2 and CO_2 within the gas phase of the TRU. Within the alveolar wall tissues, however, the low solubility of oxygen tends to limit its transport. This is not a problem for CO_2. Fortunately, the distance over which O_2 molecules have to diffuse to reach the red blood cells does not exceed half the width of the alveolar wall—1 to 4 μm.

The force (pressure difference between inside and outside of the lung, or transpulmonary pressure) necessary for lung expansion during breathing is normally quite small. The distensibility of the lung as measured by the change in lung volume for each unit change in transpulmonary pressure is called *lung compliance.* In diseases in which the alveolar structure is destroyed, the units may be more easily inflated and even remain distended during expiration. In diseases leading to fibrotic changes, the lung may resist changes of volume and is then said to be stiff or have a low compliance.

CLINICAL EVALUATION OF RESPIRATORY DISEASE

History

Of necessity, clinical evaluation of the child with respiratory disease begins with an accurate and thorough history. Careful attention should be paid to the onset of symptoms and associated signs. In cases of acute illness, the family may be able to easily elicit the beginning of respiratory distress. This may be accompanied by fever, cough, vomiting, and chest pain. The degree and character of all these symptoms should be noted. The nature of the cough, if present, should be carefully described, *e.g.,* dry, loose, productive, spasmodic. The presence of noisy breathing, wheezing, or grunting should also be noted.

The onset of chronic respiratory illness may be much more difficult to determine. Subtle events such as a sporadic cough, decreased appetite, slow weight gain, and fatigue may herald the presence of more serious respiratory disease.

Family history may also be helpful in establishing a diagnosis. The health of the family should be investigated, because there may be direct or indirect associations between the family's health and the patient's disease. Familial disease may be explained by a common genetic background or by exposure to a common group of infectious or physical agents.

Physical Examination

Careful pulmonary evaluation must include a thorough general physical examination. With this information, plus the knowledge obtained from historical and objective data, one is able to formulate a differential diagnosis. Laboratory diagnostic studies may be helpful in pinpointing a specific diagnosis, but none is as important as careful clinical evaluation and judgment.

Physical examination begins with quiet observation of the undisturbed child. Respiratory rate should be counted and the depth of the efforts noted. Look for dyspnea or labored breathing and note the character and location of retractions. Note whether other accessory muscles are used such as that which occurs with flaring of the alae nasi and head bobbing. Chest abnormalities should be noted; if present, the distribution and degree of cyanosis should be ascertained.

In addition to the respiratory rate, several objective measurements can be performed that are helpful in the clinical evaluation of a child with pulmonary disease. Height and weight should be compared with normal values as an indication of the adequacy of nutrition and growth. An obstetrical caliper and a tape measure can be used to measure the anteroposterior and lateral diameters of the thorax. The thoracic index can be calculated from this by dividing the anteroposterior diameter by the transverse diameter. As obstructive airway disease increases, the chest shape becomes more circular and the thoracic index approaches 1.0. Another measurement, useful in patients with chronic respiratory illness, is the quantitation of digital clubbing if it is present. By means of either a plaster finger cast or a shadow graph, the distal phalangeal depth (DPD) and the interphalangeal depth (IPD) are measured with a micrometer. Values of DPD/IPD greater than 1.0 at all ages are considered indicative of clubbing. All these objective measurements are helpful in clinical evaluation, but none can approach the diagnostic importance of a careful physical examination.

Evaluation of respiratory diseases requires particular attention to the upper airway, lungs, and cardiovascular system. The patency of the nose should be determined and the nature of the nasal mucous membrane noted. The pharynx should be inspected for hypertrophied tonsils, malformations, and evidence of secretions. The tracheal position should be palpated. The thorax should be lightly percussed. Dullness to percussion is often noted with pneumonia, atelectasis, and pleural effusion. Hyperresonance may be noted with pneumothorax, emphysema, and chronic obstructive pulmonary disease and air trapping.

Auscultation

Auscultation can be performed satisfactorily with either the bell or the diaphragm as long as it fits over the interspace. A knowledge of bronchopulmonary segments and lobes is necessary to record accurately the location of auscultatory findings. Breath sounds should be described as vesicular, tubular, or bronchovesicular. Vesicular sounds are normal and are heard over most of the upper chest and axilla. In this area, inspiration is a normal, high-pitched sound that is longer than expiration, which may be imperceptible. Tubular breathing is normally heard over the trachea, larynx, and upper sternum, where the expiratory phase is longer. Tubular (bronchial or tracheal) sounds are louder and more high-pitched and may be heard in parts of the lung affected by pneumonia, atelectasis, and effusion.

Rhonchi are continuous loud musical expiratory sounds produced by air moving past a fixed obstruction. This obstruction may be secretions, a foreign body, or a bronchospastic area. Rhonchi usually indicate problems in the upper airways rather than in the lung parenchyma itself. *Rales* are discontinuous, nonmusical crackling sounds produced by air bubbling through fluids in the lungs. They may be described as fine or coarse depending on the quality of the sound. Moist rales may be heard in pneumonia, atelectasis, pulmonary edema, bronchiectasis, and tuberculosis.

Another sound heard frequently is *wheezing,* which can be localized or diffuse. This high-pitched whistling sound can be heard in inspiration, expiration, or both. It is characteristic of bronchoconstriction from asthma, foreign body, and any other partial airway obstruction.

The role of pulmonary function tests should be kept in perspective. They are rarely a key factor in making a definitive diagnosis. Rather, the various patterns of impaired function overlap disease entities. Although the tests are often valuable for following the progress of a patient with continuing or progressive lung disease and in assessing the results of treatment, in general it is far more important for the student to understand the principles of how the lung works than to concentrate only on the numerical results of lung function tests.

Although the number of different pulmonary disorders is immense, the number of presenting complaints of the pediatric patient (or those presented for him by parents) is relatively few. The most common include cyanosis, rapid breathing (tachypnea), labored breathing (dyspnea), audible breathing (stridor), wheezing, and cough.

CYANOSIS

Cyanosis is a bluish color of the skin and nailbeds, attributable in most cases to the presence of an abnormally large amount of reduced hemoglobin in the capillaries. It is indicative of arterial oxygen unsaturation.

Physiology

Cyanosis appears when the absolute amount of reduced hemoglobin in the capillaries reaches 5 g/dl. An anemic patient with less than 5 g hemoglobin cannot become cyanotic. If a patient had exactly 5 g hemoglobin/dl, it would be necessary for 100% of his hemoglobin to be in the reduced form in the capillaries to produce cyanosis, a situation incompatible with life. With 10 g hemoglobin/dl of blood, 50% of the hemoglobin would have to be in the reduced form in the capillaries to cause cyanosis. If a patient had 15 g total hemoglobin/dl, only 33% of this hemoglobin in reduced form would be required in the capillaries. Thus, cyanosis appears less often in the anemic patient.

There are four primary factors that serve as the basis for a working classification of cyanosis:

1. The amount of hemoglobin unable to become fully saturated in the lung because of a variety of conditions interfering with ventilation
2. The amount of hemoglobin unable to reach the lung, passing in reduced form through veno-arterial shunts from the right side of the heart to the arterial blood
3. The amount of hemoglobin converted to the reduced form in the capillaries, *i.e.*, the extent of deoxygenation in the capillaries
4. The amount of hemoglobin in abnormal or reduced form passing through normally aerated portions of the lung

Clinical Evaluation

Cyanosis is first apparent and most evident in areas in which the epidermis is thin and capillaries are numerous: the tips of the fingers and toes (nail beds), the ear lobes, the tip of the nose, the lips and buccal mucous membrane, and, most reliably, the tip of the tongue. It may at times be difficult to ascertain clinically the presence of cyanosis, especially in darkly pigmented persons. The color of true cyanosis disappears if the blood is expressed from the capillaries by blanching pressure. Cyanosis is not necessarily accompanied by dyspnea or distress.

The distribution and duration of cyanosis should be determined. Cyanosis may be central or peripheral. The central type is characterized by cyanosis of the skin as well as the mucous membranes of the mouth and the conjuctivae. Peripheral cyanosis results from blood stasis and is usually not seen in the oral and conjunctival membranes; the systemic O_2 saturation is normal. In a newborn with immature peripheral vascular responses or a child who has been chilled from swimming in cold water too long, the cyanosis is transient and has little cardiorespiratory significance. Lasting cyanosis, however, almost always indicates a hemoglobin or cardiorespiratory abnormality and may demand emergency treatment.

The clinical assessment of oxygenation is hazardous because poor peripheral circulation may result in peripheral cyanosis when the arterial blood is well oxygenated. The amount of light available for inspection, the room temperature, the age of the patient, and the effect of various medications all contribute to the difficulty of accurately determining cyanosis by inspection alone. Comparison of the patient with normal controls is essential. When there is frank central cyanosis, arterial PO_2 almost always is below 45 mm Hg, depending on hemoglobin content and arterial pH. This is dangerously close to the level at which cell enzyme systems stop functioning normally. This is depicted in Figure 23-1.

Thus, the most reliable estimate of the oxygen content of arterial blood requires direct measurement because both hypoxemia and hyperoxemia cannot be reliably assessed by clinical observation.

Of the four primary factors potentially responsible for cyanosis, the specific cause in the individual patient should be determined first. An accurate etiology for the cyanosis can usually be established by a careful history, physical examination, and available laboratory techniques.

Conditions Leading to Cyanosis

Inability of Hemoglobin to Become Fully Saturated in the Lung. A variety of conditions leads to inadequate alveolar ventilation resulting in an increased amount of hemoglobin in reduced form passing through the lung back to the left side of the heart. On a developmental basis, there may be upper airway obstruction to adequate air entry as in atresia of the posterior nasal choanae, combinations of small jaw and large tongue (Pierre Robin syndrome), infants with poor neuromuscular control of the tongue (which becomes easily displaced posteriorly), compression of the trachea by a large mass such as a congenital goiter, laryngeal webs or cysts, tracheal stenosis, subglottic hemangiomas and vascular rings compressing the trachea inside the thorax.

Acquired airway obstruction is vastly more common. The most common cause of inadequate upper airway ventilation is accumulation of nasal mucus in the young infant, normally an obligate nose breather. Another common condition is partial obstruction because of enlarged tonsils and adenoids. Infections such as epiglottitis and acute bronchiolitis are also commonly seen. Episodes of sudden onset such as angioneurotic edema and a foreign body in the larynx

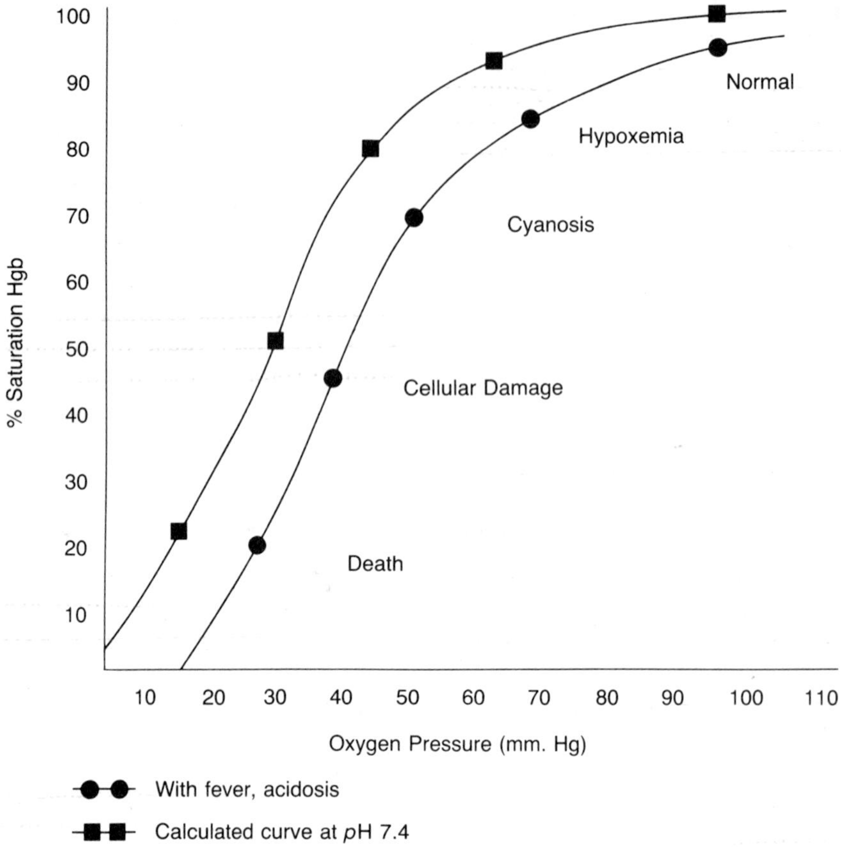

Fig. 23-1. A plotting of the oxyhemoglobin dissociation curve showing the effects of fever and acidosis compared with the curve at normothermia and *p*H 7.4.

or trachea must always be considered and require emergency treatment.

A variety of lower airway conditions interfere with the ability of adequate air to reach the alveoli. Acute bronchial asthma, smoke inhalation, bronchopneumonia, and cystic fibrosis are examples of inflammatory conditions causing intrinsic lower airway obstruction, while atelectasis, lobar emphysema, and acute pneumothorax are examples of extrinsic obstruction.

The inability of the alveoli to function properly is seen earliest in hyaline membrane disease of the newborn. Aspiration pneumonitis, drowning, parenchymal pneumonia, pulmonary alveolar proteinosis, pulmonary fibrosis, pulmonary hemosiderosis, and pulmonary edema all effectively block the diffusion of oxygen across the alveolar membrane.

Finally, the pulmonary pump may be unable to deliver an adequate volume of air to the alveoli through normal airways. Paralysis of the diaphragm, bulbar poliomyelitis, advanced muscular dystrophy, cervical cord lesions, impairment of the respiratory center—in short, any neuromuscular dysfunction may lead to alveolar hypoventilation.

It should be apparent that almost all

the above conditions are contributors to cyanosis, dependent only on the degree to which they are expressed. Few are absolutely causative of cyanosis, as are some of the cyanotic congenital heart lesions discussed next.

Inability of Hemoglobin to Reach the Alveoli. In this category, normal hemoglobin remains in the reduced form due to shunting from the right side of the heart to the arterial blood. This results in an increased level of unsaturated arterial blood distributed to the periphery of the body. Blood that does pass normally through the lungs becomes normally oxygenated and is mixed in the left side of the heart. Thus, administration of oxygen to these patients will cause only a slight decrease in the degree of cyanosis observed because the portion of hemoglobin that does pass through the lungs is normally oxygenated.

The location of the veno-arterial shunting is almost always intracardiac. There are some rare extracardiac locations (*e.g.*, pulmonary arteriovenous fistula and portopulmonary anastomoses) found in some cases of chronic hepatic disease with portal hypertension. The degree of cyanosis in the extracardiac lesions depends upon the size and number of the shunts.

As mentioned, the intracardiac shunts that produce cyanotic congenital heart disease are by far the most common cause of cyanosis in this general category. This finding of often intense cyanosis gave rise to the popular term "blue-babies." The timing of the appearance of cyanosis can vary with the lesion, some appearing at birth, some appearing later. Factors which lead to the later appearance of cyanosis include the closure of the ductus arteriosus, the presence of a patent foramen ovale, the start of exercise or exertion, and the degree of pulmonary hypertension.

Examples of conditions underlying severe cyanosis typically present from birth are: complete transposition of the great vessels, tricuspid atresia, pulmonary atresia with a ventricular septal defect, and aortic atresia. Later appearance of cyanosis is found in cases of tetralogy of Fallot, truncus arteriosus, pulmonary stenosis with patent foramen ovale, Eisenmenger's complex, and total anomalous pulmonary venous return.

Generalized cyanosis in the presence of polycythemia causing capillary stasis may be a secondary cause of cyanosis in patients with certain forms of congenital heart disease.

Increased venous pressure with resulting stasis may also produce generalized cyanosis. This is most commonly seen as a result of hard crying by an infant and may also occur during a *grand mal* seizure. A variety of heart disorders may also contribute, most notably constrictive pericarditis. Patients with cardiac failure resulting from rheumatic mitral valvular disease, left-to-right shunts, myocarditis, endocardial fibroelastosis, and infantile coarctation of the aorta may develop generalized cyanosis due in part to the increased venous pressure and stasis.

Deoxygenation in the Capillaries. Here, normal hemoglobin is converted to the reduced form while passing from the arteries to the veins. The oxygen saturation of the arterial blood is generally normal, and cyanosis is due to capillary stasis. Oxygen therapy does not reduce this form of cyanosis.

The most common clinical expression of this is the local cyanosis observed while an extremity is constricted by a tourniquet. Cyanosis of the face, hands, and feet in the first few hours after birth is another common example of local cyanosis. In older children, head and neck cyanosis because of obstruction of the superior vena cava is a rare example.

Cyanosis due to deoxygenation of the capillaries can also be generalized. Chilling of the skin from a variety of causes is the most common example. Shock, especially that associated with dehydration, is a major serious cause of capillary stasis. This may occur with severe diarrhea, acute adrenal insufficiency, and sepsis. A mottled or gray cyanosis may result from peripheral vascular collapse and pooling of blood in the skin.

Abnormal Hemoglobin Passing through Normally Aerated Lung. The most common abnormal form of hemoglobin is that found in methemoglobinemia. This condition requires spectrophotometry for diagnosis. Methemoglobinemia can be congenital, due to a deficiency of the enzyme hemoglobin reductase, inherited as either a recessive or dominant form. The ingestion of well water high in nitrates, of aniline dyes, old wax crayons, phenylhydrazine, acetanilid, primaquine phosphate, and benzocaine ointment or rectal suppositories can produce methemoglobinemia. Sulfhemoglobin is another abnormal form of hemoglobin attributed to sulfonamide administration. Since carboxyhemoglobin, resulting from carbon monoxide exposure, is bright red, it produces a reddish rather than a bluish or cyanotic discoloration of the skin. Since CO has 210 times more affinity for hemoglobin than oxygen, it is important to note that PO_2 may be normal in CO poisoning, while oxygen content is markedly reduced.

DYSPNEA

Dyspnea is a symptom, not a disorder. It can be defined as breathing that is perceived as difficult or labored accompanied by an unpleasant feeling of discomfort or distress. This may be visibly evident or it may be a subjective feeling expressed by the patient or by his parents on his behalf.

Apnea is the absence of respiratory movement. *Bradypnea* is slow respiration; *tachypnea* is a rapid or an increased rate of breathing as is *polypnea*; *hypopnea* is shallow breathing and *hyperpnea* is an increase in the depth of respiration. *Hyperventilation* is breathing in excess of the body's needs. It should be emphasized that dyspnea is *not* the same as tachypnea, hyperpnea, or hyperventilation.

It is important to be familiar with normal respiratory patterns and rates of different ages in order to recognize the abnormal states. For example, short apneic episodes and irregularity of respiration, grave signs in older children, may be normal findings in a small premature infant.

There are patterns of breathing that are related to position and to dyspnea. *Orthopnea* is a preference for a sitting position because the dypsnea is much less than that felt in the recumbent position. Children with severe dyspnea and orthopnea often find the most comfortable position is to sit cross-legged in bed leaning far forward over a couple of pillows or a bed table. *Trepopnea* is the preference for one lateral recumbent position over another, seen in tension pneumothorax and pleural effusion.

Physiology

The causes of dyspnea are very complex and not well understood. Awareness of the behavior of one's lungs and of the act of breathing is derived from several sources. These include vision, hearing, the sensation of movement and temperature change in the upper respiratory tract, sensations from vagal irritant and cough receptors, and sensations of chest wall movement.

Dypsnea occurs, in part, when the muscles of respiration perform either an unusual amount or an unaccustomed type of work. This includes all cardiopulmonary conditions in which the work of breathing is definitely increased. During normal respiration, 1.3% of the total oxygen consumption of the body is accounted for by diaphragmatic and intercostal muscles. With dyspnea, oxygen consumption by the respiratory muscles increases to 9%. This increased oxygen need may in itself contribute to a continuing respiratory distress.

Conditions in which there is an increased airway resistance commonly cause dyspnea. A normal person in whom bronchial obstruction is induced experimentally by histamine inhalation, for example, does not experience any respiratory symptoms until airway resistance is increased 3-fold or more. Severe dyspnea may not result until airway resistance is increased 5- to 15-fold.

In general, it seems likely that the sensation of dyspnea may be caused by any one or a combination of mechanisms—increased respiratory work, reduced ventilatory capacity, increased stimulation of receptors, and increased subjective sensitivity.

Clinical Perception

The sensation of dyspnea is a subjective one; therefore evaluation by the clinician is as difficult as the evaluation of other sensations, such as pain, hunger, thirst, feeling cold, and so on.

Patients may use a variety of words to describe the sensation of dyspnea. Shortness of breath, unable to get my breath, tightness, panting, wheezing, fullness, constriction are a few terms commonly used.

A history of difficult breathing should first suggest airway obstruction. Note whether dyspnea has any relation to time of day, exercise, meals, posture, and so on. Is it of relatively short term but steadily becoming worse, as in bronchiolitis, or does it seem to come and go as in asthma? Is there a seasonal variation? Diurnal? (Both suggest asthma.) Is the dyspnea of sudden onset in a previously well child? Has the child always had labored breathing, as with anomalies of the lungs or heart? Paroxysmal nocturnal dyspnea is associated classically with left ventricular failure. Exertion, if marked enough, will cause dyspnea in anyone; thus a grading system for the assessment of "dyspnea on exertion" must be used and must be age appropriate. Infants may become dyspneic while feeding from a bottle, which constitutes exercise for the infant, while an older child may develop dyspnea as a result of exercise-induced bronchospasm brought about by a vigorous game of soccer. On a +1 to +4 scale, a +1 might be the ability to keep up with peers during normal activity but inability when strenuous exercise is involved. A +4 might be shortness of breath and dyspnea at rest.

Clinical Conditions

At best, any classification of conditions that give rise to dyspnea is an arbitrary one. The following is a general outline that may be practical:

1. Mechanical factors: conditions that inhibit or restrict the normal respiratory mechanisms
   a. Upper airway obstruction (congenital, foreign body, inflammation, bronchospasm)
   b. Painful breathing, pleurisy, rib fracture
   c. Body casts
   d. Pleural effusion, hemothorax, pneumothorax
   e. Flail chest (rib fractures or costochondral junction separation)
   f. Thoracic dystrophy
   g. Elevation of diaphragm by abdominal fluid or masses

h. Extreme obesity

2. Tissue hypoxia: conditions other than those of primary alveolar or cardiac origin that result in an insufficient supply of oxygen to the tissues
   a. Anemia
   b. Overexertion
   c. High altitude
   d. Carbon monoxide exposure
3. Pulmonary insufficiency: conditions at the alveolar level that result in inadequate ventilation
   a. Atelectasis (intrinsic-obstructive or extrinsic-compressive)
   b. Alveolar flooding (aspiration, near-drowning, bleeding)
   c. Alveolar interference (hyaline membranes, alveolar proteinosis)
   d. Pulmonary edema and interstitial edema
   e. Interstitial fibrosis (alveolar-capillary block)
   f. Diseases of the pulmonary parenchyma due to inflammation
   g. Decreased pulmonary distensibility
   h. Obliterative bronchiolitis
4. Cardiac and vascular insufficiency
   a. Cardiac failure
   b. Congenital cyanotic heart disease. Depending on the degree of hypoxia associated with the cardiac lesion, dyspnea on exertion may range from mild to severe. Children, especially those in whom pulmonary stenosis is severe, may experience attacks of paroxysmal dyspnea. During these spells, the cyanosis becomes much more intense, the patient gasps for breath and may become unconscious for a time. These spells may occur spontaneously or may be precipitated by feeding, crying, or defecation. Older children learn to interrupt these spells by assuming a squatting position.
   c. Pulmonary congestion
   d. Pulmonary hypertension
   e. Decreased pulmonary circulation (congenital, embolism, thrombus)
5. Neuromuscular
   a. Unilateral or bilateral paralysis of the diaphragm
   b. Polio
   c. Guillain-Barré syndrome
   d. Muscular dystrophy
   e. Myasthenia gravis
   f. Hypopotassemia
6. Central nervous system
   a. Acidosis
   b. Drugs (salicylates, heroin)
   c. Immature respiratory center
   d. Encephalitis, meningitis
   e. Inappropriate response to hypoxia (familial dysautonomia, narcolepsy)
7. Emotional-functional

STRIDOR

Stridor is a harsh sound caused by obstruction to breathing in the larynx or trachea. Derived from the Latin, *stridulus*, meaning creaking, whistling, or grating, it is predominantly an inspiratory sound but there is often a softer expiratory element, particularly if obstruction is in the subglottic area or trachea. In some tracheal lesions, the expiratory element resembles a wheeze.

Stridor is an important indication of respiratory obstruction and should never be disregarded. The presence of stridor means that somewhere between the inlet to the respiratory tract and the outlet from the bronchi to the lungs lies a partial obstruction.

In minor degrees of narrowing, breathing may be quiet at rest, but with increased physical activity and consequent increased velocity of air flow, stridor may develop. In lesions causing narrowing at the level of the vocal cords or above, the stridor is predominantly inspiratory, but in some infants with subglottic lesions (particularly if there is involvement of the lower trachea as well), prolonged expiratory stridor is marked.

Pathophysiology

Stridor is produced by turbulence of airflow and increased velocity of air brought about by the narrowed or partially obstructed airway. A greater negative intratracheal and intrathoracic pressure must be generated to overcome the obstruction, resulting in a dynamic compression of the extrathoracic trachea during inspiration. In younger children the larynx and trachea are relatively soft and compressible, thus dynamic compression occurs more readily than in an adult and is an important secondary factor in the production of inspiratory stridor.

Three normal anatomic features lead to a greater incidence of acquired stridor in infants compared with older children and adults: (1) the small size of the infant larynx, (2) the presence of loose submucosal connective tissue in the supraglottic and subglottic regions, and (3) rigid encirclement of the subglottic area by the cricoid cartilage.

The triangular glottic opening of the infant larynx is approximately 77 mm in length and 4 mm in width at the base. In infants, edema produces a reduction in the size of this opening and signs of respiratory obstruction, but a similar degree of edema in the adult results only in hoarseness. The laryngeal mucosa is loosely fixed anteriorally to the epiglottis and laterally along the aryepiglottic folds. Collection of edema fluid in these supraglottic spaces in association with inflammatory processes leads to downward pressure on the epiglottis and to laryngeal obstruction. A similar process may occur in the narrow subglottic area with swelling of the submucosal tissue and acute respiratory obstruction. Since this area is completely encircled by the cricoid cartilage, swelling due to edema must impinge upon the airway.

History

If stridor has been present since birth, the underlying cause may be a congenital abnormality or birth trauma. In general, disorders of structure tend to be more noisy when the tissues are relaxed (*e.g.*, when the child is asleep). Disorders of function, such as paralyses, tend to produce more noise when the child is awake and active.

Any difficulty in breathing in the newborn may be accompanied by a difficulty in feedings. If the underlying cause of the breathing difficulty is a paralysis of the vocal cord, there may be paralysis of one side of the cricopharyngeal sphincter that leads to a failure of relaxation during peristalsis. This causes food to "bounce back" from the projecting shelf of unrelaxed muscle and to spill over into the tracheobronchial tree. Secondary pneumonic consolidation is not uncommon therefore, and often recurs during the early months of life.

It is a common experience in pediatrics to find several abnormalities in the same patient. Troubles rarely come singly, and the presence or absence of a second abnormality should always be kept in mind. An interval between birth and the onset of the noise suggests that the cause has been acquired. In young children common conditions which give rise to acquired stridor are inhaled foreign bodies and respiratory tract inflammation. Therefore, it is important to ask what the child was doing when the noise was first noticed; if he was playing with a toy, part of which is missing, or if he was eating, then it is wise to offer a tentative diagnosis of inhaled foreign body and to proceed with radiographic and endoscopic studies without delay.

Physical Examination

The child should be examined in a warm room because the clothes must be removed in order to observe the movements of the chest and respiratory muscles. As a consequence of increased negative intrapleural pressure during inspiration, retraction of the suprasternal tissues, sternal, costal cartilages, and intercostal spaces may occur. By applying a stethoscope to the side of the patient's neck, the position of the noise in the respiratory cycle is noted. If the noise is loud on inspiration the cause should be sought in the larynx; if the noise is loud on expiration the cause lies in the bronchial region; if the noise can be heard clearly in both phases of the respiratory cycle the obstruction lies below the vocal cords and above the bronchi. Some examiners claim to distinguish the brassy noise of subglottic stenosis, the pure tone of congenital laryngeal stridor, and the wheeze of the impacted foreign body. In certain instances the obstruction may be moved by changes of posture. In the Pierre Robin syndrome, the noise disappears altogether if the child is placed in the prone position. This provides a clue to the diagnosis and an indication of how the child may be managed. Children in whom infection has narrowed the respiratory pathway are often more comfortable when nursed sitting up.

Tachycardia, apprehensiveness, increase in respiratory rate and use of the accessory muscles of respiration indicate progression of the obstruction. Restlessness is an early indication of hypoxia and occurs before overt cyanosis. Increasing restlessness in an infant or child with respiratory obstruction may indicate the need for a tracheostomy. Since sedatives may mask the manifestations of lack of oxygen and inhibit needed accessory respiratory efforts, such medications should not be given in these instances. With establishment of an adequate airway, restlessness is followed dramatically by deep sleep.

Diagnosis

After the clinical examination is complete, it is necessary to assess the degree of narrowing and the cause of the obstruction. Almost invariably, the child with stridor must have an endoscopic and radiologic examination of the airways. The only exception to this rule is when the pediatrician is certain that infection is the cause and that endoscopy represents a greater hazard to the child's life than the infection.

Some conditions can be determined by direct examination, such as the passage of a soft catheter through the nares to detect choanal atresia or the visualization of the cherry red epiglottis characteristic of acute epiglottitis.

Anteroposition and lateral films of the neck and chest are essential to the diagnostic evaluation. The patency of the upper airway can be estimated, looking for such signs as ballooning of the supraglottic airway, compression from the retropharyngeal space, a large swollen epiglottis, subglottic narrowing, or an opaque foreign body, to name but a few patterns. The column of air in the airway can be used as a contrast medium. At times, fluoroscopy and films in both full inspiration and expiration may be helpful. The inability of one lung to empty when placed uppermost in the lateral recumbent position is very suggestive of an aspirated foreign body.

Fluoroscopy or cineradiographic studies of a barium swallow may be helpful in outlining an area of compression or displacement as might be seen with certain vascular rings or a variety of mediastinal cystic structures.

Bronchography is generally not required since the avenue of most direct diagnostic evaluation is by laryngoscopy and bronchoscopy. Bronchoscopy is indicated only when the cause of the stridor cannot be identified in the supraglottic and glottic regions.

Direct visualization of the larynx before using a general anesthesia is most important so that the movement of the vocal cords can be assessed. Accurate diagnosis of the two most common causes of stridor present since birth—congenital laryngeal stridor and paralysis of the vocal cords—can only be made by direct laryngoscopy. In children, this should be done by someone who is familiar with the characteristics of the normal infant larynx and airway and who has the necessary specialized instruments.

Etiology

Since the affected sites are hollow, the lesion responsible for stridor may lie in the lumen, in the wall, or outside the wall of the airway.

Obviously, there are many causes of stridor in infancy and childhood. For our purposes, they are best divided into those of acute or acquired origin, and those that are congenital, persistent, or recurrent.

Acute Acquired. The acute acquired causes of stridor are mainly those of infection and are discussed in more detail in the section dealing with infectious diseases.

1. Croup, infectious croup, acute laryngotracheobronchitis. The etiologic agent is most often viral, usually the para influenza viruses.
2. Acute spasmodic croup. The etiology is uncertain but may be viral, allergic, or psychological.
3. Acute epiglottitis. Usually caused by *H. influenza.* This is a potentially fatal disease and is a true medical emergency.
4. Infectious mononucleosis. Often the edema and swelling of the tonsils and adenoidal tissue can nearly occlude the airway.
5. Angioneurotic edema
6. Laryngospasm
7. Foreign bodies. The presence of a foreign body in the respiratory tract should be considered in the differential diagnosis of respiratory obstruction and of unexplained chest lesions in children.

Congenital, Persistent, Recurrent. There are a number of conditions which fall into the category of congenital, persistent or recurrent causes of stridor, the three most common of which are discussed in some detail.

1. Congenital Laryngeal Stridor. (Laryngomalacia, infantile larynx, inspiratory laryngeal collapse.) There is no satisfactory term for the most common cause of persistent stridor in infancy. The condition has been termed simply "congenital laryngeal stridor" but this describes a symptom and does not give any indication of underlying pathology.

The term "laryngomalacia" is commonly used in North America and suggests a pathologic cause, but since the condition is rarely fatal there is no good evidence that the cartilage of the larynx is abnormally soft. "Inspiratory laryngeal collapse" is a descriptive term which simply draws attention to the mechanism of the production of the stridor. "Infantile larynx" is probably the most acceptable name because the larynx, particularly the glottic region, appears disproportionately small for the child's size. Further, it does not presume to give the pathologic basis of the lesion which has yet to be determined.

The larynx is small and placed anteriorly. The epiglottis is long and omega-shaped, the aryepiglottic folds long and floppy with prominent arytenoids, and the interarytenoid cleft is deep but does not extend to the cord level. During inspiration, the epiglottis, the aryepiglottic folds, and arytenoids collapse into and over the glottic orifice leaving a slitlike opening. These floppy tissues intermittently obstruct the entrance of air and vibrate, thus causing stridor.

During expiration, the positive pressure of air from below blows them apart. The glottis is normal in size and there are no special dangers to be expected here unless an acute respiratory infection supervenes, in which case relief of the obstructed airway is urgently required.

The onset of the stridor usually occurs within the first 4 weeks of life, most often in the first week; it may even be noted within hours of birth. Occasionally parents do not become aware of the noise until the baby develops a respiratory infection as late as 6 to 8 weeks. Stridor is predominantly inspiratory, but in about 20% of patients there is a definite expiratory element. The inspiratory stridor varies considerably in intensity, being loudest with increased ventilation associated with crying or excitement. The sound varies in pitch, is often coarse and jerky or interrupted during inspiration, and varies considerably from breath to breath and when the baby is held in different positions. In some infants little or no air is heard entering the lungs during some inspiratory efforts. The cry and cough are normal.

It is rare for babies with infantile larynx to develop respiratory obstruction of sufficient degree to require an artificial airway. The stridor is more often an annoyance than a problem. If severe obstructive episodes occur in a baby in whom a clinical diagnosis of infantile larynx has been made, further investigation to determine the cause is essential.

The stridor usually lessens after the age of 12 months and may be heard only when the infant is upset or has intercurrent respiratory infections. By the age of 2½ to 3 years or before stridor usually disappears completely. A uniformly good prognosis can be given to parents of babies with this type of laryngeal malformation, provided it is the only lesion present.

2. *Paralysis of the Vocal Cord.* Inspiratory stridor, respiratory distress, and feeding difficulties are the common symptoms of bilateral or unilateral vocal cord palsy. Bilateral palsy usually results from severe malformations of the central nervous system, most often the Arnold-Chiari deformity. The stridor becomes more obvious with the development of hydrocephalus, but when the intracranial pressure is controlled it may disappear. Bilateral palsy occasionally occurs as an isolated anomaly and spontaneously improves by 2 to 3 months of age.

Unilateral palsy may occur as an isolated anomaly, in association with major malformations of the heart and great vessels, or with other neurologic disease. The lesion associated with cardiac malformations is almost invariably left-sided because of compression of the recurrent laryngeal nerve. In some babies with isolated palsy there is a history of difficult labor.

These children have feeding difficulties, too, and patchy consolidation of the lungs frequently results from inhaled milk. They are slow to gain weight, therefore, and may have to be weaned early to solid food because it is swallowed more easily. In children with paresis or paralysis, more than one direct laryngoscopy may be required in order to assess progress or resolution of the causative lesion. It is not unusual for the paralysis to clear completely, although the voice may be husky or normal. The diagnosis of cord palsy, particularly unilateral, may be difficult to establish by laryngoscopy. It is best to examine the larynx without general anesthesia. In older children, indirect laryngoscopy can be used.

3. *Subglottic Hemangioma.* It is probably more common than reported figures suggest, since the diagnosis of subglottic hemangioma may be difficult to establish during life and also postmortem. The epithelium covering the hemangioma may mask its vascularity during life, and after death it may contract so much that it can be identified only by microscopic examination.

The clinical pattern is surprisingly constant. The principal features are variable inspiratory and prolonged expiratory stridor and respiratory difficulty, a croupy or brassy cough, and normal cry. The symptoms are not present at birth but develop either insidiously or more abruptly between the ages of 1 and 3 months. There is usually progressive increase in severity of the stridor and respiratory difficulty during the ensuing few weeks or months. During the period in which the symptoms are most marked, the infant usually fails to grow. Only in mildly affected patients is normal growth maintained.

The stridor and respiratory difficulty are much worse when the baby cries or struggles due to engorgement from obstruction of venous drainage. In infants with small hemangiomas, the symptoms may be minimal when the child is breathing quietly, as when asleep. Upper respiratory tract infections aggravate the symptoms.

Other congenital, persistent, or recurrent causes of stridor are:

- Nasal polyps
- Nasal foreign body
- Laryngeal webs
- Laryngeal cysts
- Subglottic stenosis
- Tracheal stenosis
- Laryngeal papilloma
- Extrinsic airway obstruction
  - Thyroglossal duct cyst
  - Micrognathia with glossoptosis
  - Macroglossia
  - Retropharyngeal abscess
  - Cystic hygroma
  - Congenital goiter
  - Mediastinal masses
  - Vascular rings
    - Double aortic arch
    - Right aortic arch with left ligamentum arteriosum
    - Anomalous innominate artery
    - Anomalous left common carotid
    - Aberrant subclavian artery
    - Anomalous left pulmonary artery
- Neurogenic
  - Palatal control
  - Tonic contractions of base of tongue and posterior pharynx in patients with cerebral palsy

WHEEZING

Wheezing is an audible, high-pitched sound made in breathing. It is heard during expiration, but there may be an associated sound during inspiration, either stridor or a rattle, depending on the origin of the wheeze. It is frequently associated with obvious expiratory effort. Wheezing is not synonymous with bronchospasm and can result from causes of airway obstruction other than bronchospasm.

Pathophysiology

Normal breathing is not audible because, even at the maximum rate of air flow in the normal subject, the linear velocity of air flow in the tracheobronchial tree is too slow to provide a sound. Breathing only becomes audible when there is an increase in the linear velocity of air flow resulting from narrowing of the air passages.

Wheezing is produced by diseases that cause a direct or indirect narrowing of the trachea and major bronchi. The linear velocity of air flow in the smaller airways is far too low to cause any audible sound even when these are narrowed.

Narrowing of the trachea and major bronchi sufficient to produce an audible sound can occur in two types of disease processes. In one, there is dynamic narrowing of the trachea and major bronchi when the pressure outside the airways exceeds the pressure inside during expiration because of widespread obstruction of the medium and small airways. In the other, there is a localized obstruction of either the trachea or a major bronchus.

In diseases that cause obstruction in the medium and small airways, a wheeze is heard only during expiration. During inspiration the pressure inside the trachea and major bronchi exceeds that outside. An inspiratory rattle may be associated with the expiratory wheeze if there is mucus in the trachea or major bronchi. The inspiratory noise has a different quality from a wheeze.

Focal narrowing of the trachea or of a major bronchus can cause an expiratory wheeze. There is an increase in the linear velocity of airflow past the obstruction and this may produce a wheeze. If the obstruction is in the intrathoracic portion of the airways there may also be dynamic compression of the airways downstream from the obstruction if a positive pleural pressure develops during expiration. This occurs if the obstructing lesion causes a significant rise in the airway's resistance. An inspiratory stridor may also be heard if the rate of inspiratory airflow and the degree of obstruction are sufficient. The stridor heard when there is an obstructing lesion in the trachea or major bronchus is higher pitched than that produced by a laryngeal lesion, and may resemble a wheeze in quality.

In both types of obstruction wheeze may be absent during quiet breathing but it develops when the patient increases ventilation as a result of activity. With hyperventilation the linear velocity of air flow increases; if there is airway obstruction the expiratory pleural pressure becomes more positive. In many asthmatic patients, exercise-induced bronchospasm occurs, but in a patient with moderate airway obstruction the development of a wheeze after exercise may be due to increased air flow velocity without any alteration in airway resistance.

Causes of Wheezing in Children

- Obstructive disease of the small airways
  - Acute
    - Acute viral bronchiolitis
    - Hydrocarbon ingestion
  - Recurrent or persistent
    - Asthma
    - Hypersensitivity pneumonitis
    - Aspiration bronchitis
    - H type tracheoesophageal fistula
    - Subacute and chronic infective bronchitis
      - Cystic fibrosis
      - Immune-deficiency disorders
      - Nonspecific infective bronchitis
    - Alpha-1-antitrypsin deficiency
    - Obliterative bronchiolitis
    - Congenital heart disease with pulmonary hyperperfusion
- Obstructive lesions of the trachea or major bronchi
  - Acute
    - Foreign body in trachea, bronchus, or esophagus
  - Recurrent or persistent
    - Foreign body in trachea, bronchus, or esophagus
    - Vascular rings
    - Mediastinal lymphadenopathy
    - Mediastinal cysts and tumors
    - Tracheal webs, tracheal stenosis, bronchial stenosis
    - Tracheomalacia

Etiology

Chevalier Jackson is credited with the commonly quoted aphorism "All that wheezes is not asthma, and not all asthma wheezes." The important causes of wheezing in childhood fall into two main groups (see list): (1) obstructive lesions involving the smaller bronchi and bronchioles and (2) obstructive lesions in the trachea or major bronchi.

Acute Viral Bronchiolitis. Infants with bronchiolitis, usually due to respiratory syncytial virus, have marked tachypnea, dyspnea, and expiratory wheezing and grunt; they may also have cyanosis. These symptoms are associated with generalized obstructive emphysema. The differentiation between acute bronchiolitis and infantile asthma may be difficult and is discussed in greater detail in Chapter 26.

Hydrocarbon Ingestion. Hydrocarbons such as turpentine, gasoline, and lighter fluid are examples of substances which, if aspirated, cause an acute inflammatory response of the bronchial mucosa with resultant cough and bronchospasm.

Asthma. Asthma is by far the most common cause of wheezing in infancy and childhood. Obstruction occurs mainly in the medium and smaller airways as a result of smooth muscle spasm, mucosal edema, and hypersecretion of mucus. Wheezing in asthma is typically recurrent but some children develop chronic airway obstruction with persistent wheeze for weeks at a time. However, in these children its intensity will fluctuate considerably from time to time, and the fact that there is chronic obstruction can easily be missed. In very severe obstruction, wheeze may not occur owing to the very small tidal volume. Some infants under the age of 12 months also develop a persistent wheeze. Asthma is discussed in detail in Chapter 26.

Hypersensitivity Pneumonitis. A large number of conditions fall into the category of hypersensitivity pneumonitis, including pigeon-breeder's lung, farmer's lung, and humidifier disease. Exposure to doves, gerbils, and parakeets can also bring about this syndrome.

Aspiration Bronchitis. The inhalation of oral or gastric contents, especially milk, can result in a chemical bronchitis with the production of wheeze. If recurrent, an allergic component develops that is probably due to the milk protein. Poor palatal-pharyngeal swallowing coordination, and gastroesophageal reflux are often involved.

H Type Tracheoesophageal (T-E) Fistula. This H type lesion, which may be very subtle, can contribute to recurrent wheezing because of the spillover of esophageal contents into the trachea. Cough is also a prominent symptom.

Cystic Fibrosis. Many infants with cystic fibrosis have a continuous bronchiolitislike condition which may last for several weeks. Wheezing is a major component of the pulmonary symptoms, at times presenting more of a problem than the chronic cough. As the patient with cystic fibrosis reaches late adolescence, a low-grade bronchospasm becomes commonplace.

Immune-Deficiency Disorders. Immune-deficiency conditions often have a suppurative bronchiectasis resulting from the inability to properly contain infection. Cough, often producing sputum, and low-grade bronchospasm poorly responsive to bronchodilators are features of this group.

Nonspecific Infective Bronchitis. Although poorly classified and documented, there is a group of children whose symptoms resemble the chronic bronchitis of adulthood. Usually there is a history of exposure to tobacco smoke in the home. No consistent organism is isolated from these patients, who are often said to have "wheezing bronchitis" or "asthmatic bronchitis." Yet they do not have atopic disease.

Alpha-1-Antitrypsin Deficiency. Although the symptoms of dyspnea and wheezing coupled with lower lobe emphysema, as seen on radiographs, usually do not develop until the third decade of life, certain younger patients with alpha-1-antitrypsin deficiency have the persistent wheezing that is poorly responsive to treatment and characteristic of this disorder.

Obliterative Bronchiolitis. Obliterative bronchiolitis is an end-stage result of certain distal airway infections, notably influenza virus and adenoviral infections. Patchy areas of hyperinflation adjacent to areas of atelectasis result in a very uneven ventilation.

Congenital Heart Disease with Pulmonary Hyperperfusion. In congenital cardiac conditions with large left-to-right shunts, that is, VSD and PDA, the increased pulmonary arterial flow causes congestion of the capillary bed. Interstitial fluid collects in the peribronchial space, compressing the small distal airways, leading to wheezing, hyperaeration, and migratory areas of atelectasis.

Foreign Body. A foreign body is the most common cause of wheezing from large airways obstruction. Impacted esophageal foreign bodies may cause wheezing by tracheal compression.

Vascular Rings. Anomalies of the vessels originating from the aortic arch may develop true encircling rings of the trachea and cause wheezing by direct tracheal compression. Often, after surgical repair of the obstructing vessel, a defect in the tracheal cartilage may remain, resulting in continued wheezing and interference with normal cough mechanics by allowing almost complete tracheal closure to occur at the point of the cartilaginous defect.

Mediastinal Lymphadenopathy, Cysts, and Tumors. Depending on the location of mediastinal lymphadenopathy, cysts, and tumors, tracheal or bronchial compression may result, producing a persistent wheeze. Associated findings such as an irritative cough, lobar atelectasis, or swallowing difficulties may be present.

Tracheal and Bronchial Webs and Stenosis. Usually both an inspiratory and expiratory wheeze is produced by tracheal and bronchial webs and stenosis. While resting, the wheeze may be minimal or absent, but become obvious with activity, excitement, or a respiratory infection.

Conclusion

Although "all that wheezes is not asthma," asthma is by far the most common cause of wheezing in childhood; the diagnosis must be considered in every child presenting with recurrent or persistent wheezing. A chest radiograph is indicated for all children with persistent wheezing to try to exclude local bronchial compression as the cause. Further investigations, which may include radiologic screening, bronchography, endoscopic examination, and pulmonary function tests, are indicated if the clinical pattern of the wheezing is not typical of asthma.

COUGH

"The cough-reflex is the watchdog of the lung"
Chevalier Jackson

Cough is perhaps the most common symptom of acute and chronic respiratory disease in children. Because of its audible nature, it attracts considerable attention. An extravagant amount of time and money is spent on treating this symptom, one of the most important vital protective mechanisms of the body.

Purpose and Function

Cough serves to clear foreign matter and excess secretions from the air passages of the lung. This mechanism of clearance is a protective mechanism of a primitive nature used when inhaled foreign particles, noxious gases, chemical irritants, and so on, reach the tracheobronchial tree. One major function of cough is to protect the respiratory tract from inhalation of food or fluids, especially during swallowing.

Usually, the quantity of mucus secreted by the membranes lining the airway is small, and no cough is present. The action of the cilia covering those membranes is all that is needed to sweep the mucus, with any entrapped particles, up the airways into the pharynx. This mucociliary escalator extends from the terminal bronchioles of the lung; beyond that, other clearance mechanisms exist.

The fact that we normally cough little, and that persons unable to cough because of polio or spinal cord injuries may get along well for long periods of time, indicates that the normal mechanisms provide adequate clearance when they are operating properly. However, if the cilia are injured or destroyed, as frequently occurs in acute and chronic infections of the airways, or if there are excess secretions because of inflammation, cough then becomes a powerful and necessary supplementary clearance method.

Mechanism

Cough Reflex. A cough is induced by an irritation of the afferent fibers of the pharyngeal branches of the glossopharyngeal nerve, as well as the sensory endings of the vagus nerve in the larynx, trachea, and mucous membranes of the pharynx and larger bronchi. The impulses are transmitted to the cough center in the medulla and pons. Impulses from the cough center are then relayed by means of the vagus and spinal nerves from C_3 to S_2 to the muscles of the chest and larynx. A considerable amount of air is inspired. The glottis closes and the vocal cords shut tightly to trap the air in the lungs; the muscles of the chest wall, abdominal wall, diaphragm, and pelvic floor contract, pushing the diaphragm up while other expiratory muscles also contract forcefully. Pleural, alveolar, and subglottic pressures rise to as much as 200 cm H_2O, and the glottis suddenly opens. The combined effect of high intrapleural and intraabdominal pressures on expiratory volume flow rate creates a high linear velocity air stream with a high kinetic energy, which, upon opening of the glottis, makes possible the acceleration and displacement of any foreign material in the bronchi or the trachea.

It has been estimated that the linear velocities of air flow achieved in the trachea during a cough may well be as follows: in an uncompressed tracheal lumen with a diameter of 1.5 cm and a normal expiratory flow rate of 1 liter/sec, it would be approximately 15 miles per hour; at a flow rate of 7 liters/sec it could reach a hurricane velocity up to 100 miles per hour; if, in addition, the cross-section of the trachea is compressed to one-sixteenth of its normal area, the linear velocity can reach a speed of 600 miles per hour or 85% of the speed of sound.

It is important to appreciate that the cough reflex is under voluntary control and may be either inhibited or initiated at will. Voluntary inhibition because of pain prevents effective clearing of the bronchial tree of excess secretion, and central stimulation may be responsible for nervous coughing.

Not all patients nor all portions of the respiratory tree have the same stimulus threshold. Cough may be absent, at times, in a small infant with severe pneumonia or even though a foreign body is present in the tracheobronchial tree. Tolerance or decreased reflex excitability may also develop as in some patients with bronchiectasis or atelectasis where coughing is not continuous.

Clearing the Airways. The two main mechanisms by which coughing clears the airway are the "tussive squeeze" and the "bechic blast," both terms coined by the Jacksons.

Tussive Squeeze. The lung and smaller peripheral airways are compressed due to the high positive pleural pressure. Secretions and exudate are squeezed into the larger bronchi from which they can be expelled by blasts of high velocity air. The velocity of gas flowing in the alveoli and small airways is so low that little energy can be transferred to any retained secretions. During vigorous coughing, dynamic collapse of the peripheral airways due to the high intrathoracic pressure, especially at low lung volumes, may involve a large part of the bronchial tree, and the volume of air in the airways may be reduced to one-seventh the normal value. Cartilage rings in the large airways prevent complete collapse, but their lumina are considerably narrowed.

Bechic Blast. When high-velocity expiratory air flows are produced in the upper airways, some of this momentum is transferred to the foreign matter, secretions, or exudate, resulting in expectoration.

Peak velocity of gas in the trachea or larynx during a forcible cough may reach the astounding level of well over half the speed of sound or 180–300 m/sec. The rate of expiratory gas flow depends on two factors: the alveolar-to-mouth pressure gradient and the volume of gas in the alveoli at the beginning of coughing. The greater the lung volume, the greater the flow rate—hence the marked inspiratory effort which normally precedes coughing. In healthy young males an air flow volume of 12 liters/sec can be achieved easily. Deep inspiration also enables the expiratory muscles to act with greater force. At lung volumes of less than 50% of normal the maximum flow rate is halved.

The velocity of gas flow at any point in the airways depends on the instantaneous flow divided by the total cross section of all airways of that generation. As the total cross section in area of all the small airways is over one hundred times that of the trachea or larger airways, the velocity of expelled air reaches a very high level in the large airways. This velocity is further increased as the diameter of the trachea and larger bronchi is narrowed by dynamic compression due to the high positive intrapleural pressure.

Etiologic Classification of Cough

The conditions which can lead to coughing are too numerous to list in detail. Some broad areas are listed as follows:

Upper respiratory infections—acute rhinitis and/or sinusitis with postnasal drip and irritation, acute tonsillopharyngitis, epiglottitis

Lower respiratory infections—acute spasmodic laryngitis ("spasmodic croup"), laryngotracheobronchitis, measles, pertussis and parapertussis, cystic fibrosis, bronchiolitis, bronchopneumonia, tuberculosis, bronchiectasis, atelectasis

Parasitic infections—ascariasis, visceral larva migrans

Congenital anomalies—pulmonary sequestration, diaphragmatic hernia, tracheo-esophageal "H" type fistula, vascular rings, anomalous major vessels

Allergy—allergic rhinitis, asthma, hypersensitivity pneumonitis (pigeon-breeder's lung, parakeets, gerbils, and others), allergic bronchopulmonary aspergillosis

Irritants—tobacco smoke, fumes, perfumes, sprays

Pulmonary edema—congestive heart failure, hyperperfused lungs due to large left to right intracardiac shunts

Acute aspirations—hydrocarbons, talc, water, vomitus

Recurrent aspirations—palatopharyngeal incoordination, gastroesophageal reflux, mongolism, familial dysautonomia

Foreign bodies

Extrinsic irritation—retropharyngeal abscess, mediastinal cysts or tumors, enlarged mediastinal or hilar lymphnodes, pleurisy, pleural effusion, emphysema

Miscellaneous—idiopathic pulmonary hemosiderosis, chlamydial infection

Extrarespiratory—impacted cerumen in the ear, foreign body in ear, external otitis, esophageal duplication

Psychogenic or habit spasm

Special Kinds of Cough

Certain conditions, in their classic form, have characteristic coughing patterns which may be of help in diagnosis. Some examples are:

Sinusitis—particularly bothersome at night after going to bed and in the morning upon arising

Acute Spasmodic Laryngitis—rather sudden onset of a tight, harsh, barking cough, often associated with inspiratory stridor which occurs during the night and disappears the next day

Bronchitis—a deep and productive cough, especially of viral origin, which may persist 4 to 6 weeks after the associated signs of upper respiratory infection have gone

Pertussis—paroxysms of harsh, hacking cough, followed by a sudden, deep, tight, crowing inspiration or whoop

Chlamydia—occurs in infants, predominantly black, with an onset between 2 and 6 weeks of age of tachypnea and a distinctive cough. This cough is a series of harsh, staccato coughs, each separated by a brief inspiration and with no post-tussic inspiratory whoop. There are no systemic signs of illness and no fever, and the course is protracted for several weeks. A history of inclusion conjunctivitis is present in only about half the cases.

Cystic Fibrosis—should be a diagnostic consideration in infants and children who have a persistent cough and frequent respiratory infections. In infants, the cough may be paroxysmal and resemble that of bronchiolitis and not become productive until progression of the disease occurs.

Bronchiectasis—paroxysms of cough productive of purulent sputum, particularly upon arising or with changes in posture.

Nocturnal Cough—possibly a sign of bronchial asthma not associated with wheezing detectable by auscultation. The cough may awaken the child early in the morning.

Chronic Aspiration and H Type T-E Fistula—infants may cough, choke and become cyanotic when feeding, especially with milk

Postoperative Repair of T-E Fistulae or Vascular Rings—not unusual for persistence of a harsh, brassy, irritative cough for several months after surgery because of the residual area of tracheomalacia

Mediastinal and Hilar Lymph Nodes—harsh, repetitive brassy cough due to compression or infiltration of the bronchial wall

Associated Stridor—Always suggestive of laryngeal or tracheal pathology

Foreign Body—sudden onset of violent paroxysms of coughing and choking, especially in a toddler. This should be investigated. It may be followed by a symptom-free period that can delay the actual diagnosis.

Adolescent Cough—a recurrent or chronic cough in an adolescent that may be indicative of smoking

Habit Spasm—short, slight, dry cough which becomes worse when attention is directed to the cough and disappears during sleep. It frequently develops after a previous lower respiratory infection, yet persists long after any evidence of inflammation has disappeared. The cough is reinforced by the parents' concern, constant attention to and commenting about the cough, and a general level of increased anxiety in the environment.

Psychogenic Cough—nonproductive, barking, foghorn cough which older children and adolescents may delight in demonstrating, much to the irritation of teachers, parents, and physician. Its loudness and deep resonating nature are additional features. As in the habit spasm cough, no evidence of any underlying respiratory disease can be detected.

Hazards of Cough

Some hazards may arise in coughing. If coughing is severe enough, rib fractures may result. Tears at the gastroesophageal junction may produce some bleeding which can be difficult to tell from hemoptysis. Intrathoracic pressure may remain so high for a prolonged period of time with a severe paroxysm of coughing, that venous return to the heart is impeded, cardiac output falls, and unconsciousness results—*cough syncope.* Persistent coughing may interrupt sleep and this, together with the significant energy expenditure of cough, produces fatigue. In some patients, the force of the cough may precipitate vomiting, particularly when large amounts of mucus have been swallowed. Young infants may find it difficult to feed, and fluid intake may suffer. Finally, the appearance of cyanosis in patients during prolonged coughing spells is evidence of hypoxia, and is a warning to use caution and oxygen if airway manipulation is being considered.

Sneeze

The sneeze reflex is very much like the cough reflex except that it is initiated by irritation to the epithelium of the nasal passages. Afferent impulses pass through the trigeminal nerve to the medulla where the reflex is integrated. A series of reactions similar to those which mediate the cough reflex take place. In a sneeze, however, the initial air block takes place mainly at the soft palate and uvula. The uvula is suddenly depressed and a large volume of air passes rapidly through the nose, helping to clear the nasal passages of foreign matter.

Thus, the respiratory system is equipped with a series of coordinated defense mechanisms that strive to keep the tracheobronchial airways open at all times.

BIBLIOGRAPHY

Kendig EL, Jr, Chernick V: Disorders of the Respiratory Tract in Children. 3rd ed. Philadelphia, WB Saunders, 1977

This is the most comprehensive of texts dealing with the entire spectrum of clinical conditions encountered in pediatric pulmonary disease. Sixty-eight separate chapters by 52 recognized experts provide a most authoritative coverage of the material.

Murray JF: The Normal Lung. Philadelphia, WB Saunders, 1976

A current, comprehensive, readable, and well-illustrated summary of the structure and function of the lung. It has good sections on growth and development of the lung and on defense mechanisms of the respiratory tract.

West JB: Respiratory Physiology—The Essentials. Baltimore, Williams and Wilkins, 1974

This is a jewel of a book which was written as a core course for medical students. The emphasis is on gas exchange as the chief function of the lung.

Williams HE, Phelan PD: Respiratory Illness in Children. London, Blackwell Scientific Publications, 1975

Written by two well-regarded Australian pediatric pulmonary physicians, this text focuses more on the clinical pathophysiology and symptoms associated with the major areas of pediatric pulmonary disease. Very little of the text deals with neonatal pulmonary problems; its major focus is on the practitioner faced with the interpretation of symptoms characteristic of the more common pulmonary conditions.

24

Evaluation of the Cardiovascular System

Sidney Friedman

Although the format of the procedure is basically the same as in the adult, evaluation of the cardiovascular system in infancy and childhood requires unique knowledge and skills. Evaluation begins with a pertinent history based on an understanding of cardiovascular symptomatology in pediatric patients. A careful physical examination should follow, in which cardiac auscultation plays a major role. An electrocardiogram, chest radiograph, and blood count are carried out routinely in all cardiac suspects. For more complex problems, special techniques, first noninvasive and then invasive, may be required.

HISTORY

A clear description of the circumstances and reasons that bring the patient to cardiac review is helpful not only to the physician but also in orienting parents to the goals of the examination. The chief complaint in over 90% of children who appear for cardiac evaluation is the recent discovery of a cardiac murmur. Congenital heart disease and rheumatic heart disease are the two major etiologic varieties of heart disease in the pediatric age group and both are characterized by cardiac murmurs. There is also a high incidence of functional or innocent cardiac murmurs in childhood. Other less common presenting complaints are cyanosis, congestive heart failure (often precipitated by a respiratory tract infection), failure to thrive, chest pain, exercise intolerance, and occasionally the discovery of an abnormal cardiac silhouette in a chest roentgenogram or an arrhythmia.

Although congenital heart disease does not usually follow a simple hereditary pattern, the family history should be discussed. Although it is rare, there are families in which congenital heart disease is found in more than one family member, with the same lesion reappearing in two or three siblings (*e.g.*, aortic stenosis, patent ductus arteriosus, atrial septal defect, tetralogy of Fallot, and pulmonary stenosis). In evaluating the possibility of rheumatic fever, it is also important to establish a family history, since a familial pattern occurs in this disease. It should also be determined whether there is a history of streptococcal infection prior to a suspected rheumatic episode.

The time of initial discovery of a cardiac murmur is helpful diagnostically and should be established. Murmurs related to obstructive lesions are usually present at the first examination following birth. Murmurs dependent upon pressure differences between the right and left sides of the heart may not appear for weeks or months after birth. Murmurs whose intensity is related to large stroke volumes may not be appreciated to be significant for a number of years.

Evaluation of the symptoms of cardiovascular disease should include questions about cyanosis, exercise intolerance, and shortness of breath. Cyanosis related to breath-holding or exposure to cold, as with bathing, can be ignored safely. Parents are poor observers of cyanosis, particularly of the milder varieties. In persons with normal hemoglobin levels, Comroe demonstrated that only at arterial oxygen saturations below 75% is clinical cyanosis apparent to all observers in all subjects. Easy fatigability is best evaluated in the small infant by questions related to feeding patterns; this symptom may be interpreted erroneously by parents as a special need for sleep rather than intolerance to exertion. Respiratory distress is best assayed historically by questions related to the rate and regularity of respirations and the presence of retractions of the chest wall. Sighing type respirations are not cardiac in origin.

A history should include evaluation of the patient's rate of physical growth by use of one of the standard growth charts, plotting weight and height against age. A graphic expression is helpful for appreciation of gross deviations. A review of past illnesses, with particular attention to the frequency of respiratory tract infections, is usually helpful since lingering, complicated respiratory tract infections are often associated with large arteriovenous shunts due to congenital heart disease. A list of the hospitalizations and their precipitating illnesses will quickly provide information regarding serious disease.

PHYSICAL EXAMINATION

One of the chief roles of the cardiac examiner is to arrange and produce circumstances that allow the patient to be comfortable and in a favorable state of cooperation during the physical examination. Observations made with the patient struggling and crying, or even in a very fearful state, are of little value and may indeed be misleading. Infants up to the age of 6 months are readily placated with a few pleasant sounds or a bottle; between the ages of 6 months and 2 to 2½ years, a considerable effort must be made to prepare a peaceful, productive examination. First, discard the white coat. Examination on the mother's lap rather than on the examining table is very helpful. Distractions with toys, pictures, and office artifacts are sometimes successful. Perform the physical examination before subjecting the infant to the routine testing. A blood count will *not* enhance cooperation. Children beyond the age of 3 are almost uniformly won over by remarks showing interest in them as individuals, including overt flattery. Asking a preschool 3- or 4-year-old his grade in school almost always provides a cooperative subject. Another effective question is "How come you're so good?" Adolescents, particularly girls, are likely to become very apprehensive about a physical examination, especially when asked to disrobe. A private dressing room and appropriate gowns to minimize exposure are helpful measures as are verbal reassurances.

The findings of the physical examination are also profoundly influenced by the presence of fever or anemia. Both of these conditions produce high stroke volume and high cardiac output and thereby may alter the cardiac findings. Final interpretations of the cardiac examination should be deferred until anemia and fever are not present.

Vital Signs

The recorded physical examination should include *without fail* three vital measures of cardiovascular function: (1) blood pressure, (2) cardiac rate and peripheral arterial pulse rate and character, and (3) respiratory rate and pattern. Too often these vital measurements are left for the end of the examination and then omitted entirely in the recorded examination.

Blood Pressure. Measurement of blood pressure is an essential part of every pediatric examination. This determination is valid only if the infant is quiet and calm; crying, apprehension, and physical activity markedly elevate the blood pressure. Apprehension in older children can be averted by a brief period of explanation and diversion, followed by a series of measurements, with greater credence being attributed to later determinations.

Aside from the need for a basal state, a number of details of technique are important in accurately determining the blood pressure in children. The proper width of the blood pressure cuff, critical for an accurate result, is one which covers approximately two-thirds of the upper arm or thigh. A cuff that is too narrow provides falsely elevated blood pressure values that are sometimes as much as twice the normal level. A cuff that is too broad produces smaller errors, but in the direction of falsely low values. Cuffs of several sizes should be available; veterinary medical supply sources are valuable in this effort.

Blood pressure should be measured in both arms and at least one of the lower extremities. Occasional variations occur in the blood pressure level in the two upper extremities, for example, supravalvular aortic stenosis, or absence or compression of one of the subclavian arteries (post-Blalock-Taussig operation). Comparison of the upper and lower extremity blood pressure may give information leading to the diagnosis of coarctation of the aorta.

The brachial artery is used for determining pressure in the upper extremity. The cuff should be applied snugly and without bulges to the bare arm. It should be inflated rapidly to avoid venous congestion and deflated at a rate of approximately 5 mm Hg/sec. If the cuff is released too rapidly, the readings will be falsely low. If a second determination is made, the cuff should be deflated completely before restarting the second measurement.

Measurements in the lower extremities are made using the popliteal artery with the cuff applied around the thigh. After the age of 9 months, the systolic blood pressure in the lower extremities is normally higher than in the arms by about 10 to 20 mm Hg. This is due to the fact that the arterial pulse wave is agumented by the rebound wave, an effect that increases with the distance from the heart. Prior to the age of 6 or 9 months, the flush pressure in the upper extremity is higher than in the lower, usually by 5 or 10 mm Hg, due to the normal narrowing at the isthmus of the aorta. Diastolic pressures are usually equal in the upper and lower extremities.

There are several techniques available for determining the arterial blood pressure in infants and children.

Palpation. The method of palpation permits a rough estimate of systolic pressure. The cuff is inflated to a pressure above that which will cause the peripheral arterial pulse to disappear on palpation and then slowly deflated. The pressure at which the palpable pulse reappears corresponds to a level approximately 10 mm Hg below the systolic blood pressure.

Auscultation. The method of auscultation can be used for all ages, but is more difficult to apply in early infancy because vascular sounds are weak and difficult to hear. The pressure at which the first sound appears following deflation of the cuff corresponds accurately with systolic blood pressure measured intraluminally. There is less agreement concerning the indicator level which corresponds to the diastolic blood pressure. The point at which Korotkoff's sounds are first muffled or at which they disappear completely is variably taken as the level of diastolic blood pressure. Record both figures if there is more than a 5 mm difference between the two.

Flush Technique. When auscultation in infants is difficult, the flush technique may be used. A cuff is placed on the thigh or forearm and an elastic bandage is wrapped snugly around the distal extremity which is then massaged to drain the superficial blood. The cuff is inflated to a pressure above the anticipated systolic level and the bandage is removed. The skin of the hand or foot appears pale and bloodless. The pressure at which the first flush of pink color appears in the skin of the blanched distal extremity is taken as the mean arterial blood pressure. The Doppler effect and a variety of electronic methods can also be used in problem situations.

The blood pressure of a child varies directly with age. Standard normal values are available. Neonatal pressures are most variable. There is a steady increase in blood pressure throughout infancy and childhood, before stabilization at adult levels (Fig. 24-1). The pulse pressure varies normally from 20 to 50 mm Hg throughout childhood.

Cardiac Rate. Observation of the cardiac rate is also of fundamental value in evaluating the cardiovascular system. The cardiac rate can be determined prior to birth either by direct auscultation or by intrauterine electrocardiography. This type of monitoring is commonly employed during labor, particularly in high-risk pregnancies. The cardiac rate is used in determining the Apgar score after birth as a gauge of neonatal well-being. The normal fetal rate varies between 120 and 160/minute. Excessive slowing of the fetal heart is taken as a measure of fetal distress during labor. A slow fetal heart rate may also signal the presence of congenital heart block.

Newborn. The cardiac rate in a new-

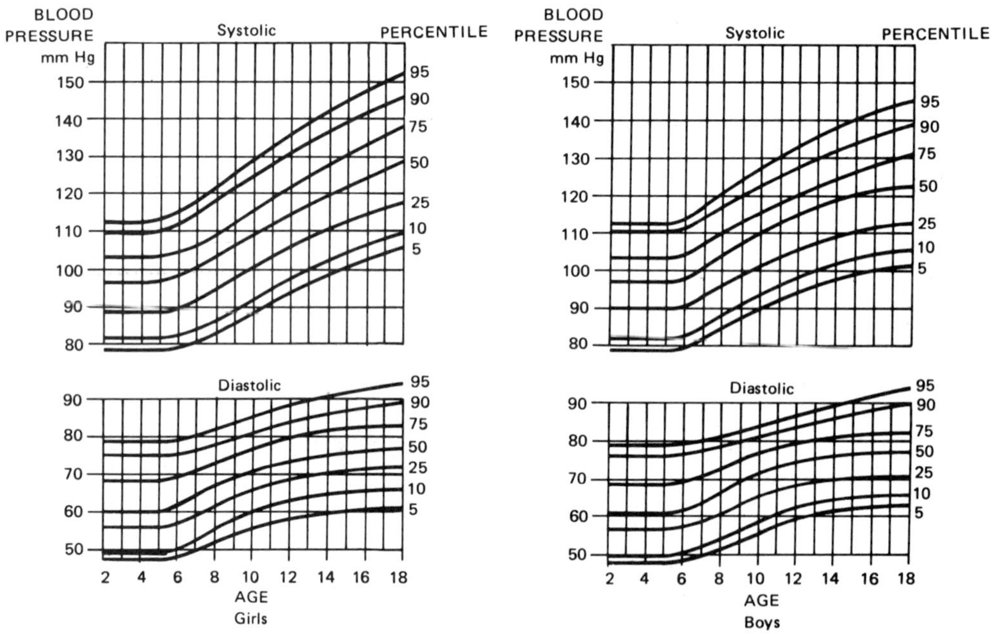

Fig. 24-1. Range of blood pressures in normal children. Percentiles for blood pressure measurement in children (right arm, seated). (Report of Task Force on Blood Pressure Control in Children sponsored by American Academy of Pediatrics. Pediatrics 59:803, 1977)

born is rapid and subject to wide variations. In small infants, the apical rate should be counted for an entire minute, rather than placing reliance on the peripheral arterial pulse. For the first 15 or 30 minutes of life, the heart rate may commonly reach a level of 180/minute. Average values for a full-term infant during the first week of life are 120 to 140/minute. The rate increases quickly with crying or feeding. A rate above 200/minute that persists when the infant is quiet should raise the possibility of a tachyarrhythmia, such as paroxysmal supraventricular tachycardia.

Respiratory variation of the heart rate is observed in many full-term newborn infants and often in premature infants. During sleep there may be periods of apnea and decreased heart rate; when respiratory movements are resumed, the rate again quickens. Cardiac arrhythmias of many types are encountered often during the neonatal period. When monitored continuously, approximately 10% of full-term newborn infants show infrequent ectopic beats, primarily premature ventricular contractions. Forty percent of premature infants studied in this way show periods of sinus bradycardia with or without nodal escape. These findings are not abnormal unless they persist.

As the infant ages, the heart rate tends to decrease. By the age of 2 years, a resting cardiac rate of 110/minute is normal. At the age of 6 years, the rate of 100/minute is normal. By the age of 10 years, the normal rate has decreased to 90 beats/minute, and in the adolescent period, values of 60 to 80 are common. Rates for males are generally below those of females.

Childhood. The cardiac rate is very labile during childhood, increasing with muscular activity and emotional stimulation, and is often higher after meals and in the afternoon. Persistent sinus tachycardia is often seen in the pediatrician's office because of fear or excitement. Parents should be asked to check the cardiac rate during sleep if there is concern about this point since tachycardia from organic illnesses persists during sleep.

Rapid heart rates may be observed secondary to anemia, shock, or fever. The heart rate usually increases 8 to 10 beats/minute for each degree F temperature elevation. In the presence of rheumatic carditis, tachycardia is present which exceeds the level to be expected from temperature elevation alone, and persists during sleep. Thyrotoxicosis is a rare cause of tachycardia during childhood. An increase in heart rate is present almost uniformly with congestive heart failure.

Adolescence. Sinus bradycardia is usually defined as a cardiac rate less than 100 beats/minute in infants, and 60 beats/minute in older children. Slow rates may be normal in states of physical training and occasionally in newborns and premature infants. Other causes of slow cardiac rates in pediatric patients include increased intracranial pressure, hypothyroidism, and increased serum potassium levels.

Sinus arrhythmia is observed most frequently in adolescence, particularly in males. It is a phasic heart rate that is often but not necessarily associated with respiration; frequently the rate speeds with inspiration and slows with expiration. Sinus arrhythmia is often seen with a slow overall heart rate, but is usually abolished by exercise. It is an early evidence of cardiotoxicity due to digitalis.

Respiration. The respiratory pattern of the newborn infant may be very irregular and variable. In premature infants, respiration may be characterized by periods of deep respiratory excursions which alternate with apnea or slow and shallow respirations. This type of irregularity in breathing usually disappears by the fourth week of life. Its presistence may indicate central nervous system disease or metabolic abnormalities which depress the central respiratory control center.

The normal range of rate of respiration varies from 30 to 50/minute at birth, to 16 to 20 at the age of 6 years, and 14 to 16 at puberty. The rate is markedly influenced by excitement or apprehension in young infants and is best determined during sleep or in a basal period. Rapid respiratory rates are observed in many pulmonary disorders and with infections, fever, poisonings (particularly salicylism), or in congestive heart failure, acidosis, or shock. Slow respiratory rates may be indicative of increased intracranial pressure, suppression of the respiratory center by sedatives, alkalosis, or poisons. The depth of respiration may be indicative of anoxia, the state of activity of the respiratory center, or the presence of acidosis or alkalosis.

The use of accessory muscles of respiration should be consciously observed and is the objective counterpart of the subjective complaint of dyspnea in adults. Flaring of the alae nasi, retraction of the intercostal spaces, other areas of retraction above and below the costal cage, and grunting with respiration represent use of accessory muscles of respiration. Respiratory distress may occur with exercise, pain, fright, anemia, cardiovascular disorders, hypothyroidism, and many other conditions. Inspiratory distress occurs more frequently with high airway obstructions and expiratory distress with low obstructions.

INSPECTION

Important information related to the cardiovascular system can be gained by simple inspection. Ease and accuracy of an examination will be abetted if pertinent clothing, necklaces, bracelets, and nail polish are removed beforehand. First, an estimate is made of the size and physical development of the patient in relationship to his age. Weight and height can be expressed in terms of percentile values. Whether the patient seems content, uncomfortable, or interested in his environment should be included in the record of general inspection. The respiratory rate and effort can be noted by simple observation.

Identification of a variety of somatic syndromes, some representing chromosomal aberrations, can help in the cardiac evaluation. The stigmata of mongolism should alert the observer to the possibility of an atrial or ventricular septal defect, perhaps associated with an endocardial cushion defect and early pulmonary hypertension. The phenotype of Turner's syndrome should raise suspicion of coarctation of the aorta; this is found in 30% to 40% of such patients. The features of Noonan's syndrome should suggest the possibility of pulmonary stenosis associated with pulmonary valvular dysplasia syndrome. Marfan's syndrome should lead to a careful search for evidence of aortic and mitral valve dysfunction. Patients with stigmata of neonatal rubella should be observed for combinations of patent ductus arteriosus, pulmonary artery stenosis, pulmonary and aortic valvular stenosis, and coarctation of the aorta. Other less common congenital somatic syndromes also have characteristic cardiac manifestations.

Cyanosis is best observed in daylight or under incandescent lighting. Exposure to fluorescent light or low intensity light, particularly with exposure to cold, will spuriously enhance the apparent degree of cyanosis. Cyanosis may be generalized or regional. A comparison of the discoloration of the nail beds of the fingers and the toes should be made by placing them side by side. The presence of a preductal coarctation of the aorta is likely to produce only detectable cyanosis of the lower extremities. A variety of other complex congenital lesions may produce regional cyanosis.

Clubbing of the fingers and toes occurs in patients with large venous-arterial shunts associated with cyanotic congenital heart disease. Clubbing is rarely present in the absence of obvious cyanosis or before the age of 6 months. A generalized redness of the fingertips may be evidence of mild arterial unsaturation, as with a large atrial septal defect. With more severe hypoxia, the angle between the base of the nail and the skin proximal to it may disappear and, still later, longitudinal curving of the nails with widening of the terminal phalanges develops. Polycythemia is almost uniformly associated with hypoxia sufficiently severe to cause clubbing. Clubbing disappears in 2 to 4 months following surgical relief of arterial unsaturation.

Inspection of the cervical veins may provide useful information concerning venous pressure. In the erect position, the external jugular vein should not be distended visibly. In the recumbent position, distention of the external jugular vein may be normal. This vein should collapse normally as the level of the patient is raised to approximately 45 degrees from the horizontal table, if the muscles of the neck are relaxed.

With each heartbeat, two small venous pulse waves can be noted: the "a wave" coinciding with right atrial contraction and the "v wave" coinciding with right ventricular contraction. These waves, at times difficult to discern, alternate with more apparent phases of venous collapse. The collapse following the a wave occurs as the right atrium becomes less distended following presystolic contraction, whereas the collapse after the v wave occurs as the tricuspid valve opens. The a wave, which occurs in presystole, can be timed with the apical impulse. A prominent a wave in presystole can be noted in patients with tricuspid stenosis or tricuspid atresia, severe pulmonary stenosis, primary pulmonary hypertension, and cor pulmonale. It may be absent with right-sided heart failure or in the presence of auricular fibrillation and other arrhythmias. The v wave may become very prominent in patients with tricuspid regurgitation and can be demonstrated by compressing the vein with the finger. The portion of the vein above the finger becomes distended from above while the portion below shows the systolic v wave as blood from the right ventricle is regurgitated into the right atrium and then refluxed into the cervical veins.

Prominent arterial pulsations can also be observed in the neck in the presence of wide pulse pressures as seen with aortic regurgitation, coarctation of the aorta, patent ductus arteriosus, and large systemic arteriovenous fistulae. A variety of congenital deformities of the chest wall can be observed in children with cardiac abnormalities. A precordial bulge may provide information concerning the size and laterality of the heart.

Edema in small infants is usually initially observed as facial and periorbital swelling. This swelling results from the loose connection between the skin and subcutaneous tissues in these areas and the head-down position of the infant. Edema rarely occurs prior to hepatomegaly in right heart failure. In longstanding right heart failure, edema of the lower extremities and ascites may occur.

Pallor and jaundice may also be observed in certain cardiac conditions. Jaundice can be the result of prolonged right heart failure and chronic congestion of the liver. Pallor may be related to severe anemia and is prominent in proportion to the hemoglobin level in patients with rheumatic fever during the active stage of the disease.

Inspection of the teeth often provides general information concerning the standard of health care provided the patient. Dental health is important in prophylaxis against subacute bacterial endocarditis. Large tonsils and upper airway obstruction may be the visible causes for chronic hypoxia leading to pulmonary hypertension and cor pulmonale.

PALPATION AND PERCUSSION

Considerable information can be gained by palpation of the arterial pulses, especially the brachial and femoral arteries. A discrepancy in the volume of the pulses between the upper and lower extremities suggests coarctation of the aorta. A strong, bounding pulse with a rapid collapse (water-hammer pulse) occurs in lesions associated with a wide pulse pressure, a large patent ductus arteriosus, aortic regurgitation, systemic arteriovenous fistulae, complete heart block, or certain high cardiac output states. In contrast, a weak pulse is palpated with severe aortic stenosis, pericardial tamponade, congestive heart failure, or cardiovascular shock. The term paradoxical pulse is applied to variations in the amplitude of the arterial pulse observed by palpation during inspiration and expiration. In pulsus paradoxicus, the pulse becomes weak or disappears during inspiration and reappears during expiration. This is observed with pericardial effusion or constrictive pericarditis, in severe primary myocardial diseases, and in frank congestive heart failure. Pulsus alternans is characterized by alternating strong and weak arterial pulses on palpation and is observed in advanced left heart failure. Pulsus bigeminus consists of a prominent pulse alternating with a prematurely occurring weaker one; this may be observed with digitalis intoxication and occasionally with no other evidence of heart disease.

Location of the apex beat is helpful in determining the spacial orientation and size of the heart. In the typical levocardia with situs solitus, the apex beat is at the point farthest to the left and downward where the impact of the heart is palpable, and indicates a leftward orientation of the heart. In dextrocardia, the apical impulse is in the fourth or fifth interspace in the right midclavicular line. Displacement of the apex beat accompanies cardiac enlargement.

Palpation permits the recognition of a cardiac thrill which is the tactile appreciation of the vibrations observed as a cardiac murmur on auscultation. The location of the thrill may suggest a specific lesion. A thrill in the second right interspace is usually associated with aortic stenosis. A thrill to the left of the lower sternum and in the xiphoid region usually signals a ventricular septal defect. In valvular pulmonic stenosis, the thrill is often to the left of the upper sternum. A palpable thrill in the suprasternal notch and over the vessels of the neck is often associated with aortic stenosis but may also be present with valvular pulmonic stenosis or other causes of turbulence in the great arteries such as a surgical systemic artery to pulmonary artery anastomosis.

The third major observation that can be made by palpation is the presence of an abnormal ventricular impulse. A sustained lift to the left of the lower sternum and in the xiphoid region indicates right ventricular overwork. In contrast, a sustained lift at the cardiac apex signifies left ventricular hypertrophy. The tactile character of the impulse varies in the right compared with the left ventricular impulse.

Varying degrees of hepatomegaly can be appreciated by palpation and percussion. In small infants, hepatomegaly is a sensitive and useful index of congestive heart failure. Massive hepatic enlargement may occasionally be observed by inspection. When the liver enlarges in a small infant, the liver edge and the anterior surface of the liver become more superficial and are palpable just beneath the anterior abdominal wall. Upon percussion, the dull note over the liver surface is also an accurate indicator of liver size.

Cardiac enlargement can at times be appreciated by palpation and percussion, particularly if more than slight. A roentgenogram of the chest is more accurate than physical examination in detecting slight changes in heart size. Detection of the left heart border by percussion or by identification of the apex beat is useful to this end.

AUSCULTATION

Successful cardiac auscultation requires favorable conditions. The patient must be relaxed and quiet. The examiner must be in a comfortable position that can be maintained without fatigue or distraction for several minutes. His stethoscope must be familiar to him and well-fitting, particularly with regard to the ear pieces and the length of the rubber tubing. While short tubing is of theoretical benefit with regard to acoustic principles, it will produce poor results if it forces an uncomfortable examining position. Finally, and most important, auscultation must be done systematically with conscious direction. Each auscultatory possibility has to be sought consciously and then noted as either present or absent. A large number of observations must be made concerning each cardiac sound or murmur. In order to make these observations accurately, the examiner must know all the acoustic possibilities beforehand, and process them through a mental checklist.

Heart Sounds

The identification of the first and second heart sounds should be the first goal of auscultation, thereby determining the two phases of the cardiac cycle: systole and diastole. The first heart sound is the louder of the two sounds at the cardiac apex and is synchronous with the apex beat. It is usually nearer to the second heart sound than the distance in time from the second sound to the first, since systole is usually shorter than diastole. The second heart sound is the louder of the two sounds at the base of the heart, and two components are often heard intermittently.

The first heart sound results from vibrations associated with closure of the mitral and tricuspid valves. Mitral valve closure usually precedes tricuspid valve closure; asynchrony results in some splitting of the first heart sound, usually with an interval of less than 0.02 seconds. This interval is difficult to appreciate. The second heart sound is due chiefly to events associated with closure of the semilunar valves. Aortic valve closure usually precedes pulmonary valve closure; this results in an easily detectable duplication best heard in the second left interspace. The degree of splitting is variable (0.04–0.06 sec), being wider during inspiration and in the recumbent position.

Evaluation of the second heart sound at the base of the heart with regard to intensity and splitting of components is one of the most rewarding efforts of cardiac auscultation in childhood. Observation of the two components of the second heart sound usually provides an accurate clue to the level of pulmonary artery pressure. The louder the second component of the second sound, the higher the pulmonary artery pressure. A reduction in the intensity of the second component in the pulmonary area suggests low pulmonary artery diastolic closing pressure, as with severe pulmonary stenosis. Accentuation of the second heart sound, especially with little or no audible duplication, usually indicates pulmonary hypertension.

A single second heart sound at the base of the heart may indicate either synchronous closure of the two semilunar valves or an inaudible pulmonary component. Wide splitting of the second heart sound is encountered with an atrial septal defect, with moderate isolated valvular pulmonic stenosis, and with right bundle branch block.

A third heart sound can be heard in approximately 25% of pediatric patients between the ages of 2 and 12 years. This third sound is found in early diastole and is coincident with the phase of rapid filling of the ventricles from the atria. It is usually heard best at or just to the right of the cardiac apex in the recumbent position. Maneuvers to increase systemic venous return accentuate the third heart sound.

A fourth heart sound is not heard normally. When present, it is due to atrial contraction and is most often heard with right atrial hypertension. Accentuation by inspiration suggests the right-sided origin of this sound.

Clicking Sounds

Clicking sounds of diagnostic significance can be heard in early systole or in midsystole. The early systolic ejection click is usually present to the left of the upper sternum and is observed in conditions associated with dilatation of the main pulmonary artery, in ascending aorta, or in semilunar valve abnormality. Prominent ejection clicks are heard with aortic and pulmonic valvular stenosis. Similar sounds can be heard with coarctation of the aorta, truncus arteriosus, severe pulmonary hypertension, and idiopathic dilatation of the pulmonary artery.

Clicking sounds that occur in the middle of systole are due to dysfunction of the mitral valve. They are found often in connection with and introducing the late systolic apical murmur of mitral insufficiency associated with papillary muscle dysfunction syndrome. The click is coincident with the maximal excursion of the mitral valve leaflet connected to the abnormal papillary muscle. Mitral valve prolapse with or without mitral insufficiency, often found with atrial septal defects, may also be associated with midsystolic clicking sounds.

Murmurs

The analysis of each cardiac murmur should include an evaluation of the following six features: (1) timing, (2) acoustic quality, (3) intensity, (4) duration, (5) location, and (6) transmission.

The timing of murmurs is facilitated by the proper identification of the first and second heart sounds. Systolic murmurs occurring between the first and second heart sound should be described with regard to the portion or portions of systole occupied. Similarly, the diastolic murmurs may be present in one or more of the three standard subdivisions of diastole (protodiastole, middiastole, or presystole). The continuous murmur overrides the second heart sounds and spills from systole into diastole.

The quality or acoustic characteristics of murmurs are usually described in a local jargon which may or may not be accurate with regard to the physical characteristics of the murmur, but which provides a group of individuals a method of communicating among themselves the acoustic characteristics of cardiac murmurs. Terms such as blowing, buzzing, musical, vibratory, harsh, rough, rumbling, expulsive, crescendo, and decrescendo fall into this category as do pitch (high, medium, and low) and the presence of peculiar overtones.

Grading the intensity of cardiac murmurs is valuable, especially for systematic comparison of murmurs in serial observations of a single patient. Levine's system, in which murmurs are graded from 1 to 6 for systolic murmurs and 1 to 4 for diastolic murmurs, was originated for use in adults. In the pediatric age group, the intensity of murmurs is not as accurately correlated with significance of murmurs as in the adult age group. Many of the functional or innocent murmurs may be louder than the apical holosystolic blowing murmur of mild mitral insufficiency.

The duration of cardiac murmurs is usually expressed in the terms suggested by Leatham. An ejection murmur is compared with a pansystolic or holosystolic murmur. The *ejection murmur* does not extend throughout all of systole but occupies a variable portion of systole starting from the first heart sound. On graphic recordings, this murmur often has a diamond-shaped or crescendo-decresendo appearance. In contrast, the *holosystolic murmur* occupies all of systole from the first to the second heart sound and usually has a plateau of intensity; it is characteristic of the murmurs observed with a ventricular septal defect or mitral insufficiency. There are rare situations in which a long ejection murmur may be indistinguishable in duration from a holosystolic murmur. Occasionally, murmurs may be heard exclusively during late systole, as with the mitral insufficiency associated with posterior papillary muscle dysfunction syndrome or mitral valve prolapse.

Determining the point of maximal intensity of a murmur is very helpful. Murmurs derived from events occurring at the mitral valve are apical in location. Sounds created at the pulmonary valve are heard in the second left interspace; at the aortic valve, sounds are heard in the second right interspace. The exception is the diastolic murmur of aortic insufficiency which is heard best to the left of the mid-sternum. Tricuspid valve deformities are reflected by sounds to the left of the lower sternum.

The degree and direction of transmission of a cardiac murmur is a useful diagnostic observation. Functional or innocent murmurs are not audible over the posterior chest wall. The murmur of mitral insufficiency is transmitted to the left axilla; the degree of transmission correlates well with the severity of the valvular insufficiency. Pulmonic stenosis produces a murmur that is transmitted to the posterior chest wall above the left scapula; aortic stenosis produces a murmur that is transmitted above the right scapula and is also carried over to the neck vessels. The murmurs generated by patent ductus arteriosus, coarctation of the aorta, and pulmonary artery stenosis are particularly heard well over the posterior chest wall; in contrast, the murmur of a ventricular septal defect is poorly transmitted to the posterior chest wall.

The following classification of murmurs has been modified from Leatham and provides a useful mechanism for categorizing both systolic and diastolic murmurs:

I. Systolic murmurs
  A. Ejection systolic murmurs
    1. Innocent, insignificant murmurs
    2. Systolic murmurs due to pulmonary or aortic valvular, infundibular or supravalvular stenoses
    3. Pulmonary or aortic systolic murmurs due to increased flow across these normal valves, as in atrial septal defect, ventricular septal defect, aortic or pulmonic regurgitation
    4. Systolic murmurs due to relative stenosis of the pulmonary or the aortic orifices, as in idiopathic dilatation of the pulmonary artery, dilatation of the ascending aorta or primary pulmonary hypertension
  B. Regurgitant systolic murmurs
    1. Systolic murmur due to mitral or tricuspid regurgitation
    2. Systolic murmur due to ventricular septal defect

II. Diastolic murmurs
  A. Regurgitant diastolic murmurs (early diastolic murmurs)
    1. Diastolic murmur in aortic regurgitation
    2. Diastolic murmur in pulmonary regurgitation

B. Ventricular filling murmurs (mid-diastolic murmurs)
   1. Diastolic murmur in atrioventricular valve stenosis, such as in:
      Mitral stenosis
      Tricuspid stenosis
   2. Diastolic murmur in relative atrioventricular valve stenosis due to increased flow and/or dilated ventricles, such as in:
      Atrial septal defect
      Ventricular septal defect
      Anomalous entrance of pulmonary veins
      Patent ductus arteriosus
      Mitral regurgitation
      Complete A-V block
      Primary myocardial disease
      Severe anemia
   3. Diastolic murmur in the presence of obstruction at the mitral or tricuspid orifices
      Tumor; ball-valve thrombi

C. Atrial presystolic murmurs (late diastolic murmurs), such as in:
   Mitral stenosis
   Tricuspid stenosis

III. Continuous murmurs, such as in:
   Patent ductus arteriosus
   Aortocardiac fistula
   Coronary arteriovenous fistulae

Pericardiac Friction Rub

A striking extracardiac sound is the pericardial friction rub. It is usually present in both systole and diastole with variable relative intensity in the two portions of the cardiac cycle. This sound may be discovered in any location over the precordium, but is heard most frequently to the left of the lower sternum. Occasionally, it is very difficult to differentiate a pericardial friction rub from a combination of a systolic and diastolic murmur to the left of the sternum. The coarse, scratchy acoustic quality of the pericardial friction rub is the best clue. Bacterial or viral infection is the most common cause of acute pericarditis and a pericardial friction rub.

Innocent Adventitious Sounds

A large number of innocent adventitious heart sounds are encountered in the pediatric age group. A variety of functional or innocent heart murmurs, the venous hum, and the physiologic third heart sound are the most common sounds in this category.

Functional or innocent cardiac murmurs are found in approximately 50% of healthy children, especially between the ages of 4 and 8 years. The differentiation of innocent murmurs from those derived from serious varieties of heart disease can be accomplished in the vast majority of instances by auscultation alone. Considerable clinical experience indicates that properly identified innocent murmurs are indeed benign. The 20-year follow-up study of Marienfeld and associates demonstrated no difference in the incidence of heart disease among a group of adult patients who as children had innocent cardiac murmurs compared with a similar group who had not shown such murmurs in childhood. Most functional murmurs disappear in later childhood; an estimated 90% of murmurs are gone by the age of 14 years. The other 10% remain for varying periods of time, but the cardiac prognosis in a child is the same whether or not the murmur persists. Two principle categories of benign murmurs are recognized: (1) the midprecordial musical murmur, or Still's "twanging-string" murmur, and (2) the basal ejection type systolic murmur sometimes referred to as a "pulmonic-systolic" murmur.

Still's "twanging-string" murmur is the most common and easily identified of the innocent murmurs. Its musical quality has been described variously as buzzing or vibratory; it occupies the first one-third or one-half of systole and in graphic recordings has a crescendo-decrescendo (diamond-shaped) configuration. It is heard best over the midprecordium with the patient in the recumbent position and often disappears or is not as loud in the erect position. The intensity is remarkably variable and is increased by exercise or other conditions associated with increased stroke volume. Intensity alone is not a useful criterion for the identification of this murmur; more important differential features are (1) the location of the point of maximum intensity over the midprecordium, that is, to the right of the apex and to the left of the lower sternum, and (2) the characteristic musical acoustic quality. Approximately 60% of innocent murmurs are Still's murmurs (Fig. 24-2).

The next most common nonpathologic murmur of childhood is the *"pulmonic-systolic"* or *basal ejection type murmur.* This murmur is best heard in the second left interspace. It too is usually confined to the first one-third or one-half of systole. The acoustic quality is less characteristic and less easily identified than Still's murmur. Its quality is

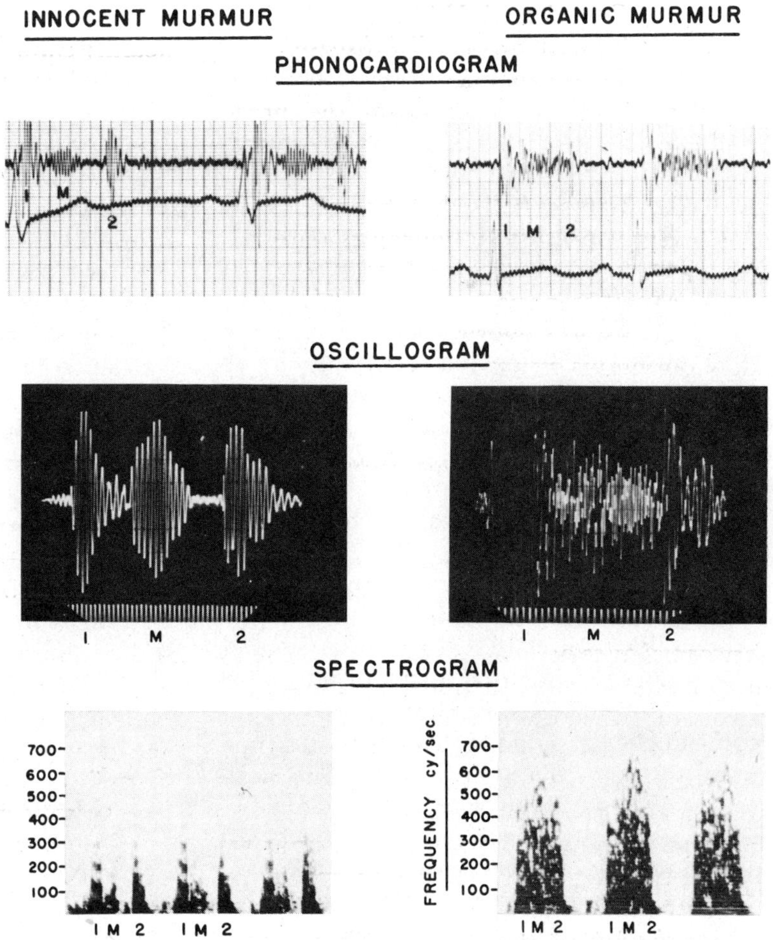

Fig. 24-2. Comparison of the phonocardiographic tracings, oscilloscopic traces and sound spectrograms of patients with innocent (functional) and organic (mitral insufficiency) murmurs. The wave form of the innocent murmur is regular and of low frequency, similar to that of a musical tone. In contrast, the murmur of mitral insufficiency has a much higher frequency of vibration and a chaotic wave form, the acoustic properties of "noise."

relatively harsh or blowing, rather than musical or vibratory, and the pitch is usually low. Because the pulmonic-systolic murmur is usually of low intensity, it is not transmitted to the posterior chest wall. A palpable thrill is never associated with this murmur. As compared with Still's murmur, it is less influenced by change in position, but is similarly accentuated by exercise. A much wider area of indecision exists with this murmur than with Still's murmur in its differentiation from significant murmurs indicating the presence of heart disease.

The basal innocent systolic murmurs are at times difficult to differentiate by auscultation from the murmurs of a small atrial septal defect, mild pulmonic or aortic stenosis, pulmonary artery coarctation, or aortic coarctation. A useful distinction is that these organic murmurs are transmitted to the posterior chest wall in a high percentage of cases. The presence of an associated thrill is also an indicator of a significant murmur. Additional evidence of organic heart disease may also help to identify the significance of the murmur.

The *venous hum* is a continuous whirring sound occupying portions of both systole and diastole, heard best beneath the right clavicle when the patient is in the erect position. This sound can be attributed to the rapid passage of blood through the cervical veins. Although occasionally there are exceptions, the venous hum usually disappears in the recumbent position. Compression of the cervical veins causes the sound to disappear abruptly while extension of the neck accentuates the intensity of the venous hum.

A positive correlation exists in the coincidence of a functional heart murmur, a venous hum, and a physiologic third heart sound. These three auscultatory findings tend to occur in the same patient, suggesting a common etiology. An increased velocity of blood flow and a high stroke volume are probably the underlying bases for all three nonpathologic adventitious sounds.

ROUTINE STUDIES

Three simple laboratory studies should be carried out routinely on all children undergoing formal cardiac evaluation: an electrocardiogram, a chest roentgenogram, and a blood count.

Electrocardiogram

The electrocardiogram provides a wide range of valuable information. Cardiac rhythm can be established and abnormalities of rhythm or ectopic pacemakers identified. Quantitative indication of right or left atrial enlargement is provided by the electrocardiogram as is the presence and severity of right, left, or combined ventricular hypertrophy. The hemodynamic mechanism of ventricular hypertrophy, differentiating pressure overwork from volume overload, may also be ascertained. The severity of such lesions as isolated pulmonary stenosis or aortic stenosis can be judged by estimating the degree of right or left ventricular hypertrophy and the presence or absence of "strain" pattern. An excellent correlation exists between the height of the R wave in lead V_1 and the intracavitary right ventricular pressure in the presence of isolated valvular pulmonic stenosis. Left ventricular "strain" pattern is associated almost uniformly with severe aortic stenosis.

A number of specific electrocardiographic patterns related to individual congenital heart lesions are recognized. These include the picture of mirror image dextrocardia, the pattern of an endocardial cushion defect or a double outlet right ventricle, and the pattern of ventricular inversion.

The electrocardiogram can provide evidence of myocardial changes as seen in myocarditis, digitalis toxicity, or ventricular "strain." These nonspecific alterations include prolongation of the P-R interval, T wave and S-T segment changes, and a variety of ectopic beats or arrhythmias.

Chest Radiograph

Cardiac size is the most useful information provided by the chest radiograph, but it is less valuable than the electrocardiogram in predicting right as opposed to left ventricular enlargement. Right atrial and left atrial enlargement are predicted more reliably by chest radiograph than is ventricular enlargement. The chest radiograph permits an evaluation of the pulmonary vasculature, both arterial and venous. The side and size of the aortic arch may be valuable information in certain diagnostic and therapeutic situations. The large globular cardiac silhouette of pericardial effusion may also be suspected from the chest roentgenogram.

The chest radiograph is particularly valuable as a diagnostic aid in the cyanotic subject with tetralogy of Fallot, transposition of the great arteries, tricuspid atresia, and persistent truncus arteriosus. A small number of specific contours may be diagnostic, for example, total anomalous pulmonary venous return of the supracardiac type (figure of eight) and total anomalous pulmonary venous drainage below the diaphragm. Corrected transposition of the great arteries and coarctation of the aorta each provide a number of valuable diagnostic signs in the plain films.

Blood Count

The routine blood count will give information concerning anemia (associated with a high cardiac output state) and polycythemia. The hematologic indices provide information concerning iron deficiency. Polycythemia is a reliable measure of chronic hypoxia due to cyanotic congenital heart disease. Relative anemia in polycythemic patients is of particular importance because treatment with iron may improve exercise tolerance and avoid the complication of intravascular thrombosis.

NONINVASIVE CARDIAC STUDIES

Phonocardiogram

The study first available historically in this category is the phonocardiogram, a graphic recording of the heart sounds and murmurs. Questions concerning the duration and timing within the cardiac cycle of murmurs, clicks and heart sounds can be readily resolved by this method. In a few instances, the quality characteristics of the wave form of the phonocardiogram may be useful, particularly in the identification of functional or innocent murmurs. A regular wave form at a low frequency (80–120 cycles/second) is seen regularly with functional murmurs and is presumed to be due to the vibration of solid structures compared with the chaotic pattern of vibrations resulting from abnormal blood flow.

Vectorcardiogram

Vectorcardiography has relatively few special applications in pediatric cardiology as a supplement to the routine scalar electrocardiogram. There are certain lesions in which the estimate of intraventricular pressure can be derived more accurately from the vectorcardiogram compared with the regular electrocardiogram. The degree of right ventricular hypertrophy in the pulmonary valvular dysplasia seen in Noonan's syndrome is an example; the level of left ventricular pressure in aortic stenosis is reflected more accurately in the vectorcardiogram than in the electrocardiogram, according to some observers. The direction of the vector loop (counterclockwise) can be helpful in identifying the presence of an endocardial cushion defect.

Echocardiogram

A more recently devised noninvasive technique, the echocardiogram, is used to determine movement characteristics of the mitral and other valves. Absence of the normal continuity of the aortic and mitral valve rings can be demonstrated supporting the diagnosis of double outlet right ventricle. Abnormalities of the interventricular septum may be established leading to such diagnoses as asymmetric septal hypertrophy or idiopathic hypertrophic subaortic stenosis. Pericardial effusion can also be detected in the echocardiogram. Future improvements in the technical aspects of scanning and recording capabilities of this noninvasive technique may indeed yield a very accurate picture of the structure and function of the intracardiac anatomy.

INVASIVE CARDIAC STUDIES

The most widely employed invasive technique is cardiac catheterization. This provides information concerning intracavitary and intravascular pressure, values of the oxygen content in blood specimens obtained from the various chambers and great vessels, the opportunity for selective angiocardiography, and finally the detection of abnormal diagnostic pathways taken by the cardiac catheter tip. The balloon catheter used in the creation of an atrial septal defect may also be employed for the purpose of carrying out a trial banding of the pulmonary artery or trial occlusion of a patent ductus arteriosus. The response of the blood pressure, particularly in the pulmonary artery, to a variety of drugs and the administration of 100% oxygen inhalation is another diagnostic method in this category. Other invasive techniques include intracavitary electrocardiography and electrophysiologic investigations with a probing catheter, including His bundle recordings. The recording of selective dye dilution curves has been used effectively as a diagnostic tool in a number of laboratories.

BIBLIOGRAPHY

Friedman S: The innocent (functional) cardiac murmurs of childhood. Clin Pediatr *4:*77, 1965

Contains a description of the common innocent cardiac murmurs of childhood by clinical and laboratory means.

Leatham A: Auscultation of the heart. Lancet *2:*703, 757, 1958

Provides a very useful classification of cardiac murmurs based primarily on timing and duration.

Levine SA: Systolic murmur: its clinical significance. JAMA *101:*436, 1933

An early reference to the use of a grading system for uniformity in expressing the intensity of cardiac murmurs.

Loggie JMH (ed): Hypertension in childhood and adolescence. Pediatr Clin North Am *25:*1978

A comprehensive review of the etiology, epidemiology pathogenesis and treatment of hypertension in the pediatric age group.

Marienfield DJ, Telles N, Silvera J, Nordsieck J: A 20-year follow-up study of "innocent" murmurs. Pediatrics *30:*42, 1962

Confirms the benign nature of functional heart murmurs by means of a long-term follow-up study.

Moss AJ, Adams, FH: Problems of Blood Pressure in Childhood. Springfield, Ill., Charles C Thomas, 1962

Cardiac Disease

25

Sidney Friedman

ETIOLOGY

Two major etiologic varieties of heart disease are encountered in childhood. These are congenital heart disease and rheumatic heart disease. Approximately 5 to 7 per 1000 newborn infants have a cardiovascular anomaly. Among school-age children, there is the same prevalence of heart disease, but increasing numbers of rheumatic subjects enter the group, reaching about 30% to 40% of the total at high school levels. The implication is that congenital heart disease is highly lethal leading to death in early childhood in almost half the cases. In addition, about 40% to 50% of children, particularly those between the ages of 4 and 12 years, have innocent or functional murmurs. Although these murmurs are unrelated to the presence of heart disease, they require accurate recognition and differentiation from the pathologic sounds.

Symptomatic Presentation

The symptomatic presentation of heart disease in childhood is quite different from that encountered among adults; chest pain is rarely evidence of heart disease. The majority (95%) of cardiac suspects in childhood are so designated because of a cardiac murmur. Cyanosis and symptoms of hypoxia are initial manifestations in many infants. Occasionally, congestive heart failure will be the initial presenting manifestation, often precipitated by an intercurrent respiratory tract infection. Failure to thrive, easy fatigability, systemic hypertension and cardiac arrhythmias are occasionally the chief complaint. Finally, the discovery of an abnormal appearance of the cardiac silhouette is not an infrequent mechanism for the suspicion of heart disease in pediatric patients.

FETAL CIRCULATION AND ITS CONVERSION TO POSTNATAL CIRCULATION

In the intrauterine circulation, the oxygen supply of the fetus is obtained from the placenta, rather than the lungs. The oxygenated blood enters the right atrium, having arrived there by means of the umbilical vein, ductus venosus, and inferior vena cava. This blood is immediately transferred to the left atrium by means of preferential streaming across the foramen ovale. The ductus arteriosus is patent and carries blood from the pulmonary artery into the descending aorta. This shunting of blood away from the pulmonary vascular bed is dependent upon the high pulmonary vascular resistance in the blood vessels of the lungs in the fetal state. The lungs receive approximately 10% of the ventricular output.

The blood in the right atrium represents a mixture of input from the superior vena cava at about 30% oxygen saturation and the blood coming in from the inferior vena cava which has an oxygen saturation of about 65%. The latter represents a mixture of fresh placental blood obtained through the ductus venosus and reduced systemic venous blood from the lower part of the body. The mixing in the right atrium is not complete. Most of the more highly oxygenated blood from the inferior vena cava enters the left atrium through the foramen ovale. Most of that from the superior vena cava enters the right ventricle through the tricuspid valve; this blood enters the pulmonary artery and more than half of it passes into the descending aorta through the patent ductus arteriosus. The remainder circulates through the lungs and eventually enters the left atrium.

Left atrial blood is a mixture of pulmonary arterial blood which enters through the pulmonary veins and the blood arriving through the foramen ovale. The oxygen saturation of the mixture in the left ventricle supplying the head and the right arm is about 60%. In contrast, the left arm and the lower part of the body are supplied by a mixture of left ventricular and patent ductus arteriosus blood with a less than 60% oxygen saturation.

At birth, a sudden decrease in the pulmonary vascular resistance occurs due to expansion of the lungs associated with the onset of breathing. There is also an increase in systemic resistance due to the collapse and cutting of the umbilical cord. As the pulmonary resistance drops, the blood is diverted from the ductus arteriosus into the lungs by the pulmonary arteries; this supply eventually arrives in the left atrium. The sudden increase in the pulmonary venous blood entering the left atrium raises the left atrial pressure and results in closure of the flap of the foramen ovale. In this way the two circuits are separated; that is, the foramen ovale is closed by the increased left atrial pressure and the patent ductus arteriosus is bypassed by virtue of the sudden fall in pulmonary vascular resistance.

Although these dramatic changes occur within a few minutes or hours, they are not completed for days or weeks. The pulmonary artery pressure drops significantly in the first day of life but a further gradual fall occurs over the next 3 or 4 weeks. The ductus arteriosus constricts rapidly within minutes after the establishment of respiration but is not anatomically closed for 1 or 2 days.

CONGENITAL HEART DISEASE

Approximately 60 or 70 different major structural abnormalities of the heart and great vessels may occur as congenital cardiac malformations. These lesions are compatible with fetal life; many others, incompatible with fetal life, result in death of the fetus. A number of malformations are not recognized at birth but become manifest several weeks later because their presenting manifestations depend upon the changes that occur normally in the conversion of the fetal circulation to the postnatal circulation.

Etiology

The etiology of congenital heart disease is largely unknown. Ingestion in early pregnancy of certain drugs such as thalidomide, LSD, and ethyl alcohol have been implicated as causes; intrauterine infection with the rubella virus is another established etiologic mechanism. Heredity seems to play a relatively minor role in the etiology of congenital heart disease in humans. However, with inbreeding in animals such as the dog, a very strong hereditary influence is demonstrable. When multiple instances of congenital heart disease occur in a single family, the specific lesions are frequently repeated.

Incidence

Congenital heart disease is the most common etiologic form of heart disease in the pediatric age group. The acquired heart disease of childhood, rheumatic heart disease, is found only rarely under the age of 4 years. The majority of those who die with congenital heart disease do so in the first weeks and months of life. In considering all the lesions of congenital heart disease, there is no predilection for males or females; in specific lesions, a sex predilection may exist. The incidence of the individual lesions is difficult to determine accurately and is dependent upon the method of data accumulation. Ventricular septal defect is the most common defect; patent ductus arteriosus is second, and tetralogy of Fallot is third. Atrial septal defect, coarctation of the aorta, aortic stenosis, isolated pulmonary stenosis, and transposition of the great vessels occur with almost equal frequency behind the first three. All other lesions are distinctly less common.

Classification

The simplest and perhaps most useful classification of congenital cardiac anomalies was proposed by Dr. Maude Abbott of McGill University in 1936 in her historic atlas reviewing 1000 autopsy specimens of congenital heart disease (see list). She suggested three categories of lesions: (1) those without shunting of blood from one side of the heart to the other, (2) those with shunting of blood from the left side of the heart to the right, (3) those with shunting from the right side of the heart to the left.

The lesions that occur in the absence of shunting are primarily mechanical obstructions and the anomalies of position. Coarctation of the aorta, aortic stenosis, and mitral stenosis are a few examples of obstructive lesions; dextrocardia, single coronary artery, a constricting vascular ring, and a right aortic arch are examples of the latter group. The name acyanotic group was used by Dr. Abbott for this category.

Clinical Classification of Cardiovascular Defects

1. *Acyanotic Group*
   Cases with no abnormal communication between systemic and pulmonary circulations.
   e.g. Coarctation of aorta, bicuspid aortic valve, isolated mitral valve deformity, congenital heart block, dextrocardia, constricting vascular ring, single coronary artery, etc.
2. *Cyanose Tardive Group*
   Cases with arterial-venous shunting with possible transient or terminal reversal of flow.
   e.g. Patent ductus arteriosus, atrial septal defect, ventricular septal defect, partial anomalous pulmonary venous drainage, aortico-pulmonary window, systemic arteriovenous fistula, etc.
3. *Cyanotic Group*
   Cases with permanent venous-arterial shunting.
   e.g. Tetralogy of Fallot, transposition of great arteries, pulmonary atresia with or without a ventricular septal defect, tricuspid atresia with hypoplasia of right ventricle, persistent truncus arteriosus, pulmonary arterio-venous fistula, etc.

Maude E. Abbott

The cardiac anomalies with left to right or arteriovenous shunts are common since they are associated with prolonged survival and successful surgical treatment. The three common lesions in this category are atrial septal defect, ventricular septal defect, and patent ductus arteriosus. A common feature of these lesions is the accentuation of the pulmonary vascular markings in the chest radiograph. Cyanosis is absent with exclusive left-to-right shunting. Less common examples of left-to-right shunting are partial anomalous pulmonary venous return, aorticopulmonary window, and systemic arteriovenous fistula.

Although the arteriovenous shunts are not associated ordinarily with cyanosis, Dr. Abbott offered the designation of *cyanose tardive* for this category. This name is the result of her observation that late in the clinical course of children with large left-to-right shunts, cyanosis did sometimes appear. She was referring to the development of pulmonary vascular occlusive disease that results in high pulmonary vascular resistance and pulmonary hypertension (Eisenmenger's complex). Under these circumstances, the pressure in the pulmonary circuit can exceed the systemic arterial blood pressure and reverse the direction of the shunt through the defect. This sequence does not occur frequently and is observed rarely in the first decade of life. Nevertheless, the consequences of such pulmonary vascular disease are devastating, since they preclude successful surgical closure of the defect and result in premature death.

The third category, the cyanotic group, consists of those lesions with persistent right-to-left or venous-arterial shunting. The most blatant right-to-left shunt occurs in transposition of the great arteries, since the entire systemic venous return enters the aorta from the right ventricle. Other common lesions of right-to-left shunting are the tetralogy of Fallot, a combination of severe pulmonary stenosis, and a large ventricular septal defect; severe valvular pulmonic stenosis with an interatrial right-to-left shunt; tricuspid atresia with hypoplasia of the right ventricle; persistent truncus arteriosus, single ventricle or single atrium; and a variety of lesions associated with pulmonary atresia.

A useful subdivision of the lesions with right-to-left shunting can be made, from a therapeutic standpoint, by use of the chest roentgenogram. One category includes the lesions with obstruction of pulmonary blood flow and, therefore, a paucity of pulmonary vascular markings; the heart is usually not enlarged. This group includes tetralogy of Fallot, tricuspid atresia with hypoplasia of the right ventricle, and pulmonary atresia with or without a ventricular septal defect. If total correction is not feasible, improvement of hypoxia can be obtained by surgical measures for increasing pulmonary blood flow. The second category includes the cyanotic lesions associated with abundant pulmonary blood flow. In these lesions, cyanosis is not as severe, but the heart is enlarged and congestive heart failure may be a presenting manifestation. Examples of this subgroup are transposition of the great arteries, persistent truncus arteriosus, and single ventricle. Finally, another very useful diagnostic finding in cyanotic infants is an extreme left-sided picture in the electrocardiogram; this is strongly suggestive of tricuspid atresia with hypoplasia of the right ventricle. Figure 25-1 presents a schema for use of various diagnostic studies in establishing a specific diagnosis of congenital heart disease.

Clinical Consequences

Pediatric cardiac supervision and treatment are focused around several unfavorable clinical sequelae which occur frequently in patients with congenital heart disease. These include (1) congestive heart failure, (2) hypoxia and its complications, (3) prevention and management of pulmonary hypertension, (4) bacterial complications of subacute bacterial endocarditis and brain abscess, and (5) syncope and sudden death.

Congestive Heart Failure. The wide variety of lesions of congenital heart disease produces a number of mechanical

Pulmonary vascular markings	Heart size	ECG	R.V. cavity* Small	Systolic murmur	Aorta ant.* from R.V.	Two* ventricles	Asc. aorta* on left	Pulses poor 4 ext.	Pulses poor legs	PA oxygen = Ao oxygen	Aorta from* rt. ventricle	Diagnosis
Decreased	Small	LVH										Tricuspid atresia
			Yes									Pulmonary atresia, intact VS (type A)
		RVH	No	Yes	Yes							TGA, VSD, PS
					No	Yes	Yes					"Corrected" TGA, VSD (single V), PS
							No					Tetralogy of Fallot
						No						Single V, PS
				No								Pulmonary atresia, VSD
	Large	LVH										Ebstein's anomaly
		RVH		Yes								Severe PS (isolated)
				No								Pulmonic atresia, intact VS (type B)
Increased	Small											
	Large	LVH										Tricuspid artresia, TGA
		RVH		Yes								TGA
				No				Yes				Aortic and/or mitral atresia
								No	Yes			Preducial coarctation
									No	Yes		Total anomalous pulmonary venous return
		BVH									Yes	Double outlet RV, subaortic VSD
						Yes						Truncus arteriosus
						No						Single ventricle

*Often can be determined by echocardiography. (Rashkind WJ: The cyanotic newborn: approach to diagnosis and treatment. Cardiovasc Clin 4:277, 1972)

Fig. 25-1. Differential diagnosis of the cyanotic newborn.

problems which may lead to congestive heart failure. In patients with severe obstructive lesions such as aortic stenosis or pulmonic stenosis, systolic overloading of the ventricles occurs. Severe degrees of systolic overloading are best reflected in the electrocardiogram in the form of right or left ventricular hypertrophy and "strain" patterns. Coarctation of the aorta and pulmonary vascular obstructive disease are other common causes for systolic overloading leading to congestive heart failure.

Diastolic overloading of the ventricle may occur in congenital heart disease as a result of the need for the right or left ventricle to handle increased volumes of blood presented during diastole. Left ventricular diastolic overloading may be associated with such lesions as patent ductus arteriosus or aortic insufficiency. Diastolic overloading of the right ventricle occurs frequently with atrial septal defect or anomalous pulmonary venous drainage. With diastolic overloading, the chest roentgenogram is most helpful in judging the specific chamber of increased volume and also the prominence of the pulmonary vasculature. A consistently accurate guide to the size of a left-to-right shunt related to diastolic overloading is the presence or absence of a mid-diastolic flow murmur, indicating augmented flow through either the tricuspid or mitral valves. In the presence of such a filling sound, a pulmonary systemic flow ratio greater than 2 to 1 can be predicted accurately.

Hypoxia. In the absence of congestive heart failure and pulmonary disease, cyanosis in congenital heart disease is related to right-to-left shunting. The peripheral cyanosis of congestive heart failure usually is recognized by the evidence of a low cardiac output. The favorable response in skin color to inhalation of 100% oxygen in patients with pulmonary disease usually differentiates this cause of cyanosis from that associated with central mixing of arterial and venous blood.

Cyanosis due to right-to-left shunting is dependent on a communication between the two circuits with a resistance to flow of blood on the right side greater than the resistance to the flow on the left side. The presence of inadequate pulmonary blood flow contributes quantitatively to the severity of cyanosis. Cyanosis is not due to diminished pulmonary blood flow *per se*. The expansion of the volume of pulmonary blood flow can favorably reduce the level of arterial unsaturation by exposing a larger volume of unsaturated blood to inspired air.

The clinical manifestations of hypoxia are clubbing of the fingers and toes, the development of polycythemia, shortness of breath on exertion, squatting, and anoxic attacks. The latter two are found almost invariably in patients with cyanotic lesions associated with inadequate pulmonary blood flow. Anoxic attacks are paroxysms of cerebral hypoxia resulting from a temporary increase in right-to-left shunting. The attacks usually occur in infancy, beyond the age of 3 months, often in the morning following breakfast. Occasionally they are associated with bowel movements or feeding. The attack is marked by increased cyanosis, increased respiratory rate and effort, and a variety of subtle or obvious changes in the state of consciousness. The latter can vary from a staring spell to rolling back of the eyes, limpness, a convulsive seizure, or death.

Pulmonary Hypertension. In patients with large communications between the pulmonary and systemic circuits, a single mean pressure must be present in the two ventricles. A systemic blood pressure level is thus established in the pulmonary circuit. Patients with this hemodynamic arrangement have a tendency to develop histopathologic changes in the pulmonary arterioles consisting initially of medial muscular hypertrophy and later of intimal proliferation. The picture of medial hypertrophy is reactive and reversible following closure of the communication; the intimal proliferation is fixed and irreversible. Wide variation exists among different subjects and lesions in the duration of pulmonary hypertension necessary for the development of irreversible pulmonary vascular changes. The factors involved in the establishment of these changes in a given patient are poorly understood. Fixed pulmonary hypertension and pulmonary vascular occlusive disease are much more likely to occur in childhood in the presence of a ventricular septal defect or a patent ductus arteriosus than in atrial septal defect. Fixed pulmonary vascular resistance below the age of 2 years is unknown in acyanotic patients. In patients with or without congenital heart disease the persistence of the fetal pattern of pulmonary vascular resistance may contribute to the presence of pulmonary arterial hypertension. Lesions associated with left atrial hypertension due to mitral valve disease may predispose to the development of pulmonary vascular disease by elevating pulmonary venous pressure. Exposure to low partial pressures of oxygen like those which occur at high altitudes may be another provoking factor. An idiopathic variety of primary pulmonary hypertension is also known to occur in which the findings of cor pulmonale follow isolated pulmonary vascular obstructive changes.

In the clinical observation of patients with pulmonary arterial hypertension, two causative possibilities must be considered: augmented pulmonary blood flow and elevated pulmonary vascular resistance. When high pulmonary blood flow produces elevated pulmonary artery pressure, successful surgical closure of the underlying communication between pulmonary and systemic circuits results in a prompt fall in pulmonary artery pressure. By contrast, in patients with elevated pulmonary artery pressure due to high pulmonary vascular resistance (intimal proliferation) closure of the defect will not result in a fall of pulmonary artery pressure and may indeed be harmful if the defect has been acting as a site of right-to-left shunting and thereby as a safety valve for the right ventricle.

Bacterial Complications. Two major bacterial complications threaten patients with congenital heart disease: subacute bacterial endocarditis and brain abscess. Both are related to transient venous bacteremia, usually involving organisms of low virulence.

Subacute bacterial endocarditis occurs less frequently in infants and children than in adults. This inverse relationship to age is related to the duration of time necessary for the development of areas of endocardial or endothelial injury. The repeated impingement of a jet of blood against a localized area of endocardium can result in the formation of jet lesions or plaques at the site of endocardial injury. The wall of the pulmonary artery opposite the site of entry of the shunt of a patent ductus arteriosus or the right ventricular wall opposite a ventricular septal defect are common jet lesion locations. The deposition of fibrin on the surface of injured endocardium permits the embedding of passing bacteria and fosters their growth and proliferation, with the eventual formation of macroscopic vegetations. Cardiac anomalies associated with turbulence and high pressure are the ones most likely to be complicated by subacute bacterial endocarditis (*e.g.*, aortic stenosis, coarctation of the aorta, ventricular septal defect, patent ductus arteriosus, mitral valve deformity and occasionally pulmonary stenosis).

When structures on the left side of the heart are the sites of subacute bacterial endocarditis, the signs and symptoms are not unlike those observed in adults with this complication superimposed upon rheumatic valvular deformity. These include high fever, weight loss, anorexia, splenomegaly, and evidence of systemic bacterial embolization such as petechiae. In children with congenital heart disease, the concept of right-sided bacterial endocarditis must also be appreciated. When the jet lesion is situated in the lesser circulation, the symptoms of embolization are related to pulmonary infarction. This may be recognized from changes in the chest roentgenogram and is manifest by chest pain and respiratory distress.

Subacute bacterial endocarditis may remain undiagnosed for several weeks. The initial fever and malaise often lead to no specific diagnosis and the administration of nonspecific antibiotic treatment. The infectious process may be temporarily aborted only to recur after cessation of antibiotic therapy. This sequence may be repeated several times before the underlying cause of the fever is established. The differentiation of a series of coincidental, self-limited infections of viral origin from subacute bacterial endocarditis is a frequent problem in patients with congenital heart disease. Withdrawal of antibiotic therapy for a number of days in order to obtain a series of blood cultures usually resolves the problem.

The organism most commonly involved in subacute bacterial endocarditis in childhood is the alpha-hemolytic streptococcus. Most but not all of these organisms are sensitive to penicillin. Acute bacterial endocarditis associated with virulent hemolytic staphylococci, or *Hemophilus influenzae*, may occur in association with septicemia. Bacterial endocarditis with organisms of low virulence may complicate cardiac surgery due to contamination from monitoring devices, intravenous tubing, and other instruments.

Treatment depends upon the organism involved and its sensitivity to antibiotics. In instances of alpha-hemolytic streptococcal endocarditis, a 4-week course of intravenous penicillin at a level of 10 to 15 million units/day is usually advised. Individualization of treatment based upon *in vitro* sensitivity studies is essential in dealing with the less common organisms.

Brain abscess in the pediatric age group is associated frequently with cyanotic congenital heart disease. The basis for this relationship is the diversion of peripheral venous blood into the systemic circulation, away from its usual pathway through the lungs. This route bypasses the filtering action of the pulmonary capillary bed, permitting the organisms of a casual venous bacteremia to find access to the arterial circulation. The poor local resistance of neural tissue to bacterial infection accounts for the predilection of the brain as the site of seeding of these organisms. The vital nature of the brain tissue and its enclosure in the inflexible calvarium accounts for the serious consequences of this complication.

The early diagnosis and successful treatment of brain abscess require a high index of suspicion of this complication in patients with cyanotic congenital heart disease. Unexplained headache, particularly if severe and unrelieved by symptomatic measures, should raise serious supicions; fever, vomiting, and changes in the state of consciousness are also common symptoms, and occasionally seizures and focal neurologic signs may be observed. Evidence of increased intracranial pressure results from the expansion of this space-occupying lesion. Once suspected, brain abscess can be sought by brain scanning techniques, including computed tomography. Antibiotic therapy occasionally can be successful in the treatment of a small subarachnoid abscess which drains spontaneously into the subarachnoid space. However, most confined abscesses require surgical drainage or total removal for cure.

Syncope and Sudden Death. A number of congenital cardiac anomalies are known to be associated with syncope and sudden death. The mechanism is the presence of a low cardiac output resulting from such causes as slow cardiac rate, serious cardiac arrhythmia, severe obstruction to left ventricular outflow, and inadequate pulmonary venous return to the left heart.

The lesion most frequently mentioned in association with syncope and sudden death is severe congenital aortic stenosis. Syncope in such patients should be taken as an indication of severe left ventricular outflow tract obstruction and should be an indication for prompt hemodynamic study and surgical treatment. In such patients, the electrocardiographic pattern of left ventricular hypertrophy and left ventricular strain is usually, but not invariably, present. In borderline instances, the T wave and ST segment abnormalities in the electrocardiogram may be provoked by exercise testing, indicating the need for measurement of the aortic valve gradient somewhat earlier.

Systolic gradients in pressure at the level of the aortic valve in excess of 70 to 80 mm Hg are sufficient to warrant surgical relief of aortic stenosis. In childhood, this is usually carried out as a palliative procedure, by aortic valvulotomy, in preference to aortic valve replacement. The opportunity for effective relief of aortic stenosis is largely dependent upon the anatomic features of the deformed aortic valve. In the case of a unicommissural aortic valve, it is particularly difficult to obtain benefit from commissurotomy. Sudden death may occur postoperatively in those patients who have had inadequate relief of aortic stenosis because of unfavorable anatomic features.

Dramatic episodes of syncope and sudden death may occur with extreme degrees of slowing of the cardiac rate. Congenital and acquired heart block may produce Stokes-Adams syncopal attacks. The cardiac rate is usually below 30/minute in patients suffering such episodes. The electrocardiogram usually shows complete atrioventricular dissociation with no relationship between the atrial and ventricular contractions. Treatment consists of the introduction of an electronic pacemaker.

The presence of severe pulmonary vascular disease may occasionally be associated with syncope and sudden death. The pulmonary venous return may be so limited by the pulmonary arteriolar occlusion that the left ventricular output is inadequate to perfuse the brain and myocardium. Syncope and sudden death may be manifestations of a variety of coordinated and uncoordinated tachyarrhythmias associated or unassociated with congenital heart disease. The ventricular tachycardias are more likely to produce serious symptoms and results than are the tachycardias of supraventricular origin.

Treatment

Definitive treatment of congenital heart disease is primarily surgical. Since 1940, an increasing number of cardiac anomalies have become amenable to successful surgical treatment; at present, almost 85% of all congenital cardiac lesions can be corrected or improved by surgical techniques.

All patients with patent ductus arteriosus or significant coarctation of the aorta should have surgical correction. Isolated atrial septal defect and ventricular septal defect should be corrected with the use of cardiopulmonary bypass, if the left-to-right shunt is significant, that is, producing a pulmonary/systemic flow ratio greater than 2 to 1. Isolated valvular pulmonic stenosis requires surgical relief if the absolute right ventricular pressure is 80 to 90 mm Hg in systole. The indication for surgical relief of aortic stenosis is a gradient in excess of 80 mm Hg at the specific site of narrowing.

Patients with cyanotic congenital heart disease and inadequate pulmonary blood flow may require palliation by creation of a systemic artery to pulmonary artery shunt. The Blalock-Taussig anastomosis (Fig. 25-2) is preferred, but in very small infants it may be necessary to carry out an ascending aorta to right pulmonary artery (Waterston) anastomosis (Fig. 25-3) because of the small size of the blood vessels involved. Patients who reach the age of 5 to 10 years with tetralogy of Fallot, with or without earlier palliation, should have a total correction of the intracardiac defects. Only by eliminating the right-to-left shunting will the complication of brain abscess be avoided.

Complete transposition of the great arteries is treated initially by creation of an interatrial communication either by balloon-atrioseptostomy or by surgical means (Fig. 25-4). After the age of 6 to 12 months, definitive treatment can be achieved by the technique of Mustard or Senning which transposes the systemic and pulmonary venous return by reorientation of the atrial septum. Combinations of lesions require individual methods of management and timing of application.

Medical management of patients with congenital heart disease consists largely in diagnostic evaluation of the anatomy and severity of the defect, timing of surgical management, advice concerning physical activity, and handling of intercurrent infections and allied medical and surgical problems. Infants with large left-to-right shunts and pulmonary

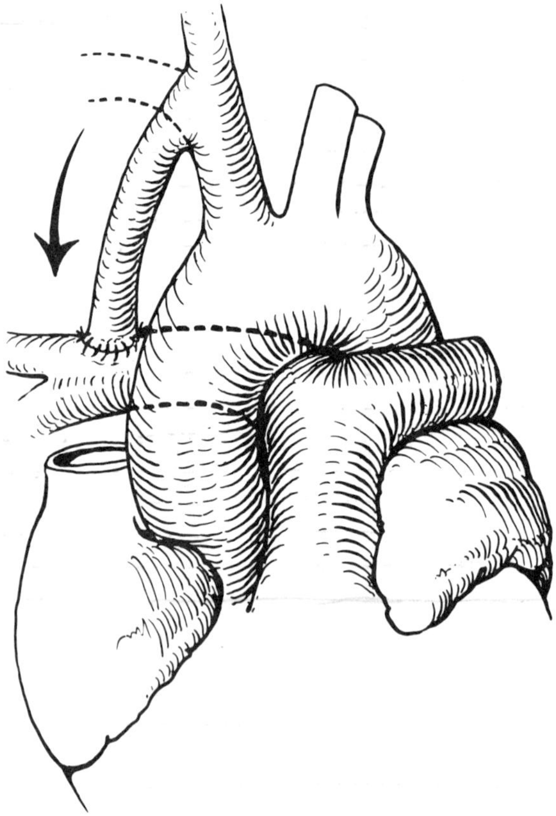

Fig. 25-2. Anatomic features of a Blalock-Taussig anastomosis created in the right hemithorax of a patient with a left descending aorta. The right subclavian artery which is a branch of the innominate artery is turned down to make an end-to-side anastomosis with the right main pulmonary artery. Arrow indicates direction of flow of unsaturated blood from right subclavian artery to right pulmonary artery, thereby increasing volume of pulmonary blood flow.

hypertension are particularly prone to atelectasis and pneumonitis, and often require repeated hospitalizations for treatment of these complications. Many patients with congenital heart disease require treatment of congestive heart failure by symptomatic measures. Most infants with congestive heart failure due to isolated coarctation of the aorta can be controlled by medical means alone. Similarly, most patients with ventricular septal defect can be successfully managed through infancy with the hope that favorable changes may occur spontaneously, either in the form of a reduction in the relative size of the defect or development of right ventricular outflow tract obstruction (self-banding). Spontaneous closure of a persistently patent ductus arteriosus may be awaited for approximately 6 months, but thereafter surgical closure is indicated.

Surgical banding of the pulmonary artery is carried out in the palliative management of patients with severe pulmonary artery hypertension. It is applicable only in

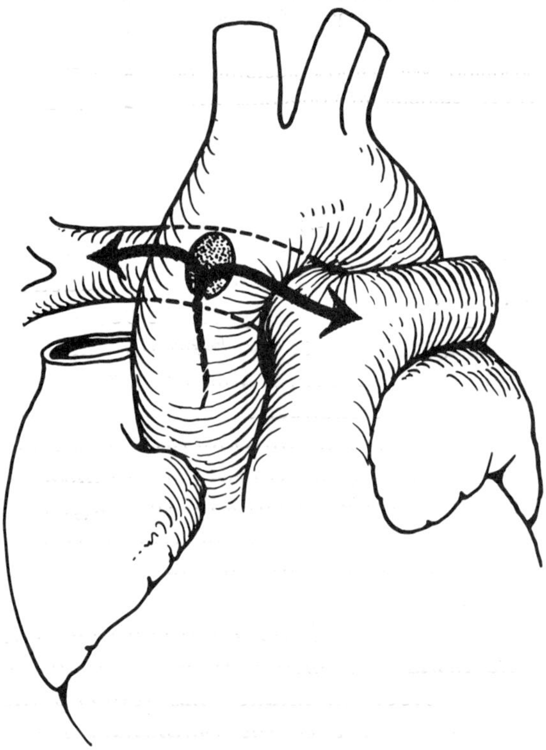

Fig. 25-3. Anatomic features of an ascending aorta to right pulmonary artery (Waterston) anastomosis, designed to increase pulmonary blood flow as a palliative procedure in infants with cyanotic congenital heart disease with inadequate pulmonary blood flow. Arrows indicate direction of blood flow through anastomosis from ascending aorta to right and left pulmonary artery branches. Volume of blood directed to right lung is usually much greater than to left lung.

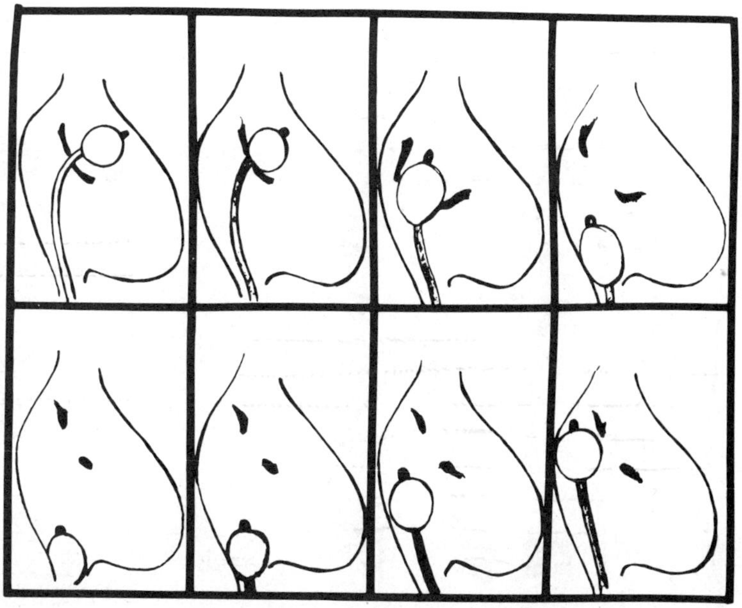

Fig. 25-4. Graphic representation of cine frames during balloon atrial septostomy. In the upper left frame the balloon is seen in left atrium inflated with contrast material with catheter coursing through foramen ovale. As balloon is abruptly withdrawn, it ruptures delicate membrane covering fossa ovalis thereby providing a significant interatrial communication which enhances mixing of blood between systemic and pulmonary circulations. In bottom frame on right balloon is seen in right atrium preparatory to deflation and withdrawal. (Rashkind WJ: Atrioseptostomy by balloon catheter in congenital heart disease. Radiol Clin North Am, 1971)

patients with a large interventricular communication or a single ventricle who have a reactive pulmonary vascular bed. Reduction of the pulmonary artery pressure beyond the site of application of the band prevents the development of irreversible pulmonary vascular occlusive changes at the pulmonary arteriolar level. The introduction of an obstruction to right ventricular outflow is beneficial in the treatment of congestive heart failure by reducing the volume of left-to-right shunting through the interventricular communication and thereby diminishing the volume load of the left ventricle. The trend toward definitive correction of intracardiac defects in infancy has reduced the need for the use of the pulmonary artery banding procedure.

Use of prosthetic valves should be avoided assiduously in childhood. Nevertheless, occasionally no other solution exists for the management of a valvular abnormality. Operations designed to patients with truncus arteriosus or pulmonary atresia (Rastelli procedure) are well developed, but the duration of effectiveness of the "valved conduit" procedures has yet to be determined. In considering the elective application of surgical treatment, an optimistic expectation that improved methods will be available in 5 or 10 years is not unrealistic when dealing with any problems for which no established procedure is now available. This has certainly been the case over the past 3 decades.

The medical management of anoxic attacks may present as an emergency situation. Use of the knee-chest position and the administration of oxygen aborts or terminates most mild attacks. In more severe instances, the use of parenteral morphine sulfate or propranolol, in that order, is effective. Oxygen and morphine should be given as promptly as possible, and thereafter the patient should be left alone to rest without further handling for 30 minutes to permit these measures to become effective.

Dramatic improvements in hypoxia can be obtained sometimes in patients by the oral administration of iron, especially if a relative anemia exists as in patients with polycythemia. The elimination of this type of anemia will also reduce the risk of intra-

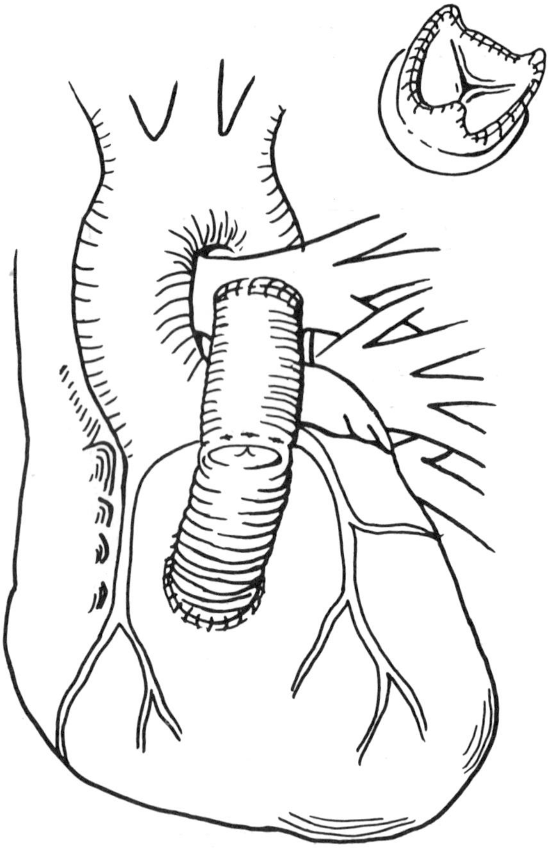

Fig. 25-5. Dacron-valved conduit (Rastelli's procedure) interposed between cavity of right ventricle and main pulmonary artery. Conduit contains porcine heterograft valve and is used to bypass obstruction at level of pulmonary valve (atresia) or to establish a right ventricular outlet where none exists (persistent truncus arteriosus).

vascular clotting that results in cerebral vascular thrombosis.

Systematic cardiac supervision in patients with mild congenital heart lesions at 6- or 12-month intervals permits (1) regulation of medications such as digitalis, (2) reinforcement of the need for prophylactic measures against subacute bacterial endocarditis and brain abscess, (3) evaluation of the degree of hypoxia by clinical and laboratory means (hemoglobin and hematocrit), and (4) the opportunity to provide advice about general health measures and activity restrictions. An annual or semiannual discussion of the patient's cardiac problem, particularly with regard to the long-range plans, the availability or lack of availability of surgical treatment, some of its details, risks, and results, make the actual encounter with these problems more bearable by parents when the hour of surgical action finally arrives.

RHEUMATIC FEVER

Rheumatic fever is a generalized inflammatory disease of unknown etiology that involves many organs of the body, but primarily the connective tissue. The organs most frequently involved in the inflammatory process are the heart, joints, skin, and brain. Rheumatic fever is primarily a pediatric disease; its etiology is related to streptococcal infection which occurs more frequently in childhood than in adult life.

Despite a decline in incidence and severity over the past 50 years, rheumatic heart disease remains the second most common etiologic variety of heart disease in childhood. Among children of school age in Philadelphia, one half of the 6 cases per 1000 with heart disease are rheumatic. During the first 3 decades of this century, rheumatic heart disease was the leading medical cause of death among school-age children. The reduction in incidence and severity of rheumatic fever over the past several decades has occurred only in the developed countries of the world; the disease continues to be rampant in the underdeveloped areas.

A vast literature based upon epidemiologic, bacteriologic, and serologic data has developed in the past 3 decades relating the beta-hemolytic streptococcus of Lancefield group A to rheumatic fever. There is considerable evidence that the streptococcus is almost uniformly related in an undetermined way to the pathogenesis of rheumatic fever. It is not directly invasive in its action in the disease. In current concepts, the streptococcus is related to rheumatic fever by an immunologic mechanism, either by a reaction of hypersentivity or by the formation and reaction of autoimmune antibodies.

Clinical Characteristics

A very high percentage of rheumatic attacks are preceded by overt or subclinical streptococcal infection. The time interval between the preceding streptococcal infection and the onset of symptoms of rheumatic fever varies between 1 and 3 weeks in the majority of cases. Most patients with rheumatic fever fall into one of three categories with regard to the persistence of their rheumatic activity. (1) In a small number of patients, an acute or fulminating course terminates in death within a few days or weeks; (2) in a slightly larger group, a chronic course of low-grade activity takes place, rheumatic activity persists over a period of months or years, never subsiding completely, and eventually death occurs from profound cardiac involvement; (3) the majority of rheumatic subjects experience a recurrent form of rheumatic fever in which individual, identifiable, self-limited episodes of active rheumatic inflammation are followed by periods of complete quiescence or inactivity of the disease. In the absence of prophylactic measures, a high percentage of such patients experiences one or more recurrences of rheumatic activity with the hazard of cardiac involvement with each episode. Within a given period of rheumatic activity, readily recognizable variations in intensity occur commonly and may produce a polycyclic course. The age range in which initial attacks of rheumatic fever occur most often is 6 to 8 years. One percent of all cases occur below the age of 4 years. Both initial attacks and recurrences occur less frequently beyond the age of puberty. Considerable variation occurs in the duration of rheumatic episodes; a range of from 2 weeks to 12 months is recognized. The majority of cases have an attack duration of 1 to 4 months. A trend exists among rheumatic patients for the occurrence of the same individual manifestations of the disease in each recurrent episode. Thus, patients with abdominal pain in an initial attack frequently manifest abdominal pain with a recurrent attack. Although this is a useful clinical characteristic of rheumatic fever from the diagnostic standpoint, exceptions to this trend occur. Of patients experiencing no evidence of carditis in the initial attack, approximately 14% manifest definite cardiac involvement in a subsequent attack.

Diagnosis

An accurate decision concerning the presence or absence of rheumatic fever is of great importance to the patient. Since no specific diagnostic test is available, the diagnosis rests in each instance on clinical judgment. Failure to recognize rheumatic carditis promptly may result in delayed treatment and increased residual cardiac damage. A false diagnosis of rheumatic fever may result in prolonged, unnecessary confinement.

An arbitrary set of diagnostic criteria was proposed by Dr. T. Duckett Jones in 1943 for the purpose of minimizing errors in diagnosis. These criteria subsequently have been modified and are widely accepted. They separate the manifestations into two categories, major and minor manifestations of rheumatic fever. The major criteria are those manifestations that occur almost exclusively in rheumatic fever, although none is pathognomonic. The minor criteria are less specific and occur in a wide variety of inflammatory diseases. In order to fulfill the criteria of Jones for the diagnosis of rheumatic fever, at least one major and two minor manifestations, or two major and one minor manifestation, must be present. The arbitrary nature of the system of Jones must be appreciated; an individual patient may have rheumatic fever with a clinical picture which does not fulfill these criteria.

The major criteria of Jones include migrating polyarthritis, chorea, subcutaneous nodules, erythema marginatum, and carditis. The presence of objective evidence of joint inflammation involving multiple joints in a migratory fashion is highly suggestive of rheumatic fever. The syndrome of *chorea* described by Sydenham in 1686 (St. Vitus' dance) represents the central nervous system involvement in rheumatic fever and has four basic features: (1) muscular weakness, (2) muscular incoordination, (3) involuntary, purposeless movements which disappear during sleep, and (4) emotional lability. The average duration of an episode of chorea is 10 weeks, although extreme variability exists. Intensification of symptoms occurs for approximately 3 weeks, followed by gradual improvement. Unilateral or hemichorea occurs in about 10% of cases; in the remainder, involvement is grossly symmetric. Chorea is more common in females than in males and rarely occurs beyond the age of puberty, except during pregnancy. *Subcutaneous nodules* are firm, round, nontender nodules which vary from 0.5 to 2 cm in diameter and are attached beneath the skin to tendon sheaths and fascia; the skin moves freely over them. Subcutaneous nodules occur in crops and are found over the extensor surfaces of the elbows, knees, and wrists, in the occipital region, and over the spinous processes of the thoracic and lumbar vertebrae. They appear most frequently at least 3 to 5 weeks after the onset of clinical manifestations, often in association with carditis. *Erythema marginatum* is an erythematous nonpruritic skin rash. It is the least specific of the major manifestations of rheumatic fever. The rash has a pink color which fades away from its sharp scalloped edges and is found mainly over the trunk, occasionally on the extremities, and rarely on the feet. The rash is recurrent and may migrate from one portion of the body to another. It is difficult to differentiate from skin rashes due to hypersensitivity to drugs.

The cardiac involvement in rheumatic fever is the most important consequence of the disease because permanent damage to cardiac tissues may occur. All three tissue layers of the heart (endocardium, myocardium and pericardium) may be involved in the inflammatory process producing the picture of pancarditis. Irreversible changes in the structure and function of the cardiac valves may result from endocardial involvement. Postinflammatory scarring of the myocardium may lead to serious impairment of myocardial function especially in the presence of superimposed degenerative (aging) changes.

The following clinical evidences of *carditis* are considered to be major manifestations, according to the criteria of Jones: (1) significant new or changing cardiac murmurs, (2) cardiac enlargement, (3) pericarditis, and (4) congestive heart failure. Evidence of cardiac involvement such as electrocardiographic abnormalities, arrhythmias, inappropriate tachycardia, and changes in the quality of heart sounds are nonspecific indications of myocardial disease and are not accepted as major criteria.

Murmurs. In childhood, endocarditis involves the mitral and aortic valves almost exclusively and the mitral valve in approximately 90% of patients with overt carditis. In approximately half of the patients with mitral lesions, the aortic valve is also involved. Isolated involvement of the aortic valve occurs in only 10% of cases. The murmur of mitral insufficiency is the most frequently heard murmur of rheumatic heart disease in childhood. It is loudest at the site of the apex beat and is transmitted in the direction of the left axilla as well as to the back on the left side where it is usually best heard beneath the left scapula. This murmur is holosystolic in duration and high-pitched and blowing in quality. Its intensity is variable; occasionally it may be of only grade I or II intensity. In the presence of mitral insufficiency, a mid-diastolic murmur may be heard at the cardiac apex with active rheumatic carditis. It is usually preceded by the appearance of a protodiastolic gallop sound.

Rheumatic involvement of the aortic valve results in the murmur of aortic regurgitation; the murmur of aortic stenosis due to rheumatic heart disease is almost never heard below the age of puberty. The murmur of aortic regurgitation is early diastolic in time, following immediately after the second heart sound. It has a high-pitched decrescendo blowing character and is best heard in the third left interspace at the anatomic position of the aortic valve (see Fig. 25-6).

Cardiac Enlargement. Evidence of increasing heart size is another clear indication of active rheumatic carditis, usually indicating severe myocardial involvement. Chamber enlargement depends in part on specific valvular deformities; but, in the presence of diffuse myocardial involvement; a generalized form of enlargement results. Cardiac enlargement associated with rheumatic carditis is almost invariably associated with the characteristic murmurs of this disease; cardiac enlargement in the absence of characteristic murmurs is not rheumatic in

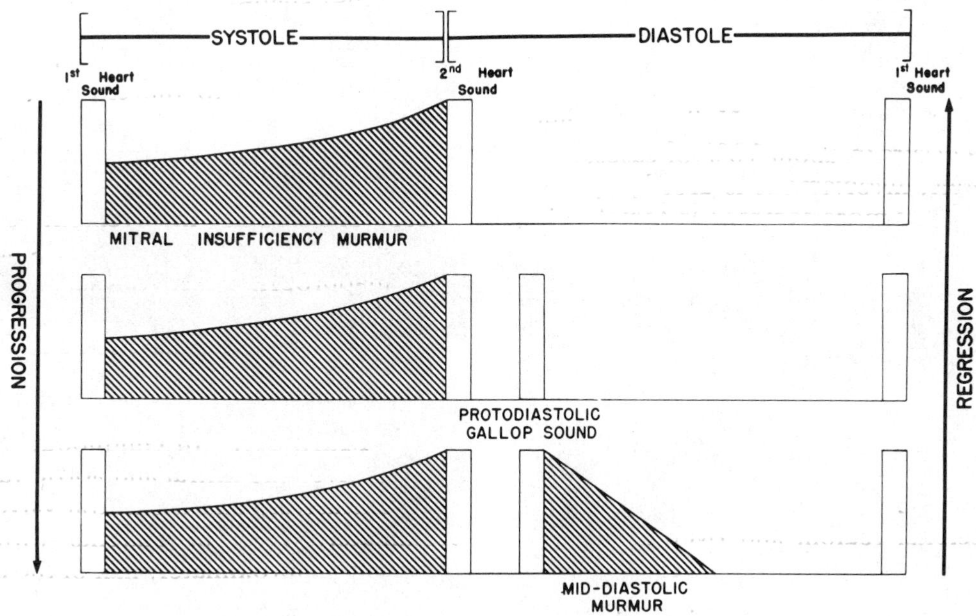

Fig. 25-6. Diagrammatic representation of auscultatory events resulting from mitral valve involvement during acute rheumatic carditis in childhood. Diagrams indicate initial appearance of holosystolic murmur of mitral insufficiency, followed by the appearance of a protodiastolic gallop sound, and of a mid-diastolic murmur. Arrows indicate the direction taken by the auscultatory events during progression and regression of cardiac involvement. (Conn HL, Horwitz O: Cardiac and Vascular Diseases, p. 773. Philadelphia, Lea & Febiger, 1971)

origin. The prognosis in rheumatic fever is related more to cardiac size than to the presence of various cardiac murmurs.

Pericarditis. Auscultatory evidence of inflammation of the visceral pericardium is another indication of the presence of rheumatic carditis. A friction rub may appear in any location over the precordium but is usually found in the left parasternal region. Frequently this adventitious sound is transient or heard intermittently. Electrocardiographic confirmation of pericardial involvement is usually available, especially in the acute stages. As in the case of cardiomegaly, a pericardial friction rub of rheumatic origin is almost always associated with the characteristic murmurs of rheumatic heart disease. The problem that occasionally arises is the need to differentiate pericarditis with effusion from the large dilated flabby heart associated with congestive heart failure. The echocardiogram may be useful in separating these two entities.

Congestive Heart Failure. Congestive heart failure resulting from rheumatic heart disease in childhood is an indication of extensive myocardial involvement. Mechanical handicapping of the heart as a result of valvular deformity is rarely of sufficient severity in childhood to account for cardiac failure. Nevertheless, as in the case of cardiac enlargement and pericarditis, this manifestation of rheumatic carditis also does not occur in the absence of one or more of the characteristic cardiac murmurs of rheumatic carditis. The manifestations of congestive heart failure in rheumatic heart disease of childhood are not grossly different from those observed in adults, but the onset may be more abrupt and the progression may be rapid. Evidence of left ventricular failure is frequently observed initially, but signs of right heart failure follow shortly thereafter. Tachycardia, tachypnea, dyspnea, and orthopnea are often the first changes noted; hepatomegaly may occur early and is a valuable index of the severity of right heart failure. It is common for peripheral edema to appear later; pulmonary edema with basilar rales appears as a very late manifestation of congestive heart failure in childhood.

The minor manifestations of Jones are nonspecific and occur in many inflammatory diseases. They provide only supporting evidence for the diagnosis of rheumatic fever and must be accompanied by at least one of the major manifestations in order to fulfill the criteria of Jones. Minor criteria include fever, arthralgia, prolonged P-R interval in the electrocardiogram, increased erythrocyte sedimentation rate or other acute phase reactants, evidence of recent beta-hemolytic streptococcal infection, previous history of rheumatic fever or the presence of inactive rheumatic heart disease. Epistaxis, pallor, anemia, abdominal pain, pneumonitis, weight loss, easy fatiguability, headache, and vomiting may also be considered minor manifestations of rheumatic fever.

Laboratory Aids

Because of the absence of any known pathogenetic agent of rheumatic fever, no specific tests for the detection or measurement of activity are available. As a result, a number of nonspecific tests have been employed for these purposes. These tests fall into two categories which differ in their purpose and in their relationship to rheumatic fever: (1) the acute phase tests and (2) the antistreptococcal antibody determinations.

The acute phase tests are entirely nonspecific in character and reflect quantitatively the destruction of tissue due to such diverse causes as inflammation, infarction, and malignancy. The test most widely used, oldest, and simplest to perform is the erythrocyte sedimentation rate. Another acute phase test recently popularized is the determination of C-reactive protein, a substance that is not normally a component of serum but is found in many states involving tissue destruction. These determinations are useful primarily in following the activity of the rheumatic process after the diagnosis has been determined from other information. In the presence of cardiac failure associated with rheumatic carditis, the erythrocyte sedimentation rate may be paradoxically decreased, often to a level that is within normal limits. In sicklemia, the erythrocyte sedimentation rate is unreliable since the shape results in failure of these cells to form rouleaux as large as would be formed by normal-shaped erythrocytes.

The second major type of laboratory determination which is useful in the evaluation of patients suspected of having rheumatic fever is the antistreptococcal antibody titer. Antibodies developed to a variety of antigenic components and products of the streptococcus reflect recent immunologic experience with this organism. The streptococcal hemolysin is referred to by the contracted term antistreptolysin-0 titer. Titers of 200 or less are commonly found in a healthy population. Values in excess of 200 may be interpreted as an indication of recent streptococcal infection. Elevated titers are encountered in patients convalescing from acute streptococcal infections as well as in patients with acute rheumatic fever (see Fig. 25-7). Among rheumatic suspects the finding of very low titers or very high titers is a more significant indication of the absence or presence of the disease than titers in the middle range. Various other antigens have been employed to measure antistreptococcal antibodies in patients with rheumatic fever. A poor correlation exists between the clinical course of rheumatic fever and the antibody titer determinations. Once elevated, titers tend to remain at high levels for 3 to 6 months regardless of the duration of rheumatic activity. Antibody titers are usually increased significantly at the time of onset of symptoms of rheumatic fever.

Treatment

Therapy in rheumatic fever is nonspecific, supportive, and symptomatic. Since only the cardiac involvement leads to permanent residua, all major therapeutic efforts should be directed toward minimizing the damage resulting from carditis. For this reason, a period of complete bedrest is essential in patients with and without obvious cardiac involvement. Effective bedrest is difficult for children and requires determined and coordinated efforts from many sources. The arthritis and fever of rheumatic fever respond dramatically to salicylate therapy in large doses. The response of arthritis and fever to salicylates is so dramatic that it represents a valuable diagnostic aid. The use of a posterior nasal pack or replacement of blood lost during epistaxis is occasionally necessary. The treatment of chorea consists of minimizing physical and emotional stimulation to the child. Sedatives and tranquilizing drugs may be of some help in the management of choreic patients but do not alter the natural course significantly. Except for the component that results from iron loss due to severe epistaxis, the anemia of acute rheumatic fever does not respond to iron therapy.

Aside from restrictions of physical activity, other therapeutic measures in patients with severe carditis and congestive heart failure include oxygen administration, diuretics, and digitalis. Salt and water restriction may also be useful in the management of heart failure due to rheumatic carditis. Patients who show progressive cardiac involvement while under observation and maximal medical support should be considered for treatment with adrenal steroids. The efficacy of such treatment is unproven in controlled studies, but temporary suppression of the inflammatory process within the myocardium usually results in a suppression of the symptoms. Anecdotal reports of dramatic, life-saving reversal of congestive heart

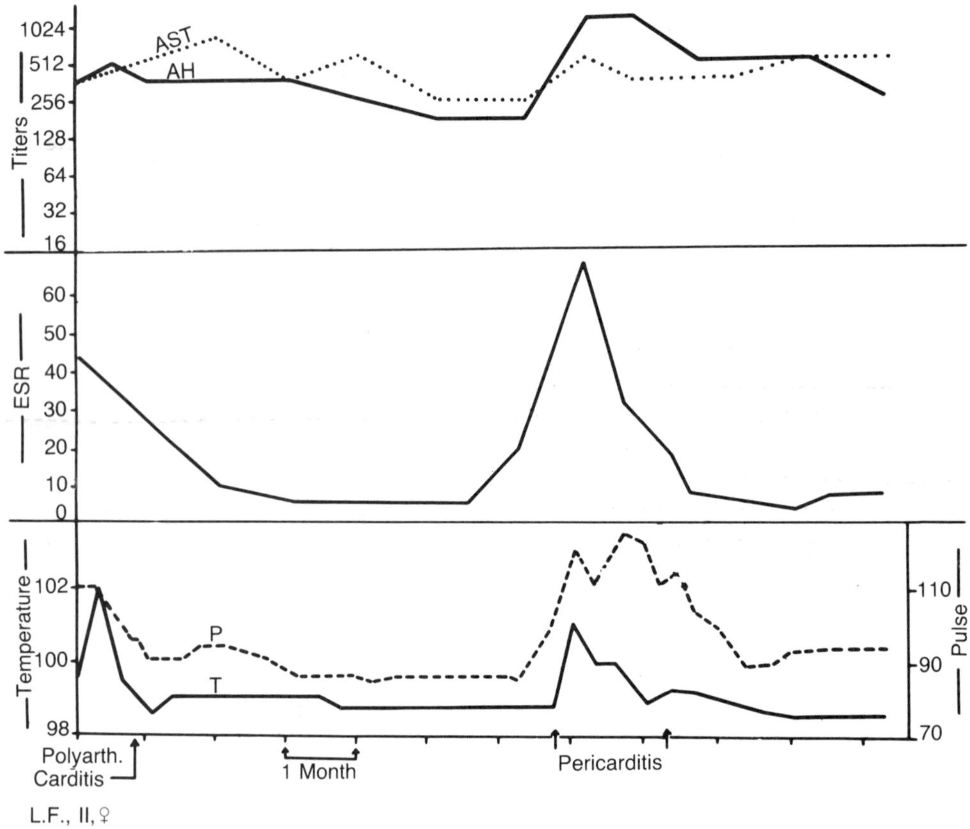

Fig. 25-7. Graphic representation of the clinical and laboratory findings in a patient with a polycyclic course of acute rheumatic fever. Lower panel depicts clinical findings. Middle panel demonstrates concurrent changes in erythrocyte sedimentation rate. Upper panel indicates antistreptococcal antibody titers which remain stable throughout fluctuating clinical course. (Harris TN, Harris S, Nagel RL: Studies in the relation of the hemolytic streptococcus to rheumatic fever. Pediatrics 3:482, 1949. Copyright American Academy of Pediatrics, 1949)

failure by adrenal steroid therapy have appeared.

The majority of rheumatic attacks end spontaneously in 1 to 4 months. Identifying the time when rheumatic activity ceases is sometimes difficult and is based on arbitrary clinical judgment. In general, the rheumatic episode may be considered terminated when all the clinical and laboratory evidence of the disease has disappeared or has reached a plateau. Further useful indications of inactivity of the rheumatic process are (1) spontaneous rise of hemoglobin, (2) spontaneous weight gain, (3) disappearance of rheumatic pallor, (4) favorable changes in the patient's personality, (5) disappearance of wide diurnal variations in body temperature, (6) nonoccurrence of tachycardia following minor trials of physical exertion, (7) disappearance of minor variations in cardiac rhythm and (8) slow sleeping pulse rate. As a general guide, patients with no overt evidence of carditis are kept at bedrest for a minimum of 6 weeks, those with overt carditis for a minimum of 3 months.

Prevention

There are two aspects to the prevention of rheumatic fever: (1) secondary prevention, the prevention of recurrences of rheumatic fever in known rheumatic subjects by the daily oral administration of antistreptococcal agents; and (2) primary prevention, the prevention of either initial or recurrent attacks of rheumatic fever by the prompt and vigorous treatment of streptococcal infection. The basis for prevention is the interruption of the relationship between infection with beta-hemolytic streptococcus and the etiologic mechanism of rheumatic fever.

All patients with a history of rheumatic fever or chorea, especially those who show evidence of rheumatic heart disease, should be placed on long-term antistreptococcal prophylaxis. The prophylaxis should be continued throughout life or until new information demonstrates that such prolonged administration is unnecessary. Prophylaxis should be continuous. For the prevention of streptococcal infection in known rheumatic subjects, the current recommended dosage of sulfonamides is 0.5 g daily for persons under 60 lb and 1 g daily for those over 60 lb. For penicillin, the recommended oral dosage is 400,000 units of penicillin G given daily on a fasting stomach. A single intramuscular injection of a slow-releasing preparation of penicillin such as Benzathine penicillin given at 4-week intervals has been demonstrated to be equally effective for antistreptococcal prophylaxis.

Penicillin is the drug of choice for primary prevention of rheumatic fever and should be continued for a period of 10 days. Effectiveness is based upon the bactericidal quality of penicillin against beta-hemolytic streptococci and is dependent upon the total eradication of streptococci from the throat. Penicillin may be administered either intramuscularly or orally. Occasionally the failure of such treatment to prevent rheumatic sequelae has been reported. In most instances, failure of the antistreptococcal treatment to completely eradicate the organism has been responsible.

CARDIAC ARRHYTHMIAS

The frequency of cardiac arrhythmias in the pediatric age group is far lower than among adult cardiac patients, in whom degenerative heart disease is the predominant pathologic process. The cardiac arrhythmias of rheumatic heart disease are benign and relatively uncommon. Temporary first-degree heart block, occasional premature supraventricular or ventricular contractions, and rare instances of complete heart block occur during acute rheumatic carditis. In rare instances in childhood, auricular fibrillation and auricular flutter may occur in the chronic active form of rheumatic heart involvement. Myocardial disease (*e.g.*, diphtheritic myocarditis, Kawasaki's disease) of any form may be an etiologic focus of arrhythmias. The cardiac arrhythmias observed with congenital heart disease are also rare and usually indicate a deteriorating state of myocardial function due to hypoxia or other deleterious causes. Arrhythmias are not unusual in patients following surgery for congenital heart disease, and they may pose a serious threat. A congenital anomaly of conduction manifest by a short PR interval and a prolonged QRS duration was described by Wolff, Parkinson, and White in 1930 and is known to predispose to tachyarrhythmias.

Benign Arrhythmias

The most common arrhythmia of childhood is *sinus arrhythmia.* This represents a phasic variation in the cardiac rate usually associated with respiration. It is a benign arrhythmia *per se* and indeed a normal variation; occasionally it occurs as an early manifestation of digitalis toxicity. *Sinus arrest* is another benign cardiac arrhythmia of childhood. Another common arrhythmia is the sporadic appearance of premature contractions originating from atrial, nodal, or ventricular foci. These occur rarely in the course of myocarditis or myocardial dysfunction and are occasionally a result of digitalis intoxication. More commonly, premature contractions from any focus occur without any other evidence of heart disease. Under these circumstances, the condition is benign, and it is safe to attempt no specific treatment and urge no restriction of physical activity.

Paroxysmal Supraventricular Tachycardia

Two serious cardiac arrhythmias are encountered in the pediatric age group, paroxysmal supraventricular tachycardia and congenital heart block. Paroxysmal supraventricular tachycardia is of special importance in young infants because it can precipitate a true medical emergency requiring prompt and precise treatment for survival. Cardiac rates between 200 and 400 beats/minute are common; congestive heart failure may develop within a few hours because of poor coronary artery perfusion and poor ventricular filling associated with extreme shortening of the diastolic interval. Many patients are not brought to medical attention until after the onset of congestive heart failure, especially the young infant who cannot transmit any feeling of discomfort. Patients first encountered at this phase of the disease may die within minutes or hours unless the tachyarrhythmia can be converted.

Many patients with paroxysmal supraventricular tachycardia are male newborn infants in whom no other evidence of heart disease can be found. The diagnosis is made by the detection of a very rapid cardiac rate and the presence of signs and symptoms of congestive heart failure, if tachycardia has persisted for more than 12 to 24 hours. Confirmation of the diagnosis requires an electrocardiogram; the tracing shows a very regular and rapid rate varying between 200 and 400 beats/minute. The QRS complexes are of normal duration and the P waves are usually not visible. The recording is also useful in ruling out the possibility of ventricular tachycardia which requires drug treatment quite different from supraventricular tachycardia.

The prognosis for infants with supraventricular tachycardia is excellent in the absence of any other evidence of heart disease. Recurrences are observed during the first year or two of life and rarely thereafter. Only in a minority of patients with paroxysmal supraventricular tachycardia is a detectable etiology manifest. The common causative factors are intercurrent infection, organic heart disease, and the abnormal conduction mechanism described by Wolff, Parkinson, and White.

The majority of patients with supraventricular tachycardia respond promptly to digitalization. A few require other medications such as propranolol or quinidine. In severe congestive heart failure and impending demise, direct current cardioversion may save the patient's life. In young infants it is wise to maintain digoxin medication for 6 to 12 months following an episode of paroxysmal tachycardia in order to defer a possible recurrence until the child is older and more tolerant of the insult of an extremely rapid heart rate.

Congenital Heart Block

Congenital heart block is a rare but important cardiac arrhythmia of infancy and childhood. Its earliest detection may occur *in utero*; the slow rate may be mistaken as a sign of fetal distress and therefore as an indication for cesarean section. Approximately half of the infants with congenital heart block have additional congenital intracardiac anomalies.

Symptoms usually are not produced by complete heart block unless the cardiac rate becomes excessively slow; this rarely occurs in infancy and early childhood. Extreme slowing of the cardiac rate may occur in the second decade of life. Cardiac rates below 40 beats/minute may lead to dizziness and syncope. Major episodes of syncope with loss of consciousness or death (Stokes-Adams syndrome) may be observed with congenital heart block. With technical improvements in pacemakers, the occurrence of even a single attack of Stokes-Adams syndrome should be considered an indication for artificial pacing.

The diagnosis of complete heart block can be made from the electrocardiogram. The tracing will show a lack of relationship between the atrial activity (P waves) and the QRS complexes representing ventricular activity. In the absence of intracardiac anomalies, the prognosis varies with the duration of the QRS complexes. The prognosis is best with a short QRS duration and least favorable with prolonged QRS duration.

HIGH CARDIAC OUTPUT STATES

A number of pathologic conditions may produce severe states of high cardiac output in the pediatric age group. Profound disturbances in cardiac function may result from the high stroke volume, increased circulating blood volume, and accelerated velocity of blood flow. Congestive heart failure, responsive only to the elimination of the cause of the high cardiac output state, may ensue.

The most common clinical state producing a high cardiac output is chronic anemia. To produce congestive heart failure, anemia must be long-standing with a level of hemoglobin below 5 g/dl. In patients with intrinsic heart disease in addition to severe anemia, congestive heart failure may appear at higher hemoglobin levels.

High cardiac output state in childhood is also that produced by a systemic arteriovenous fistula—in the cerebral circulation (vein of Galen aneurysm), in the coronary circuit, at the site of vascular tumors such as in hemangiomata of the liver, or in peripheral arteriovenous connections, either congenital or acquired (Fig. 25-8). Acquired arteriovenous connections may result from trauma, especially following arterial punctures, as in a renal biopsy. A rare cause of high cardiac output state in pediatrics is hyperthyroidism.

The physical findings in the high output states include a wide pulse pressure, with a slightly elevated systolic blood pressure and a distinctly lowered diastolic pressure. The arterial pulses are bounding in quality. A low-pitched systolic murmur of the ejection type is present over the midprecordium. A variety of graphic studies have demonstrated the physical similarity between this type of murmur and a functional or innocent murmur. Transmission of the systolic murmur to the posterior chest wall is common in the high cardiac output states. Occasionally a mid-diastolic apical murmur of relative mitral stenosis will be heard due to the accelerated velocity of blood flow at the mitral valve during the period of diastolic filling of the left ventricle. Cardiomegaly and evi-

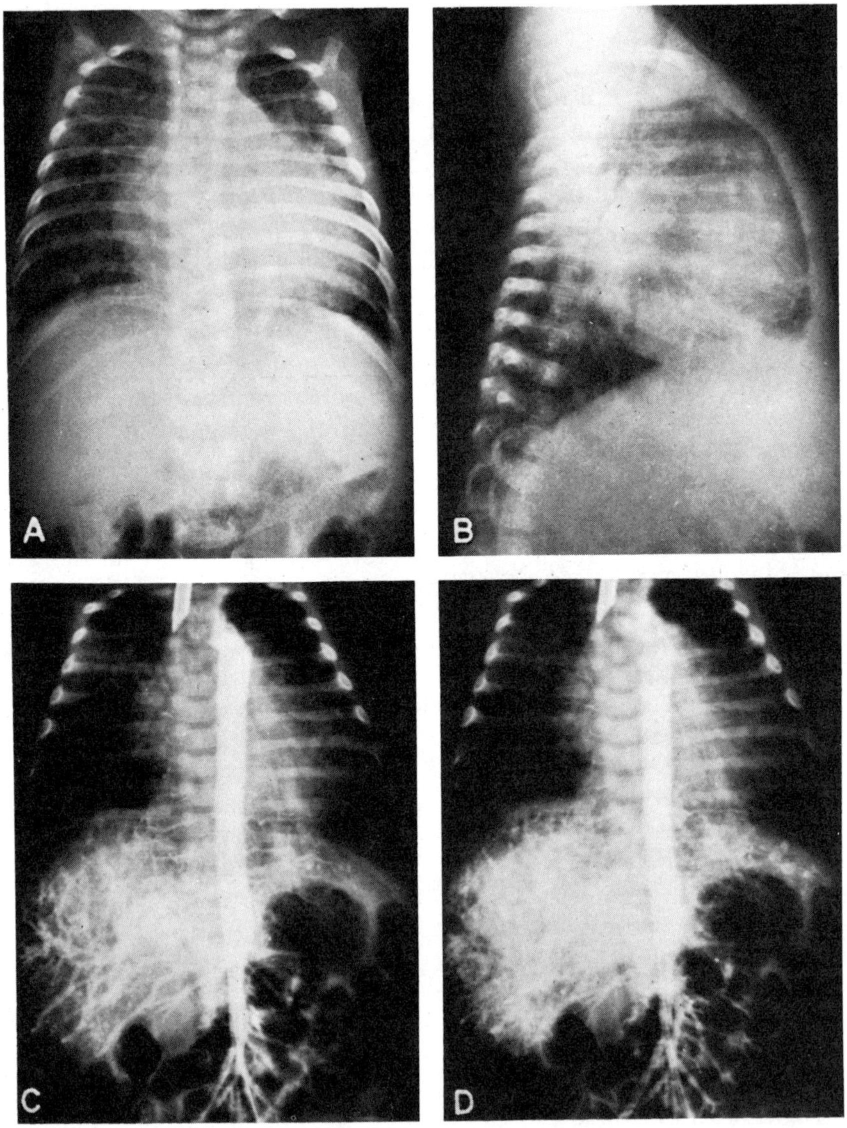

Fig. 25-8. Chest radiographs in the anterior-posterior (*A*) and lateral (*B*) views in infant with congestive heart failure resulting from multiple hemangiomata of liver acting as an arteriovenous fistula. Note cardiomegaly and prominent pulmonary vascular markings, similar to those seen with congenital heart disease. Abdominal aortogram (*C* and *D*) demonstrates multiple arterio-venous communications within the liver.

dence of left ventricular hypertrophy in the electrocardiogram complete the picture.

There may be particular difficulty in differentiating the cardiac findings in a patient with a high output cardiac state due to a hidden arteriovenous fistula from the manifestations of congenital heart disease. This problem is accentuated in early infancy and in the presence of congestive heart failure. Occasionally the diagnosis of systemic arteriovenous fistula can be suspected from auscultation if a continuous murmur is discovered that indicates a flow of blood through the fistula during both systole and diastole. Auscultation over the cranium, liver, or other suspected areas reveal the presence of a continuous murmur. Visible vascular tumors involving the skin or mucous membranes should arouse suspicion of the possibility of a generalized distribution of such tumors including hidden sites. Hypertrophy of individual extremities or portions thereof may result from vascular anomalies. Variations in surface temperature or discoloration of extremities may provide a clue to the presence of a vascular abnormality. Prominent pulsating jugular veins may be observed in the presence of a cerebral arteriovenous fistula; a loud cervical venous hum may be heard. During cardiac catheterization, the presence of highly oxygenated blood specimens from the jugular vein, superior vena cava, and right atrium compared with the inferior vena cava may result from the arteriovenous shunting within the cerebral circulation.

In radiographs of the chest obtained from patients with large systemic arteriovenous fistulas, the pulmonary vascular markings may be accentuated and mimic the plethora of pulmonary blood flow observed with intracardiac arteriovenous shunting. This radiographic feature results from an increase in circulating blood volume and the associated increase in pulmonary blood flow; mild pulmonary hypertension may also result from the overdistention of the pulmonary vascular bed.

While temporary benefit may be obtained from the symptomatic measures used in the treatment of congestive heart failure, the cardiopathy of high cardiac output states responds dramatically to the elimination of the cause. Transfusion of whole blood or packed red blood cells usually relieves the cardiac problem in chronic anemia; the surgical division of an arteriovenous fistula similarly produces a striking improvement in the cardiac difficulties in the presence of a large arteriovenous fistula. Hyperthyroidism can be treated medically or surgically or by radiotherapy.

PRIMARY MYOCARDIAL DISEASES OF INFANCY

The term *primary myocardial diseases of infancy* describes an artificial but useful category of cardiac lesions observed in small infants with cardiomegaly and congestive heart failure who have no significant cardiac murmurs and hence are unlikely to have congenital heart disease. Anemia and hypertension are absent. All these infants have evidence of left ventricular hypertrophy and left ventricular myocardial changes in the electrocardiogram.

The etiology of the lesions included in this category are not uniform: (1) interstitial myocarditis, probably of infectious (viral) origin with multiple offending agents, (2) endocardial fibroelastosis, a disease of unknown etiology which probably represents a nonspecific tissue response to injury, (3) glycogen storage disease, type II, a hereditary metabolic disorder, and (4) a congenital cardiovascular anomaly, of aberrant origin of the left coronary artery from the pulmonary artery. Each of these conditions of diverse etiology produces the same clinical and electrocardiographic manifestations, thereby constituting a useful diagnostic category. Several other vary rare conditions such as medial necrosis of the coronary arteries, involvement of the coronary arteries with polyarteritis nodosa, and amyloid invasion of the myocardium can also produce a similar picture in infancy.

Interstitial Myocarditis

Myocarditis in infancy, especially in the newborn period, is not uncommon, and is usually of viral origin. Epidemics of myocarditis resulting from infection with Coxsackie B virus have been reported from a number of newborn nurseries. The viruses of mumps, chickenpox, rubella, and the protozoan parasite, toxoplasmosis, have been implicated, but in many instances the specific agent is not demonstrable.

The manifestations of myocarditis include tachycardia, cardiac enlargement, and congestive heart failure in the absence of significant cardiac murmurs. The electrocardiogram often shows nonspecific myocardial changes including T-wave inversion, P-R interval prolongation, ST segment depression, and a variety of cardiac arrhythmias. Left ventricular hypertrophy is usually seen in the electrocardiogram, but a diffuse and balanced involvement of both ventricles may also be present.

The treatment of myocarditis in infancy is symptomatic and includes supportive measures such as digitalis, diuretics, oxygen, and salt and fluid restriction. Occasionally adrenal hormone therapy has been useful in temporarily suppressing the inflammation and edema of the myocardium. Approximately 50% of patients with myocarditis recover and show no evidence of residual heart disease. It is the lesion with the best prognosis in the category of primary myocardial disease of infancy.

Endocardial Fibroelastosis

In *endocardial fibroelastosis*, the endocardium becomes thickened and rigid; this castlike structure replaces the endocardial layer of the heart and interferes with ventricular filling as well as ventricular contractility. The left-sided chambers are involved most often although instances of 4-chamber involvement have been reported.

Congestive heart failure is often the initial manifestation, usually precipitated by a respiratory tract infection during the third to sixth month of life. Physical examination reveals only cardiomegaly in the absence of a cardiac murmur. Occasionally involvement of the papillary muscles attached to the mitral valve leaflets produce the murmur of mitral insufficiency. The chest roentgenogram shows cardiomegaly, primarily left atrial and left ventricular. The electrocardiogram provides evidence of left ventricular hypertrophy with T-wave abnormalities in the leads, reflecting left ventricular activity, leads I and V 5–7.

There is usually a favorable initial response to digitalization and other symptomatic measures. However, subsequent episodes of congestive heart failure, often precipitated by intercurrent infection, are less responsive. Death often occurs around the age of 2 years, usually with serious cardiac arrhythmias. In some instances, the process may become arrested and the child may survive for a decade or more.

In the primary form of endocardial fibroelastosis, no other evidence of heart disease is present. Secondary forms of endocardial fibroelastosis occur in congenital cardiac anomalies, usually left-sided obstructive lesions. Histopathologic examination of the endocardium permits identification of the primary and secondary forms.

Glycogen Storage Disease of the Heart and Skeletal Muscles

Type II glycogen storage disease is often referred to as Pompe's disease or cardiac glycogenosis. It is now known to be caused by the absence of a specific enzyme, acid maltase, essential for the breakdown of glycogen in striated muscle cells. When the enzyme is absent, glycogen is stored excessively in the cells of voluntary muscles and the syncytium of the myocardium. The glycogen eventually interferes with the contracting function of the involved muscles. Generalized skeletal muscle weakness and myocardial failure result.

Pompe's disease follows a mendelian genetic pattern of transmission and multiple cases may occur in a single family. Clinical manifestations include the discovery of cardiomegaly in the absence of cardiac murmurs. The electrocardiogram is striking in its demonstration of a short P-R interval (less than 0.07 sec), very high amplitude QRS complexes, and marked ST segment and T-wave changes. Left lower lobe atelectasis is very common because the enlarged heart compresses the left lower lobe bronchus. Death usually occurs in early infancy because of respiratory muscle weakness, aspiration, atelectasis, and pneumonitis. Congestive heart failure rarely is the cause of death, but marked cardiac enlargement is the rule.

Aberrant Origin of the Left Coronary Artery from the Pulmonary Artery

In this congenital cardiovascular anomaly, the left ventricular myocardium is perfused at low pressure with venous blood from the pulmonary artery by way of the left coronary which arises from the main pulmonary artery. This results in infarctlike changes in the left ventricular myocardium, often involving some of the papillary muscles attached to the mitral valve leaflets. As a result, cardiomegaly and congestive heart failure appear in the first month or two of life. Occasionally it is observed that infants with this anomaly have clinical episodes suggesting angina. In rare instances, rupture of the left ventricular myocardium may occur with the complication of hemopericardium and cardiac tamponade.

The physical findings include cardiomegaly, a prominent left ventricular impulse on palpation, the murmur of mitral insufficiency in 20% of cases, and eventually congestive heart failure. Because of the potential for surgical treatment, all patients with primary myocardial disease of infancy should be studied by cardiac catheterization with the possible exception of those with obvious glycogen storage disease. The aberrant origin of the left coronary artery should be established and the direction of blood flow in the left coronary artery determined by cineangiography and oximetry. If the left coronary artery is acting as a venous conduit in an arteriovenous connection, with the right coronary artery as the arterial source, ligation of the left coronary artery improves myocardial perfusion as does the introduction of a graft from the aorta or one of its branches to the anomalous left coronary artery. If the direction of blood flow in the aberrant left coronary artery is from the pulmonary artery into the myocardium, ligation is harmful. Intractable congestive heart failure is an indication for surgical treatment.

MISCELLANEOUS CARDIAC DISEASES OF CHILDHOOD

Some of the common varieties of cardiac disease encountered in infancy and childhood have been reviewed briefly; a large number of less common examples of cardiac involvement is recognized. Among these are the cardiac components of systemic diseases, such as the cardiac involvement in collagen diseases and rheumatoid arthritis. A serious aspect of acute glomerulonephritis is acute hypertensive cardiovascular disease. Cor pulmonale occurs in childhood; the most common causes are the chronic lung diseases of cystic fibrosis and upper airway obstruction. Cardiac manifestations are sometimes evident with hyper- and hypothyroidism. Neuromuscular dystrophies frequently include cardiac involvement. In somatic syndromes such as mongolism, Noonan's syndrome, arachnodactyly, and gargoylism, a specific cardiopathy exists. Finally, the early origins of arteriosclerosis and the prevention of this common variety of adult heart disease by measures applied in the pediatric age group are currently under intensive study.

BIBLIOGRAPHY

Abbott ME: Atlas of Congenital Cardiac Disease. New York, American Heart Association, 1936

Primarily of historical interest. The first organized treatise on congenital heart disease.

Conn HL, Horwitz O: Acute rheumatic fever. *In* Cardiac and Vascular Disease, pp 757–783. Philadelphia, Lea & Febiger, 1971

A complete treatment of rheumatic fever and rheumatic heart disease as they occur among pediatric patients.

Markowitz M, Kuttner AG: Rheumatic Fever: Diagnosis. Management and Prevention. Philadelphia, WB Saunders, 1965

An excellent review of all current considerations concerning rheumatic fever in the form of a small volume [185 pages]; includes a section on community health services.

Nadas AS, Fyler DC: Pediatric Cardiology. Philadelphia, WB Saunders, 1972

A clinically oriented reference book on entire subject of cardiac disease in infancy and childhood.

Perloff JK: The Clinical Recognition of Congenital Heart Disease. Philadelphia, WB Saunders, 1970

A complete and excellent review of the lesions of congenital heart disease with special emphasis on application of physical findings, particularly auscultation in diagnosis.

Rashkind WJ: The cyanotic newborn: approach to diagnosis and treatment. Cardiovasc Clin 4:277–280, 1972

Roberts NK, Gelband H (eds): Cardiac Arrhythmias in the Neonate, Infant and Child. New York, Appleton-Century-Crofts, 1977

A series of contributions from leaders in the field concerning the clinical problems encountered in dealing with arrhythmias of pediatric patients.

Williams RG, Tucker, CR: Echocardiographic Diagnosis of Congenital Heart Disease. Waltham, Massachusetts, Little, Brown & Co., 1977

A book which relates the clinical experience of the authors in use of the M-mode echocardiogram in solving the diagnostic problems of congenital heart disease.

Ziegler RF: Electrocardiographic Studies in Normal Infants and Children. Springfield, Ill, Charles C Thomas, 1951

A basic reference for electrocardiographic standard in pediatrics, including a careful statistical evaluation of all standard EKG values.

Bronchial Asthma

26

Eliot H. Dunsky

Bronchial asthma is a major cause of chronic disease among children. It can be defined as an obstructive airway disease characterized by recurrent episodes of bronchospasm with a significant degree of reversibility. The main pathologic features include bronchial smooth muscle spasm, mucosal edema, and accumulation of thick tenacious mucus within the bronchial lumen. All contribute toward the obstruction of the airway. The obstructive interference with ventilation produces the clinical picture characterized by coughing, shortness of breath, and wheezing. In asthmatic children, there is typically an increased responsiveness of the bronchi to various stimuli, resulting in a narrowing of the airway. The key points that differentiate bronchial asthma from other obstructive lung diseases are its "twitchy" bronchi which tend to narrow upon minimal stimulation and the characteristic reversible nature of the obstruction.

ETIOLOGY

The bronchospasm is episodic in nature, followed by asymptomatic periods of varying lengths. A smaller number of more severely affected children may have continuous symptoms with marked exacerbations of bronchospasm occurring intermittently. Clinically, these children may present with a history of recurrent paroxysms of coughing, dyspnea, and wheezing. Some authors refer to asthma as a symptom complex rather than a disease because of the diverse etiologic factors that may produce the disorder.

In recognition of the heterogeneity of bronchial asthma, attempts at classification have been undertaken. Initially, asthma was separated into two major subgroups. In one group, extrinsic asthma or allergic asthma, symptoms are caused by the inhalation of a specific allergen (*e.g.*, pollens). This reaction is known to be immunologically induced and associated with mast cell release of mediators that can produce bronchospasm. The other major group is intrinsic bronchial asthma or nonallergic asthma, in which no immunologic mechanism has been identified. Affected patients appear to have hyperirritable or "twitchy" airways. Thus, significant airway obstruction may be induced by the inhalation of nonspecific air pollutants or by respiratory tract infections. Additional types of bronchial asthma that do not fit within either one of these two categories include exercise-induced and aspirin-induced asthma.

In order to explain the diverse etiologies producing what superficially appears to be a single clinical disorder, it has been proposed that asthmatics have a common underlying defect in or partial blockade of their beta-adrenergic receptors. Stimulation of the beta-receptors produces relaxation of smooth muscle (*i.e.*, bronchodilation).

The bronchial tree contains beta-receptors which promote bronchodilation. Stimulation of these pulmonary B_2 receptors by catecholamines (*e.g.*, epinephrine, isoproterenol) activates the target organ membrane enzyme, adenyl cyclase, converting adenosine triphosphate (ATP) to 3′,5′-cyclic adenosine monophosphate (cyclic AMP or C-AMP). An increase in C-AMP results in bronchodilation as well as the suppression of certain allergic reactions. Therefore, a defect in the beta-adrenergic receptor would predispose toward the development of bronchospasm even upon modest stimulation of the tracheobronchial tree.

In addition to this postulated biochemical defect, it has long been recognized that bronchial asthma and allergy tend to occur with greater frequency in the offspring of asthmatic families. It has been suggested that asthma may be due to an autosomal dominant gene with incomplete penetrance. Up to one-half of asthmatic patients have a positive family history, while the incidence of asthma in a control population is less than 10%.

INCIDENCE

Asthma in children most frequently has its onset during the first five years. A recent United States National Health Survey reports that the overall incidence of allergy is 32.8% in children under 17. One-third suffer from bronchial asthma. Among younger children, asthma occurs about twice as frequently in males as in females. In older children, the proportion of males to females is approximately equal. The most severe forms of asthma begin very early in life and affect more males than females.

MORBIDITY AND MORTALITY

The magnitude of asthma morbidity was documented in the U.S. National Health Survey; 22.9% of all school days lost due to chronic disease was attributed to asthma. These statistics reflect only a part of the disability caused by asthma. The inability to compete effectively in sports, poor performance in school, and a general lack of energy are a few of the many sequelae of incompletely controlled bronchial asthma.

Approximately 200 childhood deaths due to bronchial asthma occur each year, yielding a mortality rate about 2 per 100,000. A much higher rate prevails in adults.

Autopsies performed on children who died of asthma reveal airway obstruction due to a narrowed bronchial lumen filled with inspissated mucus and epithelial debris. The lining of the respiratory mucosa is swollen and infiltrated with inflammatory cells including large numbers of eosinophils. Bronchial basement membrane thickening, hypertrophy of the bronchial smooth muscle, and mucous gland hyperplasia and hypertrophy are frequent findings.

Asthmatic deaths have been attributed to: asphyxia due to respiratory failure, the use of sedatives or tranquilizers that may suppress the respiratory drive, the abuse of sympathomimetic inhalers, aminophylline toxicity, and inadequate use of corticosteroid supplement in steroid-dependent asthmatics.

BETA-ADRENERGIC BLOCKADE AND CYCLIC NUCLEOTIDES

Two cyclic nucleotides, cyclic 3′,5′-adenosine monophosphate (cyclic AMP) and cyclic 3′,5′-guanosine monophosphate (cyclic

GMP), may be important in asthma since they appear to play a regulatory role in both mediator release and bronchial smooth muscle tone.

An increase in intracellular cyclic AMP suppresses the release of mast cell mediators and promotes bronchodilation. Conversely, an increase in the opposing nucleotide, cyclic GMP, promotes both the release of mediators and bronchospasm. The level of cellular cyclic AMP is increased by stimulation of the cell's beta$_2$-receptor by catecholamines (*e.g.*, isoproterenol and epinephrine). On the other hand, stimulation of alpha-adrenergic receptors on these cells by agents such as phenylephrine cause a decrease in cyclic AMP. A rise in the cellular level of cyclic GMP opposes the action of cyclic AMP. Cellular cyclic GMP is increased by stimulation of cholinergic receptors (acetylocholine) and suppressed by cholinergic blockade (atropine) (Fig. 26-1).

Additional modulation of the cyclic AMP-GMP enzymes occurs through the actions of prostaglandins E (cyclic AMP ↑) and prostaglandins F$_2\alpha$ (cyclic GMP ↑) and by the enzyme phosphodiesterase, which breaks down cyclic nucleotides. Inhibition of this enzyme appears to be the mechanism of action of the important antiasthmatic drug (theophylline) which indirectly raises the intracellular cyclic AMP. Theophylline acts by increasing intracellular cyclic AMP through inhibition of phosphodiesterase. Corticosteroids appear to enhance catecholamine effects on beta-receptors of the asthmatic, while prostaglandins have different receptors on the cell membrane.

The above factors suggest the basis on which an asthmatic patient with a partial beta blockade or stimulation of pulmonary cholinergic receptors might have a tendency to develop bronchospasm.

PATHOPHYSIOLOGY OF ASTHMA

Smooth muscle bronchospasm, mucosal edema, and the accumulation of large amounts of thick tenacious mucus diminishing the internal diameter of the bronchial

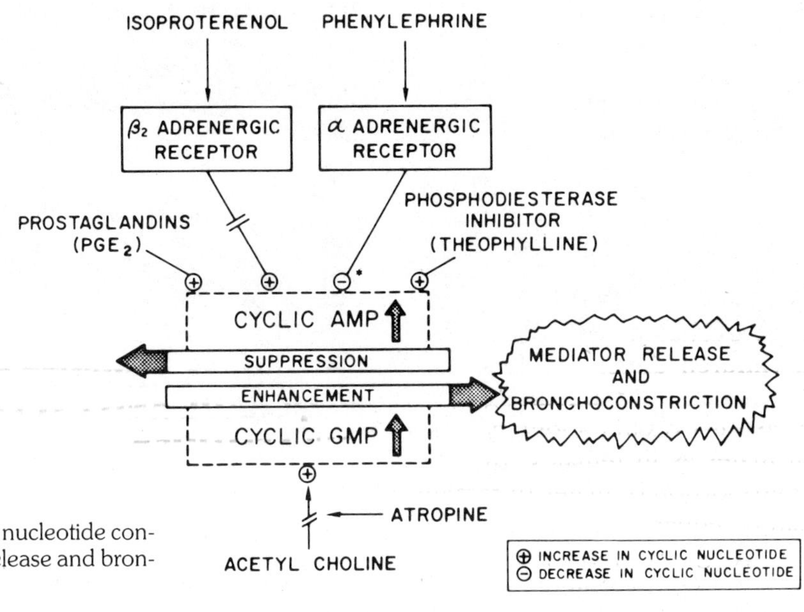

Fig. 26-1. Cyclic nucleotide control of mediator release and broncho-constriction.

lumen are the bases for the airway obstruction in bronchial asthma. Even a small change in the diameter of the lumen produces a relatively large increase in airway resistance since the latter varies inversely to the fourth power of the radius of the lumen

$$\left(R \cong \frac{1}{r^4}\right).$$

Although most of the airway may eventually be involved in severe bronchospasm, it is the small airways (less than 2 mm in diameter) that are usually affected. Since these small airways constitute only 20% of the total airway resistance, it is not surprising that when partially obstructed, few if any symptoms may be manifested. As the medium-sized and large airways become involved, airway resistance quickly and significantly increases, as do symptoms.

During normal inspiration, the bronchi dilate due to transient negative intrapleural pressure (relative to intraluminal pressure) (Fig. 26-2). This is an active process secondary to muscular effort. During the expiratory phase, the elastic tissue of the lungs and thoras tends to passively return to its original position and thus act as the driving force that expels the inhaled air. If bronchial airway obstruction exists, expiration needs to be assisted by muscular compression of the pleural cavity, including forceful elevation of the diaphragm and the use of the accessory muscles of respiration. The compression of the pleural space increases positive pleural pressure. When this transmitted pressure exceeds the intraluminal bronchial pressure, the bronchi narrow or collapse. This is seen dramatically in acute asthma as the patient uses his accessory muscles to force air out of the lungs during a markedly prolonged expiratory phase. As a consequence of the turbulent air flow through narrowed and partially obstructed airways, wheezing is heard on auscultation. As the airway obstruction proceeds, some airways collapse while others continue to function normally. To compensate for the hypoventilated area (distal to the obstructed airways), the patient increases his respiratory rate (tachypnea) and depth of respiration (hyperpnea). To produce the necessary pressure to overcome the increased airway resistance, accessory muscles of respiration are recruited, increasing the work of breathing. Even with prolonged expirations, not all the previously inspired air can be expelled, and a portion remains trapped.

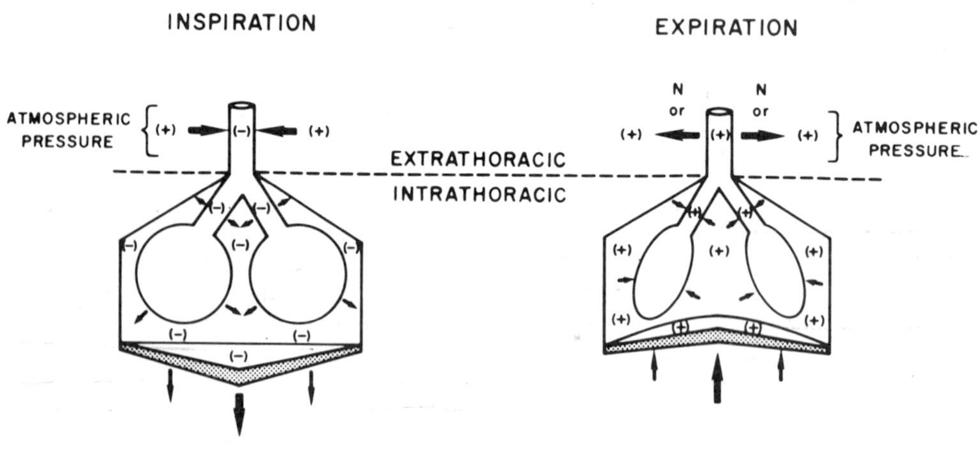

Fig. 26-2. Mechanics of obstructive airway disease.

As trapped air accumulates, the thorax becomes hyperinflated. Pulmonary function studies of asthmatic patients reveal an increase in the residual capacity (air remaining in the lung after forced expiration); these patients will ultimately have clinical and radiologic signs of pulmonary hyperinflation. In addition to increased airway resistance, the asthmatic lung has a decreased compliance, a stiffer lung. Both of these changes increase the work of breathing, which increases oxygen consumption in the already hypoxemic patient. These disturbances of respiratory mechanics are further complicated by a deranged gas exchange. Normally, each terminal respiratory unit (alveolus) is both well ventilated and well perfused. Alveolar oxygen fully saturates perfusing hemoglobin. One of the pathophysiologic characteristics of asthma is the uneven match of ventilation to perfusion. Some alveolae are well ventilated and well perfused. Some are poorly ventilated with normal perfusion, while another group may be well ventilated and poorly perfused due to pulmonary vascular constriction. In hypoventilated well-perfused respiratory units, hemoglobin can only be saturated partially with oxygen. This mismatch of ventilation to perfusion (V/Q) results in partially unsaturated hemoglobin. The remaining normal units which may be hyperventilated (due to tachypnea and hypernea) cannot saturate hemoglobin beyond its maximum carrying capacity (100%).

Partially unsaturated hemoglobin (returning from hypoventilated areas) is mixed with completely saturated hemoglobin (returning from well-ventilated areas) resulting in less than 100% saturation. This situation is analogous to a right-to-left cardiac shunt, since a certain amount of blood bypasses the functioning respiratory units of the lung. The exchange of carbon dioxide under identical circumstances in asthma is very different from that of oxygen. Carbon dioxide is 20 times more diffusible across the respiratory membrane than oxygen. Well-perfused hypoventilating respiratory units may not permit adequate local exchange of any gas including CO_2. During the mild asthma attack, in contrast to oxygen exchange, the remaining hyperventilating respiratory units may exchange (blow off) large amounts of CO_2, more than compensating for those respiratory units that are failing. Arterial blood gases confirm this phenomenon during an acute mild attack of asthma, as patients are usually hypocarbic ($PaCO_2 \downarrow$) in the face of hypoxemia. As the asthmatic attack becomes more severe due to increased airway obstruction, the minute volume (the amount of air exchanged/minute) decreases. A point is reached when the patient's remaining functioning respiratory units begin to hypoventilate and the $PaCO_2$ begins to rise. If the trend persists and medication fails to reverse the respiratory obstruction, the patient may eventually develop respiratory failure.

CLINICAL ASPECTS OF ASTHMA

Bronchial asthma may be classified into five separate groups, although a single patient may have characteristics of more than one group.

Extrinsic Bronchial Asthma

Extrinsic bronchial asthma is allergic asthma due to an IgE-mediated mechanism associated with the release of mast cell mediators. It is induced by an inhaled allergen and frequently there is a good correlation between the onset of symptoms and allergen exposure. For example, the symptoms may occur each year during the months of August and September at the time of ragweed pollination. In some patients, symptoms may follow exposure to dust, molds, feather pillows, or animal dander. Antigen exposure may also produce the signs and symptoms of allergic rhinitis and conjunctivitis. Allergic asthmatic patients usually have positive skin tests to the offending antigen as well as a positive family history for allergy. Many allergic patients with asthma respond to avoidance and specific therapy. Their prognosis is generally better than those with nonallergic (intrinsic) asthma.

Intrinsic Bronchial Asthma

Intrinsic bronchial asthma is characterized by highly irritable bronchi that easily develop bronchospasm upon exposure to nonspecific stimuli. No immunologic mechanism has been implicated. Patients develop asthmatic symptoms following exposure to various stimuli including air pollutants, respiratory tract infections, weather changes, hyperventilation, exposure to cold air, emotional stress. Allergy skin tests are usually negative. Symptoms tend to be perennial or occur mainly during the winter months when respiratory infections are frequently encountered.

Mixed Type Asthma

Patients with *mixed type asthma* have characteristics of intrinsic as well as extrinsic asthma.

Exercise-Induced Asthma or Exercise-Induced Bronchospasm

Exercise-induced bronchospasm (EIB) can be defined as acute bronchospasm following strenuous exercise. Prior to exercise, patients may be asymptomatic and have normal pulmonary functions. Five to ten minutes after strenuous exercise patients may become dyspneic, tachypneic, develop coughing or wheezing. Pulmonary functions indicate significant airway obstruction. These symptoms can be reversed quickly by beta-adrenergic stimulants or subside spontaneously, usually in less than 1 to 2 hours.

Aspirin-Sensitive Asthma

The incidence of aspirin-induced asthma is probably less than 4% among asthmatics. These patients may have a history of a triad of profuse rhinorrhea, hyperplastic sinusitis with nasal polyps, and marked bronchospasm following ingestion of aspirin. The mechanism for this reaction is unknown but does not appear to be immunologic in nature. Both aspirin and indomethacin are prostaglandin inhibitors, and this may underlie this type of asthma.

CLINICAL SIGNS AND SYMPTOMS

The presentation and course of bronchial asthma in children are variable. Symptoms may occur as acute recurrent episodes separated by asymptomatic periods. Other children have continuous symptoms with intermittent exacerbations of severe wheezing. The intensity of the symptoms may vary from mild or even unnoticed to severe, potentially fatal attacks necessitating immediate hospitalization. Asthma often mimics other respiratory diseases, but because its obstructive component is reversible, it differs from other obstructive airway disease.

Asymptomatic Interval in Asthma

The majority of children with asthma have periods in which they look and feel well. Physical examination and pulmonary function tests may be within normal limits. Other asymptomatic asthmatic children demonstrate obstructive changes in pulmonary functions suggesting persistent small airway disease. Still others claim that they are asymptomatic; yet when asked to perform a forced expiration maneuver, numerous wheezes at the end of expiration are audible. These subtle changes are an indication that at least a number of apparently asymptomatic patients have continuing obstructive airway disease and may require further therapy.

Mild Asthmatic Episode

Patients with mild episodes of asthma may develop a dry, hacking cough, mild dyspnea, and a feeling of tightness in the chest. Many may have an elevated respiratory rate. Auscultation of the chest reveals good air entry into both lungs and diffuse wheezing with a prolonged expiratory phase.

Moderate Asthmatic Episode

As the severity of the attack proceeds, the signs and symptoms of the mild attack intensify. Wheezing becomes louder and expiration more prolonged and forceful. Air entry into both lungs may be unequal, or its intensity may be diminished. The respiratory rate increases and hyperpnea develops. There may be a need for use of accessory muscles of respiration, which include flaring of the alae nasi, retraction of the intercostal and subcostal muscles, and prominent excursions of the abdominal musculature.

Severe Episode of Asthma

When tachypnea and hyperpnea become maximal, the patient is in acute respiratory distress and may assume a sitting position, grasping the edge of the bed with the hands, fostering maximal use of accessory muscles. Vomiting and complaints of chest and abdominal pain are frequently encountered. If airway obstruction progresses, breath sounds diminish, often to the point of being inaudible, and as little or no air is being ventilated wheezing may cease entirely. Under such conditions, a "silent chest" is often associated with either respiratory arrest or acute respiratory failure. In the moderate to severe attack of asthma, the physical examination may reveal an increase in the AP diameter of the chest. The shoulders are raised high and remain in a fixed position, and the chest is hyperresonant to percussion. Hypoxia may present clinically as pallor or cyanosis. The lack of oxygen may produce anxiety, irritability, restlessness, or confusion. Signs of hypercarbia include headache, muscle twitching, confusion, somnolence, and finally coma. A technique for assessing the severity of an attack of asthma is measurement of the pulsus paradoxus. The systolic blood pressure during inspiration and expiration is recorded. The greater the difference between the inspiratory and expiratory systolic blood pressures, the more severe the respiratory obstruction.

LABORATORY STUDIES

Sputum

Many asthmatic children swallow their sputum. Some can expectorate, and examination of their sputum provides useful diagnostic information. Eosinophils are often present in large numbers. Charcot-Leyden crystals, thought to be the breakdown product of eosinophils, are frequently associated with Curschmann's spirals (mucoid casts of the bronchioles). Secondary bacterial infections may be suspected when the sputum contains large numbers of neutrophils and bacteria.

Blood Studies

Asthmatic children usually have a normal hemoglobin while children with other chronic pulmonary disease may have secondary polycythemia. The total white count is frequently elevated above 12,000 cells/mm^3 during acute attacks, but is normal when the patient is asymptomatic. Peripheral eosinophilia is observed frequently in both intrinsic and extrinsic asthma. Suppression of the eosinophil count may be used as a guide to the success of drug management (*e.g.*, steroids). Asthmatics usually have normal serum electrolytes, although steroids may induce hypokalemia.

Radiographic Findings

Asymptomatic patients and those with mild asthma frequently have normal chest radiographs. In more severely affected subjects, radiographic changes include: pulmonary hyperinflation, depressed or flattened diaphragms, increase in the anteroposterior diameter of the chest, and prominent hilar bronchovascular markings. Following resolution of an acute attack, many of these findings disappear. Persistence of hyperinflation may be a sign of moderate to severe chronic disease. Some of the pulmonary complications seen on radiograph in asthmatic patients are: atelectasis, pneumomediastinum, pneumothorax, pneumopericardium, and pneumonia.

Arterial Blood Gases and Asthma

Arterial blood gases are the best means for assessment of respiratory function in acute asthma. Between asthmatic episodes, blood gases are often normal ($PaO_2 = 90 \pm 5$ mm Hg, $PaCO_2 = 40 \pm 4$ mm Hg and pH $= 7.4 \pm 0.05$). However, a small group of asymptomatic patients have a diminished PaO_2.

Hypoxemia of varying degrees is often noted in patients recovering from an acute attack of status asthmaticus for periods up to 6 weeks. During the mild paroxysm of asthma the child hyperventilates. Arterial blood gases at that time reveal a decrease in the $PaCO_2$ (hypocarbia) and a decrease in the PaO_2 (hypoxemia) (Fig. 26-3). As the attack progresses to moderate obstruction, the child can no longer hyperventilate and his minute volume decreases. Therefore, the $PaCO_2$ rises, often to a level that appears to be normal (40 ± 5 mm). Although the $PaCO_2$, in this instance, is normal, it represents a decompensatory phase and may herald subsequent respiratory failure. Finally, as bronchial obstruction becomes maximal, the muscles of respiration become fatigued, minute volume decreases further, and $PaOC_2$ continues to rise. When the $PaCO_2$ reaches 55 mm, the situation can be defined as impending respiratory failure, and at 65 mm the patient is considered in frank respiratory failure.

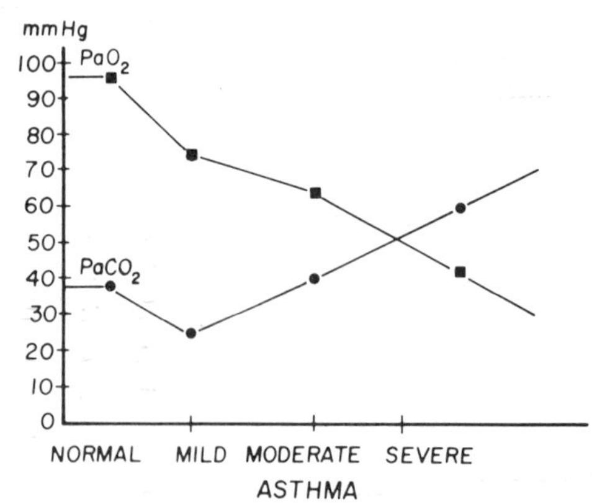

Fig. 26-3. Arterial blood gases in acute bronchial asthma.

Pulmonary function studies frequently used in the assessment and management of asthma include: peak expiratory flow rates (PEFR), vital capacity (VC), forced expiratory volume in one second (FEV_1), and maximal midexpiratory flow rate (MMEFR) (Fig. 26-4). The peak expiratory flow rate is quick and easy to perform, especially if serial measurements are required; PEFR reflects conductance in the larger upper airways. FEV_1, the amount of air that can be forcibly expelled in one second, mostly measures larger but also some small airway resistance; it is effort-dependent. Normally, the FEV_1 represents about 86 ± 7% of the vital capacity of the normal child; lower values indicate obstructive airway disease. Asymptomatic asthmatic children may have normal pulmonary function; however, some may have small airway obstructive disease not picked up in study of the FEV_1 or the PEFR. Therefore, an earlier objective sign of obstructive airway disease may be reflected in an abnormal measurement of small airway resistance such as the maximal midexpiratory flow rate (MMEFR). This value represents the mean flow rate in the middle portion of the forced expiratory volume. The MMEFR is often the earliest spirographic sign of airway obstruction and is frequently the last to return to normal after an acute attack. In addition to evaluating the degree of obstructive disease at any time, an inhaled bronchodilator will reveal the degree of reversibility of the airway obstruction. Pulmonary functions are taken before and after the administration of isoproterenol. Most asthmatics with bronchospasm have an increase of more than 15% to 20% in their PEFR or their FEV_1. Patients with chronic bronchitis, emphysema, and other obstructive diseases have less than 15% reversible obstructive airway disease. Significant reversibility of airway obstruction is the basis of the diagnosis of asthma.

Total and Specific IgE Levels

Many childhood asthmatics have an elevated total IgE which suggests the presence of allergy. Children with either historical evidence or signs of respiratory allergy require skin testing or RAST (radioallergosorbent tests, Fig. 26-5) to identify the specific allergic etiology.

Allergy Skin Testing

Scratch, prick (puncture), and intradermal allergy skin testing traditionally are used in an evaluation of specific allergy. A sensitive person has an immediate hypersensitive reaction at the punctured site. This is interpreted as evidence of specific IgE class antibodies directed against the tested allergen. Within 15 minutes, a hive (wheal and

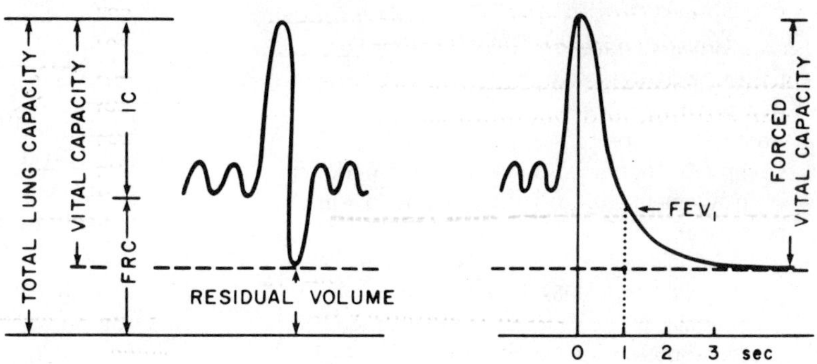

Fig. 26-4. Pulmonary spirometry and lung volumes. IC = Inspiratory capacity; FRC = Functional residual capacity; FEV_1 = Forced expiratory volume in one second.

flare) will develop. The size of the reaction is related to the degree of sensitivity.

Radioallergosorbent Technique (RAST)

The RAST test is an *in vitro* technique capable of measuring specific IgE. Specific antigen (*e.g.*, ragweed) bound to a solid disk or bead is mixed with the test serum. Both the patient's IgG and IgE antiragweed antibodies adhere to the bound antigen. After washing, radioactive anti-IgE is added to the mixture. Since the radiolabeled anti-IgE will bind only to the IgE present, there will be a correlation between the amount of measurable radioactivity and the amount of antigen specific IgE present (Fig. 26-5).

DIFFERENTIAL DIAGNOSIS

The signs and symptoms of asthma can simulate those of a variety of disease states. In the majority of instances the diagnosis is readily established.

Differential Diagnosis of Childhood Asthma

Upper Airway Disorders
- Foreign bodies
- Croup
- Laryngo- and tracheomalacia
- Retropharyngeal and peritonsillar abscess
- Aspiration syndromes

Lower Airway Disorders
- Foreign body aspiration
- Aspiration syndromes
- Vascular ring compression
- Compression of airways due to lymph node enlargement (*e.g.*, tuberculosis), neoplasm, congenital abnormalities (*e.g.*, lobar emphysema).
- Bronchiolitis, bronchitis, bronchiectasis
- Pneumonia, primary (viral, bacterial, fungal) or secondary to underlying disease
- Immunodeficiency
- Cystic fibrosis
- Hypersensitivity pneumonitis
- Allergic bronchopulmonary aspergillosis
- Alpha-1-antitrypsin deficiency
- Persistent atelectasis
- Loeffler's syndrome
- Congestive heart failure

Foreign Bodies

Foreign bodies may be lodged anywhere along the airway. A history of sudden onset of coughing, stridor, and respiratory distress are frequent. However, symptoms may develop more gradually. Foreign objects in the esophagus can cause obstruction through pressure on the trachea and may be accompanied by difficulty in swallowing. Foreign body obstruction in the upper airway may be diagnosed by a lateral neck radiograph or may necessitate endoscopy.

Croup, Bronchiolitis, and Cystic Fibrosis

Laryngotracheobronchitis, epiglotitis, and bronchiolitis are discussed in Chapter 33. Cystic fibrosis is considered in Chapter 23.

Immunodeficiency

Patients with hypogammaglobulinemia may have a history of recurrent respiratory tract infections characterized by pneumonia, coughing, and wheezing. They often have impaired lymph node, tonsillar, and adenoidal development. Quantitative immunoglobin determinations define the deficiency in most cases. Patients with defects in their cellular immune system or with severe combined immunodeficiency are fre-

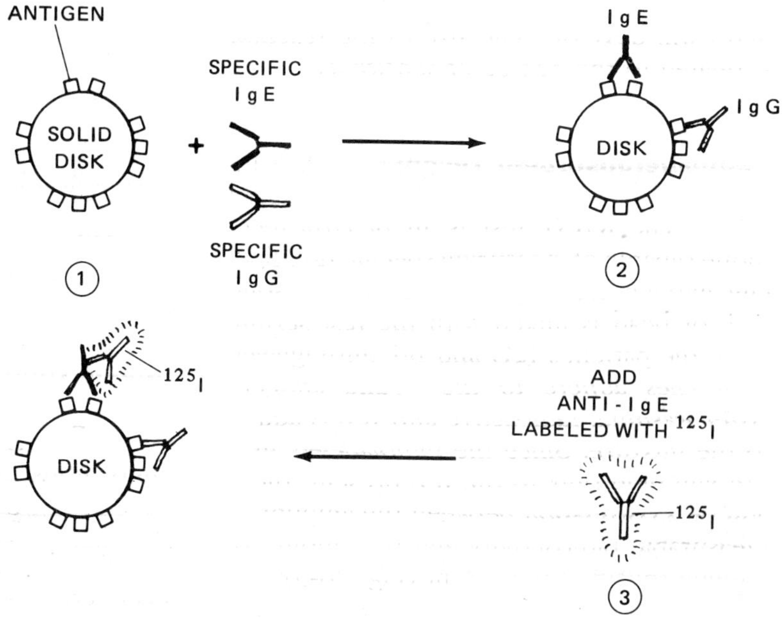

Fig. 26-5. Radioallergosorbent test (RAST).

quently so ill during the first 6 months of life that their illness is rarely confused with bronchial asthma.

Hypersensitivity Pneumonitides

Hypersensitivity pneumonitides are a group of pulmonary disorders caused by inhalation of organic dusts and proteins and characterized by recurrent episodes of coughing, fever, and respiratory distress. A few hours after exposure, fever, respiratory distress, leukocytosis, and coarse rales appear, but symptoms usually subside within 12 to 24 hours. The common bronchodilators fail but corticosteroids do suppress symptoms.

Allergic Bronchopulmonary Aspergillosis

Allergic bronchopulmonary aspergillosis may be mistaken initially for bronchial asthma. Clinical presentation usually includes recurrent episodes of coughing and wheezing, poor control of symptoms with antiasthmatic medications, fleeting pulmonary infiltrates, and the production of sputum, often brown in color and sometimes containing aspergillus hyphae. Blood studies may reveal peripheral eosinophilia and marked elevation of total IgE. Skin testing with aspergillus extract produces both an immediate (20 min) and a delayed reaction (4–8 hr). In addition, patients usually have precipitating antibodies directed against aspergillus.

Alpha-1-Antitrypsin Deficiency

Alpha-1-antitrypsin deficiency is an autosomal recessive disorder with manifestations of lung disease including coughing, dyspnea, and wheezing. This is an obstructive lung disease characterized by air trapping and poor reversibility of airway obstruction. A family history of chronic lung disease or emphysema should alert the clinician to obtain a quantitative quantitative alpha-1-antitrypsin level.

COMPLICATIONS OF ASTHMA

Status Asthmaticus

Status asthmaticus may be defined as a persistent, acute attack of asthma which does not respond adequately to treatment with sympathomimetics (epinephrine) or other commonly used bronchodilators (aminophylline). This complication can quickly result in asphyxia and therefore constitutes a medical emergency. Patients require constant monitoring and frequent reevaluation for possible modification of treatment. Predisposing factors to the development of status asthmaticus include poorly controlled asthma, abuse of sympathomimetic nebulizers, respiratory tract infections. Patients may become dehydrated because of diminished fluid intake and concomitant increases in both sensible and insensible fluid loss (hyperventilation, vomiting). Those not responding to oxygen, fluid and electrolyte therapy, and intravenous aminophylline require corticosteroid administration. The initial clinical assessment should include information about the presence of cyanosis, the quality of breath sounds on inspiration, the use of accessory muscles of respiration, the intensity of wheezing, cerebral function, the state of hydration, and the possible presence of underlying disease. Etiologic factors exacerbating or complicating asthma should be sorted out (*e.g.*, infection, atelectasis). One can estimate the severity either by using a clinical scoring system or by measuring the pulsus paradoxus. Either of these techniques afford a noninvasive method of assessment and may be used serially to judge the patient's course and response to medication. The following studies are recommended: chest radiograph (PA and lateral), CBC and differential, total eosinophil count, NP and throat culture, sputum cytology, and serum electrolytes. Arterial blood gases are drawn if clinical judgment indicates that an accurate assessment of gas exchange is required. Arterial blood gases can be interpreted as presented in Figure 2-3.

Atelectasis

In asthma, atelectasis occurs with greater frequency in the right middle lobe, possibly because its bronchus comes off at a sharp angle from the right main stem bronchus and is long and narrow. Atelectasis may cause no obvious symptoms, or a mucous plug blocking the main stem bronchus may produce massive atelectasis of an entire lung with immediate symptoms of respiratory distress constituting an acute emergency.

Pneumomediastinum

Free air within the mediastinum is thought to be the result of air escaping from ruptured asthmatic alveolae and dissecting its way along the bronchovascular tree to the hilum. Many patients are asymptomatic and the presence of pneumomediatinum is diagnosed by the radiographic finding of retrosternal free air. Signs and symptoms of pneumomediastinum include chest pain, tachypnea, and dyspnea. This complication is frequently seen in the younger asthmatic.

Pneumothorax

Pneumothorax occurs less frequently than does pneumomediastinum. However, the symptoms of pneumothorax are usually more prominent and potentially serious. They include sudden dyspnea, cough, air hunger, marked tachypnea, and frank cyanosis. Nontension pneumothoraces with free air occupying less than 20% of the hemithoracic volume are handled conservatively, while those exceeding 20% often require insertion of a chest tube and suction.

Other complications encountered include pneumonia, bronchiectasis, and, rarely, cor pulmonale. Some of the more severely affected children may show signs of inhibition of linear growth and deformity of the chest.

An important and often overlooked complication of asthma is the physical disability resulting from chronic lung disease. Frequent absences from school may interfere seriously with academic development. Poorly controlled asthmatics may be unable to participate in sports. A number of children and their families may develop significant psychopathology as a result of the problems related to asthma, or their existing psychopathology may exacerbate the asthma.

TREATMENT OF BRONCHIAL ASTHMA

The successful management of childhood bronchial asthma requires a careful assessment and identification of the type of asthma involved (*e.g.*, intrinsic, extrinsic), its duration and severity, environmental and other provoking stimuli, and a history of response and side-effects to medications. In dealing with extrinsic bronchial asthma, environmental control as well as hyposensitization should be considered.

Environmental Control

Specific allergens identified as causative factors either by history or allergy testing and interpreted as being significant etiologically should be avoided or eliminated from the immediate environment. Common allergens known to produce asthma in sensitive persons include: house dust, dog and cat dander, feathers, mold (damp basements), and bedding material (kapok and cotton fibers). Certain allergens such as dust may be partially eliminated through a concerted effort to lower its concentrations within the immediate environment.

Hyposensitization or "Allergy Injections"

Hyposensitization to various allergens may be accomplished by means of subcutaneous injections of the offending allergen administered in increasing amounts. Although the mechanism underlying successful hyposensitization is not completely clear, it appears that these injections result in increasing IgG blocking antibodies, decreased cellular sensitivity (histamine release), decreased specific IgE, and diminished allergen-induced symptoms. Indications for hyposensitization include correlation of symptoms following exposure (*i.e.*, seasonal correlation), plus positive allergy tests (skin testing or RAST). If avoidance is unsuccessful and symptoms are not easily controlled with medication, hyposensitization is considered. The following allergens are frequently used for hyposensitization in asthma: pollens, dust, and molds. The use of bacterial vaccines to treat asthma is controversial. The traditional method of selection of the appropriate antigen (skin testing) has not proven to be of value in the case of bacterial vaccines.

Ingestants in Asthma

The ingestion of certain foods has been associated with asthma in childhood. Contrary to popular opinion, foods have not been shown to be a major etiologic factor,

Of foods causing respiratory symptoms, milk and eggs are among the most common offenders. In addition to respiratory symptoms, many children have concomitant dermal (urticaria-eczema) or gastrointestinal manifestations (diarrhea or colic). Allergy skin testing for foods is far less reliable than testing with other allergens. A more accurate technique for diagnosing food allergies is an elimination diet followed by a provocation test with the suspected food. We prefer to repeat this maneuver at least three times to clearly reproduce the respiratory symptoms before incriminating a specific food. Certain drugs, including aspirin, and tartrazine dyes (yellow dye no. 5) should be eliminated if they are suspected of inducing asthma.

Medical Treatment

Theophylline, a member of the methylxanthine group, has become a drug of choice in the management of childhood asthma. Its action is accomplished through suppression of the enzyme phosphosdiesterase (preventing the degradation of cyclic AMP) with a resultant increase in cyclic AMP and bronchodilation (Fig. 26-6). The drug can be used concomitantly with beta-adrenergic sympathomimetics in a synergistic manner. The metabolism of theophylline may vary considerably among individual children. Therapeutic blood levels usually lie between 10 and 20 μg/ml. These levels are generally achieved by administering orally

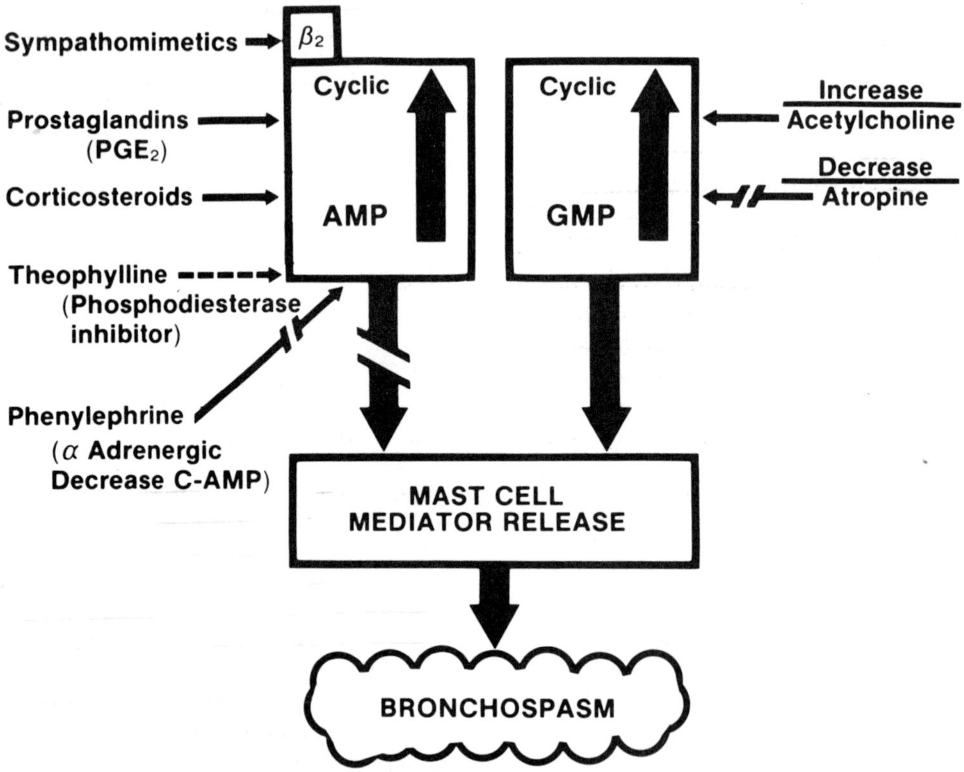

Fig. 26-6. Site of drug action in bronchial asthma.

5 mg/kg anhydrous theophylline three to four times per day. For children not responding adequately or experiencing side-effects, a theophylline blood level may be determined and the drug dosage adjusted appropriately. Most oral theophylline preparations produce adequate blood levels within 15 to 60 minutes following ingestion. Rectal preparations are less useful because of erratic absorption and possible prolonged duration of action. The intravenous use of aminophylline is limited generally to acute asthma in an emergency room or hospital setting. The toxic side-effects of theophylline overdose include nausea, vomiting, hypotension, arrythmias, hematemesis, and convulsions. Toxicity is commonly encountered when the blood level exceeds 20 μg/ml.

Sympathomimetics

Sympathomimetics act through stimulation of the beta-adrenergic receptors, producing an elevation in intracellular cyclic AMP and subsequent bronchodilatation (Fig. 26-6). Sympathomimetics used in the treatment of asthma are related to the parent compound phenylethylamine. Substitution in this compound can increase $beta_2$ activity as seen with terbutaline and metaproterenol. Certain adrenergic drugs are inactivated in the GI tract by a mucosal enzyme, catechol-o-methyltransferase. Therefore, drugs destroyed by these enzymes (*e.g.*, epinephrine, isoproterenol) are only effective when injected or inhaled. Moreover, the latter two drugs have a short half-life. Certain sympathomimetics may be administered orally, subcutaneously, by inhalation, and very rarely intravenously. $Beta_1$ drugs produce cardiac acceleration and $beta_2$, smooth bronchial muscle relaxation effects. The better known side-effects include cardiac stimulation and skeletal muscle tremor.

Ephedrine

The main advantage of ephedrine is that it is inexpensive, can be administered orally, and has a duration of 4 to 6 hours. Unfortunately, children suffer from annoying side-effects such as insomnia, headache, and other signs of central nervous system stimulation. Addiction does not seem to be a problem.

Epinephrine

The medication is not effective orally; however, it can produce dramatic relief of bronchospasm within a few minutes following subcutaneous injection. It may also be inhaled as an aerosol. Epinephrine's main disadvantages are a very short duration of action and central nervous system stimulation. It is the drug of choice for treatment of patients with acute asthma that does not respond to conservative treatment.

Isoproterenol (Isuprel)

Isuprel, an inhaled anti-asthmatic agent, has both $beta_1$- and $beta_2$-stimulating capacities. It acts rapidly (within a few minutes) and has a relatively short duration of action. One of its breakdown products, 1-3 methoxyisoproterenol, is known to be a weak beta-blocker. Therefore, it is conceivable that nebulized isoproterenol, especially when overused, may act in a paradoxical manner and produce bronchospasm. Recent developments have made available new $beta_2$ preferential stimulators including terbutaline sulfate, metaproterenol, and isoetharine. Metaproterenol (Alupent) produces prolonged bronchodilatation associated with few of the $beta_1$ side-effects. It is available in both oral and inhalation forms. Terbutaline sulfate and salbutamol are both more potent $beta_2$ stimulators than metaproterenol and may be administered by the oral, subcutaneous, and inhalation routes. One common side-effect is muscle tremor which subsides following continuous treatment.

Expectorants

Expectorants are thought to increase the flow and clearance, of the respiratory tract mucus, as well as decrease its viscosity. Acute asthma results in the production of thick, tenacious mucus that often plays an important role in the pathophysiology of the disease. Oral or intravenous fluids increase the clearance of respiratory mucus and are considered by many to be the best expectorants. Both iodides and glyceryl guaiacolate have become the primary expectorants used in the treatment of asthma either alone or in combination with other anti-asthmatic drugs. There is evidence that glyceryl guaiacolate is not an effective expectorant in the normal dosage range. Iodides also do not seem to be effective expectorants.

Cromolyn Sodium

Cromolyn sodium (Intal, Aarane), unlike the preceding medications, does not appear to affect the level of cyclic AMP or directly cause bronchodilatation; rather, it appears to prevent mast cell release of mediators through stabilization of the cellular membrane. Cromolyn sodium is inhaled as a powder which coats the respiratory mucosa. It is generally not effective when administered to patients with signs of acute asthma. When given prior to the onset of wheezing it may have a preventive action. The drug is expensive and usually requires long-term use. Efficacy may be delayed 2 to 3 weeks after treatment has been initiated. In addition, the child must be able to inhale the drug properly. Side-effects are limited to coughing, sore throat, skin rashes; pulmonary infiltrates have been reported rarely.

Corticosteroids

The mechanism by which corticosteroids produce striking relief of asthma symptoms is not well understood. Steroids appear to function in several ways including stabilization of cell membranes, prevention of lysozomal enzyme release, potentiation of sympathomimetics on the B_2 receptor with an increase in cyclic AMP, and suppression of the cellular inflammatory response. Corticosteroids do not block antigen-induced immediate type allergic asthma but can prevent the late response that is often seen 4 to 6 hours after antigen inhalation. The suppression of late asthmatic responses may be due, in part, to corticosteroid suppression of the responding inflammatory cell accumulation at the reaction site.

Certain synthetic corticosteroids such as dexamethasone have a prolonged duration of action. Steroid preparation such as prednisone and prednisolone have shorter half-lives and may be administered as a single dose every other morning in an attempt to avoid hypothalmic-pituitary-adrenal (HPA) axis suppression. In contrast, daily treatment with doses as low as 2.5 mg given on a daily basis has been shown to suppress the HPA-axis in children. An inhaled steroid, beclomethasone has been introduced for the treatment of bronchial asthma. Because of its high topical activity, a local therapeutic benefit can be derived at a dose small enough to avoid HPA-axis suppression or suppression of linear growth.

THERAPEUTIC APPROACH IN THE MANAGEMENT OF BRONCHIAL ASTHMA

Acute Attack of Asthma

The following medical regimen is used in many pediatric centers for an acute attack of bronchial asthma:

Moist oxygen is administered by mask or nasal cannula. Subcutaneous injections of epinephrine are given every 15 to 20 minutes (usually 2 but 15% need 3 injections). Most patients respond and are sent home after an injection of a long-acting epinephrine (Sus-phrine) as well as oral theophylline. Nonresponders are hydrated and are given intravenous theophylline. Patients not responding to the foregoing treatment are considered to be in status asthmaticus and are admitted to the hospital. Radiographs are taken to rule out complications of asthma. Imbalance of fluids, electrolytes, and pH are corrected. Patients not responding at this stage require intravenous corticosteroids. Children in status asthmaticus are continuously monitored using clinical scoring, arterial blood gases, and pulsus paradoxus. Asthmatic children entering respiratory failure require further therapy with either intravenous isoproterenol or artificial mechanical ventilation. As the acute attack subsides, percussion and postural drainage, expectorants, and IPPB ± Isuprel may be employed.

Subacute and Chronic Asthma

Therapy is initiated with a single oral theophylline preparation at a dose of 5 mg/kg given four times a day. Clinical response with or without serum theophylline levels indicates the need for dosage adjustment. It should be noted that the metabolism of theophylline may vary greatly from one child to another; therefore, individualization of dosage may be required.

Sympathomimetic agents are added to the regimen of nonresponders. Oral preparations such as ephedrine, metaproterenol, and terbutaline offer an oral and, in the case of metaproterenol and isoproterenol, an inhaled delivery system. Inhaled sympathomimetics often can reverse dramatically acute asthma early in the episode. The inhaler is preferably kept under parental control because of the propensity for abuse.

Children with continuing signs of asthma should receive a course of cromolyn sodium therapy. It is administered as an inhaled powder four times a day for at least a 1-month trial period. It is used solely as a preventive medication and not during a wheezing episode. Children not controlled by cromolyn inhalation may be considered candidates for steroid therapy.

Corticosteroids may be given as short-term treatment for unresponsive exacerbations of bronchospasm or as part of a long-term program to control severe chronic asthma. In either case, information on the potential side-effects of this potent medication should be supplied to parents.

Short-Term Steroid Treatment. At one time or another, a number of asthmatic children develop marked obstructive respiratory symptoms either as an intermittent paroxysm of bronchospasm or as an exacerbation of chronic asthma despite conservative treatment. Under these circumstances, a short-term (3–5-day) course of a short-acting steroid preparation (prednisone) may be administered at a dose of 2 mg/kg/day in divided doses.

Long-Term Steroid Therapy. Less frequently, asthmatic children have recurrent acute attacks or chronic disability despite the proper use of all medications. Therefore, long-term steroid therapy in addition to conservative therapy (*i.e.*, theophylline, sympathomimetics) may be necessary to control symptoms.

Beclomethasone, a highly active steroid, can be used in an inhaled form that suppresses asthmatic symptoms while minimizing systemic side-effects. Beclomethasone (Vanceril) is inhaled in very small amounts (100–400 μg/dose) up to four times per day. If the recommended dosage is exceeded, systemic side-effects may occur.

Long-term oral steroid treatment should be considered either as continuous or alternate day therapy for those failing to respond to inhaled beclomethasone. The preferred alternate day course may be instituted by administering double the daily dosage as a single dose every other morning. Those who still have persistent symptoms require daily steroid therapy with all its possible side-effects.

Partial List of Corticosteroid Complications

Cushingoid features including:
- acne, moonface, facial plethora, central obesity, striae and others

Suppression of linear growth and osteoporosis
Suppression of the HPA-axis
Muscle weakness and cramps
Subcapsular cataracts and glaucoma
Psychotic reactions
Pseudotumor cerebri
Hypertension
Peptic ulceration
Pancreatitis

Steroid-dependent asthmatics require additional steroid during stressful periods (*e.g.*, surgery, status asthmaticus) if a medical catastrophe is to be avoided. The state of steroid dependence may persist 1 year beyond the cessation of daily steroid therapy.

General Supportive Therapy

Hydration, expectorants, and percussion and postural drainage can significantly aid in the mobilization of tenacious bronchial secretions. Exercise-induced bronchospasm may be prevented with the pre-exercise use of theophylline, inhaled sympathomimetics, or cromolyn sodium. In general, the patient should receive enough therapy for him to function in a normal manner. Asthmatic children should be encouraged to participate in sports and other physical activities as long as their asthma is under control.

PROGNOSIS

Because bronchial asthma is a highly variable disease, it is impossible to accurately predict its course in any individual child. Between one-half to two-thirds of affected children will be free of bronchospastic symptoms as adults.

Children who develop severe chronic asthma often have a history of early onset of the disease (usually before the age of 3 years) and have persistent abnormal pulmonary functions. Children who "outgrow" their asthma frequently suffer persistent allergic rhinitis and conjunctivitis. Another group with a history of resolved childhood asthma experience the onset of intrinsic asthma as adults.

BIBLIOGRAPHY

Pride NB: Physiology. *In* Clark TJH, Godrey S (eds): Asthma. Philadelphia, WB Saunders, 1977

An excellent review of pulmonary function tests

and their use in the identification and interpretation of asthma.

Szentnanyi A, Fischel C: The beta adrenergic theory and cyclic AMP-mediated control mechanism in human asthma. *In* Weiss EB, Segal MS (eds): Bronchial Asthma, Mechanisms and Therapeutics. Boston, Little, Brown, 1976

A scholarly review of the beta-adrenergic blockage theory in asthma as well as a discussion of drug treatment and its effect on cyclic AMP.

Pediatric Allergy. Pediatr Clin North Am 22:1, 1975

This edition contains review articles on beta-adrenergic bronchodilators, cromolyn sodium, Beclomethasone, and the treatment of status asthmaticus.

Lichtenstein LM, Ishizaka KN, Norman PS, Scbodka AK, Hill BM: IgE antibody measurements in ragweed hayfever. Relationship to clinical severity and the results of immunotherapy. J Clin Invest 52:472, 1973

A careful study of the effects of "allergy shots" in relation to suppression of symptoms and immunologic changes.

Middleton E, Jr., Reed CE, Ellis EF (eds): Allergy: Principles and Practice. St. Louis, CV Mosby, 1978

An excellent general reference on allergic disease.

Patterson R (ed): Allergic Rhinitis: Diagnosis and management, 2nd ed. Philadelphia, JB Lippincott, 1980.

An excellent general reference on allergic disease.

Common Allergic Disorders

27

Eliot H. Dunsky

The term *allergy* or *hypersensitivity disease* includes a large and heterogenous group of immunologically-mediated adverse reactions induced by either antigens or haptens. *Antigens* are high molecular weight complexes, usually containing protein, that elicit a specific immune response involving antibodies or immune lymphocytes. *Haptens* are low molecular weight substances that become antigens only when they combine with larger "carrier" molecules. Not all antigens cause allergic reactions. Those that do are referred to as *allergens*.

Many diseases can mimic closely the symptoms of allergy, just as allergy can simulate a disease of nonimmunologic origin. In order to correctly label a child's malady as allergic in origin, an attempt to define the immunologic basis of the disease or reaction must be made. Within this context, symptoms alone may be misleading. For example, gastrointestinal symptoms immediately following the ingestion of a specific food may be due to an enzyme deficiency rather than allergy (*e.g.*, dissacharidase deficiency and milk ingestion) or "pneumonia" may be the result of allergic asthma rather than of infection.

IMMUNOPATHOLOGY OF ALLERGY

The main function of the immune system is protection. However, under certain circumstances the immune response works to the detriment of the host. In allergic disease the host suffers an adverse reaction due to an altered or hyperresponsive immune response. In autoimmunity an immune response is directed, at least in part, against the host's own tissue which has been perceived as foreign antigen.

In the human, the components of an immunologic response may be divided into two basic groups: the humoral (antibody) and the cellular (lymphocyte) systems. Characteristically, the response of either or both systems is directed against the stimulating antigen with great specificity. This highly specialized defense mechanism begins with the differentiation of a primordial stem cell in the bone marrow. The totipotential stem cell undergoes differentiation into either B cells (under the influence of the bursal equivalent) or T cells (under influence of the thymus) (Fig. 27-1). B cells further differentiate into plasma cells, which upon appropriate antigenic stimulation produce a specific antibody against a stimulating antigen. The immunoglobulins (antibodies) are plasma protein molecules composed of four pairs of polypeptide chains, two identical heavy chains, and two identical light chains. When intact, the antibody configuration appears to be similar to the letter "Y" (Fig. 27-2).

The heavy chains may have a molecular weight of approximately 53,000 and the light chain a molecular weight of 22,000 (*i.e.*, IgG). The linked heavy chain forms the entire length of the molecule, while the light chains parallel the heavy chains for only a

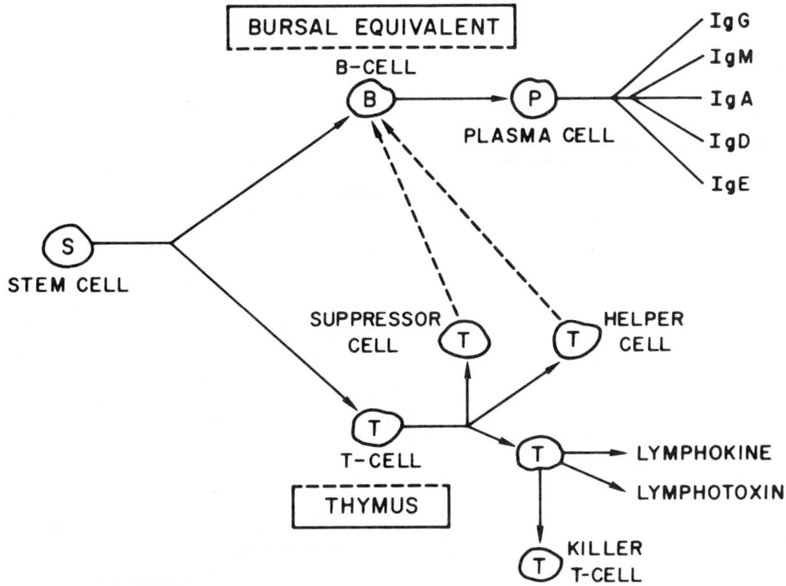

Fig. 27-1. The immune system—humoral and cellular aspects.

section of their length, forming part of the two arms of the Y. The two arms of the Y are known as the Fab fragments and act as receptor sites for antigenic determinants. The foot of the Y or the Fc portion is adapted to attach to a cell surface.

Immunoglobulins

Depending on the structure of their heavy chain, immunoglobulins can be divided into five classes (IgM, IgG, IgA, IgD, and IgE). IgM plays an important role in the primary immune response and usually is present in the form of a pentamer (5 units joined together). Although this antibody is not as selective as IgG, it is more rapidly synthesized during the initial contact with the antigenic stimulus. IgG is the major immunoglobulin of the intravascular system. It plays its most significant role during the secondary or anamnestic immune response. IgG's specificity and avidity for a given antigen is much greater than that of IgM. IgA is the major secretory immunoglobulin. Two units of IgA and their secretory piece are found in mucosal secretions and saliva; IgA is thought to play an important role in protecting the mucosal portals of entry. The role of IgD remains obscure. Immunoglobulin E plays a central role in immediate type allergic reactions. Even though it is present in extremely small amounts in the blood, it has the ability to attach selectively and remain fixed to mast cells and basophils for prolonged periods. The respiratory mucosa is richly endowed with mast cells, and as might be expected, it is one of the most common sites for allergic reactions. Children with defective antibody production, particularly with diminished IgG, suffer from recurrent bacterial infections.

Delayed Response Mechanism

The other half of the dual system of immunity is the delayed or cell-mediated response mechanism that is mediated by spe-

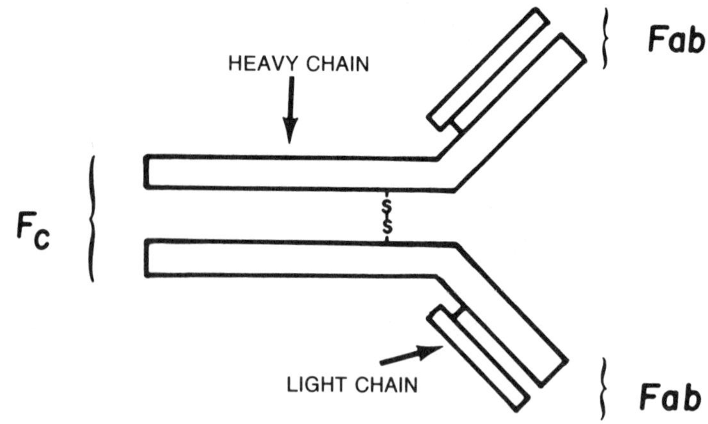

Fig. 27-2. Immunoglobulin structure.

cifically sensitized lymphocytes without the aid of immunoglobulins. Totipotential stem cells in the bone marrow circulate through the thymus, and under influence of the thymic hormone thymosin, evolve into T-lymphocytes (T cells, Fig. 27-1). In humans, these cells may be characterized *in vitro* by their ability to spontaneously form rosettes with sheep erythrocytes (E-rosettes) and undergo lymphoblastic transformation following concavalin A (con A) or phytohemagglutinin (PHA) stimulation. T-lymphocytes are responsible for rejection of foreign tissue grafts, contact dermatitis, reaction to invasion by certain bacteria (tuberculosis), viruses (measles), fungi (*Candida*), and they play an important role in the suppression of tumor growth.

In addition, T cells indirectly regulate immunoglobulin synthesis by enhancing or suppressing the B cell/plasma cell system production of antibodies (by means of T-helper or T-suppressor cells). Certain small T-lymphocytes are thought to be long-lived memory cells, which could explain the phenomenon of lifelong immunity (measles). When appropriately stimulated, T-lymphocytes can release soluble mediators that participate in the cellular defense mechanism in a number of ways. For example, migration inhibition factor (MIF) inhibits the migration of macrophages and therefore induces their accumulation at the site of inflammation. The T cell may destroy the foreign cell (killer T cell), "arm" macrophages by committing them to destroy another specific cell, or by secretion of a lymphotoxin directly kill the target cell (Fig. 27-1).

Circulating Serum Proteins

Aside from the specific sensitized responses of the immune system, there are a number of circulating serum proteins that may participate in and amplify immune reactions. A good example of this is the complement system which consists of 11 fluid phase proteins that upon activation bind to an antigen-antibody complex. Complement activation can take place by means of at least two pathways. The first or classic pathway necessitates the initial attachment of a subunit of the first component of complement (C_{1q}) to the Fc portion of the immunoglobin (IgG or IgM) in the antigen-antibody complex. The ensuing structural changes cause C_{1r} to enzymatically activate C_{1s} and the cascade begins. Activated C_{1qrs} initiates a cascade of the remaining complement components in the following order: C_1, C_2, C_3, C_5, C_6, C_7, C_8, and C_9.

The alternate pathway bypasses the classic initiation of the complement cascade via C_1. Instead, with the aid of the properdin system (that can be activated by aggregated IgA, bacterial polysaccharide, and endotoxin lipopolysaccharides), C_3 is directly activated (bypassing C_1, C_4 and C_2) and from this point the cascade continues as in the classic pathway.

Certain complement cascade products have specific biologic activities that play an important role in certain immunologic reactions in man. Soluble products of C_3 (C_{3a}) and C_5 (C_{5a}) are anaphylatoxins that cause mast cells to release histamine and can therefore simulate anaphylaxis and other immediate type allergic reactions. C_{3a} and C_{5a} are also chemotactic for inflammatory cells as is the C_{567} complex. Other functions of complement include viral neutralization and enhanced immune adherence (C_{3b}). The final attack sequence, including the activation of the terminal components C_8 and C_9, culminates in damage or lysis to the cellular membrane.

Classification of Allergic Response

To better conceptualize the various kinds of immune reactions, Gell and Coombs separated hypersensitivity responses into four basic categories (Fig. 27-3).

Type I or Immediate Hypersensitivity. Immediate hypersensitivity represents the immunologic basis of extrinsic (allergic) asthma, hayfever, anaphylactic reactions, and urticaria. Persons suffering from these diseases apparently have the genetic potential, upon exposure to the appropriate antigen, to produce a specific antibody of the immunoglobulin E class (IgE). IgE has a number of special characteristics that include the following: (1) it has the ability to passively transfer hypersensitivity for up to 6 weeks in a normal person; (2) its biologic activity is lost upon heating for 1 to 4 hours at 56° C; and (3) it does not fix complement.

IgE fixes firmly to the surface of mast cells and basophils by its Fc receptor. Mast cells are found in abundance in the respiratory mucosa, the gastrointestinal tract, and the skin. When the specific antigen binds to IgE molecules on the surface of the mast cell, a number of biochemical events occur that ultimately cause the release of biologic mediators. These events and their clinical sequelae occur within a matter of minutes and hence the term immediate hypersensitivity. Although the antigen-IgE complex initiates the mechanism of mediator release, their final release is modulated by the cell's cyclic nucleotide concentrations (*e.g.*, cyclic adenosine monophosphate) (see Chap. 26). Among the mediators released are:

1. *Histamine*—a vasoactive amine that causes increased capillary permeability, edema, increased secretions of bronchial mucosa, and smooth muscle contraction. Its action on the target organ is blocked by antihistamines.

2. *Slow reactive substance of anaphylaxis (SRS-A)*—an acidic lipid of low molecular weight, considered to be an important mediator producing prolonged smooth muscle contractions that are not blocked by antihistamines.

3. *Eosinophilic chemotactic factor of anaphylaxis (ECF-A)*—a polypeptide (molecular weight of about 500) that preferentially attracts eosinophils to the site of its release. The presence of ECF-A could explain the large number of cosinophils found at the site of an immediate hypersensitivity reaction.

Histamine and ECF-A are preformed and stored as granules within basophils and mast cells, while SRS-A is synthesized upon

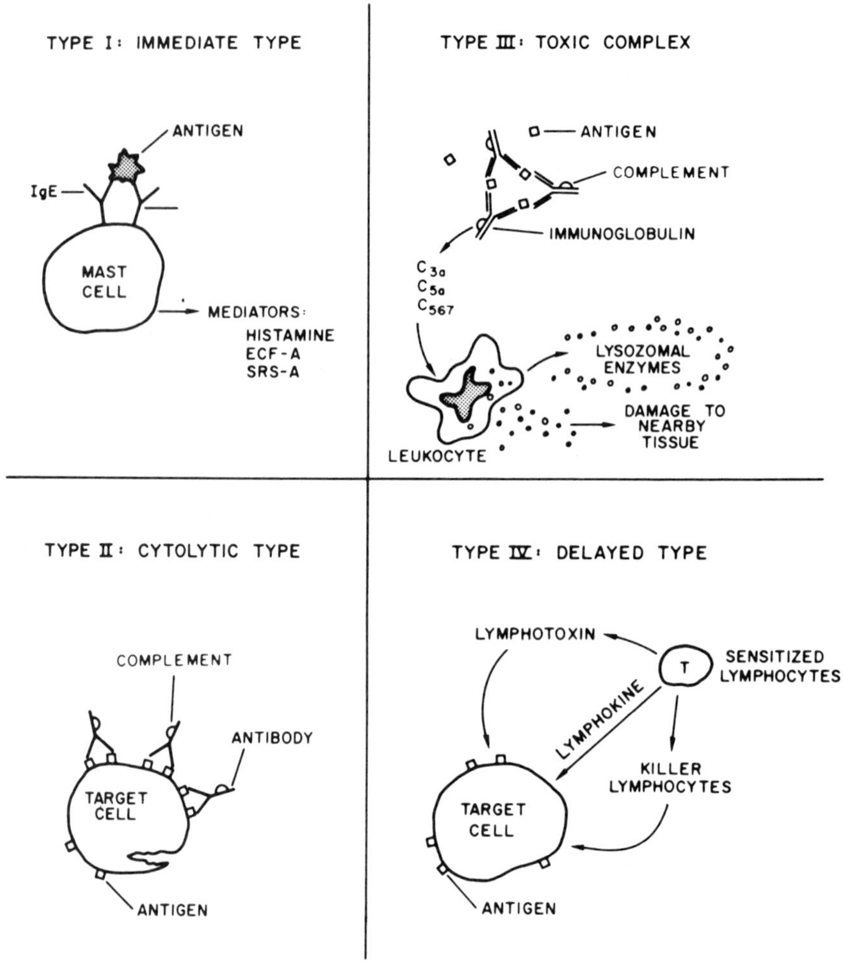

Fig. 27-3. Classification of hypersensitivity reactions.

stimulation. The release of these mediators as a group can produce prolonged bronchospasm, swelling of the bronchial mucosa, hypersecretion of mucus within the bronchial lumen, and an influx of inflammatory cells—in short, the pathology of asthma. Mediator release in the skin can cause hives, and systemic release can result in anaphylaxis.

Type II or the Cytotoxic Reaction. Type II reaction is due to antibodies, usually of the IgG or IgM class, directed against antigens or haptens on the cell membrane. These antigenic determinants may be absorbed onto the cell membrane. These antigenic determinants may be absorbed onto the cell surface or they may be an intrinsic part of the cell membrane. In type II reactions, the Fab portion of the molecule binds to the cell surface. Complement may then fix to the Fc portion of the bound antibody, and its activation under these conditions can result in damage or lysis to the cell membrane. Other cellular circulating elements so coated with antibody and fixed complement may be made more susceptible to phagocytosis and removal by the reticuloendothelial system rather than undergo lysis.

Clinical examples of cytotoxic reactions include the hemolytic anemias of the newborn (Rh and ABO incompatibility) in which maternal antibody (IgG) is directed against the newborn's RBC, transfusion reactions, penicillin-induced hemolytic anemia, and Goodpasture's syndrome. In the last example, antibodies are produced against antigenic determinants on the pulmonary and glomerular basement membranes.

Type III or Toxic-Complex Reactions. The type III reactions occur when circulating soluble antigen-antibody complexes are deposited in tissues. If the amount of soluble circulating antigen is in slight excess to the amount of available antibody (IgG or IgM), soluble microcomplexes may be formed. Although they are small enough to avoid removal from the circulation by the reticuloendothelial system, they eventually settle in small blood vessels or the glomeruli of the kidney. Following tissue deposition, complement may bind to the Fc portion of the antibody within the complex. The ensuing complement cascade causes the release of chemotactic factors (C_{3a} and C_{5a}) that attract polymorphonuclear leukocytes. The lysosomal enzymes released by these leukocytes cause the actual damage to nearby cells and tissues. In addition, anaphylatoxins, also by-products of the complement cascade, cause local vasodilation and increased vascular permeability, thus permitting further immune complex deposition and continuing local inflammation.

Type IV Reaction, Delayed or Cellular Hypersensitivity. The fourth type of reaction is referred to as delayed hypersensitivity, because the peak of the reaction usually occurs 24 to 72 hours following antigen exposure. Specifically sensitized T-lymphocytes, without the aid of immunoglobulin or complement, recognize antigens that have been processed by macrophages and react either by destroying the cell bearing these antigenic determinants or by secreting lymphokines.

Appropriately stimulated sensitized lymphocytes undergo lymphoblastic transformation and secrete soluble mediators called lymphokines (For example migration inhibition factor or MIF). Lymphokines may recruit macrophages and nonsensitized lymphocytes to the reaction site. Other lymphokines activate macrophages or lymphocytes against the foreign antigen. Still other lymphoblasts secrete lymphotoxin that directly damages the target cell.

Examples of delayed hypersensitivity are contact dermatitis, tuberculin reaction, and foreign skin graft rejection.

Atopic Disease. The term *atopy* describes a group of allergic disorders in which affected children have a predisposition to develop immediate-type hypersensitivity to various environmental antigens. Atopic diseases include asthma, hayfever, urticaria (hives), and atopic dermatitis (infantile eczema). Although there appears to be a genetic basis for the development of atopy (many patients have similarly affected relatives), the exact mode of inheritance is not clear. Atopic disorders are usually associated with increased production of IgE against various antigens and the development of immediate hypersensitivity reactions. Atopy to both ingested and inhaled allergens tends to begin early in childhood. About 10% to 15% of the population suffers from atopy. Allergic rhinitis and conjunctivitis are among the most common forms of atopy. Food allergy tends to occur early in infancy, while inhalant allergy occurs more frequently following infancy. Atopic disease, such as atopic dermatitis, is associated with a high incidence of allergic disease in the affected patient; nevertheless atopic dermatitis does not appear to be caused by an IgE mediated or any known allergic mechanism. Therefore in this latter case, *atopy* refers to the high incidence of allergy in these patients rather than the etiology of the disease.

ALLERGIC RHINITIS AND CONJUNCTIVITIS

About 10% of the population is affected at some time by the symptoms of allergic rhinitis or conjunctivitis. Symptoms may be present throughout the year (perennial allergic rhinitis, conjunctivitis), or they may have a seasonal periodicity (seasonal allergic rhinitis, conjunctivitis).

Seasonal symptoms are most often related to the release of pollen into the atmosphere during the spring and summer. The release of spores from molds growing on decaying vegetation may also produce a seasonal pattern. On the other hand, perennial symptoms may be related to allergens in the home: house dust, mold spores (released from damp basements), and animal danders.

Common Inhaled Allergens

Pollen. Only pollen that is relatively small (10–40 μm) and light in weight can become airborne and be dispersed widely. Certain trees, grasses, and weeds release such pollen, while pollen from flowers is so heavy that it does not play a significant role in inhalant allergy. Depending on geography and climatic conditions, trees pollinate in the spring, grasses in the summer, and weeds in the summer and fall.

Molds. Fungal spores are present in the atmosphere throughout most of the year except when the ground is covered with snow. They reach their peak during the late summer months when dead vegetation and a warm humid climate produce optimal growth conditions. Molds may also be found year round in the home. They tend to proliferate in damp areas (*e.g.*, wet basement, bath area). Mold-sensitive patients have either a seasonal or perennial pattern, depending on their sensitivity to specific molds and their exposure pattern.

Dust. House dust is a common indoor allergen. It is a product of partially decomposed epidermoid tissue, hair, bacteria, insects (mites), and other organic material (cotton linters from bedding).

Animal Dander. Shedded epithelium from dogs, cats, and other domestic animals can be potent allergens. Sensitive children have symptoms when exposed to the animal or the room in which the animal had been present. Even animal products such as horse hair in stuffed furniture or cattle hair in rug padding may induce symptoms.

Foods. Foods are not a common cause of respiratory allergy. In general, the few patients who have respiratory symptoms as a result of food allergy also have gastrointestinal, dermal, or anaphylactic symptoms. Food allergy will be discussed in greater detail later in this chapter.

Allergic Rhinitis

Symptoms of allergic rhinitis may vary from occasional mild nasal stuffiness to an incapacitating chronic nasal obstruction and its associated complications (*e.g.*, serous otitis media). Affected children may have a history of multiple paroxysms of sneezing, nasal congestion, nasal pruritis, and anterior and/or posterior nasal discharge. These children typically rub their noses with an upward and outward movement of the palm of the hand. In so doing, the soft anterior third of the nose bends back forming a transverse nasal crease between the rigid upper two-thirds and the soft lower third. The nose-rubbing maneuver is known as the "allergic salute," and the resulting nasal crease helps identify these allergic children. Patients may also complain of pruritis of the throat and ears. Many of these symptoms may be erroneously attributed to recurrent colds. When the obstruction is severe, the child becomes an obligate mouth breather. This may be associated with changes in phonation, post-nasal drip, sore throat, hoarseness, and chronic cough. Allergic rhinitis may also be associated with recurrent serous otitis media and hearing loss. The physical examination reveals (1) a transverse nasal crease, swollen and pale inferior nasal turbinates that may have a bluish discoloration, (2) clear mucoid discharge, (3) edema and bluish black discoloration of the skin just beneath the inferior border of both orbits ("allergic shiners"), and (4) mouth breathing and posterior pharyngeal lymphoid hypertrophy.

Allergic Conjunctivitis

Allergic conjunctivitis may be associated with allergic rhinitis or may occur independently. Symptoms are usually seasonal, but may be perennial. Affected children complain of pruritic conjunctivae, conjunctival discharge, and in some cases photophobia. The child constantly rubs his eyes. The conjunctival blood vessels are dilated and the inferior palpebral conjunctiva may demonstrate follicular lymphoid hyperplasia (which is often referred to as "cobblestoning"). Vernal conjunctivitis is a much more severe form of allergic conjunctivitis that appears each spring and summer. Patients characteristically have marked cobblestoning of the upper palpebral conjunctivae or develop an opacity at the corneal-scleral junction. Such lesions may damage the cornea and affect vision.

The diagnosis of allergic rhinitis and conjunctivitis may be confirmed with the aid of the following tests:

1. Nasal and conjunctival smear for eosinophils. Eosinophils are usually present in the secretions of the target organ. It should be remembered that eosinophils may be present in the secretions of normal infants up to the age of 6 months.
2. Allergy skin testing. This helps identify the specific offending allergen.
3. Test for IgE. An elevated total IgE would be supportive of the diagnosis; however, many patients with allergic rhinitis and conjunctivitis have normal levels.

Differential Diagnosis of Allergic Rhinitis

Vasomotor Rhinitis. Vasomotor rhinitis is a perennial rhinitis that does not have an underlying immunologic mechanism. Symptoms consist of chronic nasal congestion and rhinorrhea that is often provoked by nonspecific stimuli such as dust, chemicals, sudden temperature changes.

Foreign Bodies. Occasionally a small child puts a foreign body in the nasal passage. This soon creates a local inflammatory reaction that produces a purulent, foul-smelling rhinorrhea.

Recurrent Colds. It is not uncommon for young children to have four to six colds per year. The symptoms of rhinorrhea may be associated with fever. Eosinophils are not abundant in the nasal mucosa nor is the typical history of pruritis noted.

Rhinitis Medicamentosa. Chronic use of sympathomimetic nasal drops has been associated with a syndrome of tachyphylaxis to the decongestant requiring frequent and increased dose administration as well as worsening nasal congestion. The rhinitis eventually subsides after the medication is discontinued.

Nasal Polyps. Polyps may occur spontaneously or may be associated with chronic rhinitis of any etiology, with aspirin intolerance, or with cystic fibrosis.

Skull Fracture. A fracture involving the cribiform plate may cause persistent rhinorrhea as a consequence of cerebrospinal fluid (CSF) leakage; these cases are rare. Children may have a history of recurrent bacterial meningitis. Nasal mucus does not contain glucose, while CSF does. A dipstick indicating glucose in the nasal discharge confirms the diagnosis.

Treatment

Avoidance. Certain allergens can be completely avoided once identified. Foods can be eliminated from the diet, or a pet removed from the home. Dust control at home can significantly diminish the amount of allergen exposure. However, a number of allergens (*e.g.*, pollen) cannot be effectively eliminated and therefore treatment will be required.

Antihistamines. Many medications have antihistaminic activity; they inhibit histamine's action of increasing capillary permeability, smooth muscle contraction, and induction of pruritis by competition for the H_1 receptor site on the target organ. Antihistamines do not effect H_2 receptor sites that can control gastric acid secretion. Since histamine is a major mediator of urticaria allergic rhinitis, conjunctivitis, and pruritis in general, antihistamines are most widely used in the treatment of these diseases. The five groups of antihistamines include: (1) ethylenediamines—tripelennamine (Pyribenzamine), (2) alkylamines—chlorpheniramine (Chlor-Trimeton), (3) ethanolamines—diphenhydramine (Benadryl), (4) piperazine—hydroxyzine (Atarax), and (5) phenothiazides—promethazine (Phenergan).

Antihistamine side-effects include sedation, anticholinergic symptoms (dry mouth), gastrointestinal disturbances, central nervous system stimulation, and drowsiness.

Sympathomimetics. Sympathomimetics can be used both topically and orally. Topical therapy is generally avoided except for allergic conjunctivitis because of tachyphylaxis and rebound symptoms (rhinitis) associated with its prolonged usage. Oral sympathomimetics such as pseudoephedrine and phenylephrine hydrochloride can be used alone or in combination with an antihistamine to reduce nasal and conjunctival congestion.

Cromolyn sodium. An inhibitor of mast cell degranulation, cromolyn sodium has been used with some success in the treatment of allergic rhinitis.

Corticosteroids. Topical steroids (dexamethasone or beclomethasone) are sprayed 2 to 4 times per day onto the nasal mucosa. This is an effective form of therapy for the more severe cases of allergic rhinitis, but may be associated with a number of side-effects (*e.g.*, septal perforation).

HMS Liquifilm (medrysone 1%) and similar steroids that do not have a tendency to raise intraocular pressure are used in the topical treatment of severe allergic conjunctivitis and vernal conjunctivitis. Oral steroids are only used for short-term treatment of very severe cases. Injected long-acting depot steroids have no place in the treatment of this disease.

Hyposensitization. Allergy injection therapy is the only effective therapy that can actually cure allergic rhinitis and conjunctivitis. Indications include failure to suppress symptoms with conservative treatment (antihistamines/sympathomimetics) and intolerance or other adverse effects from these medications. This subject is discussed in greater detail in the next section.

ALLERGY SKIN TESTING AND HYPOSENSITIZATION

Allergy Skin Testing

Allergy skin testing was developed empirically long before its immunologic basis was discovered. When an allergen comes in contact with a sensitive person's abraded skin a wheal-and-flare (hive) reaction occurs within 15 minutes. The immunologic basis is an IgE-mediated immediate hypersensitivity reaction. A number of methods for the introduction of the allergen are employed.

The scratch test involves a superficial scratching of the skin followed by a drop of a concentrated allergen placed on the abrasion. The more sensitive intradermal method necessitates the injection of a minute amount (0.02 ml) of dilute antigen within the epidermis.

Both positive (histamine or histamine liberators) and negative controls are necessary for interpretation of results. The more sensitive or allergic the person, the larger the wheal and flare at a lower concentration of test allergen. However, a positive skin test only suggests the presence of specific IgE in the skin; only when positive skin tests correlate with the clinical history can the results identify the allergen as an etiologic agent in the disease.

Common allergens used for testing are trees, grasses, weeds, molds, dust, feathers, animal dander (dog, cat), foods.

Hyposensitization

When allergen avoidance is impractical and conservative medical therapy unsuccessful in the suppression of the atopic symptoms of allergic asthma, allergic rhinitis, or allergic conjunctivitis, hyposensitization to the offending allergen should be considered.

Success in hyposensitization depends upon selection of the correct offending allergen, use of biologically potent extracts, adequate dosage, and frequency of injection.

Allergy injections are initiated at very dilute concentrations and the dosage increased weekly. The dose is increased until a maintenance level is reached. Improvement of symptoms with immunotherapy is slow and often not evident during the first 6 months. Side-effects include both local and anaphylactic reactions.

Persons with symptomatic improvement also undergo immunologic change including a rise in IgG-blocking antibody, loss of sensitivity to antigen-induced basophil histamine release, a decline in the level of specific IgE after a number of years of treatment, and suppression of the rise in specific IgE that occurs with each new seasonal exposure to the antigen.

In addition, recent studies have shown that hyposensitization induces the proliferation of T-suppressor cells that may ultimately be responsible for the suppression of the antigen-specific IgE production.

URTICARIA AND ANGIOEDEMA

Urticaria (hives) is a disorder of the skin characterized by transient, erythematous, pruritic, superficial eruptions usually associated with an elevated central wheal. *Angioedema* is similar to urticaria; however, the deeper subcutaneous tissues are also involved.

Urticaria may be acute or chronic. Acute urticaria is usually of short duration, often less than a week. Persistence beyond 6 weeks is considered chronic. The hive itself is transient and often lasts less than 24 hours.

It may be a discrete wheal-and-flare reaction taking a circular form, or hives may coalesce to cover a large area of skin.

Angioedema usually involves swelling of the skin and subcutaneous tissues. The mucosal lining of the gastrointestinal tract as well as the upper airway may be affected. In the latter case, death may occur due to asphyxia.

Immunologic Mechanism

An intradermal injection of histamine or a mast cell degranulator elicits the formation of a hive within 15 minutes. Histamine is an important vasoactive mediator stored in dermal mast cells and released during certain immunologic reactions. The IgE-mediated immediate hypersensitivity reaction (type I) has been implicated in many cases of urticaria. Dermal biopsies often reveal an eosinophilic infiltration. Histamine may also be released from mast cells during the complement cascade by the action of anaphylatoxin (C_{3a}, C_{5a}). Complement can be activated during type II and type III reactions or by the alternate pathway. However, many cases of urticaria have no clearly defined immunologic basis; therefore, urticaria appears to be heterogenic in origin.

Etiologic Factors

Allergens either ingested or injected are often the cause of urticaria, while inhalant allergens are uncommonly involved. Drugs are among the most frequent etiologic factors. Lesions may appear within minutes following exposure or after days or weeks. Frequently implicated drugs are: penicillin, sulfonamides, and mast cell degranulators (*e.g.*, codeine). The ingestion of foods can be associated with allergic urticaria, including milk, egg, cola drinks, peanuts, citrus fruits, chocolate, fish, seafood, and strawberries. Food coloring (tartrazine yellow dye), preservatives (benzoic acid) and aspirin can cause hives on a nonimmunologic basis. Injectable drugs and vaccines as well as insect stings and bites may result in urticaria. Infections including viral (infectious hepatitis, infectious mononucleosis), bacterial (abscess, UTI), and fungal (tinea pedis), as well as parasitic infestations are documented causes of hives.

Cholinergic urticaria is characterized by multiple tiny hives often provoked by exercise, overheating, sweating, and emotional stress.

Physical urticarias are hives induced by cold, heat, pressure, stroking (dermatographism), and light (actinic urticaria).

Urticaria may be the initial manifestation of an underlying disease state such as malignancy (*e.g.*, Hodgkin's disease) or connective-tissue disorder (*e.g.*, systemic lupus erythematosus or periarteritis nodosa).

Differential Diagnosis

Urticaria Pigmentosa. Hives associated with a local dermal accumulation of mast cells resulting in slightly elevated brown pigmented macules or placques are known as urticaria pigmentosa. When the lesion is stroked, hives appear locally.

Papular Urticaria. These are small pruritic papules that may present initially as a hive following an insect bite. Lesions usually last a number of days and have a telltale puncture in the center of the lesion.

Erythema Multiforme. Although hives may be present, other target or iris lesions usually characterize erythema multiforme.

Hereditary Angioedema. An inherited disease characterized by recurrent episodes of angioedema is known as hereditary angioedema. Swelling can involve skin, GI tract (abdominal cramps), respiratory mucosa (upper airway obstruction). There may be a family history of angioedema or of family members who died of asphyxia. Lesions are often precipitated by minor trauma. The disease is due to a deficiency of C_1-esterase inhibitor.

Treatment

Identification and elimination of the etiologic antigen of urticaria would be ideal. Unfortunately, no etiology is found in up to three-quarters of patients with chronic urticaria. Therefore, treatment is symptomatic. Antihistamines (hydroxyzine or chlorpheniramine) often provide some relief. Most cases of acute urticaria subside without an etiologic diagnosis.

Extensive urticarial lesions (giant urticaria) and angioedema may require treatment with epinephrine. Steroids are indicated only under extraordinary circumstances

ANAPHYLAXIS AND INSECT STING ALLERGY

Anaphylaxis is a systemic form of immediate hypersensitivity. Most of these reactions are believed to be an IgE-mediated (type I) reaction associated with release of vasoactive substances. Other immunologic reactions (type II and type III) are capable of fixing complement and releasing anaphylatoxins (C_{3a} and C_{5a}) as well as kininlike substances (C_{2b}). The systemic release of vasoactive mediators can produce increased capillary permeability, peripheral vasodilation, bronchospasm, and severe hypotension.

Etiology

Almost any allergen can cause an anaphylactic reaction. The route of allergen administration is important. Injection is more likely to cause anaphylaxis than oral or topical administration of the same allergen.

Drugs. Drugs are among the most common causes of anaphylaxis, with Penicillin and its derivatives as prime offenders. Injected drugs such as intravenous radio contrast material, foreign serums, hyposensitization serum, vaccines, enzymes, as well as other proteins, are particularly potent inducers of anaphylaxis.

Chemical Histamine Releasers. Certain drugs such as codeine, morphine, and d-tubocurarine are chemical histamine releasers that cause anaphylactoid reactions.

Foods. Foods can induce anaphylaxis in sensitive persons. Among the common foods implicated are egg white, nuts, and seafoods.

Insect Stings. Bees, wasps, yellow jackets, and hornets (hymenoptera species) are common causes of insect sting anaphylaxis (see below).

Clinical Features

Systemic anaphylatic reaction often begins within a few minutes following exposure to an allergen. The earlier the onset, the more severe the reaction. The patient suddenly feels weak and ill, is pale and diaphoretic, and suffers from vertigo. Cardiovascular symptoms are caused by a combination of systemic vascular dilatation and fluid loss through transudation, resulting in hypovolemia and hypotension. Patients can develop the signs and symptoms of cardiovascular shock (pallor, diaphoresis, cold extremities, hypotension, weak, thready pulse, and so on). If not treated promptly such an anaphylactic response may terminate in fatal irreversible shock. Respiratory signs and symptoms include dyspnea, chest tightness, wheezing, and asphyxia due to edema of the mucosa of the upper airway. Some patients develop generalized urticaria or angioedema. Edema of the gastrointestinal mucosa causes abdominal cramps and nausea. Severely affected patients may lose consciousness and become incontinent.

Treatment of Anaphylaxis

The best treatment for anaphylaxis is prevention. Previous drug reactions as well as adverse reactions to environmental antigens should be assessed carefully and the appropriate avoidance measures recommended.

Treatment for an acute reaction is subcutaneous epinephrine (0.01 ml/kg of 1:0 1000 epinephrine). Patients in shock may require cautious intravenous administration of epinephrine (1:10,000).

If the allergen is an injectant or insect sting in an extremity, a tourniquet should be placed proximal to the site of entry. Patients with signs of shock require administration of large volumes of intravenous fluids. Resistant hypotension requires intravenous vasopressor treatment: metaraminol (Aramine) or levarterenol (Levophed). Oxygen can be delivered by means of a face mask or nasal prongs. Following these urgent procedures, antihistamine can be administered; however, its efficacy in anaphylaxis is not clear.

Patients with bronchospasm need oxygen and intravenous aminophylline, as in acute asthma. Those with laryngeal edema that produces obstruction of the upper airway should undergo tracheostomy. Corticosteroids can be helpful in the treatment of anaphylaxis; because their biologic action is delayed for a number of hours, they are not the first drugs administered.

Insect Sting Reactions

Over the past 10 years, 300 to 400 deaths have occurred in the United States as a result of insect stings. Anaphylaxis is most often associated with the stings of insects from the order of Hymenoptera (bees, wasps, hornets, and yellow jackets) and the fire ant. Anaphylaxis from insect sting does not differ from anaphylaxis from other causes. Although atopic persons have a greater tendency to develop anaphylactic reactions, they also occur in nonatopics. Most insect stings result in a local reaction. In addition to bites and stings, the inhalation of insect products or parts (*e.g.*, caddis fly and cockroach) has been associated with respiratory allergy. Identification of the insect may not be possible. Allergy skin testing with whole insect body extracts can identify the offender. Skin testing with the insect venom alone seems more reliable in identifying the hypersensitive patient.

Treatment of Insect Stings

Anaphylaxis following insect stings is treated the same as anaphylaxis from other causes. In addition, patients with positive skin test correlating with history are given hyposensitization beginning with a very low dose of insect extract. Allergy injections are usually carried out for no less than 10 years. This therapy is satisfactory in the majority of cases. Patients are instructed to carry an insect sting kit containing epinephrine. Avoidance measures include:

Not using perfumes or scents
Not wearing bright-colored clothes
Wearing shoes outdoors
Avoiding outdoor picnic and garbage areas

ATOPIC DERMATITIS

Atopic dermatitis or *infantile eczema* is a common skin disease affecting 1 to 3% of all children. The skin lesions are highly pruritic, erythematous eruptions with a symmetric distribution. Persistent scratching may induce exudative lesions in the acute stage or lichenification during the chronic stage. Often there is a positive family history of eczema. The lesions usually appear during the first 6 months of life and usually resolve between 2 and 4 years. However, some patients continue to have exacerbations or persistence of lesions throughout childhood and occasionally into adulthood.

Atopic dermatitis was thought to be an allergic disease because of its frequent association with other atopic disease (*e.g.*, hayfever and asthma) but it does not appear to be caused by an IgE-mediated mechanism. Nevertheless, these patients do have a number of immunologic abnormalities including a partial T cell defect and a markedly increased level of IgE. How these findings relate to the etiology of the skin rash is not clear. An important characteristic of atopic dermatitis is the skin's low threshold for pruritis. Also characteristic are abnormal blanching following stroking of the skin and delayed blanching following intradermal injection of acetylcholine. The significance of these dermal vascular changes is not clear.

Clinical Course

During the first few months of life, symmetric dermal lesions often appear as fine pruritic papules over the cheeks or the extensor surfaces of the extremities. As the infant matures, the rash tends to localize over the flexural areas (anticubital fossa and popliteal fossa). Abrasion of lesions due to rubbing and scratching can produce a wet eczemoid lesion. When infected, heaped up crusts filled with bacteria develop. The exudative stage may become generalized involving most of the body, skin, and scalp. In time, the chronic irritation of the skin produces a lichenified (thick, leatherlike) lesion. Lesions often exacerbate during the dry winter months. The epidermis of these patients is delicate, has a marked tendency toward dryness and pruritis and is easily irritated by soaps, detergents, and rough or tight clothing (particularly wool). In the young child and infant certain foods may exacerbate lesions. Elimination diets generally have not been successful in suppressing the lesions.

Treatment

Treatment is primarily directed at suppression of pruritis which often occurs following drying or irritation of the skin. Dry skin can be hydrated with the use of a hydrophilic ointment (*e.g.*, Eucerin). Bathing is limited and a gentle soap (*e.g.*, Dove) is used. Fingernails are cut short to minimize traumatic scratching. Clothing should be soft (cotton) and loose-fitting. Rough sweaters and bedding are avoided. Persistent pruritis is treated with antihistamines (hydroxyzine) and topical steroids. Infected lesions are treated with wet compresses and systemic antibiotics. The key to successful management is in-depth parental counseling in topical care of their child's skin.

Complications

Secondary bacterial infection of generalized eczema can lead to erythroderma. Patients exposed to herpes virus or smallpox vaccination may develop severe generalized viral lesions, known as Kaposi's varicelliform eruption. This complication has a 5% mortality. Therefore, contact with herpes lesions and smallpox vaccination must be avoided by patients with atopic dermatitis.

FOOD ALLERGY

The ingestion of a specific food can cause a variety of symptoms in the hypersensitive child, including anaphylaxis, urticaria, gastrointestinal disorders, wheezing, changes in personality, headaches, and eczema.

Food allergy is seen more frequently in children than in adults. Foods commonly associated with allergic reactions are milk, egg, wheat, chocolate, corn, citrus fruits, nuts, legumes, berries, and seafood. Cooking or processing of the food reduces its allergenic capability. Allergic reactions to foods may be either immediate or delayed. The immediate type of reaction appears in many cases to be IgE-mediated. The mechanism for the delayed reactions are difficult to define immunologically. Unfortunately, a poorly defined reaction which may or may not be related to the food ingestion, may be ascribed to food allergy or to an immunologic mechanism.

The allergens in foods are usually proteins or polypeptides. When a food is suspected of being an allergen, an attempt at documentation must be made. Skin testing with food antigens is not always reliable since food extracts may be poor allergens. In addition, food additives, coloring, or contaminants may actually cause the reaction, rather than the food itself.

Of all the foods allergenic in childhood, cow's milk is most frequently incriminated. The casein and lactalbumin of cow's milk are the offending allergens. A history of atopic reaction shortly after ingestion with positive skin tests confirms the diagnosis of immediate hypersensitivity. Gastrointestinal complaints, colic, and so on, may be related to disaccharidase deficiency rather than milk allergy. Gastrointestinal allergy is often associated with eosinophilia and eosinophils in the feces. Milk ingestion can be associated with respiratory symptoms similar to asthma, pulmonary infiltrates, iron-deficiency anemia, and diarrhea (Heiner's syndrome). The affected child has high titers of antimilk precipitating antibodies. Symptoms subside on a milk-free diet.

Although food allergy often provokes cutaneous and gastrointestinal symptoms, respiratory symptoms are far less common, and when they occur, are usually accompanied by dermal or gastrointestinal symptoms.

Diagnosis of food allergy can be aided by repeated (3 times) elimination and challenging diets. If the history suggests a violent reaction, this technique should be avoided.

Aspirin, food dyes, and preservatives are discussed in the following section.

DRUG ALLERGY

Almost any drug can cause an immunologically mediated adverse reaction in a sensitized person. Certain drugs are frequent sensitizers (penicillins) while others are rarely allergenic (erythromycin). For a reaction to be classified as allergic, some evidence suggesting its immunologic mechanism must be present.

Drug reactions can be divided into two major groups.

Drug Reactions

In Nonallergic Persons. The first group of drug reactions includes those that normally occur in many nonallergic persons: toxic effects, side-effects, and secondary effects.

Toxic effects or overdosage occur when the drug is taken in amounts greater than necessary to achieve a pharmacologic effect, or there may be a decreased requirement because of drug clearance abnormalities (*e.g.*, kidney or liver damage).

Side-effects are undesirable properties of a drug that can occur when the drug is administered at appropriate dosage. These adverse effects often are not related to the therapeutic function of the drug (*e.g.*, drowsiness following antihistamines, tremor, and excitement with sympathomimetics).

Secondary effects include reactions that are not directly caused by the drug's pharmacologic action, but may result as a consequence of the drug's action—superinfections following antibiotic treatment.

In Sensitive Persons. A second category of drug reactions is related to a person's special sensitivity to a particular drug or drugs. This includes drug intolerance, idiosyncrasy, and allergy.

Drug intolerance is an adverse reaction related to the pharmacologic action of the drug even in small dosage. An example is drowsiness from antihistamines when only a fraction of the recommended dose is administered.

Idiosyncrasy is an adverse reaction due to a person's individual biochemistry. For example, hemolytic anemia occurs in glucose 6-phosphate dehydrogenase (G-6-PD)-deficient persons when treated with nitrofurantoin.

Allergic reactions or *hypersensitivity reactions* occur in immunologically sensitive persons and are unrelated to the drug's pharmacologic action. Examples are penicillin-caused anaphylaxis and neomycin-induced contact dermatitis. Most drugs are low molecular weight haptens that become allergens when combined with larger carrier molecules. Allergy to drugs occurs in only a small percentage of patients taking a certain medication. The reactions may occur 1 to 2 weeks following initiation of therapy in a previously unsensitized child. Once the patient is sensitized, the allergic reaction may occur immediately following exposure.

Mechanism

The mechanisms of drug allergy vary and may include any or all of the previously described four types of immunologic reactions. For example, type I reaction (anaphylaxis) can occur with penicillin therapy, as can type II (hemolytic anemia). Type III or toxic-complex reactions (serum sickness) can occur following foreign protein administration, as with antisnake venom treatment. Type IV or delayed hypersensitivity can present as cutaneous contact dermatitis following topical neomycin administration.

Allergic reactions to drugs include cutaneous reactions, anaphylaxis, serum sickness, pulmonary reactions, liver disease, renal disease, hematologic abnormalities, drug fever, and allergic vasculitis.

Cutaneous Eruptions. Allergic dermal drug reactions include urticaria, angioedema, erythema multiforme, erythema nodosum, exfoliative dermatitis, and others. "Fixed drug eruption" describes the recurrence of a rash in the same area following reexposure to the sensitizing drug (frequently barbiturates). Photoallergic reactions on the exposed skin can occur in patients taking sulfonamides following activation of the drug by the sun's radiant energy. Contact dermatitis occurs as a delayed reaction to topical medication resulting from sensitivity to a drug (*e.g.*, neomycin) or a preservative in the medication (*e.g.*, parabens).

Most allergic cutaneous lesions are highly pruritic, possibly their one clinical common denominator.

Anaphylaxis. Almost any drug can cause an anaphylactic reaction; however, penicillin and its derivatives are among the most common offenders during childhood (see section on anaphylaxis earlier in this chapter).

Serum Sickness. Serum sickness is an allergic reaction to injected foreign protein (*e.g.*, equine-derived antisera). Symptoms include rash, fever, joint pain, lymphadenopathy, and nephritis. This is a type III (toxic-complex) reaction. Symptoms appear 7 to 10 days following administration of the medication. Today, equine-derived sera are rarely used, with the exception of antisnake venom, but a similar response occurs with other drugs (*e.g.*, penicillin).

Pulmonary Disease. Bronchospasm may occur as part of anaphylaxis or as a consequence of aerosolized antibiotics. The inhalation of pituitary snuff in the treatment of diabetes insipidus may cause asthma or a hypersensitivity pneumonitis. Nitrofurantoin, penicillin, and sulfonamides have been associated with pulmonary infiltrates, systemic illness, and eosinophilia.

Liver Disease. Allergic reactions to salicylates, isoniazid, phenothiazines, and halothane can result in liver disease.

Kidney Disease. Administration of methicillin has been associated with the development of antitubular antibodies and interstitial nephritis.

Drug Fever. Patients receiving drugs can develop a persistent high fever, often with leukocytosis. Symptoms usually appear about 1 week following the initiation of therapy with drugs like penicillin and the sulfonamides.

Vasculitis. Some patients initially develop fever and/or erythema multiforme, progressing to a generalized vasculitis as a result of drug treatment. Others develop vasculitis without other manifestations.

Hematologic Disorders. Hemolytic anemia, thrombocytopenia, and granulocytopenia are hematologic disorders caused by allergic drug reactions.

Diagnosis

The history is of primary importance in the diagnosis of drug allergy. In certain instances, laboratory studies are very helpful (*e.g.*, Coombs' positive hemolytic anemia, complement consumption in serum sickness). Immunopathologic studies may occasionally be of aid. Allergy skin testing has only been of value in penicillin allergy in predicting immediate type reactions.

In vitro tests for drug allergy have been disappointing with the exception of the radioallergoabsorbent test (RAST) for penicillin allergy, probably because most offenders are haptens or metabolic products.

Treatment

The offending drug is discontinued unless required for a life-threatening illness. Treatment following drug removal is symptomatic and includes the use of antihistamines, topical antipruritics, aspirin for systemic symptoms, and occasionally steroids for severe reactions.

Desensitization consisting in injections of the offending drug beginning with minute amounts followed by frequent (every 15 min) and cautious progressive increments has had some success in treating penicillin allergy.

BIBLIOGRAPHY

Blanti JA (ed): Immunology II. Philadelphia, WB Saunders, 1978

An excellent general reference on immunology.

Connel JT: Allergic rhinitis. In Weiss EB, Segal MS (eds): Bronchial Asthma, Mechanisms and Therapeutics. Boston, Little, Brown & Co., 1976

The pathologic mechanisms, clinical evaluation, differential diagnosis and treatment of allergic rhinitis are discussed.

Fudenberg HH, Stites DP, Caldwell JL, Weils JV (eds): Basic and Clinical Immunology, 3rd ed. Los Altos, Calif, Lange Medical Publications, 1980

Reviews clinical immunology including cellular and humoral mechanisms, immediate hypersensitivity and complement.

Norins AL: Atopic dermatitis. Pediatr Clin North Am 18:801, 1971

A review of atopic dermatitis including etiologic, clinical, and therapeutic considerations.

Parker CW (ed): Clinical Immunology. Philadelphia, WB Saunders, 1980

An excellent general reference on immunology.

Sheffer A: Urticaria and angioedema. Pediatr Clin North Am 22:193, 1975

Immunologic and nonimmunologic mechanisms in urticaria, hereditary angioedema, physical urticaria and aspirin intolerance are discussed.

The Skin

28

Paul J. Honig

Dermatologic disorders occur in up to 30% of patients seen by pediatricians. Familiarity with frequently occurring skin problems is required. Patients presenting with rare or perplexing problems can be evaluated in cooperation with a pediatric dermatologist.

EVALUATION OF THE SKIN

The skin measures between 1.5 and 4.0 mm in thickness, of which the epidermis comprises 0.05 to 0.1 mm (Fig. 28-1). Basal cells divide and differentiate into keratinocytes, the predominant cell of the epidermis. The renewal process of the epidermis occurs every 28 days, as indicated by the time required for tritiated thymidine-tagged basal cells to reach the stratum corneum (where they are flattened and without nuclei).

The skin functions as a protective barrier for the body. Skin color is produced by melanin, carotene, and hemoglobin. The melanocyte, which produces melanin, is derived from the neural crest and migrates to the basal cell layer of the epidermis. The function of melanin is to protect the skin from injury by ultraviolet radiation.

The dermis is composed mainly of collagen and elastic fibers, acid mucopolysaccharides, blood vessels, and neural elements. It functions as the nutritive bed for the epidermis and is involved in the regulation of heat loss and host defenses.

History

Some rashes are classic and easily diagnosed by observation. A variety of pathogenic mechanisms or agents can cause identical rashes. A careful history is most important in evaluation of dermatologic problems. In addition to the routine history, particular emphasis should be given to the following questions:

1. Does the child appear toxic or sick?
2. Has the child been sick in the recent past?
3. Has the child had contact with someone who has been ill (family or friends)?
4. Where did the rash begin and how did it spread (distribution)?
5. Does the rash itch?
6. How has the rash been treated? Medication history, current skin care.
7. Is there a prior history of immunizations?
8. Is there a past history of illness?
9. Is there a family history of allergies?
10. Has the child had contact with pets?
11. Has the child been on a recent hiking, camping, or picnicking experience? What are his common play areas?
12. What is a description of the child's bedroom and home environment?

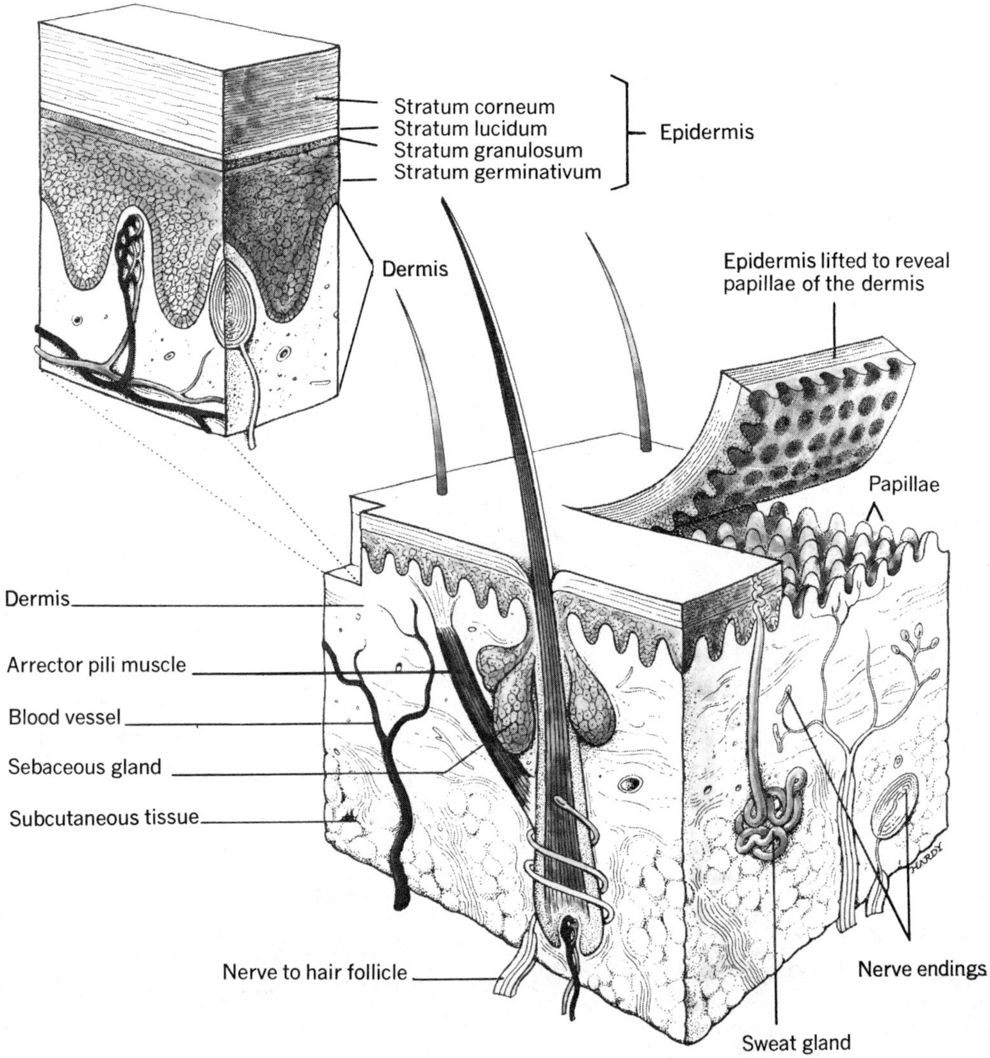

Fig. 28-1. Histology of the skin. (Chaffee EE, Lytle IM: Basic Physiology and Anatomy, 4th ed.) Philadelphia, JB Lippincott, 1980.

Basic Skin Lesions

The ability to make diagnoses of skin lesions comes about as the result of retrieval of historical information surrounding the problem, recognition of patterns of distribution, clues of configuration and grouping, and prior visual experience. Written descriptions are not an adequate substitute for pictures or personal experience. The following definitions are important:

Macule—a small, flat, colored spot which when palpated cannot be distinguished from the normal surrounding skin

Patch—the result of coalescence of several macules

Papule—small, palpable, elevated, solid

lesions of various colors, less than 1 cm in diameter
Plaque—result of the coalescence of papules
Vesicle—small, elevated, translucent, thin-walled, fluid-containing lesion, less than 1 cm in diameter
Bulla—a large vesicle greater than 1 cm in diameter
Pustule—vesicle whose fluid has become cloudy
Nodule—large papules greater than 1 cm in diameter
Wheal—elevated lesion, at times with irregular margins, produced by collection of dermal fluid
Crust—collection of dried serum, blood, or pus
Scale—adherent flakes
Erosion—superficial loss of skin, epidermal loss as occurs in nonscarring abrasion
Ulceration—significant loss of skin, including entire epidermis plus part of dermis resulting in scarring
Atrophy—loss of tissue resulting in a sunken appearance of the skin

BASIC LABORATORY TESTS

Skin Biopsy

A circular plug or excised portion of skin is removed for study by light or electronmicroscopy. The histologic diagnosis is used for confirmation of a clinical diagnosis or delineation of an unknown or suspected clinical entity.

Special stains can be used to identify various substances in the tissue sample, such as mucopolysaccharides, lipids, collagen fibers, elastic fibers, nerves, melanin, iron, calcium. In addition, skin specimens can be incubated with fluorescein-conjugated antisera in certain suspected autoimmune disorders (*e.g.*, systemic lupus erythematosus, diskoid lupus erythematosus).

Cultures

Bacterial
Fungal—special media such as Sabouraud's agar (with antibiotics to inhibit bacterial overgrowth)
Viral

Potassium Hydroxide Preparations

Using a no. 15 blade, the leading edge of a lesion is scraped. Ten percent potassium hydroxide is mixed with the scales which have been put on a glass slide. After covering this suspension with a glass coverslip, gentle heating dissolves the epithelial cells quickly. This preparation is then examined under a microscope with magnification ×10 for hyphae and spores.

Tzanck Test

The Tzanck test is used for rapid cytologic examination. The process is valuable when trying to prove the presence of herpes simplex or other herpes viruses. A smear is made by scraping the base of a freshly opened vesicle. The material obtained is stained with Giemsa's stain and examined under the microscope for the presence of multinucleated giant cells (Fig. 28-2).

Wood's Light Examination

The Wood's light is a filtered mercury lamp which emits light in the range of 3600 Å. It is useful in the diagnosis of entities that produce material that fluoresces

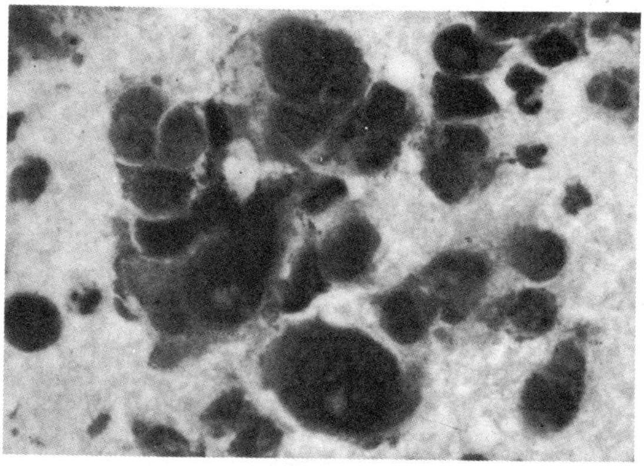

Fig. 28-2. Multinucleate giant cell.

when exposed to light (*e.g.*, blue-green fluorescence of tinea capitis, orange-red fluorescence of urine from patients with erythropoietic porphyria).

Patch Test

The patch test is used when testing skin for contact sensitization to various chemicals, by applying the material to be tested to the skin and covering it for 48 hours with an airtight patch. After exposing the test area to air for 20 minutes, the skin is examined for erythema and vesiculation.

NEWBORN

Transient Skin Lesions of Newborn

Milia
Sebaceous gland hyperplasia
Erythema toxicum
Miliaria
Mottling
Skin trauma

Milia are 1-mm white papules occurring in 40% of newborns. They are frequently seen on the forehead, cheeks, and nose. Within a few weeks of birth, these epidermal cysts exfoliate spontaneously. *Sebaceous gland hyperplasia* is seen in full-term infants as a heavy concentration of minute white or yellow papules over the nose and cheeks. These spontaneously disappear over several weeks or months. In 30% to 70% of full-term infants, scattered white papules or pustules on an erythematous base appear at 24 to 48 hours. These lesions are termed *erythema toxicum*. The presence of these lesions correlates directly with maturity (not seen in infants less than 30 weeks; seen in up to 60% of infants at 42 weeks' gestation). The lesions are differentiated from staphylococcal infections by the presence mainly of eosinophils rather than polymorphonuclear cells in the infiltrate of the pustules. Heat rash or *miliaria* is the result of blocked sweat ducts. The lesions appear on the head, face, and in the intertriginous areas as vesicles, papules, or pustules. With air conditioning this problem is less common. *Mottling* or *cutis marmorata* results from the response of the infant's skin to cooling. The bluish marbling or lacklike pattern of the skin of the extremities and trunk disappears with rewarming of the infant. At times, infants who have had intrauterine monitoring with a scalp device or have been delivered with forceps may manifest abrasions, bruises, or the depressed skin lesions of fat necrosis.

Congenital Pigmentary Changes

Mongolian spots
Pigmented nevi
  Systematized
  Sebaceous
  Giant hairy
Cafe au lait spots
Ash leaf macules
Congenital adrenal hyperplasia
Urticaria pigmentosa

Infants may be born with multiple types of pigmentary variations. Some of these are of no consequence, while others may indicate the presence of underlying disease.

Areas of slate blue to gray pigmentation (indicating dermal melanocytes) occur very frequently in Negro, Oriental, and Indian infants. They have been termed *Mongolian spots* and occur in any part of the body. They usually disappear in one to two years; however, some may persist.

Flat, *melanocytic nevi* occur in 1% to 3% of newborns. There is some controversy about the premalignant potential of these lesions because of reports indicating a slight risk of conversion to malignant melanoma. It is not practical to remove all melanocytic nevi.

Another lesion with similar potential is the *giant hairy nevus.* Present at birth, it can occupy a large area of the skin surface. The lesion is usually unevenly pigmented, somewhat elevated, and eventually covered with long, dense hairs. Because of the low incidence of conversion to melanoma, small lesions should be removed. Those lesions covering a large surface area are impossible to remove completely and therefore, must be followed carefully for changes in color, ulceration, or nodularity.

Another nevus is the elevated, linear, *widespread epidermal nevus.* This lesion, usually an autosomal dominant, can be associated with various skeletal, vascular, and central nervous system anomalies.

Cafe au lait spots are sometimes found in the newborn. They are flat, nonpalpable, coffee-colored lesions. They vary in size and shape. When six or more are present, greater than 1.5 cm in size, neurofibromatosis or gonadal dysgenesis should be suspected.

The *ash leaf macule* is a flat hypopigmented (whitish) spot that is present in more than 90% of patients with tuberous sclerosis. In Caucasian patients, the macules are more easily seen by shining a Wood's light on the skin.

Another sign of systemic disease is the pigmentation associated with *congenital adrenal hyperplasia.* Affected children have increased skin pigmentation around the nipples, umbilicus, and perineum.

Collections of mast cells can appear as light, brown macules or elevated plaques, known as urticaria pigmentosa. Stroking these lesions causes release of histamine with resultant erythema and swelling (Darier's sign). In infants, irritation may induce blister formation. At times the process is diffuse and systemic signs of histamine release occur.

Congenital Vascular Changes

Nevus flammeus
Sturge-Weber syndrome
Capillary and cavernous hemangiomas
Lymphedema (Turner's syndrome)

Two common vascular lesions in the newborn are the *macular hemangioma* (salmon patch) and the *capillary hemangioma.* Salmon patches occur on the nape, the eyelids, and the glabella. Nearly half of newborns have a Salmon patch. Those on the face usually fade, while those at the back of the head and neck persist. When the lesion is large and intensely red, it is called a *nevus flammeus* or *port wine stain.* This type of lesion localized in the distribution of the trigeminal region of the face can be associated with seizures and hemiparesis (*Sturge-Weber syndrome*).

Capillary hemangiomas frequently begin as macular white lesions which then elevate into red, raised, spongy tumors. They are vascular lesions which are common and disappear with time. Another variation of this lesion is the *cavernous hemangioma.* This vascular tumor is deep, large, and bluish. It also feels spongy. Thrombocytopenia can be associated with this lesion.

Lymphedema is a vascular abnormality. When swelling is limited to the legs and feet and transmitted as an autosomal dominant condition it is called Milroy's disease. When swelling of the hands and feet occurs in females, gonadal dysgenesis must be considered.

Congenital Infections

Rubella
Herpes simplex
Cytomegalovirus
Sepsis
Toxoplasmosis
Syphilis
Varicella

COMMON DERMATOSES

Acne

Acne vulgaris is a disorder of adolescence. It begins with stimulation of the sebaceous glands by androgen. Testosterone is converted by the enzyme 5-alpha reductase to dihydroxytestosterone, the hormone apparently responsible for sebaceous gland hypertrophy and increased production of sebum (Fig. 28-3). This normal physiologic process occurs in all children. Those who are predisposed probably have the abnormalities which lead to acne formation. First, abnormal keratinization within the follicular canal leads to obstruction of the pilosebaceous unit and accumulation of sebum and distention of the unit. The whitehead (closed comedo) is a papule formed by the obstructive material bulging just below the skin surface. When this material protrudes above the skin surface, the blackhead (open comedo) is formed. The black color is due to melanin, not dirt. Second, there is increased colonization with *P. acnes* which contains lipases that hydrolyze sebum to free fatty acids causing a severe inflammatory response when pilosebaceous units are disrupted. This releases the substance into the surrounding tissue. The free fatty acids are walled off by an inflammatory response, producing the red papules and pustules characteristic of acne.

Therapy is aimed at relieving the obstruction of the pilosebaceous unit and decreasing colonization with *P. acnes.* Correction of both abnormalities is necessary for complete control. Topical retinoic acid (vitamin A acid) is the most effective agent used to reduce obstruction of the pilosebaceous unit. This medication inhibits formation of tonofilaments and reduces adhesiveness between keratinocytes. The secondary irritant effect of retinoic acid also accelerates healing of inflammatory lesions by increasing local blood flow. Colonization of the pilosebaceous unit with *P. acnes* can be reduced by the use of systemic antibiotics (*e.g.*, tetracycline, erythromycin), topical antibiotics (*e.g.*, erythromycin, tetracycline, clindamycin), and benzoyl peroxide. Topical benzoylperoxide is bacteriostatic and, like retinoic acid, produces increased local blood flow. Since rupture and release of free fatty acids from the pilosebaceous unit results in inflammatory lesions, avoidance of trauma to the acne-prone areas is also important.

Diaper Dermatitis

A rash that occurs on the skin below the area covered by the diaper is called *diaper dermatitis.* Differentiation of the various types of diaper dermatitis is difficult. Clues from history and physical examination are necessary when characterizing the etiology of this rash. The different types of diaper rashes include:

TABLE 28-1. Congenital Infections

Etiology	Clinical Findings	Significant Perinatal History	Smears from Skin Lesion	Cultures
Herpes simplex	Grouped vesicles on an erythematous base. May become pustular. Frequently appears on presenting part (i.e. head in vertex delivery, buttocks in breech delivery.	Frequently none. Mother or father with genital herpes simplex.	Tzanck test of base of unbroken vesicle demonstrates multinucleated giant cells.	Viral culture positive for herpes simplex
Syphilis	As in the adult, mucocutaneous lesions appear in a variety of forms; most common are papules or even plaques. Lesions may occasionally be pustular or vesicobullous.	Syphilis	Darkfield examination positive for spirochetes. Also in nasal discharge or moist periorificial lesions.	
Varicella	Generalized eruption which progresses from papule to vesicle to crust. Occasional pustule formation. May have erythematous base or can become hermorrhagic.	Mother with chicken pox shortly before delivery of infant	Tzanck smear same as herpes simplex.	May be cultured on special viral medium (human fetal diploid kidney cells or monkey kidney cells)
Cytomegalic inclusion disease (CMV)	Vesicles	Usually not helpful	Not helpful	Cytopathic effects characteristic of CMV in WI-38 cells (human fibroblasts)
Sepsis	Pustules, lethargy and so on	Amnionitis	Helpful at times	Blood cultures positive
Rubella	Purpura—"blueberry muffin" lesions. Cataracts, deafness, congenital heart disease, microcephaly, mental retardation.	Maternal infection with rubella during pregnancy especially first 8 weeks		Viral culture positive for many months
Toxoplasmosis	Generalized maculopapular eruption in 25% of infants. Lasts only two weeks. Choreoretinitis, cerebral calcifications, mental retardation, hydrocephalus or microcephaly.	Maternal infection during pregnancy. Usually no clues.		Innoculation of mice with body fluid or tissue (Sabin-Feldman dye test or specific IgM valuable)

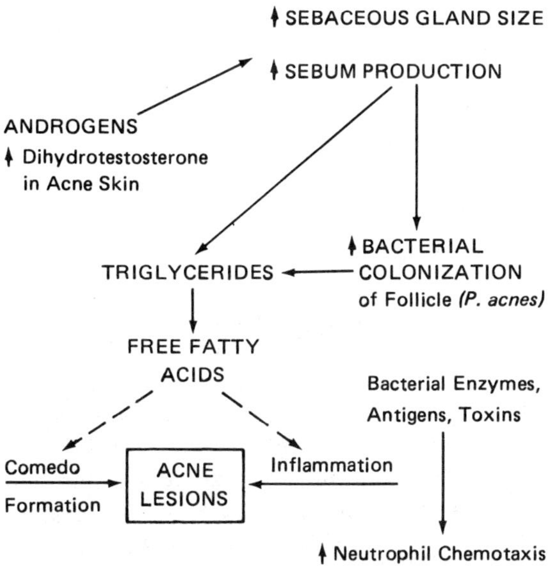

Fig. 28-3. Proposed mechanisms of pathogenesis of acne. (Esterly NB, Furey NL: Acne: current concepts. Pediatrics 62:1044, 1978. Copyright American Academy of Pediatrics, 1978)

1. *Chafing dermatitis.* Rash occurs only in that portion of the diaper area in which friction is greatest (inner thighs, genitals, buttocks, abdomen). The rash waxes and wanes and often has a shiny, glazed surface appearance. There are occasional associated papules.
2. *Atopic dermatitis.* Examination can disclose lesions on other body surfaces, such as the cheeks, typical of atopic involvement. There is often a family history of allergy.
3. *Moniliasis.* Moniliasis is the most characteristic of the diaper rashes; usually intensely red and confluent with a sharp border beyond which there are satellite papules and pustules.
4. *Seborrheic diaper rash.* Generally this rash has an erythematous and scaly appearance most pronounced in the creases of the groin and buttocks, retroauricular area of the neck, axillae and limb creases.
5. *Mixed or undiagnosible rash.* Often one cannot categorize some of the rashes that occur in the diaper area including mixtures of the above rashes.

Treatment for diaper dermatitis is determined by the diagnosis. In general, proper skin care, which includes a mild soap, decreased frequency of washing, and keeping the diaper off as much as possible will lead to resolution of the problem. When atopic dermatitis is present, the use of topical steroids is necessary and when candida albicans has been incriminated, an antifungal agent such as mycostatin should be used.

Contact Dermatitis

The appearance of the rash is the major clue to diagnosis of contact dermatitis. When the sensitized skin comes in contact with an external antigen, an allergic response occurs. Linear or geometric areas of erythema, vesiculation and oozing occur. The shape of the eruption often coincides with the shape of the offending material. Allergic contact dermatitis is a cell-mediated delayed hypersensitivity reaction.

Two examples seen in childhood are the contact dermatitis following exposure to poison ivy and acquired nickel dermatitis. Streaks of vesiculation appear after a child brushes against an ivy poison plant. The offending agent is an oleoresin, urushiol, which contains the chemical pentadecylcatechol. Nickel dermatitis is frequently seen in the female as a response to nickel-containing jewelry. Earlobes are commonly involved because of the popularity of pierced ears.

Shoe contact dermatitis usually begins on the instep and dorsal aspect of the toes. The offending antigens are usually rubber, glues, and dyes used in making the shoes. Patch tests with the suspected substances confirm clinical suspicions.

Xerosis

Xerosis means dry skin. It is a more common problem during wintertime. The rash is pruritic and appears as rough, red, dry, scaly skin. It is similar in appearance to "chapped hands or cheeks" seen in cold weather. Decreased bathing and application of external oils may be beneficial.

Seborrheic Dermatitis

Yellow, oily scales with a background of erythema appearing on the scalp, face, chest, back, axillae, and perineum in infants and children is designated *seborrheic dermatitis*. The pathogenesis is unknown. Cradle cap is the term given to the temporary scaliness that occurs in the scalps of infants. In most instances, seborrheic dermatitis is responsive to mild topical steroids.

Dandruff

Dandruff in children may occur with several conditions:

1. seborrheic dermatitis
2. atopic dermatitis
3. tinea capitis
4. psoriasis

Differentiation is aided by clinical appearance, cultures, and response to therapy. *Seborrheic dermatitis* responds readily to antiseborrheic shampoos and topical steroids. *Atopic dermatitis*, however, is frequently made worse with harsh shampoos and responds very slowly to topical steroids. The diagnosis of *tinea capitis* is best made with cultures. If steroids are used in the presence of tinea capitis, there is frequently increased scaliness of the scalp because of suppressed local immunity of the skin and increased growth of the fungus. *Psoriasis* is usually recognized by the thick scales which are piled on an erythematous base. The margins of the scalp line are frequently heavily involved.

Nummular Eczema

Nummular eczema is an eruption that differs from atopic eczema in that the lesions are circular, erythematous, and scaly, and they consist of crusted patches or plaques. Affected children usually do not have an atopic background and IgE levels are generally not elevated.

Viral Exanthems (See Chap. 34.)

Urticaria

The causes of urticaria are legion. Almost anything can induce the typical lesions including infections, drugs, foods, insect bites, and physical factors. The lesion itself is caused by vasodilatation and leakage of fluid and red blood cells from involved blood vessels. The vascular damage can be caused by such mediators as histamine, complement, and immune complexes. IgE can attach to and cause degranulation of mast cells in sensitized individuals with resulting histamine release. Urticarias are usually acute and transient, but at times they are chronic and recurrent. They rarely accompany serious disease such as hepatitis or collagen vascular disease. A benign form of urticaria is *papular urticaria*. It occurs in young children who become sensitized to insect bites. The bites generally occur in exposed parts such as the face, arms, and legs. With sensitization, urticaria occurs on the trunk or other sites distant from the insect bite.

Pityriasis Rosea

Pityriasis rosea is thought to result from a viral infection, although no agent has been isolated. In 80% of children, a large, oval, solitary lesion appears on the trunk (herald patch) prior to the eruption of multiple lesions, which follow the cleavage lines of the skin. When looking at patients' backs, the term christmas tree distribution has been used. The rash lasts 4 to 8 weeks, is pruritic early in the course, and then becomes asymptomatic. Individual lesions are oval or round, slightly raised, pink to brown, and peripherally scaly. When the pityriasis rosea lesion appears in adolescence, it must be differentiated from secondary syphilis.

OTHER GENETIC DISORDERS

Ichthyosis

There are four major forms of *ichthyosis*. Dominantly inherited ichthyosis vulgaris and sex-linked ichthyosis are considered to be retention keratoses secondary to increased adhesiveness of the stratum corneum with a normal epidermal proliferation rate. Two other forms are dominant-inherited epidermolytic hyperkeratosis and recessive-inherited lamellar ichthyosis. In addition to increased adhesiveness, these conditions also have an increased epidermal proliferation rate. Other uncommon forms of ichthyosis include: erythrokeratodermia variabilis, ichthyosis linearis circumflexa, Rud's syndrome, Refsum's syndrome (metabolic disorder involving phytanic acid), Sjögren-Larson syndrome, and Netherton's syndrome. To describe and differentiate all these syndromes is beyond the scope of this chapter (see Biblio.). Families of patients should be given genetic counseling when the specific type of ichthyosis has been identified.

Epidermolysis Bullosa

Epidermolysis bullosa is a rare congenital and hereditary blistering disease which occurs in various forms:

1. epidermolysis bullosa simplex—autosomal dominant
2. epidermolysis bullosa letalis—autosomal recessive
3. bullous eruption of the hands and feet—autosomal dominant
4. dystrophic epidermolysis bullosa—dominant
5. dystrophic epidermolysis bullosa—recessive

In all forms, friction or trauma results in the formation of blisters. Pathologic differentiation by electronmicroscopy is sometimes helpful. Experimentally induced blis-

TABLE 28-2. Differentiation of Pityriasis Rosea from Syphilis

Findings	Pityriasis Rosea	Syphilis
Herald patch	+	−
Ovals following dermatomes	+	−
Lymphadenopathy	−	+
Mucus membrane lesions	−	+

ters are biopsied and sent for analysis. Cleavage planes are helpful in this differentiation as seen in Figure 28-4.

BACTERIAL INFECTIONS

Impetigo and Ecthyma

The most common infections of the skin involve *Staphylococcus aureus* and group A beta-hemolytic streptococcus. Superficial denudation with resulting yellow crust generally indicates infection with *Staphylococcus aureus*. Frequently group A beta-hemolytic streptococcus is also cultured from these lesions. Usually, when bullae alone are formed as in bullous impetigo, only *S. aureus* is cultured.

Ecthyma is the term used for deeper skin infections with group A beta-hemolytic streptococcus. *S. aureus* is frequently cultured from these lesions. Ten days of antibiotic treatment is recommended to prevent spread of the infection on the affected child and onto contacts. Unfortunately, when nephritogenic strains of streptococcus are involved (types 1, 4, 25, 49, and so on), glomerulonephritis may occur despite antibiotic treatment; however, spread of the skin infection to others is prevented.

Cellulitis

Cellulitis is a deeper infection of the skin generally due to streptococcus, *S. aureus*, or *Hemophilus influenzae*. The typical presentation is an area of tender, warm, swollen, indurated erythema with ill-defined borders in a child with fever and regional adenopathy. With *H. influenzae* cellulitis, or, rarely, pneumococcal cellulitis, the skin color of the affected area may appear blue. Complications are due to direct extension to surrounding tissues (arthritis, osteomyelitis)

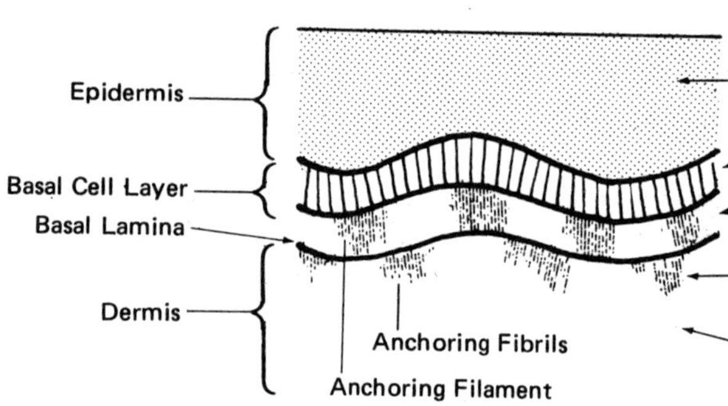

SPLIT LOCATION	TYPE	GENETICS
Upper Epidermis	EB hands and feet	Dominant
Basal Cell Layer	EB Simplex	Dominant
Between Basal Cell Layer and Basal Lamina	EB Letalis	Recessive
Between Basal Lamina and Anchoring Fibrils	Dystrophic EB	Dominant
Below Anchoring Fibrils in Dermis	Dystrophic EB	Recessive

*Epidermolysis bullosa.

Fig. 28-4. Experimentally induced blisters. Separation points as seen by electron microscopy.

or septicemia. Isolation of the offending organism can be accomplished by blood culture or injection and aspiration of sterile saline at the leading border of involved skin.

Meningococcemia, Gonococcemia, *Pseudomonas septica*

Meningococcemia, gonococcemia, and *Pseudomonas septica* may present with erythematous macules, papules, or pustules caused by bacterial emboli to the dermal blood vessels. These lesions usually become palpable and purpuric. At times, the centers become black and ulcerated (septic infarcts) due to total occlusion of the vessels by the septic emboli.

The skin lesions of gonococcemia are often associated with tenosynovitis (dermatitis-arthritis syndrome). The hemorrhagic vesicopustule (dirty pustule) generally develops on the distal extremities. The organism is not easily cultured from the lesion.

Pseudomonas infections commonly produce hemorrhagic necrosis. The eschar is usually surrounded by bright erythema (ecthyma gangrenosum).

VIRAL INFECTIONS

Herpes Zoster

Herpes zoster is caused by a DNA (varicella-zoster) virus. Most patients have a past history of chickenpox. Tingling or pain occurs along the involved dermatome in the preeruptive stage. The child feels ill and may be febrile. The lesions first appear as red papules near the central nervous system and spread out along the nerve distribution, then vesiculate, desiccate, and scab over in 7 to 10 days. Herpes zoster may be contagious (causing chickenpox in susceptible persons). When it occurs in adults, it may indicate an underlying malignancy. This is not generally true in children.

Hand-Foot-and-Mouth Disease

During spring and summer, children affected with hand-foot-and-mouth disease present with papulovesicles on the palms and soles, and ulcers in the mouth. The children are usually afebrile and nontoxic. Coxsackie virus A 16 is often isolated.

SUPERFICIAL VIRAL INFECTIONS OF SKIN

Molluscum Contagiosum

The lesion produced by the pox virus, molluscum contagiosum, is a papule with a white center that can be expressed. Since the virus is contained in the white core, its removal results in healing of the lesion. Lesions can be single or multiple and they favor intertriginous areas such as the axillae and groin. The following are important features of molluscum contagiosum:

1. It has pox virus etiology.
2. It is common in swimmers and wrestlers.
3. It is not always umbilicated.
4. It is associated with immunosuppression.
5. Its duration is 6 to 9 months.
6. It may become inflamed.
7. Eczematoid patients are especially susceptible.

Verruca Vulgaris

The common wart resembles a tiny cauliflower. It may be long and slender (filiform wart), flat (verruca planus), located on the soles (plantar warts), and it may be venereal (condyloma acuminata). The lesions are produced by a DNA virus (papova virus), which resides in the epidermis. Therapy is difficult at best. Important facts about verruca vulgaris include the following:

1. It is caused by papova virus located in the epidermis.
2. It is unusual in early infancy.
3. Its peak incidence occurs between 12 and 16 years.
4. It is transmitted by direct contact.
5. Trauma such as nail biting and increased perspiration favors inoculation.
6. Sixty-five percent of warts disappear spontaneously within 2 years.
7. Thirty to fifty percent of plantar warts disappear within 6 months in prepubertal children.

FUNGAL INFECTIONS OF THE SKIN

Tinea Corporis

The center of the circular patch generally clears as the leading edge spreads out. The lesions are most frequently confused with nummular eczema. Diagnosis can be made by scraping the active outer rim of papules and examining the scales with a KOH preparation under the microscope. The lesions do not fluoresce under Wood's light. The most common offending fungi are *Microsporum canis* and *Trichophyton mentagrophytes*.

Tinea Capitis

Although tinea capitis was commonly caused by the species of genus *Microsporum* in the past, it is now most commonly caused by *Trichophyton tonsurans*. The two forms have different clinical appearances. The *Microsporum* genus generally causes round patches of scaling alopecia. Shining a Wood's light on the lesions yields a blue-green fluorescence. Kerion formation can occur as a swollen, boggy abscess. The *Trichophyton* genus usually causes scattered alopecia. The alopecia is not always oval or rounded and is irregular in outline with indistinct margins. Normal hairs grow within the patch of alopecia. At times the hairs break off at the surface of the scalp, leaving a "black dot" appearance. Diffuse scaliness may simulate dandruff where minimal hair loss is not noted. Wood's light examination of the lesions does not produce fluorescence. The organism can cause a folliculitis, suppuration, and kerion formation. Treatment in both cases consists of orally administered griseofulvin. Diagnosis is made by culturing the affected scalp area.

Tinea cruris is generally caused by *Trichophyton mentagrophytes* or *Epidermophyton floccosum*. Tinea pedis which is usually due to *T. rubrum* or *T. mentagrophytes* is an infection occurring only in postpubertal children. The cracking and peeling of the skin simulating tinea pedis in prepubertal children is generally a manifestation of atopic eczema or hyperhidrosis.

Tinea Versicolor

Tinea versicolor, a superficial fungal infection of the skin caused by *Pityrosporon orbiculare* derives its name from the fact that it produces color changes of the skin including hypopigmentation, hyperpigmentation, and redness. Wood's light usually causes yellowish-brown fluorescence. Moisture promotes growth of the organism. Therefore, exacerbations occur in summer or in athletes who sweat excessively. The infection is difficult to eradicate and frequently recurs. A KOH preparation shows large spores and short stubby hyphae frequently referred to as "spaghetti and meatballs" (see Fig. 28-5).

Chronic Mucocutaneous Candidiasis

Children with chronic mucocutaneous candidiasis have immune deficiencies and experience persistent involvement of the skin, tongue, and lips. These children also are troubled with chronic paronychia.

BITES AND INFESTATIONS

Children are often bitten by insects, especially mosquitoes and fleas. The papules, urticaria, blisters, and hemorrhagic lesions produced are frequently misdiagnosed. The season of the year, the grouping of the lesions, the central punctum, and the distribution on exposed surfaces provide the clues for diagnosis. With sensitization, a condition termed papular urticaria can occur. (urticaria is discussed earlier in this chapter.) Unfortunately, no treatment for insect bites exists. Prevention by insect repellents offers relief.

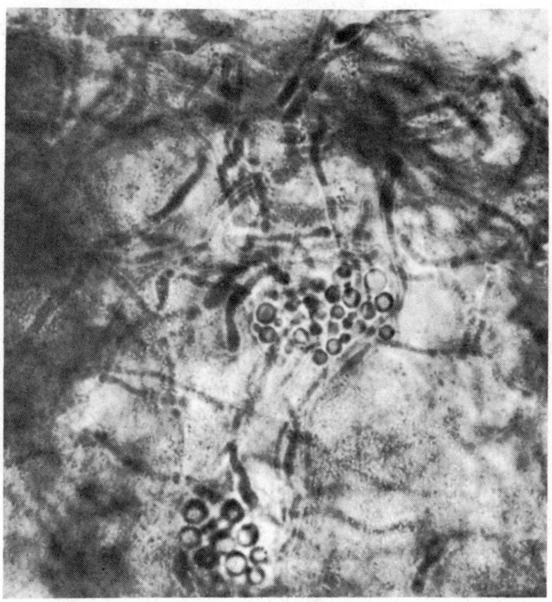

Fig. 28-5. Malassezia furfur. Note blunt-edged hyphae and clusters of spores that form "spaghetti and meat balls" pattern. (Domonkos AN (ed): Andrews' Diseases of the Skin, 7th ed, p 374. Philadelphia, WB Saunders, 1982)

Scabies

The cardinal sign of scabies is pruritis. Infants and children excoriate themselves to the point of bleeding. There are two clues to diagnosis: (1) distribution on the hands, feet, and folds of the body, especially the finger webs, and (2) common occurrence in other family members. Infants may develop blisters and involvement of the head and face, in contrast to the manifestations in adults.

Diagnosis of scabies is made by scraping involved skin and looking for the mite under the microscope objective 10× (Fig. 28-6). Once infestation occurs, it usually takes one month for sensitization and pruritis to develop. Although the use of lindane is an effective treatment, it should not

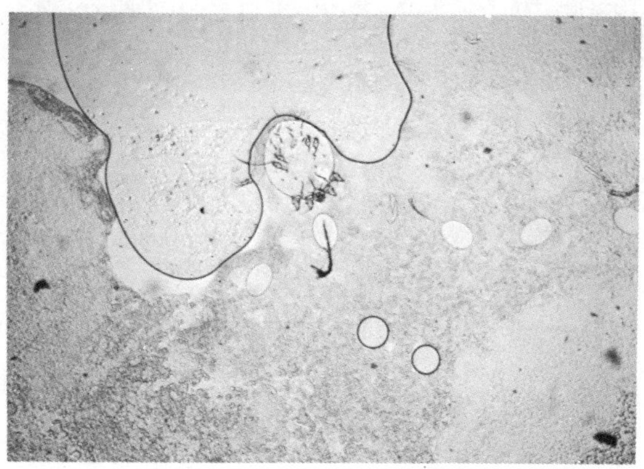

Fig. 28-6. Adult female *Sarcoptes scabiei.*

be used in children under 5 years of age, and especially in those under 1 years of age. Because of a large surface area in young children and transcutaneous absorption, significant blood levels may occur. The toxin can be concentrated in the central nervous system producing seizures. Use of crotamiton is recommended as an alternative therapy.

Pediculosis

The major louse infestation (pediculosis) in children is in the scalp. The infestation has the appearance of "dandruff" in the hair behind the ears. Pruritis of the scalp is common. The female attaches her eggs to the hair shaft. The egg hatches and the nit is left behind. Numerous nits attached to the hair resemble dandruff. Lindane shampoo is the recommended treatment.

Cutaneous Larvae Migrans

Migration of the dog or cat hookworm *(Ancylostoma braziliense)* in the superficial layers of the skin causes the characteristic serpentine red skin tracks. Topical thiabendazole has been effective therapy in some cases. Severe symptoms may be relieved by corticosteroids.

Spider Bites

The spider *Loxosceles reclusa* (brown recluse spider) found most commonly in south central United States, is responsible for most reactions caused by the bite of a spider. The spider is quite small, only 8 to 10 mm long, and bears a violin-shaped band over the dorsal cephalothorax. The venom contains necrotizing, hemolytic factors and spreading factors. The initial symptoms include mild stinging or pruritis. A hemorrhagic blister then appears which can develop into a gangrenous eschar. Severe bites can cause a generalized erythematous macular eruption, nausea, vomiting, chills, malaise, muscle aches, and hemolysis. Treatment includes oral corticosteroids within 6 to 12 hours after the bite, antibiotics, and surgical removal of the necrotic area to prevent spread of the toxin.

HAIR AND NAIL PROBLEMS

Alopecia Areata

Alopecia areata is hair loss in circumscribed areas. Ten to twenty percent of patients have a family history of the disorder. Nail pitting may accompany the problem. The prognosis varies, with 95% of children regrowing their hair within one year. An immune mechanism for this disorder has been proposed because of the dense, lymphocytic, perifollicular infiltration that exists on biopsy specimens. Diffuse hair loss may occur, including eyebrows and eyelashes. In those cases, the prognosis is poor. Treatment of the condition is usually not successful; most cures are spontaneous.

Trichotillomania

Some children develop the habit of rubbing, twirling, or playing with their hair. This is known as trichotillomania and can cause hair breakage or irregular patches of hair loss. Occasionally, the patches show complete loss. Most physicians regard this problem as a "nervous habit." Regrowth of hair can occur but occasionally the hair is permanently lost.

Hair styles which cause excessive tension on the hair shafts can also cause hair breakage and loss (traction alopecia) or folliculitis when the skin is broken (traction folliculitis).

Two disorders termed ectodermal dysplasia show scant hair growth. The hidrotic type is an autosomal dominant. These children have scant hair, severely dystrophic nails, teeth abnormalities, and normal sweat glands. The anhidrotic type is x-linked and associated with hypoplastic or absent sweat glands, defective or absent teeth, and frontal bossing.

There are many varied nail disorders and variations of normal in children. These include scattered pitting, white spots, and longitudinal ridging. Some children are born without nails. Others have thickened, yellow, crumbling nails, as in psoriasis. Others have heavy pitting as in lichen planus or psoriasis. Dystrophic nails (20-nail dystrophy) has no known etiology. Spoon-shaped (concave) nails have been reported in children with severe iron-deficiency anemia. Dystrophic nails can be secondary to chronic infection of the posterior nail bed (paronychia). Longitudinal pigmented (brown) bands occur secondary to melanocytic nevi of the nail beds. The nail-patella syndrome occurs rarely and includes dystrophic nails and absence of the patella.

Albinism

Children with albinism have fair skin, fine silky hair, blue sclera, nystagmus, strabismus, and refractive errors. Three types of albinism exist. Tyrosinase is inactive in one type, or the permease is absent. In both cases, melanin and pheomelanin are not formed. When the enzyme-mediating dopa quinone conversion to melanin is absent, melanin is not formed but pheomelanin synthesis is maintained.

Partial Albinism

A dominant form of partial albinism exists in which localized areas of skin and hair are devoid of pigment. Ocular albinism also occurs. Two syndromes with albinism are Waardenberg's syndrome (white forelock, heterochromia of the iris, sensorineural hearing loss) and Chédiak-Higashi syndrome (immune defect, leukocytes with giant granules).

Hypopigmentation

Loss of pigmentation can be due to absence of melanocytes as in vitiligo and halo nevus. *Vitiligo* is a symmetric, patchy loss of

Disorders of Pigmentation

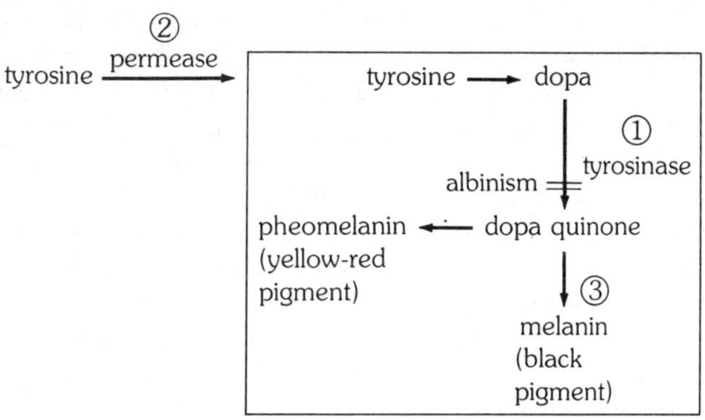

pigmentation. Hair located in areas of vitiligo is often white. It can be associated with alopecia areata, pernicious anemia, Addison's disease, hypothyroidism, diabetes mellitus, hypoparathyroidism, and other endocrine disorders. Vitiligo and some of the diseases associated with it may be autoimmune disorders. Antibodies directed against melanocytes have been detected. An example of this mechanism is the halo of depigmentation surrounding a regressing intradermal nevus in childhood (halo nevus).

Suppression of melanocytic pigment production can cause loss of pigmentation, as in postinflammatory hypopigmentation. An example of this is the white patch of hypopigmentation and scaling frequently seen on the face, trunk, or extremities of children with atopic eczema. At times, inflammation can produce increased pigmentation, secondary to stimulation of pigment formation by the melanocyte.

Pigment deep in the dermis appears gray or blue at the surface of the skin. Mongolian blue spots are an example. The nevus of Ota is dermal pigment in the distribution of the ophthalmic branch of the fifth nerve. This pigmentation can involve the sclera and palate as well.

Certain syndromes are associated with pigmented skin lesions. The Peutz-Jeghers syndrome is a dominantly inherited syndrome which includes frecklelike lesions of the lips, nose, buccal mucosa, fingertips and subungual areas associated with polyps occurring in the small intestine, stomach, or colon. Melena and intussusception are the chief complications that may develop in the second decade. There have been some reports of malignant transformation of the intestinal polyps. Albright's syndrome should be suspected when there are unilateral *cafe au lait* spots with irregular borders occurring in the lumbosacral area. Included in this syndrome are bony abnormalities and precocious puberty.

Single or multiple red-brown papules or nodules occurring on the extremities or face of children may have a confusing histology. Although the lesion is benign, it has been frequently misdiagnosed as malignant melanoma. Therefore, the name, benign juvenile melanoma, was assigned to it (other names include Spitz nevus or spindle-and-epitheliod nevus). True malignant melanomas are rare in childhood. They usually arise from congenital pigmented nevi.

Diffuse hyperpigmentation is associated with Addison's disease, acromegaly, and hemachromatosis.

MISCELLANEOUS DISORDERS

Erythema Multiforme

Erythema multiforme is often secondary to infections (echo virus, Coxsackie virus, *Mycoplasma pneumoniae*, influenze type A, herpes simplex) or to drugs (penicillins, sulfonamides, hydantoins, barbiturates). It is a self-limited, hypersensitivity disease. When mucous membranes are involved, the term Stevens-Johnson syndrome is used.

Toxic Epidermal Necrolysis

Children with toxic epidermal necrolysis first present with marked tenderness of the skin when touched. A "sunburned" erythema then follows, which spreads involving various portions of the skin surface. With mild involvement, superficial desquamation (flaking) occurs as following a sunburn. Severe involvement leads to shearing away of large sheets of skin leaving a denuded, oozing surface, similar to that which occurs after a burn. Often the skin can be rubbed off, leaving a raw surface (Nikolsky's sign).

The process occurs most frequently in young children (less than 6 years) and is secondary to an epidermolytic toxin released by *Staphylococcus aureus* bacteria (phage from group 2), or other noninfectious toxins. Antistaphylococcal therapy is administered until an etiology is ascertained.

Drug Rashes (See Chap. 27.)

Erythema Nodosum

The lesions of erythema nodosum appear as deep, tender, erythematous nodules or plaques on the extensor surfaces of the extremities. They are thought to be hypersensitivity phenomena secondary to infections (streptococcal infections, tuberculosis, coccidiomycosis, histoplasmosis), inflammatory bowel disease, sarcoidosis, malignancies, and drugs. The exact immunologic mechanism has not been clarified.

Psoriasis

The skin lesions in psoriasis vary in size and shape. They are usually erythematous, sharply marginated, elevated plaques with adherent white scales, which when removed result in pinpoint bleeding (Auspitz sign). Areas of involvement are predominantly the scalp, elbows, knees, and intergluteal region. The nails are often deformed, with pitting or other dystrophic changes. Teardrop lesions (guttate) may occur over a large area following streptococcal respiratory infections.

The etiology of psoriasis remains unknown but there is a familial predisposition. Certain histocompatibility loci occur frequently in those patients with a positive family history (HLA B 17) and in those children with psoriasis following a streptococcal infection (HLA B 13).

Granuloma Annulare

Granuloma annulare is thought to be a result of trauma, usually beginning as a module which spreads peripherally with central clearing. It appears as a ringlike group of small flesh-colored or pale red papules. It is frequently confused with tinea corporis. Unlike tinea corporis, scaliness is absent. The problem lasts for several years and then spontaneously disappears. Local or diffuse lesions may occur on any portion of the body, especially the ankles, instep, wrist, and back of the hands, elbows, and knees.

Pyogenic Granuloma

Another lesion seen in children at sites of trauma (frequently insect bites) is pyogenic granuloma. The lesions rapidly grow to about 0.5 cm in diameter and then stabilize. They have the appearance of a pedunculated capillary hemangioma and bleed easily. Histologically, dilated capillaries with prominent epithelial cells are embedded in an edematous stroma. Treatment is surgical removal.

Kawasaki's Disease

Mucocutaneous lymph node syndrome is of unknown cause. The diagnosis is made in children with four of the following criteria: (1) fever of more than 5 days' duration, (2) inflamed conjunctivae, (3) polymorphous rash (frequently morbilliform or scarlatiniform), (4) nonsuppurative cervical adenopathy, (5) edema of the hands and feet with intense palmar and plantar erythema, and desquamation which begins periungually, (6) fiery-red lips that fissure and crust, and a strawberry tongue.

Acrodermatitis Enteropathica

Acrodermatitis enteropathica has an insidious onset. Early (average age 9 months), the child fails to thrive. An eczematous, moist eruption appears around the mouth, eyes, perineum, hands, and feet. Next, hair is lost and diarrhea begins. The dermatologic findings are similar to moniliasis. *Candida albicans* is frequently present as a secondary invader. The syndrome is rare, inherited, and responds to zinc administration.

Child Abuse

The physician must be constantly aware of the skin manifestations of child abuse. Bruises in unusual locations and at various stages of healing are suspicious. Bite marks, unexplained burns (especially circular scars from cigarettes), and geometric scars are worrisome. Frequently the scars conform to the weapon used, for example, strap marks, belt buckle scars, curved or linear coat hanger marks, and so on. Any child with these findings should have a skeletal survey and be reported to a child protection agency (see Chap. 30).

Pyoderma Gangrenosum

Pyoderma gangrenosum is a lesion that develops in 10% of children with ulcerative colitis. It can also be found in patients with regional enteritis, and rheumatoidlike arthritis. First, a pustule or papulovesicle appears and becomes necrotic. The lesion extends and develops into an ulcer with undermined necrotic bluish margins. The lesions are sterile and the histology is nonspecific. Improvement with steroids suggests an immune pathogenesis.

Cold Panniculitis

During the cold of winter, infants and some older children develop red, indurated nodules and plaques on exposed skin (especially the face). Apparently, the subcutaneous fat in infants and some children solidifies more readily at lower temperatures because of the high concentration of saturated fats. Infants who hold ice popsicles in their mouths are also susceptible to cold panniculitis.

Necrobiosis Lipoidica

Patches of yellowish atrophic skin with telangiectasias can appear on the skin of children, usually females, with diabetes mellitus. Vascular changes may cause necrobiosis of collagen in the lesion. Treatment for necrobiosis lipoidica is symptomatic and difficult.

THERAPY

Great strides have been made in understanding treatment modalities for skin problems. Proper skin care is as important as any medication. Unfortunately, many patients feel the need for better hygiene when a pruritic rash appears. This leads to overwashing, using of harsh soaps, and thus worsening of the rash. In any situation, a moderate frequency of washing and the use of mild soaps (*e.g.*, Dove, Tone, Caress) is beneficial.

A group of medications used in dermatology is the topical steroids. These steroids are rated according to potency (low = hydrocortisone; moderate = fluocinolone acetonide, triamcinolone, betamethasone valerate; high = fluocinonide, halcinonide). In general, high-potency steroids should not be used in children. Fluorinated steroids should not be used on the face because of the risk of atrophy, erythema, telangiectasia, and acne. A moderate-potency steroid may be used for an acute eruption, with a changeover to a low-potency preparation when improvement occurs. Systemic effects have been reported with the use of topical steroids on rare occasions; usually, patients systemically affected have had a severe unrelenting dermatosis that has been treated for a prolonged period of time.

Greater detail on the use of dermatologic medications and other treatment modalities appear in the bibliography.

BIBLIOGRAPHY

Domonkos AN (ed): Andrews' Diseases of the Skin, 7th ed, p 374. WB Saunders, 1982

Eaglestein WH, Pariser DM: Office Techniques for Diagnosing Skin Disease. Chicago, Year Book Publishers, 1978

Ellerstein NS: The cutaneous manifestations of child abuse and neglect. Am J Dis Child 133:106, 1979

Depicts specific skin findings in abused children.

Esterly NB, Furey NL: Acne: current concepts. Pediatrics 62:1044, 1978

Best current review article available.

Fitzpatrick TB: Dermatology in General Medicine, 2nd ed. New York, McGraw-Hill, 1979

The bible for dermatologists. Very comprehensive text on all subjects in dermatology. Not limited to pediatric problems.

Solomon LM, Esterly NB: Neonatal Dermatology. Series, Major Problems in Clinical Pediatrics. Philadelphia, WB Saunders, 1973

The best reference for skin findings in the newborn.

Weinberg S, Hockelman RA: Pediatric Dermatology for the Primary Care Practitioner. New York McGraw-Hill, 1978

Another general reference for the primary care physician.

Weston WL: Practical Pediatric Dermatology. Boston, Little, Brown, 1979

A fine general reference for nondermatologists delivering primary care to children and adolescents.

Normal and Abnormal Emotional Development

29

Herman S. Belmont

ASSESSMENT OF THE TOTAL CHILD

A thorough foundation in the fundamentals of child and adolescent mental health sciences is an integral part of the pediatric student's armamentarium. The more familiar the physician is with all areas of the child's development, the easier it is to treat the rapidly and constantly changing child patient as a total person. There is an ordered sequence of progression in such areas as physical, cognitive, social, moral, and emotional development, all proceeding concurrently and mutually influencing one another. Within each of these, there are multiple lines of development.

One of the most difficult questions that the student must deal with concerns the boundaries of normal developmental manifestations for a particular child. A study of accumulated knowledge about development is helpful but the best aid is an extensive experience with large numbers of children whose developmental manifestations are carefully observed. From the beginning, the pediatric student should make it a habit to carefully assess the patient's developmental manifestations in relation to his chronologic age. Gradually, the student accumulates a reservoir of information about the expectations of a particular child's development. The student must ask now not only what is normal but what is normal for a given chronologic age and stage of development.

Changing manifestations of development are sometimes referred to as "phases" and reflect what is going on intrapsychically as well as externally. The idea of phases has been exploited to rationalize many deviations and problems in the development of the personality that would hardly fall into the category of normal healthy development. Many parents have concluded a description of a chronically provocative and disobedient child with the question, "But don't you think it's only a phase, doctor?" or "He'll grow out of it, won't he?" Whether he'll grow out of it is, of course, an important question.

A second consideration is discerning whether a particular form of behavior at a given time is dynamic, flexible, changing, and temporary, that is, an expected behavioral response to problems the child is normally struggling to master within himself, or whether the behavior is rigid and persistent, preventing the child from growing and advancing to later stages of development and adaptation appropriate to his situation. A form of behavior is no longer a phase if it persists, and no longer a dynamic surface manifestation of the child's current adjustment efforts, but rather a fixed and lasting handicap preventing his growth and advancement to later stages of development and adaptation.

In differentiating between a normal and a pathologic manifestation, consider the parent and his experience. Sometimes a parent is either inexperienced or biased. The mother of a firstborn child may think that each developmental phasic manifestation is an abnormality; or she misjudges an abnormality as "just a phase." With the second and third children she has learned what to expect. On the other hand, the parent of a handicapped, retarded, or psychotic child may be the last to recognize abnormal behavior because it is too painful.

Sometimes a physician may see an opposite kind of bias. For example, parents of an adopted child who was conceived illegitimately may worry about the child's entirely normal phasic genital handling at ages 4 and 5. They may be convinced that he is a potential sex degenerate who has inherited a natural "weakness." What they see and interpret is probably a product of their worst fears rather than an objective view of what is happening. Similar factors operate in the physician.

The physician, however, should be careful not to regard every mother of a firstborn as lacking objectivity and all adopted parents as biased.

Through understanding the parents and their position, it is often possible to favorably influence their role in the child's development. For example, the parents' acceptance or rejection of pregnancy and other attitudes prior to and during pregnancy may be determining factors in the subsequent parental input to the child's development. Reactions to a newborn child following a series of miscarriages or the loss of a child may result in overprotection. A new mother may experience a letdown, predisposing her to a subsequent postpartum depression associated with cessation of previous intense investments and focus of her family on her welfare and well-being. Throughout pregnancy, a parent may have counted on the child being born a certain sex; this could result in serious interference in parenting. The physician should be sensitive and alert to the fact that parents may demonstrate the same degree of variability in personality, attitudes, and emotional responses as their children.

Do not attribute to the parent the sole responsibility for all that takes place within the child's development. Many parents naturally attribute such power and responsibility to themselves, and when their physician mirrors this tendency they become burdened with feelings of guilt and self-criticisms. Genetic and constitutional factors as well as environment go far beyond specific parental influences. The role of sociologic, cultural, economic, and geographic influences, in addition to a host of potential acts of fate, must be considered. Inheritance of human traits does not preclude environmental influences.

Identical twins may show a higher concordance than fraternal twins in such characteristics as independence, capacity for enthusiasm, guilt, introversion, and tendency toward genetic psychopathic disorders. In other twin studies that contrasted identical and fraternal twins, identical twins showed greater concordance in timing, quality and quantity of smiling, vocalizing, attending to the mother, as well as timing and intensity of fear of strangers. There is also evidence for a genetic component for characteristics of approach—withdrawal and adaptive behavior of children. These factors, however, are subject to subsequent environmental influences. A healthy respect for the multiplicity of determinants in development and psychopathology enables the student to acquire a more mature and comprehensive approach to the specific problems of an individual child.

Even today physicians tend to dichotomize the etiology of most illnesses, as either organic or psychologic. Just as all development is multidetermined and physical development cannot be isolated from all other concurrent lines of development, similarly so-called physical pathology cannot be isolated from all the other determinants of pathology. A spectrum ranges from those conditions which appear to have a predominant psychological etiology, to those in which there is a balance of psychological and physical factors, to those in which the organic etiology appears predominant. Since developmental and pathologic processes are never static and the effects of influencing factors are cumulative in any particular instance, it is difficult to distinguish where the psychological factors and physical factors begin and end. For example, mothering experiences in early infancy, the nature of stimulation and handling, and the psychological state of the mother have been correlated with developmental manifestations ordinarily regarded as "organic." The establishment of respiratory equilibrium, vocalization, extent of cerebral-neuronal dendrite development, susceptibility to infection, and cognitive development are examples of areas that appear directly responsive to early experiential input.

STAGES OF EMOTIONAL DEVELOPMENT

Development differs from growth. Growth means an increase in physical size either of the total organism or of its parts, involves relatively permanent tissue changes, and is part of the progress toward physical maturity. Maturation, on the other hand, refers to those aspects of physical and psychological progression that relate to intrinsic sequential patterning of specific steps toward maturity, appearing on a built-in timetable based on largely biologic or inborn sources. The concept of development encompasses the interaction of growth and maturational patterns and the total of past and present experience.

First Year

Although development generally progresses through recognizable stages, "nature" and "nurture" make each child unique. Through genetic and constitutional endowment, some infants are extremely active and restless and respond vigorously to stimuli. Others are inactive and have to be prodded and urged to suck. Some children are born with a deficiency of phenylalanine hydroxylase and can become hopelessly retarded or relatively normal, depending upon how much phenylalanine is ingested during their early years. But every child is born dependent and helpless, requiring supplies from the outside, usually at the mother's hands, for nutrition, sensory experience, and care.

In the beginning, physiologic and psychic needs are not differentiated; the child has no real psychic structure, few memory traces, and no concept of awareness of objects or of himself. Only through his repeated contact with the outside world to fulfill basic needs, do his primitive psychic functions, encompassed in the hypothetical term "ego," gradually develop.

During feedings, the child experiences sensations of taste, temperature, mother's warm arms and breasts, firmness, gentleness, or even mother's awkwardness. Continuous circular interactions between the child and the mother occur during the first months of life. With the routine sequence of hunger, discomfort, crying, and finally the appearance of mother to gratify him, the child gradually distinguishes parts of the outside world from himself.

The hungry infant, in response to the sounds of mother approaching or preparing for feeding, appears momentarily comforted, as if having activated a memory of gratifications or sensations associated with being fed, and feels momentarily relieved. This form of imagery is a first step in mental functioning. Soon he cries, eventually realizing that only a real person gratifies him and he begins to differentiate reality from his own images of satisfaction. As his interactions with the outside world continue, action and trial action lead to the beginnings of thinking; more memory traces are laid down, and he acquires knowledge. His perceptual-motor capacities grow and he begins to form concepts. He starts to develop a sense of identity, reality-testing capacities, and relationships with objects. He learns gradually to control and regulate the discharge of his drives, to postpone immediate satisfaction for future gain, to integrate and synthesize stimuli from all sources. He experiences anxiety and establishes psychic mechanisms for defending himself against anxiety. He adapts to and makes changes in the external world.

These are all functions in his developing ego, and they continue throughout his childhood. They evolve especially as a consequence of the repeated interactions between the child and the most important aspect of his environment, his mother, as she responds to his expressed needs.

The progress of development is irregular; with forward spurts, regressions, and plateau periods in which consolidation of advances is taking place. Developmental changes are irregularly distributed among the cognitive, social, emotional, and sensory motor areas.

Sometimes inner developmental changes manifest themselves in behavior that is characteristic of the period; this is identified as a "phase" or landmark in the course of development. The social smile, a highlight in the mother-child relationship and psychic development of the child, appears around the second or third month but may come as late as the sixth month. The child sees a face and smiles. We assume an association has been made between any face and pleasurable gratification (by now he is capable of following a face with his eyes)—the child's beginning capacity to recognize visually and respond to a gestalt previously associated with pleasure. This response is a precursor of a true object relationship. In blind children the smile response may be delayed until the 4th to 6th months (holding and talking to the child are also associated stimuli contributing to the smile response). There is an important feedback factor here; when the infant smiles the mother responds to him. (Institutionalized children may have a delayed smile response.) It is significant that any face moving to and fro elicits the same response. It is only through the child's repeated experience with the mother that over an additional period of months her face (and their relationship) assumes a specificity.

Gradually, the child's sensory and motor functions become more developed. Some surface manifestations of underlying development are so widely understood and accepted that they are taken for granted and not labeled as phases. The infant several months old tends to try to put everything he can into his mouth: food, an arm, a piece of clothing, or a blanket. The progressively developing hand, eye, and mouth integration reflects the tremendous focus on the mouth during this period.

At around 5 to 7 months and for several months afterward, we see a change in many babies, that is a period of fearing strangers. During the preceding months, as a result of repeated feeding and care from his mother and others, the child's powers of perception and recognition have developed. He recognizes his mother and sometimes his father, as differentiated from other people. We assume that he senses that when he is hungry or uncomfortable or has other needs, his mother alleviates them. We assume that along with this he is confronted also by his first great fear—that these needs may not be fulfilled. Consequently, he cries when he is separated from his mother or doesn't see her. He also cries when a stranger tries to pick him up. He knows this is not his mother, and if his mother is there he clings to her, denying the stranger's existence. This is evidence of healthy normal development in the child, who can now discriminate between mother and non-mother (object awareness). The potential for further development is established. An abnormally persistent fear which is no longer a phase, but intense, inflexible, and exaggerated, indicates psychopathology.

Similarly, the child cries when the mother disappears; this should not be regarded as evidence of his being "spoiled." His crying is a reflection of his fear of desertion and helplessness, and of his fear that fulfillment of his needs will go unnoticed if she is not there. In general, with every advance in development there is an associated threat or demand. The newborn does not psychically perceive any threats; he has no object relationships, no perception of reality, and as yet no fears of desertion. The 5- to 7-month-old child can distinguish the mother from strangers, but he is not yet aware of her continuing existence when she is not in view (object awareness but no object constancy).

During this time the child continues to integrate his experiences into sets which hold together associatively, for example, pleasant, unpleasant; self, others; strange, familiar; real, imagined. He distinguishes emotions and uses them more appropriately, with greater specificity.

Throughout the child's development, particularly during the early months and years, the mother's role is crucial and we must understand her needs and capacities for this role. Various members of the extended family, particularly the father, also contribute to the "mothering" function.

During the child's initial stages of differentiation from his surroundings (the early months), there is a progressive development of more complex locomotor functions, growing through circular reactions. Sensory investigations in which sensory experiences are associated with specific kinds of stimuli develop. After the first 6 months, the child may become attached to some inanimate object, for example, a diaper, a blanket, a stuffed fuzzy toy, which he finds to be a source of comfort. It is thought that such a "transitional object" serves as a bridge in the course of the child's differentiation of and separation from his mother. The object (*e.g.*, a piece of blanket) simultaneously bears characteristics of both the mother (soft, warm, familiar odor) and the child himself. The transitional object may not be given up until grade school. Some children, such as recent generations of Japanese who have had more continued closeness and body contact with the mother, seem to have a lesser tendency to become involved with such transitional objects.

Second Year

Before the second year, objects were explored with the hands, eyes, and mouth. Hands were brought to the mouth, at first accidentally and then intentionally as certain actions became associated with particular effects. There was a constant striving toward mastery, such as climbing over objects, learning to back out, and standing up. The infant's sensory perceptions occurred in a nonspecific and visceral fashion, as with primitive sensations of equilibrium, tension, temperature, vibration, movement, and the rhythm of rocking. At approximately 6 months, more discrete, graded, and specific sensations appeared with a gradual reduction of intuitive sensitivity in which the child became less responsive to autonomic sensations.

Toward the end of the first year, in a progressive movement toward separation and individuation, as described by Margaret Mahler, there is a period of active practicing of motor skills and exploration of the environment. Words may begin to be used and identified with objects as well as being related to needs. There are sharper sensory discriminations. The child practices moving away from the close tie to the mother; at times he crawls away from her and then returns to "refuel." Other times the child seems almost oblivious to her. At around this time, many children are weaned from the breast. The child is influenced by a wide variety of maternal practices, ranging from sudden and abrupt interruptions of gratification to prolonged indulgence.

By the last two-thirds of the second year, in a stage which Mahler refers to as a "rapprochement stage of the separation individuation progression," the child appears to become closer to the mother and wants to share experiences with her.

At about this time also, the child becomes more aware of himself and the things he can do, feel, and perceive in the world around him. He is pleased with himself and his newly acquired abilities, and he repeats them over and over, wanting to guard them jealously. When he is put to sleep, he is asked to relinquish his actions, perceptions, and fresh conceptions of being a going concern. He fights it. He doesn't want to go to sleep and would rather stay up and play. He is not flexible about it, not having the wherewithal to reason and plan.

At about the same time, the child may become negativistic, refusing to do as he is told. He does this not because he is stubborn or mean, but apparently because he wants to assure himself about something of which he is uncertain, that he is a capable person with thoughts of his own. Without this progression and its consequences, he would never give up being a dependent nonentity. The sooner he develops this assurance that he can operate independently, the sooner he is able to abandon the earlier fear of being deserted in his helplessness. In a few months, this phase subsides normally if he is helped to develop more and more assurance of his capabilities and independence; therefore, he has less need to prove them negativistically. If the child's behavior at this time is dealt with too punitively, the child may regard his independence as dangerous and therefore not worthwhile. He may retreat to a continuing dependent behavior.

As the child grows a little older, more is required of him and he soon finds himself in the midst of a struggle between his own strong wishes and the expectations of those around him, particularly his parents. It is no longer a matter of proving himself an entity in his own right but rather a contest between his own strong wishes and those of his demanding parents. He is torn between gratifying himself, for example, by scribbling on a wall with a crayon, and losing his mother's approval and love. Depriving himself of gratifications in order to retain her love and approval is crucial to the child's future evolution and socialization. Children unable to work out these problems in relation to a loving, guiding, interested mother develop considerable potential impairment of this capacity.

Conflict over toilet training is typical in the second year and temper tantrums increase, reflecting inner struggle. It is hoped that the child will resolve his second major fear, that of losing his parents' love and approval, by taking over many of their expectations as his own. He masters his toilet functions and tantrums subside, and there is a greater degree of social compliance in the mastery of his impulses.

During the second year, if the mother leaves a child who has been successfully trained, he may regress and need complete retraining. This is because he has not yet internalized controls over these functions but carries them out to obtain the mother's approval and love as long as she is present and available. Eventually, when the child incorporates his mother's prohibitions and assumes her attitudes, he remains trained even if they are separated.

For children taken into a foster home at this time, there may be a deficit in the new mother-child object relationship. The child is often so slow in toilet training that the foster mother may become exasperated and have the child transferred to another foster home. Subsequently there is regression, infantile destructiveness, misbehavior, soiling, and poor control of impulses. This may become a vicious cycle in which each new foster parent reacts similarly and the child never has the opportunity for a satisfactory object relationship. The same situation may arise in the child of a working mother who is constantly shifted from one caretaker to another. Without a satisfactory object relationship, the child may not be trained until later in childhood.

Preschool Years

During the child's third year of life he gradually accepts separation from his mother and masters the concept of her permanency even when she is out of his presence for longer periods of time. The child develops a greater interest in other adults, a sense of time, an increasing tolerance of small frustrations, and a capacity to delay gratification for some future goals.

Moving through the preschool years, the child achieves a greater mastery of his more impulsive desires, and his drives find expression in progressively more socially adaptive activities. He is less helpless and dependent and participates more actively in the mastery of his inner demands and his environmental expectations. Between ages 3 and 6, new behaviors reflect the child's further development. There is a beginning awareness of boy-girl differences, a greater familiarity with various body parts and the pleasurable sensations derived from them, an activation of competitive and possessive drives, and an expression of feelings of love and possessiveness, particularly for the parent of the opposite sex. The result of these developmental struggles is that the child appears concerned with another fear. This threat may be understood as a symbol of the punishment the child fears for his emerging forbidden aggressive and rivalrous love feelings. He tries to cope with these dangerous (to him) impulses and the anticipated punishment in ways which give rise to certain behavioral manifestations of this period.

The fear which characterizes this period is of injury and mutilation with overreaction to minor hurts. He may respond to his fear and anxiety by becoming babyish, whiny, peevish, and overly sensitive to the least hurt, thereby arming himself against a greater and more dangerous injury. Or, he may assume the opposite attitude of extreme defiance and irritability. These are two principal methods that many children (and adults) use to cope with a great threat, such as serious illness or hospitalization—they either become overly fearful and helpless or uncooperative and rebellious, thereby denying the situation.

In addition, the child may try to handle a danger he senses from those immediately around him in his family as punishment for his forbidden feelings and desires by displacing the danger onto some distant and more easily avoided object, thereby developing a "phobia." It may be a frightening picture in a book, a dog, or an imaginary monster that is the "danger." Such fears are common at this time and are simply a surface reflection of a normal developmental struggle. It is only when these fears become fixed and intense, and prevent further progression in development that they are pathologic.

Similarly, sleep disturbances may develop. When the child gets into bed, he tries to stay awake and be on guard against dangerous and frightening thoughts. He fights going to bed and sleeping, and often sleeps fitfully and restlessly, awaking frequently. Night terrors and bad dreams are more common for the same reason. At this time, a child is apt to be cowardly and overly sensitive to the slightest injury, crying and screaming over a tiny splinter. He is overly aware of defects and injuries in others. The child can ordinarily master this developmental hurdle with the help of understanding, kind, and supportive parents until he reestablishes a more satisfactory equilibrium of the various forces within him and gains satisfactory control of his forbidden desires. The child ordinarily accomplishes this by age 5 or 6.

School-Age Child

The manner in which a child makes the transition from home and his parents to school and a greater involvement with other adults and children reflects the success of his developmental progress during the preceding years. With children of latency age, roughly 5 to 12, social, mental, and emotional growth is favored by an opportunity to actively master and take over personal responsibility for what had previously been passively experienced (because the parent had assumed this function). This was also true of the preschool child. Children need an opportunity for progressive and successful mastery and achievement of tasks which tax their capacity, but neither frustrate them nor prove beyond their ability. They do better with gradual and modulated exposure to change, and subsequent development is best built upon previous favorable growth.

The child of 5 to 12 has a basic need for a continuing relationship with specific parent figures or their surrogates who provide some continuing point of reference in the process of personality growth and development. These parent figures offer the child reasonable assurance of fulfillment of basic needs deriving from the reality of his dependence on outside supplies. This means "home," food, clothing, and affectional investment. Parents also serve as a model or standard of behavior with which to identify, by their function as individual persons and in interrelations with spouse and children, as well as by their mediation of stimulation and establishment of limits for the child's behavior. Parents also should allow the child an opportunity for working out male or female sex role identifications and therefore both a male and female parent figure optimally should be present during this time, as in the preceding years. There is continuing need for the parents to provide adequate support and understanding as the child moves through progressive developmental phases.

The crucial role of the continuing "parent" is supplemented by significant experiences with figures outside the home who serve as ego ideals for identification, sources and objects of affection, sources of stimulation and creativity, sources of patterns of limit and control, models for sex role identification, and the means for acquisition and development of many ego skills. For these experiences outside the home to be meaningful and to contribute effectively to development, they must be sufficiently associated in nature to the child's experience in his own home. Too abrupt a contrast renders the additional experience relatively less usable. To promote the most favorable experience with figures outside the home, the school seems to be the most fertile and readily controlled source for the greatest number of children.

Every child, especially during his school-age years, needs continuing peer group relationships, continuing over time and not interrupted by forces outside his control; this is an important factor in achieving ego growth. Peer relationships are important in facilitating separation from parental dependency, in firming up the child's own sense of identity and self-concept, in developing the capacity for socially acceptable aggressiveness and group cooperation, and in functioning within the more extensive social system. During this period, we see an expansion in the child's intelligence and a broadening of his social understanding and capacity for empathy and altruism. He displays a progressively better mastery of his environment, and he is less apt to regress and disintegrate under the impact of crises. He shows progressively more effective synthesis and integration of external demands.

The school-age child notably acquires a better capacity for coping with his earlier and more directly manifested drives and impulses. He does this in several ways. Through *sublimation*, a child may express these drives with a changed aim. Thus, a child who was sexually curious, a peeper with a desire to search and see, now diverts his expanded curiosity to many different areas. He also develops reaction formations, attitudes which are the antithesis of his earlier drives. The child who had little concern about nudity now becomes more self-conscious about his body, not wanting to expose himself indiscriminately to others. A child who earlier expressed certain cruel and destructive drives now turns to kindness and a degree of social regard. The child who had been self-centered, now becomes less possessive and more generous.

For the school-age child, play takes on a rapid pace and there is more involvement in games. There is a marked increase in motor discharge of the child's energies as a means of coping with forbidden drives. He uses his muscular system to discharge these strong drives and tensions; however, when he gets too tired to do so, he becomes irritable, cranky, and unhappy. Generally speaking, this is a period of steady and progressive development in many areas rather than abrupt and erratic change.

Adolescent

Starting with the junior high school years, the child comes to a period in development which at first glance appears to have no rhyme or reason. This is especially true because the adolescent seems to be changing constantly. Adolescence is characterized by rebelliousness, search for independence, volatile emotions, trouble in handling sexuality, questions and confusion regarding values and ideas, and search for identity. These manifestations reflect underlying dynamic, complicated transitional changes from childhood to adulthood.

There are important and difficult tasks which the adolescent has to achieve. Continuing the trend of latency years, he must establish a considerable degree of detachment from his parents, releasing himself from emotional dependence; as he gets older this can become confused with his continuing economic dependence. Often the parental ties are too threatening, too stimulating, and too frightening, and when they are abruptly interrupted, the teenager may shift his feelings with the same intensity toward some other leader or peer group. He may deal with his feelings by turning them into their opposite. Frequently, an adolescent moving toward independence, with great love for his parents, acts in a reverse behavior pattern and begins to demonstrate feelings of intense hate, contempt, and revolt.

Another task of the adolescent is to clarify his personal identity. He literally goes around at times asking "Who am I?" "What is the meaning of existence, of life?" He reads and engages in philosophical discussions, searching for knowledge. He has to come to terms with his drives, his feelings of inferiority and inadequacy. He has to master his relationships with his own and the opposite sex. He must be able to move from selfish, self-centered love to tender object-oriented love, to understanding and valuing the love object for the object itself. He has to achieve a sense of responsibility toward himself and other persons, to find a career and some direction.

During the child's early adolescence, the pediatrician should be particularly aware of the marked disparities among different parts of the child's physical development as well as disparities between his development and that of his peers. This is important in the psychological development of the child.

Size and relative development of arms, legs, breasts, nose, genitals, secondary sex characteristics, are a source of great concern for young teenagers. They often feel inferior and ashamed and try to fight against feelings of clumsiness, awkwardness and inadequacy. They may withdraw or try to overcompensate to get the admiration of others, or they may express complete denial of their situation by exaggerating their defects and trying to make themselves look as ugly and clumsy as possible. At this time parents need help in knowing how to support the teenager's vulnerable ego; the pediatrician can assure the parents that patient understanding and time accomplish more than long lectures and nagging.

Teenagers have a shaky self-esteem even though they may act unconcerned and indifferent. There is an ever-present fear of loss of ego control in the management of drives which have become intensified and at the same time he desires independence of parents and their supports. With the reactivation of forbidden drives and their intensification, there is a resulting fear of the possible consequences if he fulfills these desires. As part of the struggle for control of drives, the adolescent may fear losing his mind, may fear dying, and may become preoccupied with life, questioning whether he will ever reach adulthood.

One way the teenager handles the intensified and reactivated drives directed toward the parent, and his emerging struggle between his conflicting dependent and independent wishes in relation to his parents, is to put some distance between himself and his home. Often the adolescent looks to the peer group for a sense of belonging and sharing of its power. Closeness is achieved by conformity of dress and constant telephone communication. These supports are used to bolster the threatened ego controls as the young person moves further from the parents.

Around the ages of 14 to 16, it is not uncommon to see regressive manifestations as a defense against the anxieties derived from the strongly emerging forbidden drives of childhood. An anxious young man can suddenly behave like a dependent baby in the classroom, at home, or outside among his friends. He is sensitive, vulnerable, and given to crying easily. Paradoxically, when help is offered, he is resentful and rejects it perhaps because this makes him feel too much like a baby. He struggles back and forth. He doesn't want to be a baby; he wants to grow up. At the same time, when you deal with him man to man, he is unable to handle it and retreats. There may be regressions in eating habits during this time and even to transitory wetting, soiling, and anal masturbatory activity. If the regression does not elicit an overreaction from those around him, the adolescent generally swings back and forth, and gradually winds up ahead.

Menstruation plays an important role in the fantasy life of early adolescent girls. For some the significance of the menses is that female genitalia are dirty and malodorous. They may then react with extreme cleanliness; others may be haphazard and negligent about their physical appearance. For some, menstrual bleeding means damaged genitals, castration, a preview of the vulnerability of female genitals in heterosexual activity. For others, awareness of the menses is a very welcome indication of having reached womanhood and the potential for adult female sexuality, pregnancy, and eventual motherhood. This ushers in a more receptive and soft feminine attitude toward the opposite sex.

When acne appears, the teenager becomes sensitive. In his mind it may be connected with constipation or masturbation, and discussion is distasteful. Often he does not follow the recommendations of the dermatologist because he "knows what it is really all about."

Also as part of the regressive reactivation of earlier drives, there is a good bit of exhibitionism, peeping, showing off, and exposure of parts of the body. There may be some normal fleeting transvestitism, perhaps as a regression to the period when the child at 4 or 5 placed great emphasis on who had a penis and who did not. During this time also, the boy has trouble coping with erections because they occur easily, often at the wrong time and place. He becomes easily excited in response to slight stimuli.

Almost all boys and some girls become occupied with masturbation in early adolescence, but they engage in masturbatory activity with considerable guilt and anxiety. In spite of some factual knowledge of sex, their emotional reactions may be quite intense. Fantasies deriving from early development color and distort current conflicts and guilt feelings. Concerns and myths about the effects of masturbation continue to be amazingly similar from generation to generation. The fears remain the same—impotence, loss of pleasure, infertility, damaged children, injured genitals, weakness, stupidity, recognizable telltale evidence on the skin, neck movements, jerkiness of hand activities, and so on. Masturbatory activity in the boy, like menstruation in the girl, may also contribute to a sense of adequacy in genital function, a feeling of mastery of the sexual process and a solid masculine orientation to heterosexuality.

Changes in the adolescent occur not only in instinctual manifestations but in the level of ego function. He may regress to the period during which he did not internalize prohibitions and all limits came from the outside (parents). The teenager, therefore, at this time often views the adult as potentially punitive and judgmental. He feels that the doctor will be critical and he may be guarded and secretive when they meet.

Object relationships during early adolescence seem directed toward the opposite sex more for narcissistic gratification than for any interest in the object itself. Once dating begins, there is a tendency to collect as many "scalps" as possible. The teenager samples and explores a wide variety of social interests and activities. If parents try to force the child into a particular niche, he may become fixed at a narrowly restricted orientation and lose his potential for development in different directions.

As we move into the postpubertal period, around age 15 to 19 or 20, we see the adolescent searching for a greater degree of stabilization. Now he has to solidify and synthesize his ideals and contradictions, his identifications with the peer group, and his values, and to precipitate out of that a composite that works for him. Also, he must discover a way of coping with any forbidden sexual feelings that are directed toward his immediate family and find other outlets for his sexual drives and fantasies.

Much of this takes place as part of the loosening of the adolescent's ties to his parents and a gradual reduction of the focus on himself. He develops an interest in social matters, values, and various religions and ideologies. He weighs and evaluates different ideals and values from his peer group, from teachers and authors, and from his parents. He is often more cynical about and critical of his parents and previously idealized institutions. He sifts and blends these in various ways most appropriate to his own needs, in terms of past, present, and future perspective. In this process, he elevates certain ideas, objects, and persons and invests them with special importance and loving feelings. They become his ideals and help substitute for the previously idealized parents. Ordinarily, given the opportunity to freely explore and sample ideas and values from multiple sources, he identifies with ideal objects, with the peer group, and with parents. A healthy identity prevents the teenager from rejecting parental attitudes totally and yet allows him to resemble yet differ from his parents. The truly healthy and workable identity is an amalgam of many different sources and not confined to one source only.

Finally, what started out as a helpless

and dependent nonentity psychically now has emerged into a complex and independently functioning late adolescent. Thus, he may once again find some kind of suitable working relationship with his family, comfortably relating to them as one person to another. He gradually comes to terms with his own ideas about religion, his personal philosophy, his potential vocational strivings, and the reality of where he is and where he's going.

Among the many developmental changes, a fundamental component is the progression from narcissistic, self-oriented sexuality to romantic love with a mixture of both sexual and tender feelings, shared with the loved person. Just as there are variations in growth rates in adolescents, so too does the readiness for engaging in active sexual expression of these feelings vary. Crises may result when teenagers who are not ready find themselves prematurely pushed by group pressures from those who are more precocious sexually. Not infrequently, the physician is sought out for counseling regarding conflicting individual and cultural values surrounding sexual behavior.

Finally, the adolescent becomes an adult when he has achieved a solid identity, a responsible vocational orientation, a capacity for both tender and heterosexual love, a functioning set of values, and independence. Once more he is able to maintain a reasonable state of equilibrium between his instinctual drives, his superego, and the outside world, using adaptive and flexible ego functions.

WORRISOME DEVELOPMENTAL MANIFESTATIONS

Various developmental manifestations can present problems for those dealing with children. Here, the physician is helpful to both the child and the parents because he has a greater developmental perspective and a multidimensional approach.

A parent's concern about a child's thumbsucking—an entirely normal manifestation of early strong sucking needs—cannot be dealt with arbitrarily. Some parents regard thumbsucking as an offensive and disgusting habit that results in dental malformations. In some cases, the physician must evaluate whether the parent indirectly encourages the child to use sucking satisfaction as a form of universal gratification whenever he has a need that is not gratified. Such a parent puts a nipple in the child's mouth each time he cries. The physician must teach parents the role of constitutional variations in sucking needs of different children. For example, an infant whose hunger needs are satisfied before his strong sucking needs are fulfilled during a feeding has to do some supplementary sucking.

Early in the child's development, when object relationships are not yet established, parents may observe occasional rhythmic genital stimulation during feeding. This normal activity may become the focus of especially sensitive and overly watchful parents. Timely, supportive reassurance for the parents may forestall complicating overreactions. Most children engage periodically in masturbatory activity, and unless this persists as a fixed and all-encompassing activity, it may be regarded as a normal manifestation of development.

Children during the first year may show disturbance at bedtime, with restlessness and crying as soon as the mother leaves the child's bedroom. These manifestations are understandable because in the child's normal development, he gets a feeling of helplessness in the absence of his newly recognized source of gratification. Some parents respond by holding the crying child and carrying him throughout a large part of the night, so that he won't be anxious about his parents' absence. Others try to "break the habit" by leaving the child to cry himself to sleep over long periods. In the first instance, aside from making the parents angry with the child, he becomes a participant in a ritual which, if continued long enough, can interfere with the entire process of separation—individuation. In the second instance, his basic trust in the newly emerging environment may be threatened. The pediatrician might help the parents resolve the dilemma by suggesting a modified approach. For example, the parent may allow the baby to cry for 4 or 5 minutes, return to the room to comfort and quiet him, and leave again. If the crying is resumed, the entire procedure is repeated, and as many times as necessary. If the crying continues, in a few days the period is increased to 5 or 6 minutes and so on without permitting the crying period to last beyond a 10-minute period, which appears to be too anxiety-producing. Through such an approach the parents can appreciate the young infant's need for gentle support, without interfering with the gradual progression of growth and mastery. Sudden and excessive interruptions of the mother-child relationship may, on the other hand, result in prolonged developmental regressions and feeding disturbances.

We have referred briefly to transitional objects, negativism of the early second year of life, and temper tantrums. With patient and understanding responses to these temporary surface manifestations of underlying developmental changes, they soon pass. With overly severe responses, these manifestations may be compounded and persist. Appropriate support by the physician helps to ameliorate such excessive responses.

We know that many transitory forms of behavior in the school-age child and adolescent reflect the ebb and flow of dynamic development. These do not constitute a problem unless they become marked and persistent, either because of constitutional variations in the child, developmental interferences such as a marked parental overreaction, or a combination of these.

Sometimes the child shows a lag or precocity or unevenness in maturational steps. This can be a problem, particularly if the environmental responses and supports do not help the child to achieve satisfactory mastery. Children are born with different degrees of capacity for eating, speech development, control of bowel and bladder functions, and sleeping. Some children show long continued hyperactivity or hypoactivity; some are significantly precocious or mildly retarded in cognitive development. There are variations in achieving autonomy from parents. Some children have significant delays in speech development and disorders in articulation and language comprehension. These deviations in maturational patterns can complicate a child's development, adding a special quality and cast to what he brings into the child-environment interactions. What evolves in their subsequent development also depends on the ability of the parents and other environmental resources to cope with the deviations and to move them toward an adaptive integration with the child's other capacities.

DEVELOPMENTAL INTERFERENCES

Every child, in addition to showing behavioral manifestations of underlying developmental changes which are ordinarily transitory, also experiences conflicts inherent in the process of development, such as his need to adjust to the relinquishment of breast-feeding or the struggles between indulgence of his wishes and fear of losing his parents' love. What must be considered constantly is whether external interferences disturb the "typical unfolding of development." In other words, to what extent are unjustified demands being made of the child that do not take into account his capacity to cope with them?

Parental Interferences

External interferences include parental over-or-under-reactions at specific developmental phases, inadequate supplementary or auxiliary supports of development by the environment (mother), noxious attitudes and orientations of significant persons in the child's environment, and any acts of fate. The young infant needs protection by a person who is capable of nurturing both the child's mind and body. If the person caring for the child's bodily needs deals with him in a warm, tender, and feeling way, interacting and responding appropriately, the child's emotional needs are also being fulfilled. Serious developmental interferences result from a lack or a deficiency of a need-satisfying adult, with whom the child can interact on a continuing basis, and who responds to his signals of distress and calls for comfort and gratification, establishes an emotional communication with him, and eventually becomes someone he can love and trust.

Similarly, the child's development throughout is favored by adult figures who can relate to him and provide him with appropriate developmental necessities. Unfortunately, many children are unwanted and in homes in which the adult responsible for their care lacks the capacity to fulfill their needs. This is often true in children born out of wedlock, children of young and immature parents, children of parents badly handicapped by serious problems such as alcoholism, drug addiction, and mental illness, and children of working mothers with no adequate mother substitute. Children experiencing severe forms of neglect exhibit failure to thrive without sufficient organic disease to account for it. This is characterized by failure to grow and gain weight, developmental slowness, occasional vomiting or diarrhea, feeding difficulties, and weakness, fatiguability, and irritability. Lesser degrees of deficiency and deprivation in mothering are common developmental interferences.

Qualitative inadequacies in maternal attitudes act as interferences with child development. Spitz has related infantile neurodermatitis, fecal play, persistent hypermotility and rocking in children, to characteristic and specific maternal attitudes. Tens of thousands of children are victims of severe child abuse. Parents who abuse their children frequently have severe social problems and marital discord, as well as financial difficulties. Many of these parents are in a state of continual anger and the only stimulation needed to express this anger violently may be some difficulty in child rearing.

A number of so-called acts of fate modify and interfere with development. Divorce and separation of parents disrupt the family structure, with emotional repercussions in the parents, varying degrees of object loss for the child, sometimes questions of placement, involvement of the child in extensive unpleasant legal contests, problems of divided loyalties, and many other associated difficulties. Also included in acts of fate are death, serious illness, prolonged absences, and working habits of parents. Even the timing, spacing, number, and sex distribution of the child's siblings, as well as the child's ordinal position in the family, may affect him directly and indirectly through the parents. The nature of the extended family—their illnesses, deaths, and demands on the parents—may be crucial interfering determinants in the child's development. When a family moves frequently and the child's object ties with peers and his familiar environment are interrupted repeatedly, when he is subjected to sexual abuse or seduction, when he is regularly exposed to the authority of a humiliating and ridiculing or physically abusive adult, such as a parent, teacher, or sitter, the child's ego capacity may be unable to cope with such interferences.

The more thoroughly the pediatrician has mastered the developmental vicissitudes of children, the more effectively he strives to soften the impact of developmental interferences, to give the parent insight into the child's needs at these times, and to bolster a badly fractured or strained ego in the child.

DEVELOPMENTAL ARRESTS

Disorders in children can be the result of a lack of progress in the development of certain ego functions or in the advancement of the drive development, rather than manifestations of internal psychic conflict or a conflict with the environment. Children may retain feeding habits from earlier periods, restricting their diet to particular foods or foods that do not require chewing. Some children show persistent enuresis, soiling, and immaturity inappropriate for their age. Not every instance of these manifestations are examples of developmental arrest, since they may also be expressions of other forms of psychopathology. Children exhibiting developmental arrest appear overly oriented toward personal gratification without an appropriate balance in relation to the expectations and requirements of society; these children are more self-centered and less object-oriented and tend to readily deny the demands of reality. The capacity to postpone immediate gratification for future gain is not well developed. The result is that these children have not been able to relinquish gratifications associated with soiling, wetting, and impulsive discharge. Similarly, some children continue in later years to express directly drives which were normal and expected at early periods in development (*e.g.*, exhibitionistic and voyeuristic [peeping] tendencies).

Developmental arrests can be serious handicaps to effective function. When it becomes evident that the behavior is fixed and unchanging despite early modifications in child-rearing practices or other factors which appear to contribute to them, it is advisable to seek consultation and treatment, if necessary, before these problems are further compounded. Simply eliminating the behavioral manifestation through threat or prohibition may lead to more serious problems. For example, a child of school age was a severe stutterer. His mother related that he had been enuretic since infancy and that she had "cured" this by placing a meat cleaver on his night-table, threatening to chop off his penis if he wet again. He had stopped wetting that night but from that time on began to stutter.

Hospitalized Child

A most important interference with the child's development may be illness or hospitalization. These experiences are often referred to as "traumatic," stimuli that come in such abundance, intensity, and unfamiliarity that he cannot assimilate and master them. The age and stage of developmental progression of the child at the time of his illness or hospitalization is of fundamental significance in understanding the meaning of these experiences for him.

Infancy. Up to the age of 6 months, a hospitalized child tends to show varying degrees of agitation in response to changes in his customary environment and differences in patterns of handling him. After 6 months, having a degree of ego and object differentiation, the child shows manifestations of stranger and separation anxiety upon removal from regular contact with his mother. The child's beginning basic trusting relationship with her has been jarred and disrupted.

Between the ages of 6 and 18

months, the child is working through his "differentiation" and "practicing" stages of separation-individuation. Disruptions of the child's delicately established identity and object relationships that result from abrupt separation from his mother, may cause regression and retreat to earlier levels of development with sleep and feeding disturbances.

Ages $1\frac{1}{2}$ to 6. In the period from $1\frac{1}{2}$ to 2 years, the child is extremely sensitive to the threat of separation or desertion. He is now working through the *rapprochement* stage of the separation—individuation process—where he has moved into a closer interaction with his mother. The child is trying to develop a sense of autonomy which is seriously threatened by the enforced separation and restrictions of movement associated with hospitalization.

In the third year, hospitalization may be viewed as a punishment for forbidden activities or even wishes. This is understandable in view of the child's struggle between the gratification of his own wishes and the fear of loss of his parents' love and approval. He may respond with a rigid reinforcement of control of all of his impulses or else turn in the other direction and yield to all the partially repressed and recently abandoned pleasures and forbidden activities, such as wetting and soiling and babyish demanding behavior. There may be reactivation of whining and clinging, crying, temper tantrums, and destructive behavior.

From ages 3 to 6, mutilation anxieties are high and although separation anxiety is diminished at this stage, there is a real threat of loss of physical integrity and a sense of intiative. The child is apt to interpret all forbidden actions and thoughts as punishable by physical mutilation and even castration, and so may react to hospitalization and threatened procedures by denying his anxiety through acting completely contrary to what might be expected to someone who was ill. He may refuse to cooperate or accept any limitations. Another form of response is to submit completely and become a perfect patient. At times some children retreat to earlier levels of functioning.

School Age. The child in the early school-age years, from 6 to 8, continues to have a high degree of mutilation anxiety and fear of loss of control and mastery. Since his superego has by now been fairly well established and functions with some degree of severity, he may interpret the hospitalization punishment for all his wrongdoings. As the child gets older, the effects of hospitalization reflect his current problems. A young teenager may regard hospitalization as threatening to expose his masturbatory activities. In the midst of a dependence-independence struggle, removal to a hospital bed in which he is bathed, nursed, and at times even fed, may be unbearable.

Physician's Role

The physician can play an important role in ameliorating developmental interference in the ill child. He can strive to keep to a minimum the changes in the child's living situation. For example, can the child be treated at home? If the child has to enter the hospital, can the parents be with the young child or visit the older child frequently? Are medications administered by the least traumatic route and frequency? Are medical and surgical procedures, laboratory studies, restrictions of diet and movement, length of hospitalization, and restriction of activities kept at the necessary minimum. Finally and most important, does the physician make an effort to reduce the traumatic impact of these experiences?

The physician has the responsibility to communicate at the child's level of understanding and to prepare him for each new experience. If he receives in advance an explanation of a laboratory procedure, a restriction in activity, and a separation from home, the experience may still be unpleasant, but is likely to be less upsetting. When the child is unable to master the situation, he resorts to less satisfactory responses, to earlier seemingly less threatening levels of development, to denial of painful aspects of reality, and to arrests and fixations in development which may serve as foci for later neurotic development or character changes.

There is an advantage in preparation for procedures, and in simple clarification as they are being carried out, thereby reducing the completely helpless, dependent and passive aspects of these experiences. It is important that the child be given an opportunity after hospitalization to discuss and understand fully all that has happened and its significance for him. He may be confused about the meaning of his experiences, or he may have distorted reality with his own personal and age-appropriate fantasies. Ample discussion of misconceptions can be invaluable in enabling a child to master the trauma inherent in most medical experiences.

PSYCHOPATHOLOGY DERIVING FROM INTRAPSYCHIC CONFLICT

The personality structure of the preschool child is fundamentally different from that of the school-age child. How the preschool child's needs and wishes are dealt with is to a greater degree determined by the expectations, prohibitions, and threats of the world around him. For the young child, the parents constitue the principal representative of the external environment. During the preschool years of development, the child's behavior reflects change in parental expectations. Even in these early years, his personality begins to take over some of the functions of regulating and controlling instinctual wishes. However, these controls continue to bear a close relationship with the external world. The controls are not firmly established, are readily influenced from the outside, and require continuing support from the parents in order to be maintained.

As a consequence of developmental changes during the latter part of the preschool period, the child in grade school adopts within his own psychic structure many of the prohibitions and controls previously applied from without by the parents. He has established identifications with important child-rearing figures and has internalized their prohibitions and controls. From this point he deals with two authorities, one within himself and the other, external and parentlike.

The child's behavior is responsive not only to continuing external threats and influences, but there is a continuing potential for conflict of an intrapsychic nature, between the child's wishes and his own prohibitions as embodied in his superego structure. The superego continues to retain the punitive qualities and characteristics it held at the time the superego was laid down around the age of 5 or 6. This is why the child can develop a conflict that is not understandable rationally in terms of current environmental circumstances. Such a conflict is intrapsychic among several personality structures, and has a pathology that cannot be resolved by altering the current environment. This is evidenced by the continued existence, and even the development of symptomatology, often in the face of optimal environmental circumstances. This intrapsychic pathology often requires intensive psychotherapeutic intervention beyond the scope of the pediatrician.

On the other hand, children at any age may develop symptomatology when confronted with an overly stressful environment and show improvement when the environmental stress is alleviated. Here, the therapeutic approach may involve environmental modification as well as some kind of support for coping.

The school-age child continues to be dependent on his environment, so that there is an overlap and interplay between intrapsychic and environmental factors; both must be evaluated carefully in assessing psychopathology and determining the appropriate therapeutic approach. Although the final eruption of psychoneurotic symptomatology may be precipitated by some environmental circumstance, the symptomatology is characteristically well rooted in earlier predisposing developmental fixations and intrapsychic conflict. It is not likely to be very responsive to environmental changes. Specialized psychiatric intervention is necessary for the various psychoneurotic problems.

PROBLEMS IN EGO FUNCTION

Certain children show significant disturbances in one or more of the principal functions of the ego, that hypothetical portion of the psychic "structure" which mediates and integrates internal drives and external reality. Some of the functions of the ego have been indicated in the review of the young child's development. They consist of perceptual-motor functions, memory, thinking, object relations, reality testing, a sense of identity, defense, and integration and synthesis of stimuli from all sources. Serious disturbances of one or more of these crucial functions markedly impair the child's developmental progress. Impairments are seen in organic brain syndromes, in childhood psychoses, and in ego weaknesses of lesser degree. Mental retardation also constitutes a type of ego disturbance, namely, that of noticeable impairment of the ego's cognitive functions.

Children with attention deficit disorder (also referred to as minimal brain dysfunction or hyperkinetic syndrome), either of organic etiology or from severe developmental deprivation, may show a wide constellation of characteristics, in addition to localized manifestations of a neurologic nature. In addition to a persistent reluctance to let go of a situation once it has been structured, a perseverative quality, often there is increased irritability, excessive reactions of rage and despair, excessive crying, or withdrawal due to frustration.

Children with attention deficit disorder tend to be overly talkative and repetitive, somewhat awkward and deficient in perceptual-motor function, clumsy, and therefore somewhat destructive. They overreact to frustration, to which they are easily susceptible. They are also somewhat guileless with a capacity to misjudge social situations; they miss the point and therefore tend toward social immaturity. They are often not accepted by their peers, are excluded, and lack adequate social experiences. These characteristics further contribute to difficulties in school adjustment and performance.

A severe form of ego disturbance is the *pervasive developmental disorder* (also referred to as childhood psychosis). Here there is a marked impairment of the child's sense of identity, reality testing, and object relationships, including interpersonal communication. One type of pervasive developmental disorder, infantile autism, first described by Kanner, consists of a caricature of the earliest levels of psychic development that continue to manifest themselves. Afflicted children appear to be living completely detached from the world around them and the circular interactions between child and parent are broken down.

As described by Mahler, the child seems never to have mastered the separation-individuation process. He relates in a seemingly satisfactory way with his mother until a point somewhere in the second year or first months of the third year when special ego adaptations are required of him in response to special demands or stressful circumstances; he responds with a markedly disturbing reaction. The child either clings desperately to his mother searching for some kind of union with her or easily slips back into a regressed level of isolated, detached, and autistic function. It is as though in the face of some external demand, the resources of the ego are incapable of coping and resort either to progressively increased demands on his mother as an auxiliary ego or to severe regression. The child's capacity for functioning in any of the ego areas is thus seriously impaired.

There are also children who from time to time show rather erratic pictures of development, with onset after 30 months of age *(childhood onset pervasive developmental disorder)*. On examination, they evidence combinations and degrees of disturbance of several of the ego's functions, including impairment in social relationships. These children remind one of the extreme examples of developmental deviations referred to earlier, with excesses and deficiencies in development of sensory function, motor movement, speech, self-mutilating activities, constricted or inappropriate affect, sudden excessive anxiety, and resistance to change in environment. It is as if the executive apparatus of the psychic structure were out of commission and the various functions of the ego were being expressed without appropriate modulation and integration.

Children with ego disturbances are both distressing and markedly distressed. They exhibit degrees of disruption and disorganization of the core aspects of the entire psychic function; the roots of these difficulties are often inborn or the product of early environmental insults and require long, intensive, and sometimes heroic therapeutic efforts.

The subject of mental deficiency, a special type of ego disturbance of complex etiology, is discussed elsewhere in this book.

The preceding brief accounts of pathology have featured predominant characteristics and etiologic determination. Many behavioral manifestations are determined in a composite fashion. In some instances the same symptomatology may have different causes in different people. Delinquent behavior in children, learning and reading disorders, and chronic hyperactivity are examples of conditions which may derive from multiple etiologies separately or in combination. Any of these conditions could result from a developmental deviation, or from various developmental interferences which have been described as modifying the child's optimal development.

Similarly, arrests in instinctual and ego development, psychosis, organic brain syndrome, various ego weaknesses, mental retardation, or psychoneuroses may be the major causative factors in any of these pathologic categories. For example, a delinquent child may be performing antisocial acts out of a sense of overwhelming guilt and a search for punishment, whereas the same antisocial act might be a consequence of his limited cognitive development, psychosis, or severe weakness in reality testing and internal controls, either organically or functionally determined.

REFERRAL

It is the primary care physician and not the child psychiatrist to whom parents and community turn for early guidance and understanding of healthy child development and rearing, as well as for a comprehensive approach to the ill, hospitalized, and even dying child. He is the key mediator and instructor in child and adolescent mental health. Only after the physician has thoroughly explored questions about the child's development or problems in his "total" development, will he turn to a child psychiatrist or other mental health specialist for consultation. This procedure would be reserved for certain cases in which the problem exceeds the experience and realm of comprehensive pediatric practice.

BIBLIOGRAPHY

Freedman D: Hereditary control of early social behavior. In Foss BM (ed): Determinants in Infant Behavior, III. London, Methuen & Co, 1965

Kanner L: Autistic disturbances of affective contact. Nervous Child 2:217, 1943

Mahler MS: Of Human Symbiosis and the Vicissitudes of Individuation. New York, International Universities Press, 1968

Mahler, MS: On child psychosis and schizophrenia: autistic and symbiotic infantile psychoses. The psychoanalytic study of the child 7:286, 1952

Nagera H: Early Childhood Disturbances, the Infantile Neurosis, and the Adulthood Disturbances. Monograph Series of the Psychoanalytic Study of the Child, #2. New York, International Universities Press, 1966

Ribble M: The Rights of Infants: Early Psychological Needs and Their Satisfaction (2nd ed). New York, Columbia University Press, 1965

Rosenberg LE: A geneticist's approach to the vulnerable child. In Anthony EJ, Koupernik C (eds): The Child in His Family: Children at Psychiatric Risk, pp 133–137. New York, John Wiley and Sons, 1974

Spitz RA: The First Year of Life. New York, International Universities Press, 1965

Thomas A, Chess S, and Birch HG: Temperament and Behavior Disorders in Children. New York, New York University Press, 1968

Child Abuse and Neglect

30

Howard L. Weinberger

A 3-month-old infant is admitted to the inpatient unit weighing less than his birth weight; he gains weight rapidly in the hospital.

A 6-month-old boy is brought to the Emergency Room with a history of irritability for 24 hours and is found to have a fractured femur.

A 2-year-old is seen in the office for a checkup and is noted to have multiple bruises on his face and trunk.

A 3-year-old dies of head injuries after a history of falling from her bed.

These patients are examples of infants and children suffering from child abuse and neglect. How does the physician recognize this condition? What risk factors are involved? What are the responsibilities of the health professional in the management of this problem?

HISTORICAL BACKGROUND

Attitude of Society Toward Children

Children are often called our nation's greatest natural resource. Unfortunately, they are not always treated as such. The protective attitude of society toward children in western cultures has evolved very slowly. Infanticide and human sacrifice are described in the Bible and in Greek and Roman literature. Until the last century, the child was viewed as property in many western countries. Charles Dickens was an outspoken critic of the way children were treated in England in the latter half of the 19th century.

In the United States, Child Labor Laws were instituted in the early part of this century to protect the welfare of children who were being exploited by their families and society. The earliest record of a child abuse case in the United States (1874) was instituted under the auspices of the Society for the Prevention of Cruelty to Animals to gain protection for a young girl.

Recognition of Child Abuse by Health Professionals

The health professions have been particularly slow in recognizing the problem of child abuse. The first reported cases were brought to the attention of the medical community by radiologists in the late 1940s and early 1950s. They identified radiographs of young children who had suffered subdural hematomas and multiple fractures of long bones. The physicians caring for these patients had no ready explanation for these findings, and made efforts to determine their etiology, looking for vitamin deficiencies, defects in metabolism of calcium and phosphorus, and underlying skeletal disease.

There were additional examples of children who had suffered multiple episodes of trauma (fractures in various stages of healing) without a concomitant history to explain the trauma. Careful assessment failed to reveal underlying organic pathology, and the only conclusion was that these youngsters had suffered unreported physical trauma at the hands of their caretakers.

Throughout the 1950s and early 1960s, recognition of instances of child abuse was rare, and the scattered reports in the literature were met with disbelief. When one investigator estimated that as many as 10,000 abused children might be identified each year, many professionals, both in the medical and social service communities, assumed this to be an exaggeration.

To this day, there are wide discrepancies in the reporting of cases of child abuse—discrepancies by region and community and discrepancies within a community as discussed in the section on Incidence and Demography.

DEFINITION OF CHILD ABUSE AND NEGLECT

Earlier descriptions by Kempe and others used the term "battered child syndrome" but more recently the concept of physical abuse has been broadened to the term, "child abuse and neglect," which is more inclusive and under which an entire spectrum of conditions may fit.

The definition of child abuse and neglect which was part of Federal legislation passed in 1974 (*Child Abuse Prevention and Treatment Act*, PL93-247) is as follows:

> The physical or mental injury, sexual abuse, negligent treatment, or maltreatment of a child under the age of 18 by a person who is responsible for the child's welfare under circumstances which indicate that the child's health or welfare is harmed or threatened thereby.

An even broader definition, developed by the New York Family Court, expands the concept of the "maltreated child" even further:

> A "maltreated child" is a child under eighteen years of age who has had serious physical injury inflicted upon him by other than accidental means.
>
> A "maltreated child" is a child under eighteen years of age impaired as a result of the failure of his parent or other person legally responsible for his care to exercise a minimum degree of care:
>
> (1) in supplying the child with adequate food, clothing, shelter, education, medical or surgical care, though financially able to do so or offered financial or other reasonable means to do so; or
> (2) in providing the child with proper supervision or guardianship; or
> (3) by unreasonably inflicting, or allowing to be inflicted, harm or a substantial risk thereof, including the infliction of excessive corporal punishment; or
> (4) by using a drug or drugs; or
> (5) by using alcoholic beverages to the extent that he loses self-control of his actions; or
> (6) by any other acts of a similarly serious nature requiring the aid of the Family Court.
>
> A "maltreated child" is also a child under eighteen years of age who has been abandoned by his parents or other person legally responsible for his care.

INCIDENCE AND DEMOGRAPHY

Estimates of the true incidence of child abuse vary, but nationwide it is thought to be about 1 million maltreated children each year. Of these, 30,000 to 40,000 children are severely injured and 2000 to 3000 are killed.

In New York State alone, there were more than 50,000 children reported as abused or neglected in 1979.

Age

The average age of the abused child is under 4 years, and the majority of instances occur in the young child under 2 years.

Although abusive parents may come from any age group, the average parental age is the late 20s.

Marital Status of Parents

The majority of abusive parents are married and living together at the time of the abuse.

Socioeconomic Status

It is clear from a variety of studies that child abuse and neglect occur in every socioeconomic stratum. Families living in poverty are more inclined to experience a wide variety of crises which place their children at greater risk than middle-class children.

The recognition and reporting of suspected child abuse and neglect has lagged in the private practice community. Reports of suspected abuse and neglect tend to emanate from emergency rooms and public health clinics, although increasing numbers of reports come from schools, public health nurses, and the community at large. A number of explanations have been offered for this lag in reporting from the private practice population such as:

Continued belief that parental rights outweigh the child's rights
Continued lack of awareness of the reality of child abuse and neglect by practicing physicians
Denial and disbelief that "my patient could do this"
Attempt to protect family from publicity
Lack of social service support. The physician may have a tendency to try to do it alone. (Rescue fantasy: "I'll provide all the services for this family.")
Physician's reluctance to get involved.

Unfortunately, the practicing primary care physician is rarely in the position to be able to provide the time and services needed to respond adequately to a family in crisis. Most states and communities require that a case of suspected abuse and neglect must be reported before social services are made available.

PHYSICAL ABUSE

The extent of physical injuries suffered by children ranges from superficial bruises on the skin to murder. Since the physician is rarely a witness to the actual event leading to the injury, it is incumbent on him to be highly suspicious, yet sensitive to and compassionate about the overall situation. Certain examples should be emphasized:

Unexplained Death of a Child

The unexplained death of any infant or child is a great tragedy to all involved. Although it is possible that the death may have resulted from child abuse, one should consider the possibility of SIDS (sudden infant death syndrome). This condition occurs most frequently in infants less than 6 months of age (peak 3–4 months). Affected infants generally have no cutaneous physical findings and were apparently healthy and "thriving" until the fatal episode. Parents demonstrate appropriate levels of anguish, grief, and often self-recrimination. Soon after an infant's death, it is probably better to err by assuming the death is due to SIDS rather than to accuse the parents of abuse.

Multiple Fractures

Multiple fractures can occur as a result of a major traumatic accident such as a fall from a second-floor window or an automobile accident. However, the majority of falls in children do not result in fractures. Some estimates are that 80% of infants and young children will sustain a fall in the first year of life, but few will result in significant injury.

Multiple fractures in various stages of healing should be suspect. In the differential diagnosis, one should consider osteogenesis imperfecta, but this is a rare condition generally recognized from birth along with other findings such as blue sclerae.

Any fracture in a child under 6 months of age should be suspect. A self-induced fracture is almost impossible, though it is often the presenting complaint (*e.g.*, "the baby twisted his leg in the crib").

Subdural Hematoma with Retinal Hemorrhage

The so-called "shaken baby" syndrome —subdural hematoma with retinal hemorrhage—may occur with or without an associated skull fracture. These injuries are due to violent shaking motions, creating shearing forces on the bridging veins over the cerebral cortex. One may also note associated skin bruises under the axillae or other parts of the body where the baby was held and shaken.

Multiple Cutaneous Lesions

A variety of cutaneous injuries may be noted including:

Ecchymotic lesions in various stages of healing

Unusually shaped bruises such as rope burns around wrists or ankles, looped cord (so-called omega-shaped lesions), cigarette burns, "branding" injuries from irons, hair curlers

Bruises in *unusual positions* such as across the back or "slapped-hand" outline over the face

Human bite marks—may be caused by other children or adults

Usually these lesions can be easily differentiated from the typical black-and-blue marks noted over the dorsum of the lower extremities in many toddlers who "bump into everything." Parents may complain about "easy bruisability" and some consideration should be given to the possibility of a mild coagulation defect, such as Willebrand's syndrome. However, it is important not to be drawn into unnecessary hematologic studies.

Burns

Burns may be accidentally incurred or intentionally induced, or they may be the result of neglect or inappropriate attention. Children may be punished for a variety of "infractions" by being burned or branded. Thus, the shape, position, and timing of the burn should be considered in differentiating accidental from intentional injury.

Poisoning

There are approximately 1 million incidents of poisoning in young children each year, the majority of which are due to errors of omission rather than to intentional poisoning by parents. On the other hand, inappropriate or inadequate limit setting may contribute to the etiology of a significant number of accidental ingestions.

Sexual Abuse (Including Rape and Incest)

The magnitude of the problem of sexual abuse of children has only recently begun to be recognized. Its true incidence is impossible to obtain, since the problem is so overshadowed by cultural taboos.

Preliminary studies in a number of programs have served to invalidate several myths about sexual abuse. These studies show

First, that sexual abuse including incest occurs more often than health professionals would like to believe,

Second, that the assailant is known to the victim in the majority of cases and is most often a parent, friend of the family, or relative,

Third, that the assault occurs in the child's home or in the assailant's home in about two-thirds of the cases. In most instances, the mother is absent from the home at the time of the incident, and in some cases, the mother is actually compliant in the incident.

As in other examples of child abuse and neglect, the majority of families of victims are economically deprived, with a high incidence of unemployment.

Most workers now view sexual abuse as a form of child abuse, rather than as a variant of adult sexual crimes. The role of the physician in the management of sexual abuse is thus very similar to his role in the management of any case of child abuse: recognition, protection of the child, advocacy for the child and family to improve their functioning.

Injury in Which Physical Findings Do Not Coincide with the Account of the Injury

In summation, the health professional should be suspicious of child abuse and neglect whenever the history of the injury does not coincide with the physical findings noted.

CHILD NEGLECT

Child neglect is more difficult to define, to diagnose, and to prove than child abuse. Neglect and emotional abuse may occur in any age group.

Since parents are responsible for the care and protection of their children, they are accountable for errors of omission —neglecting the child's needs—as well a errors of commission—physical abuse.

Parents who are chronically under the influence of alcohol or drugs are not capable of providing protection for their children. Inadequate limit setting may result in falls, drownings, burns, and auto injuries, and may account for some of the numerous instances of "accidental" poisoning which occur to children in the United States each year.

Some aspects of child neglect may be explained by poverty, such as inadequate clothing, food, or shelter. In most instances, however, poverty alone is not the major factor in instances of neglect.

Educational Neglect

School children may be kept at home because of parental illness, or other needs perceived by the parents. All youngsters have the right to an opportunity for public education until they are 16 years of age and if they are prevented from making use of this opportunity, the school system or a public social agency may have to resort to reporting the family for educational neglect.

Medical Neglect

All children should be healthy and have their health needs met. Some health clinics assume the responsibility for ensuring follow-up of children with chronic diseases and even for evaluation of well children. Situations may arise in which the health professionals appear to be more concerned with follow-up than the parents. This may result from inadequate information being provided to the parents or from hostility or fear directed toward the health care provider. The child with undue lead absorption may require multiple courses of chelation, but because he is asymptomatic, parents may not see the need for treatment with the same degree of priority that the clinic does. When repeated efforts at arranging follow-up fail, reporting the parents for medical neglect may be the only recourse.

Multiple Emergency Room Visits

Kempe has suggested that any child brought to a hospital emergency room three times in one week should be hospitalized, the implication being that whatever the chief complaint, the parental message is clearly a "cry for help."

Repeated visits to *different* emergency rooms in a community are often difficult to identify. They may reflect "doctor-shopping" and distrust by the parents or unhappiness with the care in a particular institution. However, they may be an attempt to cover up and protect the family from being recognized as abusive or neglectful.

A new mother, isolated and afraid, may bring her healthy infant to a hospital emergency room with multiple complaints. This is not malingering but rather may be another example of the "cry for help" alluded to above.

Appropriate recognition and management depend on a staff that is alert and sensitive to these cries for help, a staff that is not uncomfortable looking beyond the surface of the initial chief complaint for the "hidden agenda."

Psychologic/Emotional Abuse

Disturbances of parenting have become recognized as contributing factors in many instances to their children's behavior problems. Some of these disturbances are amenable to change. Others result from transgenerational patterns of behavior that are less easily changed.

Deprivation of emotional support has been well documented as the cause of marasmus in hospitalized or institutionalized infants. These infants are recognized by their apathetic, staring appearances; they may ruminate when left alone and show little "reaching out" to the surrounding environment.

The syndrome, "failure to thrive" (FTT) may result from parental deprivation. *Failure to thrive* is defined as a condition occurring in an infant or young child whose growth is 3 standard deviations below the mean for age or whose growth falls progressively through several percentile curves. FTT can be the result of a variety of biomedical problems such as chronic renal disease, cystic fibrosis, and severe congenital heart disease. The biomedical causes of FTT are readily identifiable.

When no biomedical etiology is recognized, failure to thrive may be a result of parental deprivation. Affected infants and children classically gain weight rapidly in the hospital situation. Linear growth delay may be part of this picture and "catch-up growth" is a feature following separation from the depriving environment.

In some families, more than one child demonstrates failure to thrive. In other cases, a mother who has been successful in parenting one child may be taxed beyond her limits to provide sufficient emotional support when a subsequent child is born.

ETIOLOGIC FACTORS IN CHILD ABUSE AND NEGLECT

Three essential elements come together to produce the pattern of abuse and neglect: the abusive parent, the special child, and the crisis which "ignites the spark."

Characteristics of Abusive Parents

Parents of abused or neglected children may exhibit any of the following characteristics:

Isolation. Abusive parents may have a lack of contact with an extended family, may undergo multiple moves (*e.g.*, carnival family) or repeated relocations, even within the same community, may live in a community of transient people, or may live anonymously in a large city.

Poverty. Naturally, poverty brings its share of pressures on a family.

Poor Parenting Experience. In their own childhood, a parent may have had a lack of experience with a nurturing parent, a lack of development of a trusting relationship, and a history of abuse/neglect as a child. He often believes in harsh punishment.

Psychological Factors. Less than 10% of abusive parents are overtly psychotic. Borderline or low intelligence is noted in some instances. There is a history of lack of control or poor impulse control.

Drug Addiction/Alcohol Abuse. Parental addiction leads to inappropriate limit setting and an increased risk for "accidents"—ingestions or injuries.

Unrealistic Expectations. Lack of understanding about normal child development leads to expectations beyond the ability of the infant or child to perform.

Inappropriate Response to Seriousness of Injury. An inappropriate parental response to his child's injury may manifest itself in delay in seeking medical care, emergency room shopping, poor explanation or no explanation for child's injuries, and detachment, overreaction, or hostility.

Characteristics of the Abused or Neglected Child

Special. Often one child in a family is selected for abuse for no apparent reason. Sometimes a prolonged stay in a neonatal intensive care unit without parental involvement may lead to poor maternal-infant bonding.

Different. A child who is "different" may have slow or retarded development with poor emotional feedback to the parent or a high level of intelligence in a low IQ family, or he may be hyperactive.

Irritable. An irritable child may be one who cries a lot or is colicky. A high-pitched cry may be a sign of brain damage.

Compliant. The child who is missing his childhood because of being forced to accept responsibilities early may be a compliant child. He may exhibit "very good" behavior during painful procedures in the hospital and he may have an undue fear of his parents. This child prefers the hospital to home. (These characteristics may be noted as an effect of living in an abusive environment.)

Crisis (or series of crises)

Precipitating events and stresses may be exacerbated by poverty. The precipitating event may be a major life crisis, such as a move to a new community, a parent losing a job, or a divorce or separation; or, it may be a seemingly minor event (the straw that broke the camel's back) such as the washing machine breaking down in a family with an enuretic child.

Resolution of one stress may not resolve the entire problem. Unless the family receives some help to resolve underlying problems, abuse may recur with any subsequent crisis.

Child abuse in a family may be of two types: one in which there is a single isolated episode and the other in which a repetitive pattern of poor parenting exists.

Helfer has developed a theoretical construct which helps to explain the etiology of child abuse and neglect as a multigenerational phenomenon. WAR or the World of Abnormal Rearing is outlined in Figure 30-1. This schema conceptualizes a number of critical points in the development of the milieu in which child abuse is likely to occur:

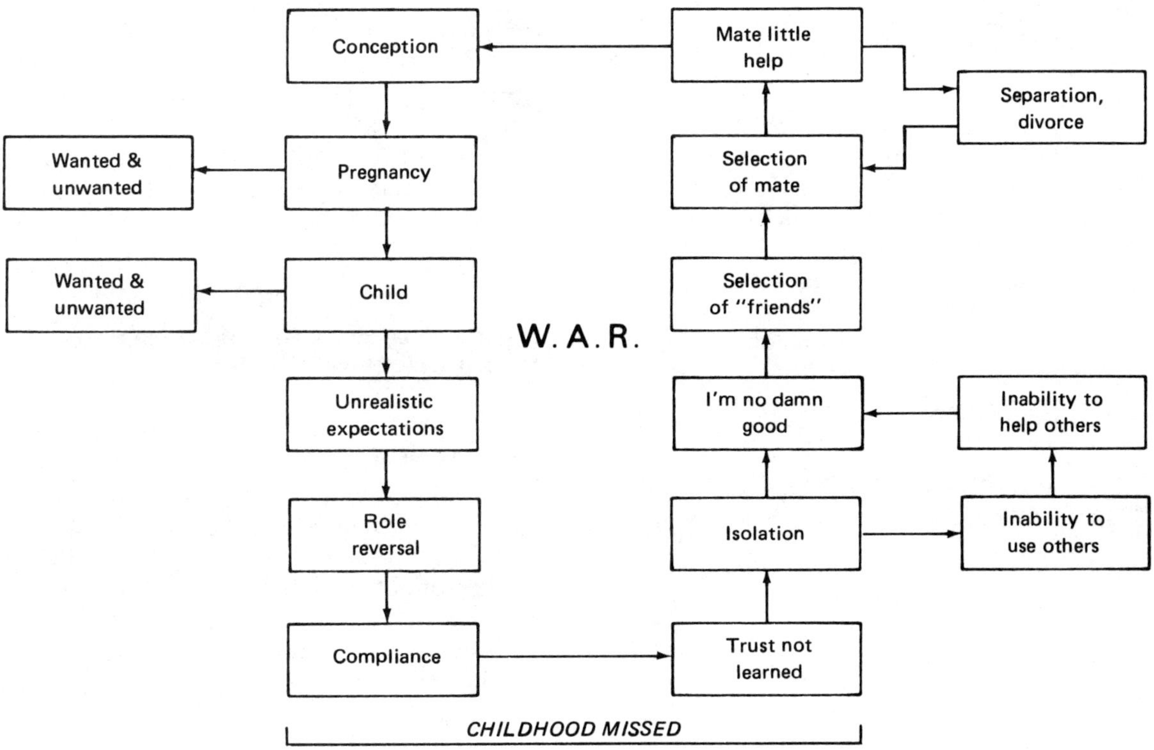

Fig. 30-1. World of abnormal rearing cycle. (Helfer RE: A Self-Instructional Program on Child Abuse and Neglect (in cooperation with the Committee on the Infant and Preschool Child of the American Academy of Pediatrics and the Staff of the National Center for the Prevention and Treatment of Child Abuse and Neglect, Denver), 1974)

Conception may lead to an unwanted pregnancy and an unwanted child.
Unrealistic expectations lead to role reversal in which the child takes on the parenting role.
Lack of development of trusting relationships leads to an inability to help or use others for help.
Friends and a mate tend to be selected from people with a similar background.

This cycle is not necessarily inexorable, and the chain of events may be broken at any point. For example, parenting classes may be helpful in providing more realistic expectations of children's developmental levels: a parent aide or family member may intervene at the right time to provide respite to an overwrought parent; a spouse with positive parenting experiences may counterbalance the poorer experience of the other parent.

When the cycle does follow this construct, however, it serves to provide an understanding of how this problem could develop. It also may be helpful to those providing services to the family to realize that in addition to the abused or neglected child who needs care and services, there is also a parent who once may have been a victim as well.

RESPONSIBILITIES OF THE PHYSICIAN

Prevention

1. Maintain a High Level of Suspicion. Especially when the history does not coincide with the physical findings of injury or neglect, maintain a high level of suspicion.

2. Recognize the Risk Factors. The physician should be suspicious of the *risk* of child abuse and neglect in certain instances. The following are situations in which the physician should be concerned:

The pregnant woman who continues to express denial, anger, or depression about her pregnancy into the third trimester
The mother who does not seek to make eye contact with her newborn infant in the delivery room
The mother who has not accepted the gender of her infant by the time of the first office visit
The parent who cannot "stand the sound of the baby's cry"
The mother who leaves her 2- to 4-month-old on the examining table unattended and stares out of the window during your examination of her child.
The parent who has unrealistic expectations of the young child's developmental level, who expects the child to "act like an adult"
Multiple office visits or emergency room visits or calls for seemingly insignificant problems or concerns.

Approach to the Child Who Has Undergone Abuse/Neglect

1. Make the presumptive diagnosis. After making the presumptive diagnosis, document all physical findings carefully in the medical record. Photographs should be taken whenever possible to have a record of external bruises or other injuries, the state of dehydration, or weight loss or inanition. Radiographs of long bones and ribs should be ordered to reveal evidence of older fractures and to "date" their stages of healing.

2. Intervene. The primary responsibility for the physician is the appropriate medical management of any injuries which are found. If the potential for abuse and neglect can be recognized and effective intervention can take place, the abusive incident may be aborted. Kempe has demonstrated in Denver that the introduction of skilled, successful parents or parent aides can serve the twofold purpose of modeling appropriate parenting behavior and avoiding predicted incidents of abuse and neglect.

3. **Separate the child from the environment.** Serious consideration should be given to separating the infant or child from the offending environment. This can be accomplished by identifying alternate caretakers in the family or by short-term foster care at the discretion of the social services personnel. Physicians should not be reluctant to hospitalize for immediate relief, even if the child is not seriously ill or injured.

Separation serves several purposes; first and foremost, it protects the child and in some situations is actually life-saving. It serves to give everyone "breathing room." The parents are often relieved that someone has responded to their "cry for help." They will rarely refuse a recommendation of hospitalization for observation, although many parents are reluctant to agree to voluntary foster home placement. It also gives the helping professionals time to gather additional information from the family and other interested parties.

Inform the Parents

When child abuse or neglect is suspected, it is incumbent upon the physician to call together a conference which includes the parents, a social worker, and nursing personnel involved in the child's care.

The parents should be informed tactfully and dispassionately of the findings and the concerns regarding the child's well-being. They should be told, for example, that the physical findings are not consistent with the history provided. A brief explanation should be offered about the legal responsibilities to report instances when the health professional suspects abuse or neglect.

Report to the Appropriate Agency

Most states require reporting within 24 to 48 hours of all suspected cases of abuse and neglect, usually to the Children's Protective Services of a Department of Social Services. Police agencies need not be involved unless there is a death or serious threat to the life of the child.

Ideally, the call should be made while the parents are present so that they may hear what is being said. This helps avoid misunderstandings and maintains communication on an open and honest level between parents and health professionals.

It is important to note that there is a legal responsibility to report cases of child abuse and neglect. In addition, there is a potential penalty for *not* reporting. Recently, courts have ruled that physicians and hospitals may be held responsible for failure to report suspected cases of child abuse and neglect, especially if subsequent harm is incurred by the child.

The physician is *not* expected to be a defense attorney, prosecuting attorney, judge, or jury in these cases, but he has the responsibility to report *suspected* cases of child abuse and neglect. It is up to the Children's Protective Services to do the additional investigation and up to the courts to resolve issues while protecting the rights of all involved.

Play the Role of Advocate

Whenever possible, the physician should try to play the role of advocate for the family as a whole. In all instances, the goals of intervention are to protect the child, while at the same time to help the family remain together as a unit and to ensure that necessary support services are provided. It is important to note that although the primary physician is not in a position to provide all the services necessary to help a family in need, he can often maintain a continuing relationship with the family if appropriate communication is initially established.

BIBLIOGRAPHY

Elmer E: A followup study of traumatized children. Pediatrics 59:273, 1977

Fontana VJ: The Maltreated Child: The Maltreatment Syndrome in Children, 2nd ed. Springfield, Ill, Charles C Thomas, 1971

Friedman SB, Morse CW: Child Abuse: A five year followup of early case finding in the emergency department. Pediatrics 54:404, 1974

This report and that of Elmer are two follow-up reports of cohorts of abused children and control children who had suffered accidental injury. A wide variety of problems existed in both groups five and eight years after the initial study, suggesting that poverty may have as powerful an impact as abuse itself.

Helfer RE: A Self-Instructional Program on Child Abuse and Neglect (in cooperation of the Committee on Infant and Preschool Child of the American Academy of Pediatrics and the Staff of the National Cnter for the Prevention and Treatment of Child Abuse and Neglect, Denver). 1974

This material is coordinated with audiotapes wich provide an opportunity for self-instructin of a wide variety of health professionals, including medical students.

Helfer RE, Kempe CH (eds): The Battered Child, 2d ed. Chicago, The University of Chicago Press, 1974

Kempe CH: Sexual abuse, another hidden pediatric problem: the 1977 C. Anderson Aldrich lecture. Pediatrics 62:382, 1978

Presents an overview describing the characteristics of the abused child and the abuser, and a review of the management of this problem.

Kempe CH, Helfer RE: Helping the Battered Child and His Family. Philadelphia, JB Lippincott, 1972

The three books of Fontana, Helfer and Kempe, and Kempe and Helfer provide extensive background reading on the etiology and management of the entire spectrum of child abuse and neglect.

Mental Retardation

31

David Baker

Mental retardation (or subnormality) is a major chronic handicap with profound implications for total life adjustment. The modern definition of *mental retardation* (significantly subaverage general intellectual functioning originating during the developmental period and associated with impairment of adaptive behavior, learning, and social adjustment) views broadly not only cognitive ability (as measured by "intelligence tests") but the total resultant summation of a person's competency in social adaptation. The term "mentally retarded" is limited to those persons who have inherent mental deficiency as a result of anatomic, physiologic, or biochemical impairment of central nervous system (CNS) function. Those who are unable to function intellectually or socially at the level expected by their chronologic age as a result of non-CNS disability, sensory deprivation, social-cultural deprivation, or emotional disturbance, can best be described as having *pseudoretardation.*

As noted in Table 31-1, the majority of retarded people fall into the "mild" or "borderline" groups. Opinion is divided whether persons who appear normal on physical and neurologic examination are retarded because of polygenic inheritable factors (familial retardation) or sociocultural determinants. Siblings of mildly retarded patients show a higher frequency of *mild retardation* when compared with siblings of severely retarded patients, who are likely to be normal in intelligence. The mildly retarded are *educable*, that is, capable of learning elementary reading, spelling, arithmetic; with modern educational and vocational training and community-based supportive programs, they are capable of being employed and becoming independent and self-sufficient.

The *moderately retarded*, in educational terms, are *trainable* and have potential for self-care and activities of daily living. These patients need supervision. Employment in a sheltered workshop while maintaining residence at home or in a group home is a feasible goal.

The *severely* and *profoundly retarded* are unable to provide for their own needs and are dependent upon others for care. In this group are seen the various morphologic stigmata of congenital malformations, as well as the signs of severe neurologic damage from pre- and perinatal insult to the CNS.

The prevalence of mental retardation (IQ less than 70) is estimated to be about 1% of the adult population, but 3% of newborns will be identified as retarded at some point in their lives. In children, mental retardation is second only to learning disabilities in frequency, and it is more often seen than cerebral palsy (0.5%) or epilepsy (0.5%–1%). More children are found to be mentally retarded during the school years because tests require greater comprehension for children of increasing age, and also because the child fails to cope with the de-

TABLE 31-1. Characteristics of Varying Degrees of Mental Retardation

IQ = MA/CA		SD	Function	Physical Findings	Family History of Mental Retardation	Socio-cultural Factors	Prevalence (%) MR	Pop	Therapeutic Goals
Borderline	70–84	−1.01 to −2.00	Basic academic skills "slow learner"	Essentially normal	+	4+	67	13	Basic academic and social skills to be capable of self-support and independent living in community
Mild	55–69	−2.01 to −3.00	Educable (vocational training)	Essentially normal	+	3+	22	2.7	Same as above
Moderate	40–54	−3.01 to −4.00	Trainable	Increasing frequency of neurologic deficits. Stigmata of dys-morphism	Only in cases due to genetic disorders	0	6	0.2	Self-care skills involving activities of daily living and sheltered workshop
Severe	25–39	−4.01 to −5.00	Dependent		Same as above	0	3	0.1	Protective care at home or group home
Profound	<25	−5.00	Totally dependent		Same as above	0	2	0.05	Custodial care

mands of the school. The child who can learn by rote and can manage tasks requiring only concrete thinking may fail a test requiring abstract conceptualization, yet the "6-hour retarded child" (in school) may show good adaptive ability in a social setting other than school.

ETIOLOGY

Infection

Prenatal infection includes the various intrauterine infections such as rubella, syphilis, cytomegalic inclusion disease, toxoplasmosis, and infection due to herpes virus. Postnatal infections that cause mental retardation may be due to bacteria or viruses, including postinfectious encephalitis and meningitis.

Toxic Agents

Mental retardation may be induced in the perinatal or neonatal period by maternal ingestion of such agents as alcohol, phenytoin, trimethadione, lead, and mercury; toxemia of pregnancy, and kernicterus associated with hyperbilirubinemia related to blood group incompatibility and various other causes. In older infants and children, retardation can be a result of postimmunization toxicity after administration of pertussis and smallpox vaccines and a result of ingestion of lead and other toxic agents, causing encephalopathy.

Trauma or Physical Agents

Trauma or physical agents include interferences with fetal circulation, birth injury, anoxia at birth, radiation and postnatal injury due to cranial trauma or battered-child syndrome.

Disorders of Metabolism, Growth, or Nutrition

Among the etiologic agents are the various metabolic disorders related to lipid, protein, and carbohydrate disorders. Among the important causes are hypoglycemia, PKU, galactosemia, homocystinuria, and protein/calorie malnutrition. Endocrine disorders such as hypothyroidism are estimated to occur in 1 of 3000 to 4000 newborns. Neonatal screening tests for PKU and hypothyroidism are mandatory in most states.

Other Causes

Mental retardation may also be associated with multiple congenital defects, gross postnatal brain disease syndromes, chromosomal abnormalities, prematurity, degenerative CNS disorders, major psychiatric disorders, and psychosocial environment factors such as deprivation and cultural-familial retardation. Children suffering cultural-familial retardation usually suffer only mild impairment, while environmentally deprived children have more severe retardation. The relative incidence of chromosomal disorders and inborn errors of metabolism as causes of mental retardation is 14% but estimates of genetic causes range as high as 50% to 70% (see Smith, Opitz in biblio.; Table 31-2). Emphasis on good prenatal care and nutrition, prevention of accidents, abuse, neglect, and poisoning are likely to result in decreased incidence of retardation. Advances in methods of immunizations and treatment of infectious diseases also contribute.

TABLE 31-2. Relative Incidence of Causes of Mental Retardation

Etiology	Percent
Inborn errors and hereditary disorders	4
Early influences on embryonic development (chromosomal changes; multiple congenital anomalies, prenatal infections	33
Maternal and perinatal causes (fetal malnutrition, 1%; prematurity with hyperbilirubinemia, hypoglycemia, trauma, hypoxia, 11%)	12
Acquired childhood diseases	4
Environmental and social problems	19
Cause unknown	28

Recently, from the population of nonspecific or undifferentiated MR, a syndrome has been described termed the "fragile X" syndrome or nonspecific X-linked MR. The frequency is one-half that of Downs' syndrome. There is a family history of affected males disproportionate to females. A narrowing or breakage in band Xq 27 or 28 near the distal end of the long arm of the X chromosome has been found in affected male patients and in carrier female relatives. One-third of hemizygous females may show MR, but of a milder degree than the male counterpart. Phenotypic correlates are: increase in testicular size, prominent symphysis of the mandible, large ears, and head circumference normal to increased.*

PREVENTION OF MENTAL RETARDATION

Even before pregnancy, prevention of mental retardation is possible. All women of childbearing age should be immunized

* Gerald PS: X-linked mental retardation and the fragile-x syndrome. Pediatrics *88*:594, 1981.

with rubella vaccine. Family planning education can be helpful in avoiding high-risk and unwanted pregnancies. Genetic counseling and prenatal diagnosis by amniocentesis have provided a powerful technology to detect the affected fetus.

With pregnancy, efforts should turn toward preventing contamination of the fetal environment with bacteria, viruses, and teratogenic agents. Good prenatal care ensures that the fetus is monitored for intrauterine growth impairment and for the ill effects of maternal toxemia or diabetes. Close monitoring during labor and delivery allows early detection of fetal distress.

Recent advances in neonatology have resulted in improved care for high-risk newborns, including early detection of metabolic defects. Proper therapy of infantile diarrhea and avoidance of hypertonic dehydration can minimize mental impairment from those sources.

In older children, good nutrition and good medical care are of particular importance. A consistent immunization series should be given to each child. Parents should be educated on safety measures to prevent accidents, trauma, and poisonings. Medical practitioners should be alert for signs of child abuse and neglect.

EARLY IDENTIFICATION AND DIAGNOSIS

Regular developmental assessments should be performed, especially in high-risk infants and children. This includes regular measurement of growth parameters, including head circumference. Examinations should be performed to detect sensory handicaps as part of the routine child-care program.

Once signs of mental retardation are noted, a complete diagnostic workup should be pursued to determine the etiology (both primary and contributing) and to make a functional assessment of the degree of retardation in various aspects of development (Tables 31-3 & 31-4). The reader should consult the articles by Smith and Optiz for a practical approach to diagnosis (see biblio.) The physician should refer the patient to subspecialists if he wants to coordinate the workup himself, or he should refer the patient to a center that offers complete diagnosis and evaluation services by team approach. In any event, the primary physician should take the responsibility for ensuring that the diagnostic services are completed satisfactorily, that the family is thoroughly informed, that the genetic aspects of the problem are addressed, and that parents have adequate opportunity to ask questions, ventilate their concerns, and assume that there will be a planned comprehensive program for follow-up care and supervision.

The primary physician is most likely to make the initial identification of the severely to moderately retarded child who presents with craniofacial abnormalities, microcephaly, neural tube defects, or other dysmorphic birth features, or who shows rather clear-cut developmental delays early in infancy and childhood. The mildly retarded to borderline retarded group may not be recognized as early, especially if these children get poor or sporadic medical supervision. They are often referred from day-care centers, preschool nursery programs, or, unfortunately, later in elementary schools.

Attention to developmental assessment (as outlined in the chapter on *Motor and Intellectual Development*) should enable the physician to detect children with milder degrees of retardation prior to school entrance. These children usually exhibit delays in development, particularly in language and personal-social and adaptive behavior, and they may show unusual degrees of responsiveness in terms of being hypoactive; on the other hand, they may be hyperkinetic.

TABLE 31-3. Basic Metabolic Screening Tests

	U Benedict's Clinitest	U Glucose oxidase Clinistix Tes-Tape	U $FeCl_3$	U 2,4 DNP	U&P AA Chr.	U Berry	Specific Test
Amino Acids PKU	±		+1	+	+		Serum phenylalanine
Homocystinuria					+		U Nitroprusside cyanide
MSUD*			+2	+	+		Enzyme assay WBC
Histidinemia			+3		+		
Carbohydrates Galactosemia	+	0					Enzyme assay RBC
Mucopolysaccharides Hurler's syndrome, and others						+	U Mucopolysaccharides
Hypothyroidism							T_4, TSH

U = urine
P = plasma
2,4-DNP = 2,4-Dinitrophenylhydrazine
AA Chr = Aminoacid chromatography (qual.)
*Maple syrup urine disease

1 green or blue-green, fading to yellow
2 gray with green tinge
3 green or blue green

MANAGEMENT

The physician must face the problem telling the parents that their child is retarded and helping them provide for the needs of the child in order to stimulate maximum developmental potential while they are rearing their other children and dealing with their own wounded feelings. The physician must recognize the parents' right to complete, accurate information and their responsibility to make major decisions affecting the child in the context of their own family situation. Physicians do not realize how much influence they have on the family and how much their support can help the family cope with these difficult situations.

Parental reactions to the diagnosis of retardation initially are shock, depression, and disbelief. It is important to tell *both* parents the diagnosis at the same time and to plan several sessions after the initial statement so that they can air their feelings and questions. Often the parents do not hear the entire message the first time because they are emotionally upset and cannot focus on the issues. The diagnosis should be validated in an authoritative fashion. Anticipate that the parents may have doubts and may want other professional opinions; indeed, the physician should encourage them to seek the opinions of a competent specialist rather than to let them "shop around" and perhaps fall into the hands of charlatans.

Do not give false reassurance ("The

TABLE 31-4. Checklist for Remediable Conditions

Condition	Procedure
Specific sensory deficit: vision hearing	Careful examination; oto-audiologic and ophthalmic evaluation
Seizure phenomenon including "convulsive equivalent"	EEG
Metabolic and endocrine disorders	Metabolic screening tests, T_3, T_4, GTT*
Systemic disease including failure to thrive	Appropriate workup
Toxic (exogenous factors)	Pb and EPP† levels
Increased intracranial pressure	Funduscopic examination; skull film, CT scan
Ongoing active and progressive disease	Tests for metabolic disorders affecting CNS, CSF exam, CT scan, EEG
Other specific etiologic factors	Serology for rubella, herpes virus, cytomegalic inclusion disease, toxoplasmosis, STS
Genetic factors	Family history, buccal smear, karyotype, biochemical and enzyme studies, examination of other family members, genetic counseling
Learning disability	Psycho-educational evaluation, educational programming
Speech and/or language disorder	Language/speech/hearing evaluation and appropriate therapy

*Glucose tolerance test
†Erythrocyte protoporphyrin

child will grow out of it") in an effort to spare their feelings. Yet, be sympathetic and recognize that the parents are experiencing a loss and going through a period of grief and mourning during which they may have difficulty relating to the physician who bears the bad news. The parents often view themselves as being damaged since they have given birth to a damaged child.

When the diagnosis of mental retardation is made in the postpartum period, the problem can be especially distressing, as in the case of a newborn with Down's syndrome or other genetic or congenital defects, as in the case of Down's syndrome infant of older parents, and especially as in the case of the first baby. During pregnancy, the parents usually anticipate the possibility of the child being abnormal and the first question asked is in regard to that. Do not delay telling the parents that the child is abnormal, and help them make an identification with and attachment to the baby to help them cope with the problem.

In the case of the child who has a gradually evolving picture of retarded development, the initial attachment of the child to the parents has been made; the problems of coping with the diagnosis will then include denial and ambivalence. After the initial shock, the parents often experience feelings of rejection, or they may compensate and overprotect the infant. Often, excessive coercive pressure is placed on the child, who is viewed as "lazy." In any event, parental attitudes of coercion, rejection, or overprotection complicate and interfere with further development of the child.

The basic goal of the physician is to help the child achieve his maximum potential. Secondary emotional problems are frequently encountered. Therefore, close follow-up with anticipatory guidance and counseling should be planned. A long-term longitudinal "life-cycle" follow-up will enable the physician to deal with problems presented at each stage of the child's development. It is also necessary to deal with the significance of mental retardation to the parents. Parents often view the child as having no potential and fail to recognize that the child will make developmental progress following the usual sequence, though at a slower rate than normal children. Often young parents do not inform other family members or their other children of the situation; they should be encouraged to do this promptly because they need the additional support of their extended family.

During early infancy, problems center around basic home care such as feeding, sleeping, and other problems familiar to physicians who take care of infants. Later, concern will be focused on motility, toilet-training, and still later on language development, socialization, and the need for a preschool stimulation program.

It is important to convey the value of the child to the parents. The child should receive regular immunizations and care of intercurrent illnesses. Conditions which interfere with development (*e.g.*, serous otitis media with hearing loss) should be prevented or treated promptly. It is important to let the parents know what to expect and to set up goals for the next epoch of development. Parents should be praised and reassured for doing a good job in taking care of their children. The positive aspects of the child should be stressed, but in a balanced, realistic fashion. The opportunity to talk with other parents who have had similar problems and who have learned methods of coping is a therapeutic experience.

In the past, institutionalization of the mentally retarded had been recommended freely. It has been shown that a nurturing, stimulating home environment can provide the opportunity for maximal development, and no effort should be spared to build into the program support for the family to rear the child at home. Indications for institutionalization are highly selective and should be reserved when other measures fail and the family cannot cope with the child. However, it must be recognized that the care of an extremely handicapped child can be a tremendous burden. Many programs are being offered for respite care or part-time placement; in this way, the family can have a vacation knowing that the child will receive care. This may be necessary at times when there is a breakdown in the family's capacity to meet the child's needs and should be looked at as part of a positive therapeutic program rather than a negative event.

Community Mental Health and Mental Retardation Centers offer counseling including home visits from mental health workers and from parents of retarded children. These services should be used freely. Parents should be encouraged to join and participate in parents' organizations for the benefit of group therapy, to be actively involved and to effect change in the local community to improve the care of the retarded.

The history of mental retardation illustrates the relationship between society and an underprivileged minority. Indeed, the way in which a society deals with its handicapped is a measure of its level of civilization with respect to moral and ethical matters.

In the early part of the century, "scientific" ideology and the eugenics movement were well-intended but misguided forces in segregating the retarded (including many who are now viewed as socioculturally deprived) into institutions, where they languished. The efforts of organized parents' groups (The National Association for Retarded Citizens) with the help of visionary humanistic professionals (such as Grover Powers, former professor of pediatrics at Yale University) were instrumental in changing this picture and are part of the story of a broad movement for human rights and the dignity of the individual.

One may view parental counseling in terms of phases in which crucial decisions are made in the course of development. The major phases include care during infancy (including infant stimulation programs), preschool programs, school-age programs, problems related to pubertal and adolescent development, and vocational training. Adolescents with emerging sex drives and poor self-control present many problems. Recreational and social programs are needed for the retarded who have problems being accepted by other children and being isolated from the community.

The *Right to Education Act* (PL92-142) mandates an individualized appropriate educational program in the least restrictive environment to all children over 3 years of age. The physician must be familiar with resources within his community which offer services to the retarded. Furthermore, he should make efforts to improve the quality of these services by supporting parents' groups and to establish educational programs, and community mental health/mental retardation centers. His influence in the community is considerable, something which physicians often underestimate. His involvement in giving support to child abuse programs, immunization programs, and supportive services to the school are also important with respect to the problems of mental retardation.

BIBLIOGRAPHY

Barlow CF: Mental Retardation and Related Disorders. Philadelphia, FA Davis, 1978

This is a highly informative, clinically oriented approach, written in excellent style.

Milunsky A: The Prevention of Genetic Disease and Mental Retardation. Philadelphia, WB Saunders, 1977

The author, a geneticist, writes knowingly of the recent advances in this rapidly growing area. The ratio of information acquired to time expended reading this work is very high. A wide range of topics is covered, including the causes and prevalence of mental retardation, principles of genetic counseling, prenatal diagnosis, prevention of prematurity and perinatal morbidity, lead intoxication, infectious diseases, and early intervention. Legal, economic, and eugenic issues are discussed.

Opitz JM: Mental Retardation: Biologic Aspects of Concern to Pediatricians. Pediatrics in Review, Vol. 2: 41, 1980

A highly concentrated overview with classification and logical scheme of diagnosis.

Richmond JB, Tarjan G, Mendelsohn R (eds): Mental Retardation: A Handbook for the Primary Physician, 2nd ed. Chicago, American Medical Association, 1974

This is a brief overview of the subject and is useful as a desk reference.

Smith DW, Simons FER: Rational diagnostic evaluation of the child with mental deficiency. Am J Dis Child 129:1285, 1975

This article clearly presents a practical approach for diagnostic procedures and data illustrating the relevance of various studies in relation to the history and physical examination.

Seizures and Other Paroxysmal Disorders

32

Charles B. Brill
Michael A. Mitchell

Paroxysmal disorders are recurrent, reversible alterations of brain function. Several occur frequently in children, particularly syncope, migraine, breath-holding, and seizures. Although not discussed in this chapter, recurrent neurologic dysfunction also characterizes certain other diseases such as drug abuse and rare inborn errors of amino acid and urea metabolism.

Paroxysmal Disorders

- Seizures
- Migraine
- Syncope
- Breath-holding spells
- Paroxysmal vertigo
- Others
  - Hypoglycemia
  - Psychiatric disorders
  - Drug abuse
  - Certain inborn errors of metabolism

SEIZURE DISORDERS

Seizures are clinical manifestations of hypersynchronous firing of cerebral cortical neurons. They are more frequently seen in children than in adults and are among the most common neurologic disorders in pediatrics. It is stated that 4% to 8% of *all* children experience one or more seizures between infancy and adolescence. This higher incidence of seizures in childhood reflects a greater seizure susceptibility in the immature brain which many children eventually outgrow, particularly when they are otherwise neurologically normal.

The stage of cerebral development strongly influences seizures. Examples discussed later in this chapter are neonatal seizures, infantile spasms, and febrile convulsions in which the onset, types, and duration of seizures are remarkably age-dependent. Cerebral maturation and the presence or absence of demonstrable brain pathology are major factors determining whether seizures will be outgrown, will change in type, or will persist to become epilepsy in adulthood.

DESCRIPTION AND CLASSIFICATION OF SEIZURES

Hughlings Jackson's 1880 definition of seizure remains one of the best: "A seizure is an occasional, excessive and disorderly discharge of neurons resulting in an excess, distortion or deficit of central nervous system function. These disruptions of CNS function will vary according to the area of seizure onset and pathways of spread within the brain."

Our description of seizures (Table 32-1) is derived from the International Classification, which is based on both clinical and electroencephalographic (EEG) abnormalities. This description successfully characterizes most childhood seizures.

Epilepsy, a Greek word meaning "seizure," is a heterogenous group of disorders having in common a susceptibility to recurring seizures caused by intrinsic congenital or acquired brain abnormalities which may or may not be demonstrable by present-day diagnostic techniques. The types of seizures and the presence or absence of nonseizure abnormalities such as mental retardation, or physical deformities greatly depend on what brain disease is present in each case. Frequently, seizures occur in children who are otherwise neurologically and developmentally normal. When seizures are com-

TABLE 32-1. Seizure Classification with Examples of Clinical and EEG Findings

Seizure Type	Examples of Seizure Activity	Typical EEG Findings
Partial seizures	Some memory or consciousness maintained	
Motor (Focal motor)	Jacksonian march, adversive, speech arrest	1. Focal abnormality* 2. Normal†
Sensory (Focal sensory)	Localized cutaneous, visual, auditory, smell, taste, or vertiginous sensations	
Complex (Psychomotor)	Impaired consciousness, visual or auditory misperceptions or hallucinations, anxiety, automatisms, *déjà vu*, visceral sensations (typical postictal lethargy and headache)	
Multifocal	Multiple partial seizures	Multifocal abnormalities
Generalized seizures	Memory and consciousness lost	
Major motor ("Convulsion" or *grand mal*)	Tonic-clonic. Sometimes purely tonic or clonic. "Secondary generalized major motor seizures" are very common, e.g., those with an aura, preceding partial seizure or localized EEG abnormality	1. Focal abnormality* 2. Normal† 3. Bilaterally synchronous discharges‡
Absence (*Petit mal*)	Brief loss of consciousness with or without eye-blinking, automatism, clonic jerks or changes in tone (no postictal symptoms)	Bilaterally synchronous discharges especially 3/second spike-wave
Myoclonic	Massive or localized single jerks, often occurring in clusters. One characteristic type is infantile spasms	Various bilateral discharges‡ (hypsarrhythmia in infantile spasms)
Atonic (Astatic or "drop seizures")	Abrupt loss of tone, resultant fall frequently causing facial injury. Often associated with myoclonic seizures	

*Focal paroxysmal discharges or disturbances of background rhythms (see Fig. 32-1)

†EEG may become positive with special techniques (*e.g.*, sleep recording or nasopharyngeal leads)

‡Such as spike-wave, polyspike, or paroxysmal slow waves (see Fig. 32-3)

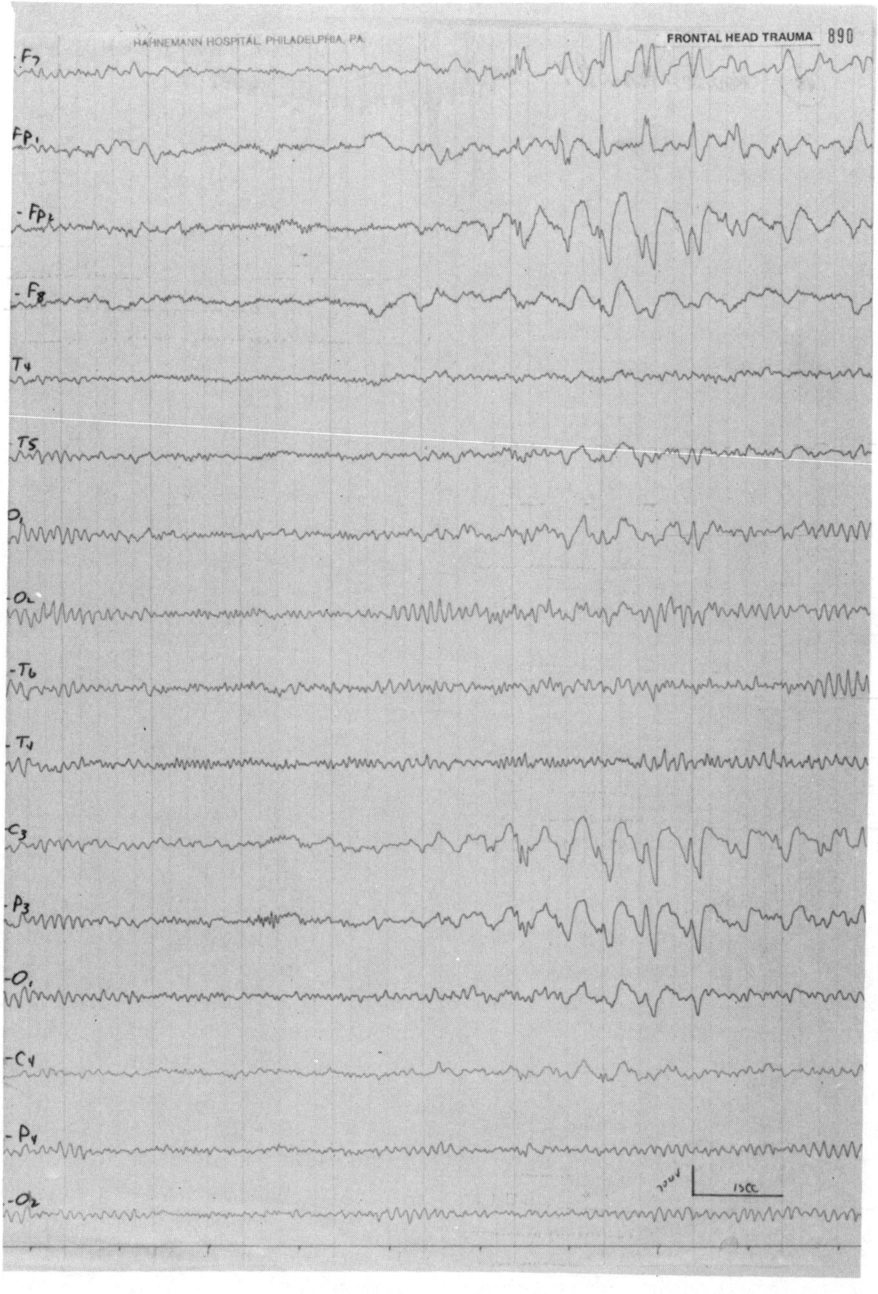

Fig. 32-1. EEG of 15-year-old girl who suffered severe head trauma with loss of consciousness and seizures. There was a frontal lobe contusion. EEG shows left frontal spike and spike-wave abnormality (T_3-F_7, F_7-FP_1, FP_1-FP_2 and F_3-C_3, C_3-P_3). Note that the location of the abnormality is more important than the configuration of the abnormality—spike-wave. This case also shows that the spike-wave abnormality is seen in focal epilepsy, and not only in absence seizures.

pletely or nearly completely controlled through good medical management, a large proportion of epileptic children live unhampered lives, do well in school, get a driver's license, and pursue a satisfying adult career. Although we do not ignore the terms "epileptic" or "epilepsy," we prefer the official label "seizure disorder," which is more objective, more comprehensible to laymen, and far less prejudicial when it appears in the child's school or medical records.

In nonepileptics, sudden onset of seizures frequently indicates such serious acute brain diseases as intracranial infection, head injury, and various toxic/metabolic disorders. Also, about 5% of small children have seizures triggered by high fever (see Febrile Convulsions); epilepsy affects only 0.5% of children in the same age group.

Partial Seizures

Partial seizures is a relatively new term encompassing manifestations of localized seizure involvement of the brain (Fig. 32-1). The cerebral localization can be inferred by history or observations of the initial symptoms or motor phenomena. Often a description by the parent or other observer must be sought since the patient may have partial or complete amnesia for the attack. Sometimes the history will give a better localization for the origin of partial seizures than the EEG.

Partial Motor Seizures. The most typical "focal" or partial motor seizure is tonic stiffening and/or clonic jerking of the face or extremity contralateral to the cerebral focus. Most often the initial involvement is rather diffuse, for example, an entire extremity or the face and upper extremity. Relatively rare are *Jacksonian seizures*, which begin in a highly localized part and then "march" in a way predictable from the functional anatomy of the motor strip, for example, an initial twitching of the thumb spreading to the fingers and then simultaneously to the face and lower extremity. These seizures, especially the jacksonian, indicate a focus in or near the contralateral precentral gyrus (motor strip).

Adversive seizures are also common. The head and eyes are turned contralaterally from the focus and the extremities on both sides may assume characteristic postures, particularly extension of the contralateral and flexion of the ipsilateral extremities in a manner similar to the infantile tonic neck reflex. Sometimes the contralateral rotation of the head and trunk is so strong that the patient actually turns in circles. Adversive seizures usually arise from contralateral cerebral foci but they may arise anywhere in the hemisphere, particularly in frontal, temporal, or occipital areas.

Purely inhibitory seizures causing only temporary paralysis of the affected part are rare. When the hemisphere dominant for speech (usually left) is involved, speech arrest or aphasia may accompany partial seizures. *Postictal (Todd's) paralaysis* of the parts involved may follow a partial motor seizure and usually clears within several hours.

In children, partial motor seizures, focal or multifocal, often accompany acute diffuse disturbances in brain function such as meningitis or hyponatremia or reflect underlying diffuse brain damage. Although each case must be evaluated carefully, partial seizures in these situations do not indicate permanent localized brain damage. Epileptic children with stereotyped partial seizures and well-defined EEG foci (see Fig. 32-1) can be assumed to have a cortical lesion, but it is remarkable how often one fails to demonstrate the lesion by sophisticated tests. When demonstrable, examples of lesions causing chronic partial seizures are cysts, vascular anomalies, other cerebral malformations and brain tumors.

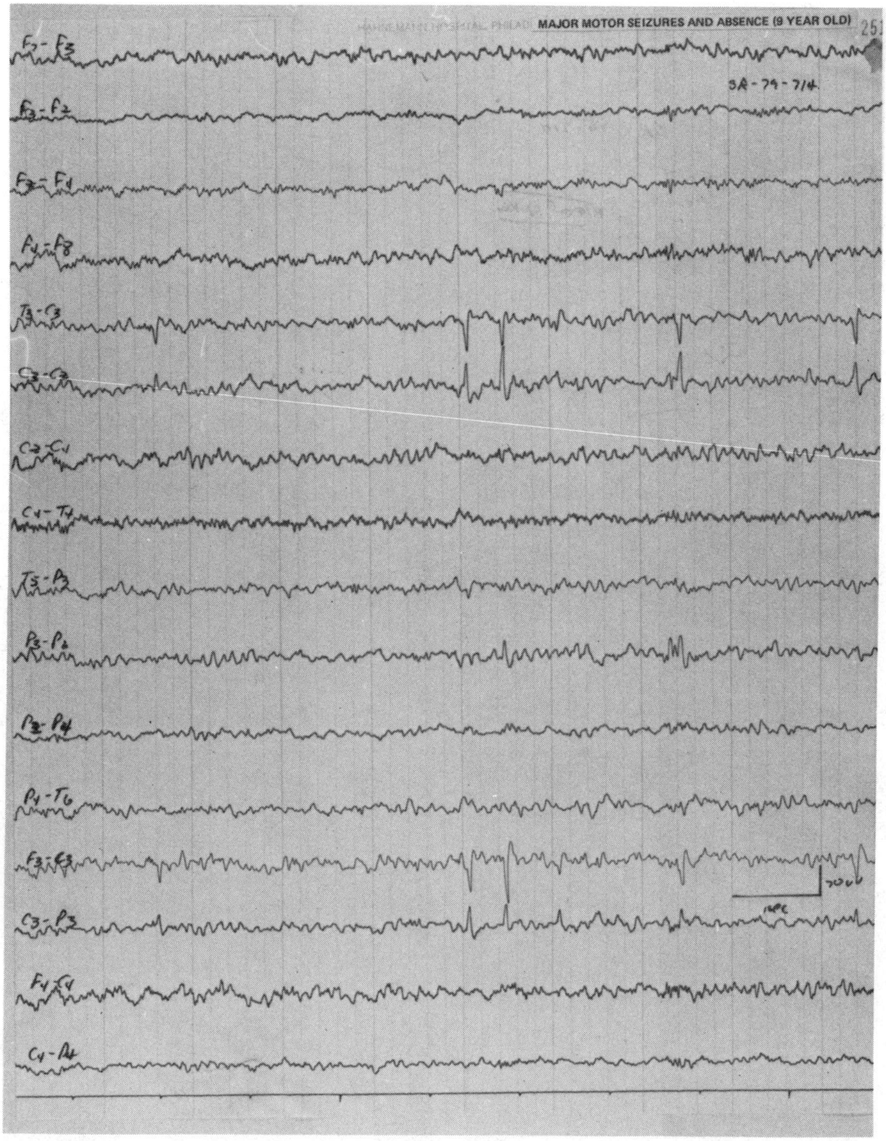

Fig. 32-2. EEG of neurologically normal 9-year-old, with infrequent major and absence seizures. EEG shows rolandic vertex spikes (T_3-C_3, C_3-C_2 and F_3-C_3, C_3-P_3). Note that there is a small wave following each spike. Slow waves are inhibitory.

Partial Sensory Seizures. *Partial sensory seizures* occur when irritative foci affect cerebral cortical sensory areas; thus, they can be categorized as somatic and special sensory seizures. *Somatic sensory seizures* arise from the contralateral postcentral gyrus (sensory strip) and are most frequently described as a numbness or tingling, although pins and needles, movement, warmth, and other sensations may be felt in the body part

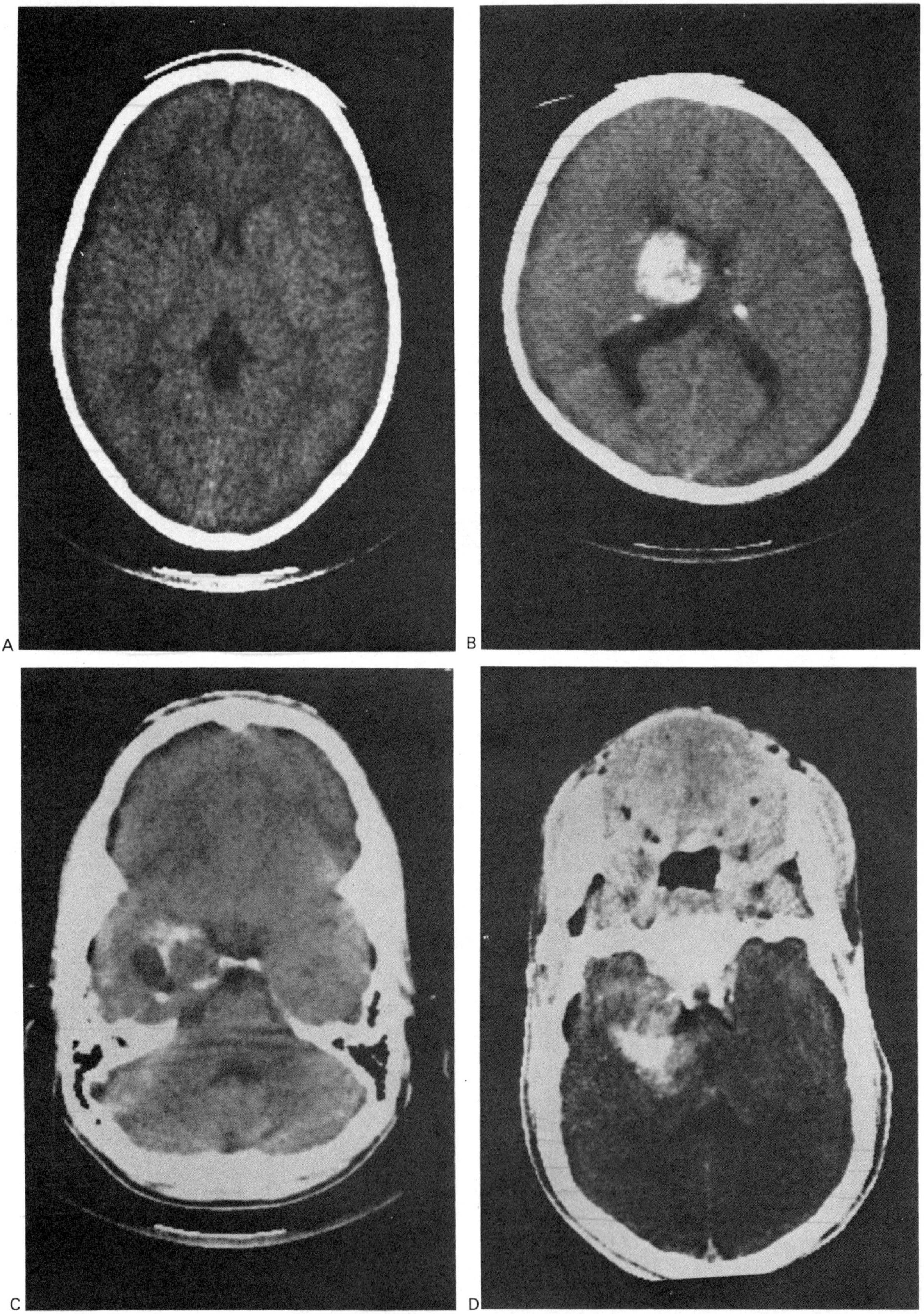
A
B
C
D

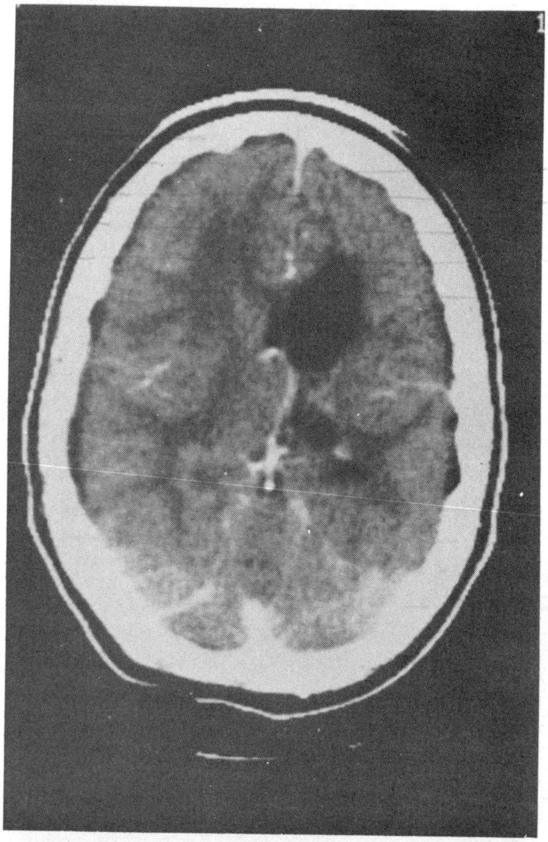

E

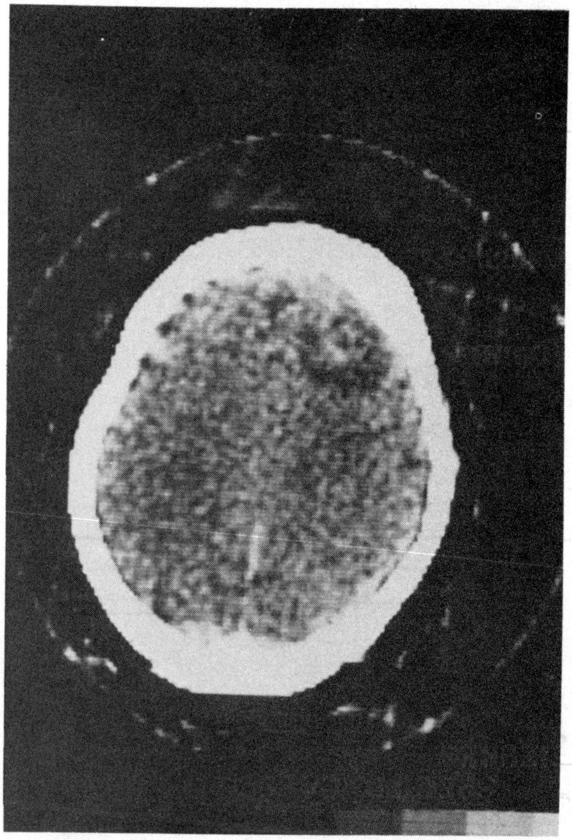

F

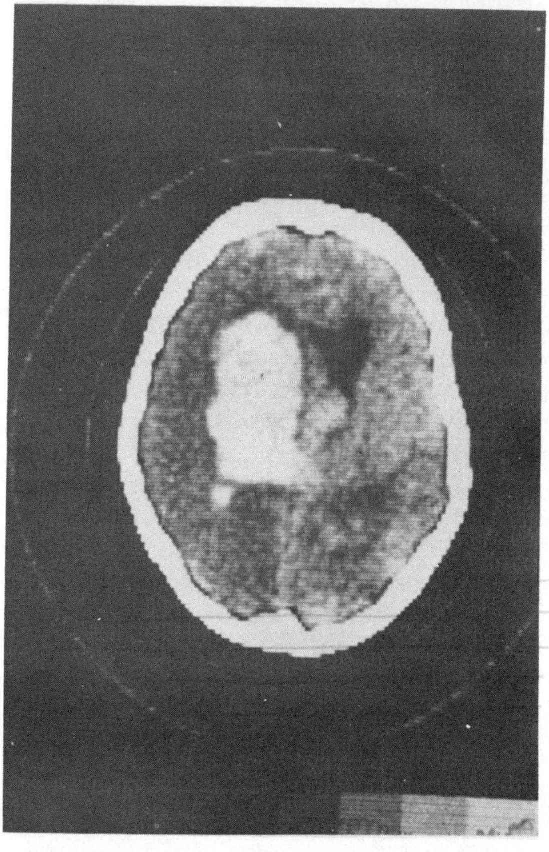

G

Fig. 32-3(*A* to *G*). Computerized tomography in seizure patients. (*A*) Two-and-one-half-year-old boy with developmental delay and hypotonia had a 12 minute generalized seizure associated with a fever of 102°F. CT scan was normal. Note that this is a symptomatic seizure, and not a simple febrile seizure, because of the prolonged duration, low fever, and abnormal neurodevelopmental status. (*B*) CT scan of an 8-year-old boy with severe, mixed seizure disorder, mental retardation, and hypotonic quadriparesis. Skin showed multiple vitiliginous spots and sebaceous adenomata. CT scan, without contrast, shows multiple subependymal calcific masses, with a large mass in the region of the right foramen of Monro. Diagnosis is tuberous sclerosis. (*C* and *D*) Twelve-year-old boy with a severe behavior disorder and generalized seizures, preceded by an aura of vague upper abdominal discomfort. CT scan, done in the axial plane, without contrast enhancement (*C*) shows a densely calcified, partly cystic temporal lobe tumor. Views in the coronal plane, done with contrast enhancement (*D*), show extension into the thalamus and hypothalamus, with slight midline shift, and compression of the ipsilateral lateral ventricle. (*E*) Twelve-year-old girl with spastic right hemiparesis and brief right focal seizures, both with and without loss of consciousness. CT scan shows a porencephalic cyst of the frontal horn of the lateral ventricle. The entire left hemisphere is smaller than the right. (*F*) Fourteen-year-old boy with cyanotic congential heart disease. Fever, obtundation, and a left focal seizure. Examination showed a left hemiparesis and papilledema. CT scan showed a right frontal contrast enhancing lesion, with central lucency and surrounding edema. Surgical diagnosis was brain abscess. (*G*) Eighteen-year-old girl with a history of right focal seizures. She had the sudden onset of a similar seizure with headache, right hemiparesis, and coma. CT scan without contrast showed a large thalamic hemorrhage. Postmorten examination showed an AVM as the cause of the hemorrhage.

affected by the seizure. The initially localized sensations may spread on the involved side as does a Jacksonian motor seizure. Due to the proximity and overlap of the Rolandic motor and sensory strips, motor seizure phenomena often occur concurrently.

A common type of partial sensory or motor seizure is the *benign focal* with Rolandic spikes. The sensory aura or motor activity frequently involves the facial structures. These seizures often occur during sleep. The EEG shows Rolandic or midtemporal spikes (Fig. 32-2). The benign nature of the partial sensory seizure is shown by the fact that the seizures can be brought under excellent control with anticonvulsants and also that they can disappear with normalization of the EEG in the early teens.

Special sensory seizures arise from the occipital visual, temporal auditory-vestibular and olfactory, and Sylvian taste areas. *Occipital visual seizures* are usually elementary phenomena such as flashing lights and should be differentiated from migraine attacks. More complex visual seizures, such as change in size or color of objects seen, usually arise from temporal lobe association areas. Seizures from the other sensory areas produce hallucinations of sound, motion, smell, or taste which, because of their close proximity to other temporal lobe structures, are very frequently the aura to a complex seizure.

Complex Partial Seizures. *Complex partial seizures* (also called "psychomotor" or "temporal lobe" seizures) are fascinating, particularly because they affect areas of the cerebral cortex serving such complex functions as emotion, memory, and other intellectual activities, and the highest levels of autonomic system integration.

Although the pattern of seizure phenomena varies greatly from patient to patient, the attacks are usually characteristic and indicative of origin in one or the other temporal lobes, especially the anterior and medial "limbic" portions. Adolescence and young adulthood are particularly important times for the development of complex partial seizures, most likely due to the combination of preexisting lesions and maturational characteristics of the temporal lobe.

Complex partial seizures can be described as five general types: (1) arrest of activity with staring only, (2) arrest of activity with staring followed by automatisms, (3) psychic seizures, (4) seizures with visceral phenomena, and (5) progression to secondary generalized seizures. These seizures are frequently considered in the differential diagnosis of childhood behavioral and psychiatric disorders.

Attacks causing *arrest of activity* with staring typically last 1 to 2 minutes, rarely more than 5 minutes. Consciousness is impaired and the patient usually cannot remember the attack. These "psychomotor lapses" are frequently misdiagnosed as simple absences (*petit mal*), but they are different due to their longer duration, postictal confusion, and EEG findings. Arrest of activity with staring followed by simple or complex automatisms is similar with the additional phenomenon of *automatisms*, which are repetitive, automatic-looking movements. Simple automatisms include various orofacial movements such as lip-smacking, chewing, or mumbling, and movements of the hands like pulling at clothing, rubbing the face, or fumbling with objects. Because simple automatisms also occur in absences, there is further potential confusion between these two very different seizure disorders (see also Generalized Seizures).

Complex automatisms encompass more integrated motor activity such as running in circles, removing clothing, or continuing in a rather aimless way some voluntary activity that was in progress before the seizure. Often the automatic behavior reflects a partial awareness of the environment.

Psychic phenomena are consciously experienced by the patient. Affective components are common, usually fear or anxiety, and are generally recognized by the patients as not being real. Only a few patients describe the affective experiences as being pleasant. Memory phenomena include the famous *déjà vu* (a peculiar and inappropriate sense of familiarity), a sudden feeling of strangeness of the current environment, or a recollection from the past. Perceptual distortions of sight or sound can be striking such as the "zoom lens" phenomenon where objects in the environment seem to shrink or enlarge. Hallucinations, such as formed visual or auditory images or reliving a past experience, may be stereotyped or may vary from attack to attack.

Visceral phenomena, both subjective and objective, frequently occur. The olfactory hallucinations (usually distinctly unpleasant odors) are often associated with other phenomena such as *déjà vu*, or they may simply be the aura to a major motor seizure. Visceral sensations are quite common—frequently a peculiar abdominal distress which may become a "rising sensation" of abdominal discomfort moving upward in the trunk to the throat or head. *Abdominal epilepsy* refers to paroxysmal abdominal pain as a seizure manifestation, although epilepsy is a rare cause of the syndrome of recurrent abdominal pain in children. Objective autonomic changes include pupillary dilatation, tachycardia, hypertension, changes in visceral motility, and irregular respirations. The external autonomic changes may suggest rage or panic to an observer but usually the patient's mobility and consciousness are impaired.

Multifocal Seizures. Children with multifocal seizures fall into two large groups. The first group includes those with acute brain disturbances such as anoxia, bacterial meningitis, encephalitis, hypoglycemia, hyponatremia, hypocalcemia, and lead intoxication. Clearly their prognosis depends on whether the acute cerebral insults are fully reversible. The second group is composed of epileptic children who usually have other signs of diffuse brain injury, particularly mental retardation. The seizures are often difficult or impossible to fully control and consist of various partial motor types such as jerky eye movements, tonic adversive posturing, and localized clonus. These children may also suffer generalized attacks such as major motor, myoclonic, atypical absence, and atonic seizures.

Generalized Seizures

The several types of generalized seizures imply diffuse discharges that occur synchronously in both cerebral hemispheres. Apparently all of us have cerebral mechanisms for the most common type of generalized seizure, the *major motor seizure*, so it is not surprising that major motor seizures are common and occur in many different clinical settings. Probably most major motor seizures are secondary generalized seizures resulting when initially localized discharges rapidly become diffuse. On the other hand, certain epilepsies, particularly typical absences and certain major motor seizures, are called primary generalized seizures because at present no localized "generator" has been found to explain the bilaterally synchronous EEG discharges in these cases.

Major Motor Seizures. After early infancy major motor seizures are by far the most common type of seizure, occurring, for example, in about 80% of epileptic children and in most children with febrile convulsions. Among epileptic children with major motor seizures, about half also have other types of seizures. When parents say "convulsion" they usually mean a major motor seizure and, when asked, usually recall their fear that their child was dying when the convulsion began.

The attack may occur abruptly or it may be preceded by an aura or by nonspecific prodromal behavioral changes such as irritability. When an *aura* is experienced beforehand, there definitely is a focal origin of the convulsion. Basically, auras are initial partial sensory seizures progressing immediately to a secondary generalized major motor seizure.

Next, there is a sudden loss of consciousness, a fall if the child is not supported, and a generalized muscle contraction resulting in the *tonic phase* of diffuse rigidity, arrest of breathing, cyanosis, and upward deviation of the eyes. Sometimes there is a piercing cry, biting of the tongue or cheek, and loss of urine. The tonic phase is followed by a *clonic phase* of repeated flexor spasms of the entire body. Jerking respirations now resume and the intervals between clonic jerks lengthen until clonus ceases. Pooling of pharyngeal secretions is prominent. Autonomic phenomena also occur, including pupil dilatation, skin vasomotor changes, piloerection, sweating, tachycardia, and hypertension.

The clonic jerks are followed by the *postictal phase* with unconsciousness, flaccid muscles, absent tendon reflexes, and extensor plantar reflexes. As patients awaken, they are confused and frequently so irritable that they become combative if restrained. Often there is a postictal headache and a desire to sleep. Unfortunate consequences can occur if the postictal state is mistaken for intoxication or some sort of antisocial behavior. The patient cannot remember the attack, but knows that it occurred because of postictal discomfort.

In children there is considerable variation in the severity and duration of the convulsive phase as well as the length of postictal CNS depression. Typically, the tonic and clonic phases together last about 2 minutes, but often are shorter or longer, lasting up to 5 minutes. Although most children suffer no discernible brain injury from occasional brief major motor seizures, there is always the risk of anoxia, especially if status epilepticus develops. *Major motor status epilepticus* refers to convulsions prolonged over 15 minutes or recurring so frequently that the patient does not recover consciousness in between; it is a true medical emergency.

Besides typical tonic-clonic major motor seizures, there are purely tonic or clonic vriants. As a rule, tonic seizures are brief and often occur during sleep. Purely clonic generalized seizures occur mostly in small children, especially in febrile convulsions.

The EEG during a major motor seizure reveals generalized high-frequency discharges during the tonic phase and spike-wave discharges in the clonic phase. During the postictal phase, brain waves are initially depressed in amplitude and then abnormally slow. This postictal slowing subsides gradually and sometimes requires 7 to 10 days to fully disappear.

Absence Seizures. *Absence* or *petit mal seizures* are in essence "blank stares" with sudden, brief interruption of consciousness.

Typical absences form a relatively distinctive, and well-known entity in epilepsy which is largely confined to children over 5 years of age and adolescents. However, it is found in only 5% of all childhood epilepsy patients. The term *petit mal* should probably be avoided because many laymen and some physicians use it to describe any seizure other than a convulsion.

Absences commonly last less than 10 seconds and infrequently more than 30 seconds. They are subdivided into simple and complex forms; both can occur in the same person. In a simple absence the patient suddenly stares blankly, stops verbal or motor activity, and is unconscious but does not fall. The attack begins and ends abruptly with the patient fully alert afterward. Occasionally during the seizure, the patient continues some simple motor activity such as walking.

Although the patient is typically unaware of the seizure itself, he or she frequently detects it from the interruption of ongoing events. Those attacks that last over 10 seconds tend to be complex with additional features such as eyelid fluttering, drooping of the head, myoclonic jerks, or automatisms. Typical automatisms are fumbling of the hands, lip-smacking, or verbal stuttering.

In the untreated patient with typical absences, the attacks are extremely frequent and the EEG is virtually always abnormal. Twenty to forty attacks per day are common, and there may be hundreds. The EEG displays sudden generalized bursts of 3 per second spike-wave complexes (see Fig. 32-4) during and between attacks. Clinical attacks and EEG discharges can often be induced by asking the patient to hyperventilate by using stroboscopic light stimulation or emotional tension (*e.g.*, the normal anxiety of being called on in class). When the EEG discharges last 4 seconds or more, consciousness is transiently impaired even though a clinical attack may not be obvious. Since absences typically begin between age 5 and 10 years, teachers or parents frequently misinterpret them initially as daydreaming or peculiar mannerisms.

Another feature of children with typical absences is that except for their "spells," they are usually neurologically normal. A few show learning disabilities, particularly when seizure control is difficult. Less than 5% are retarded. In many patients, a positive family history suggests an autosomal dominant genetic etiology.

Finally, it is important to differentiate absences from brief, complex partial (psychomotor) seizures because of the occurrence of staring and automatisms in both. As opposed to absences, brief psychomotor seizures generally last more than 30 seconds, are often preceded by an aura, may cause only partial alteration of consciousness, produce postictal confusion and often headache, and usually show localized EEG abnormalities. This differentiation is important because of significant differences in drug therapy. Usually, the prognosis for seizure control and outgrowing the seizures in adolescence or young adulthood is good. However, about 50% of patients have one or several major motor seizures during their course, and a minority remain epileptics in adult life.

Atypical absence seizures do not differ much clinically from typical absences but are very different in the total clinical picture and EEG findings. Children in this category are heterogeneous but the majority are retarded or borderline. One large group, called "*petit mal* variant" or Lennox-Gasteaut syndrome, exhibits mental retardation, "slow" (2/second) spike-wave discharges, and multiple types of seizures including absences, tonic seizures in sleep, and myoclonic/atonic seizures (discussion follows).

Petit mal status or spike-wave stupor is a prolonged confusional state lasting hours or even days with associated continuous spike-wave discharges. This may occur in atypical or typical absence seizure states. The diagnosis is confirmed by obtaining an immediate EEG.

Myoclonic and Atonic Seizures. Myoclonic and atonic seizures are a difficult topic in childhood epilepsy because affected children (1) are often hard to classify, (2) have seizures that vary greatly in severity, type, and causative factors, and (3) have a high incidence of other neurologic problems, particularly mental retardation. Many patients with myoclonic/atonic seizures experience other types of seizures as well, particularly atypical absences and multifocal and major motor seizures.

Myoclonus is a sudden involuntary jerk which may be generalized or localized to one body part. Patterns of myoclonus vary; some forms of myoclonus are not seizures, such as the normal myoclonic jerks that occur when one is falling asleep.

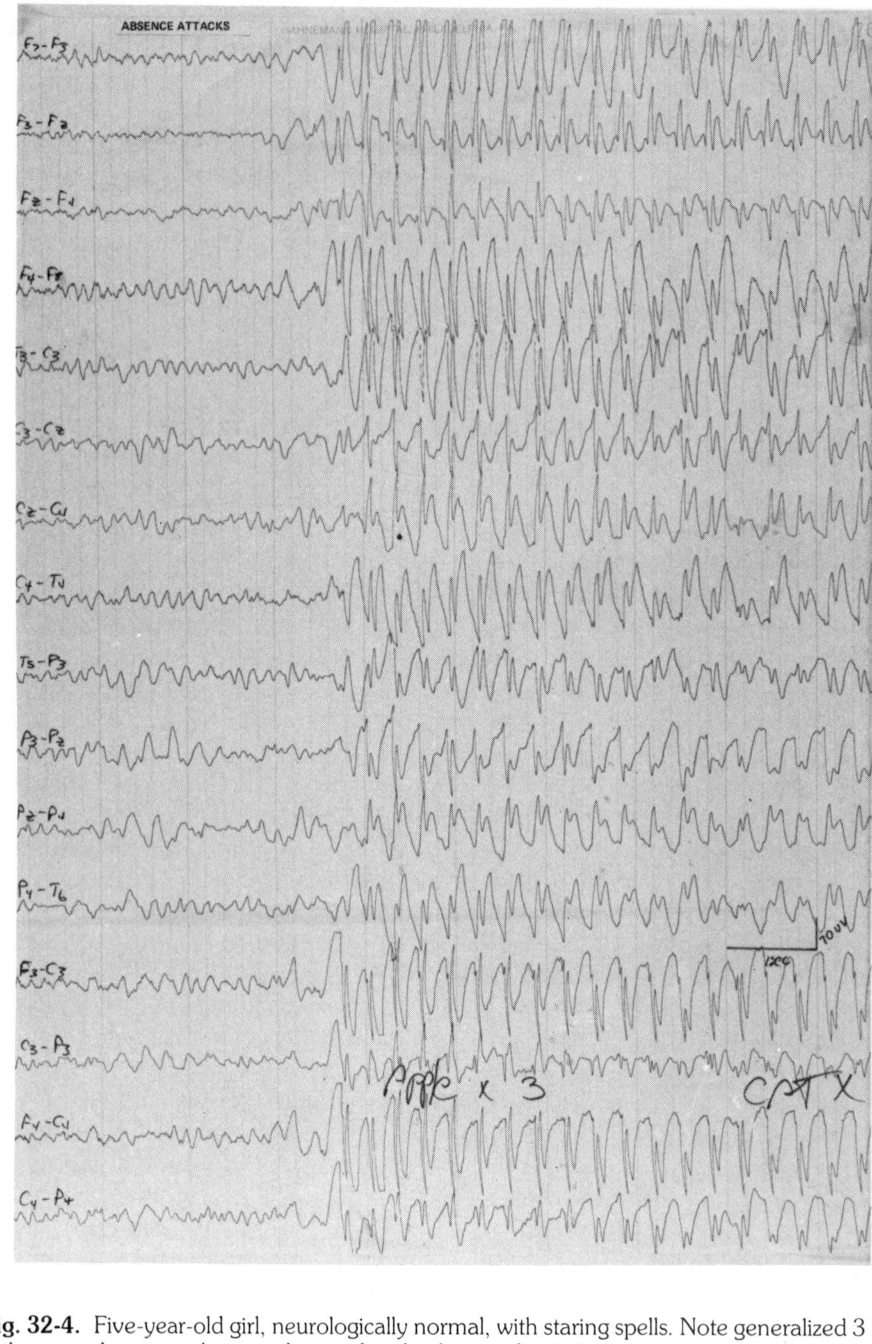

Fig. 32-4. Five-year-old girl, neurologically normal, with staring spells. Note generalized 3 hertz spike-wave bursts, with normal preceding background activity.

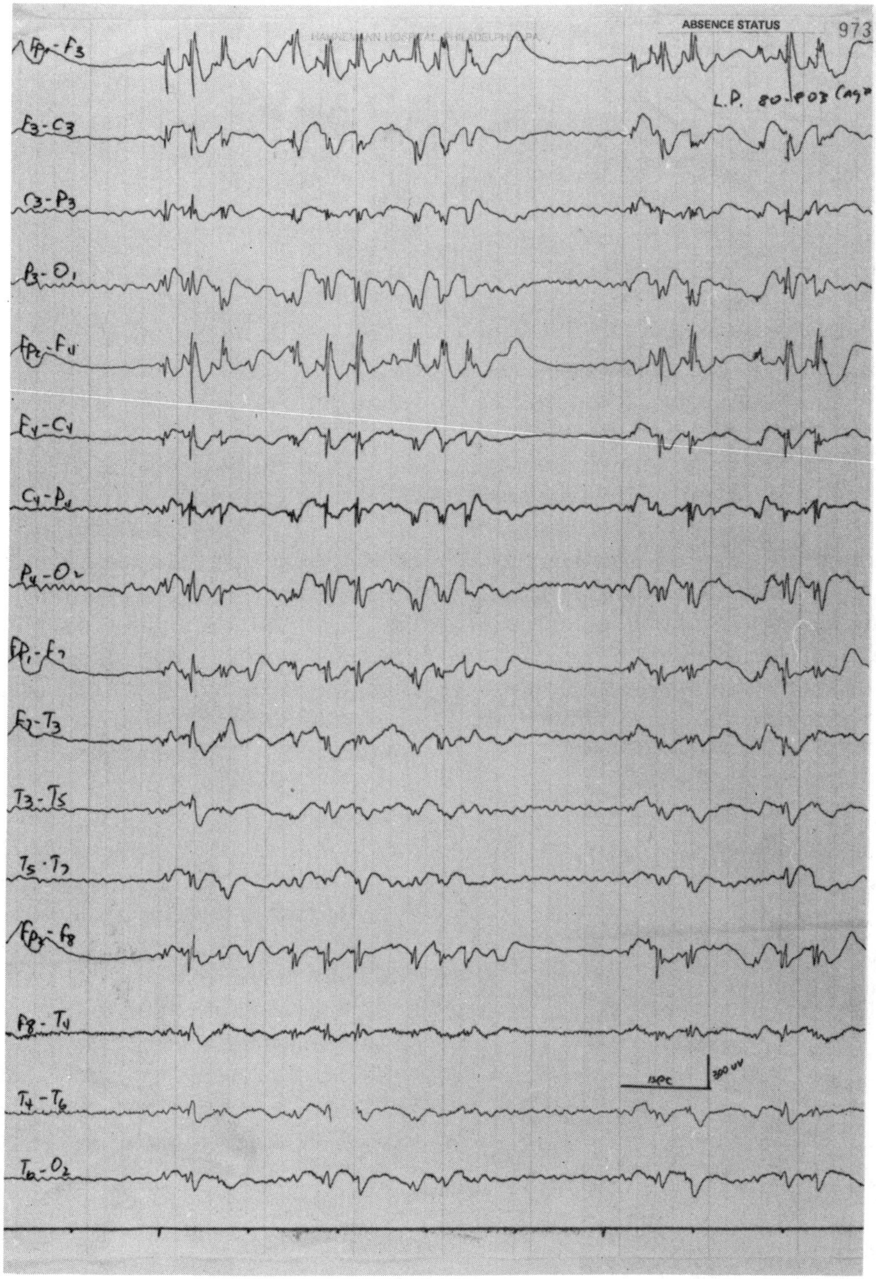

Fig. 32-5. Twelve-year-old girl with stupor and eyelid twitches. EEG shows trains of generalized, irregular spike-wave bursts, consistent with absence status. Patient responded promptly to intravenous diazepam.

Atonic seizures cause a sudden loss of tone of a few seconds' duration. As "epileptic drop attacks," atonic seizures often result in serious facial injury because of their sudden, unpredictable onset.

Infantile spasms are the most characteristic syndrome of myoclonic epilepsy in infancy. They are often the first recognized neurologic symptoms in a baby who will later be retarded and are frequently responsive to a unique treatment, *e.g.*, ACTH or corticosteroids. Infantile spasms characteristically begin around the sixth month and have usually ceased by the second birthday. The attacks are a 2- or 3-second generalized muscle contractions causing flexion of the trunk and extension of the arms—hence descriptive names like infantile spasm, "salaam attack" or "lightening spasm." Like other myoclonic seizures, infantile spasms tend to occur in clusters, particularly during drowsiness or arousal. Usually, the EEG shows a continuously abnormal pattern called "hypsarrhythmia."

SPECIFIC CAUSES OF SEIZURES

Table 32-2 lists causes of seizures in three critical age groups. This diversity of causes emphasizes the importance of considering seizures as symptoms of CNS involvement and the need to treat the underlying cause, if possible, as well as the symptom.

PATHOGENESIS OF SEIZURES

Metabolic Factors

Neurons function by conducting electrochemical impulses along their membranes and affecting other neurons through synaptic neurotransmitters. Derangement of these neuronal membrane functions is the physiologic hallmark of seizure activity. Normally, the central nervous system depends on a continuous blood, oxygen and glucose supply because CNS stores of glycogen and high-energy compounds are very limited. During a prolonged major motor seizure, cerebral energy metabolism increases while blood oxygen and glucose supplies tend to decrease due to impaired cardiorespiratory function from the convulsive activity. Cerebral anoxia, acidosis, and circulatory disturbance pose serious threats of further brain damage during convulsive status epilepticus.

Normal neuronal energy metabolism produces high-energy compounds, particularly ATP, which maintain the neuronal resting potential and repolarization through the Na^+-K^+ ATPase membrane "pump." During both normal and seizure-induced neuronal depolarization, Na^+ rushes into the neuron and then repolarization is rapidly accomplished by curtailment of the Na^+ influx and a transient K^+ outflow. The Na^+-K^+ ATPase pump then reestablishes the resting ion gradients (low intracellular Na^+, high intracellular K^+). Other factors influencing depolarization/repolarization include: (1) Ca^{++} and Mg^{++}, which seem to modulate Na^+-K^+ permeabilities, (2) neurotransmitters, such as the excitatory transmitter acetylcholine which increases Na^+ permeability and the inhibitory transmitter gamma-aminobutyric acid (GABA), which appears to increase Cl^- permeability, (3) Cl^-, which affects membrane potentials, (4) glial cells, which may stabilize neurons by taking up excess extracellular K^+, and (5) many other poorly elucidated factors including structural characteristics of the membrane macromolecules, actions of other neurotransmitters, and influences of trace metals such as zinc and manganese.

A number of systemic metabolic disturbances are routinely complicated by seizures. Anoxia and hypoglycemia, destabilize neuronal membranes through impaired en-

Table 32-2. Causes of Seizures by Age Group*

Newborn Period	Infancy-Childhood	Adolescence
Anoxia or ischemia	Febrile convulsions	Unknown
Antepartum	Unknown	Trauma
Intrapartum	Perinatal insult	Anoxia or ischemia
Postpartum	Cerebral malformation	Infection
Infection	Trauma	Drug abuse
Meningitis	Accidents	Perinatal insult
Sepsis	Child abuse	Genetic
Encephalitis	Anoxia or ischemia	Brain tumor
Herpes simplex	Infection	Vascular malformation or disease
Enteroviruses	Meningitis	
Metabolic derangement (see Table 32-3)	Encephalitis	
Prenatal abnormality	Brain abscess	
Cerebral malformations	Reye's syndrome	
Intrauterine infections: rubella, cytomegalovirus, toxoplasmosis, syphilis, and others	Genetic	
Neurocutaneous syndromes	Nondegenerative, *e.g.*, classic absences	
Tuberous sclerosis	Neurocutaneous syndromes	
Birth injury	Inborn errors: aminoacidurias, hypoglycemias, lipid storage diseases, hemoglobinopathies, etc.	
Drug withdrawal	Metabolic derangement	
Barbiturates	Hypocalcemia	
Narcotics	Hypoglycemia	
Unknown	Hyper- and hyponatremia	
Inborn errors of metabolism (see Table 32-3)	Uremia	
	Intoxication	
	Drug ingestion	
	Lead poisioning	
	Brain tumor	
	Vascular malformation or disease	

*Listed by approximate order of frequency

ergy metabolism. Seizures typically accompany states of hyponatremia, hypocalcemia and hypomagnesemia. Striking seizures and EEG changes occur in infants who are vitamin B_6-deficient probably through insufficiency of GABA whose synthesis is B_6-dependent. Experimentally, poisoning of the Na^+-K^+ ATPase pump produces seizures.

Epilepsy: Cellular and Physiologic Factors

The intrinsic cerebral abnormalities underlying chronic seizure states appear variable, especially when the great diversity of epilepsy in childhood is considered. Many theories suggest defects in neurotransmitters and synapses, such as: (1) a genetic deficit of inhibitory neurotransmitters like GABA causing abnormal cortical excitability, (2) neuronal groups becoming hypersensitive as the result of loss of afferent connections, (3) abnormal postsynaptic receptors, and (4) mechanical distortion of neuronal processes. Other theories attribute neuronal hyperirritability to disturbed membrane depolarization/repolarization from defects in cellular energy metabolism of Na^+-K^+ ATPase pump function. Another theory suggests a glial cell abnormality such as defective glial K^+ uptake, resulting in neuronal depolarization from excessive extracellular K^+.

In humans and in experimental animals, much is known about the epileptic focus. The foci commonly show glial cell proliferation, partial loss of neurons, and partial loss of synapses from the remaining neurons. In some patients the focus is a definite pathologic lesion (see Fig. 32-2), examples of which are (1) localized malformation of cortical blood vessels, (2) scars from old injuries such as trauma, hemorrhage, anoxia or infection, (3) cysts, (4) foci of active infection, (5) malformations from neurocutaneous disease such as tuberous sclerosis, and (6) space-occupying lesions such as brain tumors, abscesses and subdural hematomas. Virtually all epileptogenic foci lie in the cerebral cortex, although foci can occur in deep neuronal groups.

Electrical recordings from cortical foci reveal characteristic autonomous, rhythmic, highly synchronized discharges which represent bursts of action potentials and activity of both inhibitory and excitatory synapses. If the firing of these cells becomes sufficiently synchronized, then the scalp EEG shows typical discharges such as spikes, as in Figure 32-1. However, the scalp EEG will fail to record some foci because of remote location or insufficient synchronization. Through their axonal processes, the neurons of the focus propagate their abnormal discharges to other areas of the brain (see Fig. 32-1), and it is the balance of inhibitory *versus* facilitatory responses of the neurons outside the focus that determines whether a clinical seizure results. Present evidence indicates that partial seizures and secondary generalized seizures occur when an excitatory feedback circuit is set up from the focus to other cortical neurons and deep neuronal masses such as the thalamus and basal ganglia.

The *primary generalized epilepsies* are less common and not as well understood than focal epilepsy. The most characteristic generalized epilepsy in childhood is typical absences (*petit mal*) in which genetic and maturational factors suggest a neuronal biochemical disorder.

Genetic and Maturational Factors

Genetic influences can be principal or contributing causes of seizures and are of greater importance in children than adults. Autosomal dominant inheritance, with incomplete penetrance, is implicated in typical febrile convulsions and classic absences. In EEG studies of nonepileptic relatives of children with typical absence seizures, the 3/second spike-wave discharge is asymptomatically expressed in an autosomal dominant fashion. Genetic predisposition is also seen in post-traumatic epilepsy in which the likelihood of a seizure disorder resulting from serious head injury is up to five times greater in those patients with a positive family history of epilepsy.

Maturational factors strongly influence the type of seizure that appears in the neonatal period and infancy. (See Neonatal Seizures, Febrile Convulsions, and Table 32-2.) Adolescence is also a critical time for the expression of maturational factors; a long-standing cerebral lesion may first manifest itself with seizures, or a preexisting seizure disorder may be "outgrown" or may become worse.

Cerebral Damage from Seizures

It has already been emphasized that anoxic brain damage may occur when ventilation is impaired, as in prolonged major motor seizures or newborn apneic seizures. Another concern is that the abnormal neuronal activity of seizures might injure brain cells, particularly in infancy when cell maturation and growth are very active. In neonatal rats, brief electroshock seizures (less than $\frac{1}{2}$-second of convulsive activity once daily for 10 days) reduces brain size, cell number, and rate of early motor-reflex development. In animals, normal neuronal groups can be induced to become "epileptic cells" after frequent low-intensity stimulation (kindling) or after bombardment from a distant epileptic focus (mirror focus). Both these phenomena can be prevented by treatment with phenobarbital.

In humans, seizures and the continuous subclinical cerebral discharges of infantile spasms may contribute to the associated mental retardation. In poorly controlled seizure patients, the neuronal and glial abnormalities seen in epileptic foci may reflect progressive deterioration. One hopes that adequate anticonvulsive therapy can not only save children from anoxia but also prevent other potential adverse effects of seizures upon cerebral development and subsequent seizure susceptibility.

Factors Triggering Seizures

Although most epileptic seizures seem to happen spontaneously, there are many patients who are apt to have attacks under certain conditions. Sometimes this is characteristic of the type of seizure disorder, like the induction of absences by hyperventilation, photic stimulation, and anxiety. Many patients with various types of seizures are sensitive to one or more of the following:

1. Diurnal cycle—sleep deprivation often induces seizures and some patients only have attacks, asleep, awake, drowsy, or on arousal.
2. Emotional stress—many completely controlled patients start having seizures again when under stress.
3. Menstrual cycle, particularly the several days before each period.
4. Infections—even without fever, infections often exacerbate childhood seizure disorders.
5. Alcohol and illicit drugs—seizures may occur as the patient recovers from a "high" and there is often sleep deprivation and failure to take anticonvulsant medication as well.
6. Medication—occasionally an anticonvulsant paradoxically *worsens* a seizure disorder (*e.g.*, phenytoin in absences), and convulsions can be induced by many commonly used drugs, such as phenothiazines, butyrophenones, antihistamines, local anesthetics, theophylline and penicillin, chiefly when they are given in large parenteral dosages.

SEIZURES IN NEONATES

Due to nervous system immaturity, seizure manifestations in neonates are very different. Often they are fragmentary and subtle, especially in premature infants. Apneic spells can be caused by seizures. Sustained tonic seizures are relatively uncommon but can seriously impede ventilation. The EEG is helpful in confirming the presence of seizures and estimating prognosis.

The principal causes of neonatal seizures are summarized in Table 32-2. The major cause is hypoxia and/or ischemia occurring during labor or in the early newborn period from conditions such as premature placental separation, breech delivery, meconium aspiration, or respiratory distress syndrome. In premature infants, severe hypoxia is often associated with intracranial hemorrhage and seizures.

Metabolic disturbances are frequently involved in neonatal seizures. Severe systemic neonatal conditions such as anoxia or sepsis are very often complicated by varying combinations of acidosis, hypoglycemia, and hypocalcemia. Significantly less common are "pure" states of hypoglycemia, hypocalcemia, or hypomagnesemia. Though rare, inborn metabolic errors must be considered since some are treatable (*e.g.*, vitamin B_6 dependency and several of the amino acid disorders). Hyperbilirubinemia and intrapartum physical brain injuries are now less frequent due to improvements in obstetric and neonatal management. Since some congenital brain anomalies are not recognizable on physical examination, they may be responsible for otherwise unexplained neonatal seizures. When the mother is a drug addict or otherwise on large doses of medication, the infant may demonstrate withdrawal symptoms such as irritability and seizures.

As in other ages, seizures in the neonatal period must be considered symptoms of brain involvement; prognosis for the future brain development depends largely on the cause of the seizures. Overall, roughly 1% of all newborns have seizures and of these, one-half to two-thirds will subsequently be normal. As examples of prognosis determined by cause, seizures from hypoxia-ischemia and intracranial infection carry a very high risk for subsequent brain impairment while those due to "benign neonatal tetany" (primary or uncomplicated type of hypocalcemia, hypomagnesemia, or hyperphosphatemia) generally have an excellent prognosis for subsequent normal brain development.

Metabolic Causes of Neonatal Seizures

Anoxia
Acidosis, hypoglycemia and/or hypocalcemia complicating neonatal stresses such as anoxia, ischemia, sepsis, or birth trauma
Primary hypoglycemia: small-for-dates babies, infants of diabetic mothers
Primary tetany (benign neonatal tetany) due to hypocalcemia, hypomagnesemia, or hyperphosphatemia, usually around the second week of life
Hyponatremia: inappropriate ADH syndrome
Hypernatremia
Kernicterus: hemolytic disease, liver dysfunction
Inborn errors of metabolism: maple syrup urine disease and other amino- and organic acidopathies, B_6 dependency

---

FEBRILE CONVULSIONS

Fever-induced seizures occur in about 5% of all young children and are therefore about 10 times more common than afebrile seizures in this age group. Although the pathophysiology is poorly understood, an age-dependent sensitivity of the nervous system allows triggering of the seizure by fever (Fig. 32-4). Also, the family history is often positive in a parent or sibling; this indicates a genetic factor.

Over three-fourths of patients have *typical febrile seizures* (also called simple, benign, or uncomplicated). The child, who is neurologically and developmentally normal, experiences a single, brief (less than 10 minutes; frequently less than 2 minutes), clonic or tonic-clonic (nonfocal) seizure with a temperature of 102°F or above, usually within a few hours after onset of the fever. A few children become briefly unconscious without tonic or clonic activity. The peak age is 18 months, and the range is 6 months to 5 years (Fig. 32-4). Fever is usually from upper respiratory infection, less often from gastroenteritis, roseola, pneumonia, and others.

The remaining one-fourth of fever-triggered seizures are *atypical febrile seizures* because (1) the child is not neurodevelopmentally normal or (2) the seizure is "complicated," that is, over 10 minutes' duration, focal or multiple, or with minimal temperature elevation. The diagnosis of febrile convulsions always excludes other primary CNS disorders and therefore tests appropriate to the individual case must be carried out to rule out CNS infections such as meningitis, encephalitis, and brain abscess, metabolic disturbances such as hypoglycemia and electrolyte imbalance, and intoxications such as lead poisoning, vascular insults, and unreported head trauma due to child abuse. Also, the many epileptic children whose seizures are exacerbated by infections are not considered to have "febrile convulsions syndrome."

Sequelae of Febrile Convulsions

The majority of children with febrile convulsions will subsequently be normal. Those with *typical febrile seizures* have about a 1% risk for later epilepsy—about twice the risk in the general population. The risk for another febrile seizure is age-dependent (see Fig. 32-6).

However, children experiencing an *atypical febrile seizure* (neurodevelopmentally abnormal child or complicated seizure) may have a risk approaching 1% for death or permanent neurologic residua. For example, older children or adolescents developing complex partial seizure disorders rarely have a history of prior febrile status epilepticus which may have left permanent temporal lobe damage. In general, the child with an atypical febrile seizure is at a greater risk for subsequent epilepsy (up to 15% when both the neurodevelopmentally abnormal and complicated febrile seizure risk factors are present), and here the febrile seizure appears to be the initial manifestation of a preexisting epileptogenic CNS abnormality.

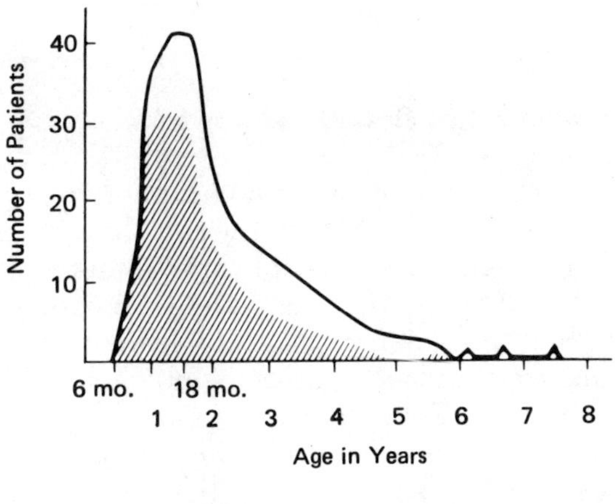

Fig. 32-6. Age when febrile convulsions occur. Upper curve: all attacks, initial and recurrent. Shaded area: initial attacks only. (Based on 200 children with initial and recurrent febrile convulsions reported by Frantzen E, Lennox-Buchthal MA, Nygaard A: Longitudinal EEG and clinical study of children with febrile convulsions. Electroencephalog Clin Neurophysiol 24:197, 1968)

Management

After a febrile seizure of short duration, the physician's concerns are diagnosing and treating the febrile illness and deciding whether to give prophylactic anticonvulsants.

Diagnosis requires careful examination and clinical assessment to find any systemic or intracranial disease capable of causing the seizure. Lumbar puncture should be performed with even a slight suspicion of intracranial infection, and glucose, calcium, and electrolytes should be checked in most instances. In patients with typical febrile seizure, other studies such as CT or isotope brain scans re usually not necessary, and the value of electroencephalography is controversial since normal and abnormal EEGs do not correlate with subsequent epilepsy. Fever is controlled by tepid baths, salicylates, and treatment for the infection.

Because so many attacks occur soon after onset of fever, antipyretics are of limited value and anticonvulsants are of no value when given at onset of fever for preventing recurrences during subsequent febrile illnesses. In general, the *initial typical febrile seizure* does not require prophylactic anticonvulsant treatment in view of the extremely low risk for subsequent CNS injury and the significant side-effects of medications. The indication for preventing recurrences with phenobarbital, 3 mg/kg/day (2 divided daily doses, blood phenobarbital of at least 15 μg/ml) include: (1) less than one year of age at onset, (2) a second typical febrile seizure, and (3) all cases of *atypical febrile seizures*, since atypical patients seem to be at a higher risk for febrile status epilepticus and subsequent epilepsy. In the first two instances, treatment, if well tolerated, may be stopped at age 24 to 30 months. Since side-effects of phenobarbital are relatively common, the indications for this and alternative drugs should be carefully considered. In atypical patients, treatment should be started and neurologic consultation obtained.

DIAGNOSIS OF SEIZURE DISORDERS

Diagnosis of seizures requires a careful history of the events which preceded the seizure and the phenomena observed, usually by the parent. Since most seizures have terminated by the time the child is seen by a doctor, the physician is heavily dependent on a description of prodromata (aura), abnormal movements or behavior, incontinence, tongue-biting and postictal drowsiness, confusion, and weakness. Sometimes a recurrent, paroxysmal event proves to be nonepileptic (see list, Paroxysmal Disorders in beginning of this chap.). Careful physical, neurologic, and developmental examinations must be done, with particular attention to searching for evidence of other neurologic dysfunction, such as signs of meningitis in a child with fever and seizures or signs of cerebral palsy and developmental delay in a child with seizures and a high-risk birth history. A careful examination of skin may reveal *cafe au lait* spots of neurofibromatosis or hypopigmented spots of tuberous sclerosis.

The principal laboratory test is the EEG, but since it can be normal or nonspecifically abnormal in children with or without seizures, it cannot replace good clinical judgment in seizure diagnosis. Occasionally a child is found to have an "epileptiform" EEG without having epilepsy, for example, siblings of children with absences. The yield of EEG abnormalities can be increased by "activating" techniques, such as hyperventilation flashing light (photic) stimulation, recording during drowsiness and sleep, and the use of nasopharyngeal or sphenoidal electrodes. In special laboratories, simultaneous video and EEG recordings of attacks can be helpful, for example, in documenting hysterical seizures.

Other diagnostic tests are directed to the cause rather than the physiology of seizures. CT scan (see Fig. 32-3B) is a revolutionary advance in the diagnosis of brain diseases. Indications for CT scanning in seizure patients are partial (focal) seizures, signs suggestive of focal or progressive CNS disease, and seizure refractory to therapy. CT scanning largely replaces skull radiographs and isotope brain scans. Other tests which should be done in most patients are serum glucose and calcium and screening tests for inborn metabolic errors and intoxication with drugs and lead.

Treatment of Seizure Disorders

Comprehensive management for seizure disorders should start with a discussion of the diagnosis and plan for treatment with the family, including the patient if possible. Proper first aid for seizures (airway maintainence, avoidance of placing objects in the mouth) should be discussed as well as prognosis for seizure control which is good in many instances.

Long-term oral anticonvulsant medications are the mainstay of seizure therapy. Even if a brain lesion is found and removed, the patient still has to take drugs for a prolonged period. The goal of drug therapy is complete seizure control with no significant drug-related side-effects. This can be attained in a majority of children, but in a sizable minority one must compromise between incomplete seizure control and drug side-effects. Unfortunately, a few children are inadequately controlled even with toxic doses. The choice of drug depends on seizure type (Table 32-3), and dosage is a function of body weight (Table 32-4). The least toxic drug likely to be effective should be started in conventional doses, and blood levels checked whenever seizures fail to respond or drug side-effects occur. Whenever possible, a single drug rather than combinations should be used.

TABLE 32-3. Drug Indications by Seizure Type

Disorder	Drug (in order of probable usefulness)
Convulsive seizure disorders	
Major motor	
Partial	carbamazepine
motor	phenobarbital or
sensory	primidone*
complex	phenytoin
Multifocal	carbamazepine phenobarbital or primidone phenytoin valproate
Nonconvulsive seizure disorders	
Absence	valproate ethosuccimide clonazepam
Myoclonic/atonic	valproate clonazepam ketogenic diet
Infantile spasms	ACTH, corticosteroids clonazepam valproate
Febrile seizures	phenobarbital*
Neonatal seizures	phenobarbital phenytoin valproate

*particularly when low doses are effective and behavioral side-effects are absent or minimal

Note. In individual cases, other drugs not listed here may prove to be more useful.

Blood anticonvulsant levels are widely available and a cornerstone of good management. Levels should be checked (1) whenever side-effects develop, such as sedation or incoordination, and (2) when seizures relapse, fail to respond, or change in type. Other laboratory tests should be done periodically to monitor possible toxic effects of each drug, the appropriate tests varying with the drug. The frequency of anticonvulsant dosage depends on the drug half-life (see Table 32-5). Most anticonvulsants are best given twice daily, except carbamazepine and sodium valproate whose shorter half-lives may require 3 or 4 daily doses.

After early infancy the use of tablets, chewable tablets, and capsules is encouraged for more accurate dosage, provided that the pills are crushed beforehand for infants to prevent aspiration. Liquid phenytoin (Dilantin) is particularly prone to dosage errors due to incomplete shaking of the suspension. When immediate "therapeutic coverage" is desired, an oral loading dose of twice the maintenance dose for 2 days or a parenteral loading dose should be given (Table 32-5).

In many patients, psychological stress increases seizures and *vice versa.* Intervention by a properly *trained counselor or psychiatrist* often improves seizure control when emotional conflicts improve.

Other modes of therapy include (1) ACTH or corticosteroids for infantile spasms, (2) induced ketosis for refractory myoclonic seizures using a ketogenic or medium-chain triglyceride diet, and (3) surgical excision of epileptogenic foci in carefully selected patients.

Treatment failures may result from problems other than the epileptogenic disorder itself: (1) medication noncompliance, (2) improper seizure classification and medication choice, (3) misdiagnosis of disorders such as syncope or breath-holding as epilepsy, (4) injudicious drug usage such a sudden discontinuation (which may trigger status epilepticus), underdosing, failure to

TABLE 32-4. Doses and Pharmacologic Data of Major Anticonvulsants

Drug	Possible Routes for Administration	Total Daily Dosage: Infants and Toddlers (mg/kg/day)	Total Daily Dosage: Older Children (mg/day)	Therapeutic Blood Level (ug/ml)	Average Half-life (hours)	Number of Daily Doses	Common Side-Effects (and serious Toxic Effects)*
Phenobarbital	Oral IM, IV	3–8 10–15	45–120 (10 mg/kg)	10–40	96	2	Sedation, hyperactivity, learning and behavior disorders, respiratory depression, (allergic rash)
Primidone (Mysoline)	Oral	15–25	250–1500	(phenobarbital level of 5–15)	96	2	Similar to side-effects from phenobarbital
Cabamazepine (Tegretol)	Oral	10–20	200–1600	4–12	12	2–4	Diplopia, dizziness, sedation, (blood dyscrasia, hepatopathy)
Phenytoin (Dilantin)	Oral† IV†	4–10 10–20	100–400 (10–20 mg/kg)	10–20	24	2	Gum hyperplasia, hirsuitism, ataxia, sedation (blood dyscrasia, hepatopathy, allergic rash, rickets, pseudolymphoma, lupuslike reaction, neuropathy)
Valproate‡ (Depakene)	Oral	30–60	750–3000	50–100	10	3–4	GI irritation, sedation, hair loss, (hepatopathy)
Ethosuccimide (Zarontin)	Oral	20–40	500–1500	40–100	30	2	GI irritation, sedation, (blood dyscrasia)
Clonazepam (Clonopin)	Oral	.03–0.2	2–20	0.01–0.05	30	2–3	Very sedative, ataxia, hypotonia

*See *Physician's Desk Reference* or drug literature for more extended lists of toxic and side-effects
†Phenytoin should not be given IM due to poor absorption. Chewable tablets (Dilantin Infatabs) should be used in preference to liquid phenytoin due to potentially serious dosage errors with phenytoin suspensions.
‡Other generic names are sodium valproate, valproic acid, and dipropylacetate
NOTE: The "therapeutic" blood level varies greatly among different patients.

obtain drug levels, drug toxicity (which may actually increase seizures), and unnecessary polypharmacy, (5) failure to deal with emotional disturbances, (6) inadequate patient-family instruction, (7) failure to diagnose an epileptogenic systemic disease such as hypoglycemia, phenylketonuria, or pyridoxine dependency, and (8) unrecognized progressive CNS disorder such as tumor, neuronal degenerative disease, or vascular malformation. All patients with unusual or refractory seizure disorders should be evaluated by a consultant experienced in pediatric seizure diagnosis and management.

Status Epilepticus

Major motor *status epilepticus* is a medical emergency in which convulsions continue for more than 15 minutes, or recur so rapidly that the patient does not recover consciousness in between. This is in contrast to the typical major motor seizure which averages 1 to 3 minutes. In status epilepticus, the child becomes hyperthermic, acidotic, and hypoglycemic after approximately 25 minutes of continuous seizures. After this period, cerebral blood flow and oxygen and glucose delivery to the brain can no longer keep up with the increased cerebral metabolic rate. Therefore, increased brain damage or death may ensue.

Status epilepticus occurs most commonly in an epileptic patient who suddenly discontinues medication or develops an acute infection. When status epilepticus develops without a previous history of seizures, it implies a very serious illness, such as encephalitis, electrolyte disturbance, hypoglycemia, head trauma, or vascular insult. The mortality rate in the group of patients with prior epilepsy is quite low, 0 to 3%. In the group without a prior seizure history, the mortality rate is 10% to 20%, related as much to the underlying disease as to the seizures themselves.

See list for the principles of treatment of status epilepticus. The physician should try to control the seizure with one drug, if possible, use the drug with which he is most familiar in large enough doses that high drug levels are quickly achieved. A common error is to use small doses and repeat them frequently; this may preclude the achievement of adequate levels.

Emergency Treatment for Convulsive Status Epilepticus

Initiate treatment immediately and move to Intensive Care environment as soon as possible.

Maintain vital functions, especially *respiration*. Assure airway by
- Proper positioning and removal of secretions
- O_2 administration
- Intubation, if necessary.

Check vital signs. Remember, a few more seizures are less harmful than brain anoxia.

Perform a rapid neurologic and general physical examination, checking in particular:
- Signs of infection, trauma, dehydration, intoxication, papilledema, and focal neurologic dysfunction.
- Status of brainstem function—spontaneous respiration, pupillary responses, extraocular movements.

Insert an intravenous line

Draw baseline glucose, electrolytes, blood gases, CBC.

Administer glucose 25–50 g immediately.

Administer anticonvulsant drug immediately.

1. Diazepam (Valium) 1–20 mg IV *slowly* (1–3 mg/minute). Note very short action (about 20 minutes) and potential respiratory depression.
2. Phenytoin 20 mg/kg IV *slowly* (50 mg/minute). Use immediately after diazepam to provide long-lasting treatment, or use as initial drug. Hypotension and cardiac arrythmia may occur, especially during too-rapid administration.
3. Phenobarbital 10 mg/kg IV *slowly* (100 mg/minute)—long-acting alternate or adjunct to phenytoin. Respiratory depression may occur, especially after diazepam or with too-rapid administration. Give phenobarbital 10 mg/kg IM when IV medications cannot be immediately given.

4. If diazepam, phenytoin and phenobarbital are ineffective paraldehyde drip 1% to 10% in dextrose 5% in water. Dilutional hyponatremia may occur. Induction of coma may occur with phentobarbital curarization and intubation with ventilator support.

Avoid excess fluid administration which may result in hyponatremia and brain edema.

Initiate maintenance anticonvulsant medication

Phenytoin 5–10 mg/kg/day and/or phenobarbital 5–15 mg/kg/day (initially IV in divided doses)

Follow blood anticonvulsant levels closely and adjust doses accordingly.

In infants or in dehydrated children, it may be very difficult and time-consuming to achieve an intravenous injection. Here, intramuscular phenobarbital 10 mg/kg often is effective within 15 minutes and allows the nurse or assistant to administer the medication while the physician concentrates on establishing good ventilation and other essential supportive measures.

A continuous partial motor seizure is called *focal or partial status epilepticus* and may result in depression of consciousness and respiration, particularly in infants and small children. It is treated in the same way as major motor status. *Petit mal* status epilepticus, discussed under Absences, usually responds well to intravenous diazepam (5–10 mg).

MIGRAINE

Migraine refers to chronic, recurrent, often pulsatile headaches, accompanied by visceral symptoms and sometimes neurologic signs. Migraine is very common in childhood, particularly between age 5 years and adolescence. Younger children may also have migraine, but headache is less typical at this age, and the clinician may have difficulty making the diagnosis.

Clinical Manifestations

The well-known *classic form* of migraine, which comprises only 10% of cases, displays the characteristic "aura" of visual disturbances such as flashing lights, colors, or blindness, followed by the intense throbbing unilateral pain of "hemicrania" in the eye, forehead, and temple with associated photophobia, nausea, vomiting, and abdominal distress. Sometimes the patient experiences the aura without proceeding to headache. Occasionally the aura is other focal symptoms such as parasthesias or aphasia.

Common migraine is far more frequent but less characteristic, having diffuse rather than unilateral pain and frequently no visual aura. The prodrome of common migraine is more apt to consist of personality change, lightheadedness, or nausea. Typically, attacks of both types of migraine last several hours, inducing the child to retire to a dark room to "sleep it off."

Light and sound make the child with a migraine attack more uncomfortable; therefore they do not want the TV or stereo on during an acute attack. The headache usually lasts for one to several hours, very rarely for days. In a younger child recurrent car sickness, abdominal pain, nausea, or vomiting may be a harbinger of migraine. Alternating hemiplegia may be a migranous manifestation.

In complicated migraine, hemiplegia, ophthalmoplegia, or other focal signs accompany the attack. Vertigo, ataxia, dysarthria, and vomiting are attributed to basilar artery migraine. Episodic confusion, macropsia, or micropsia (Alice-in-Wonderland syndrome) are behavioral or perceptual manifestations. These deficits or signs usually clear rapidly during the first several such attacks. With repetition the signs may persist for longer periods, hours to days, and may even be permanent, representing ischemia infarction.

In classic migraine, the side of the headache and the auras are likely to vary in different attacks; if these symptoms are persistently unilateral, an arteriovenous malformation should be ruled out.

Pathogenesis

The pathogenesis of a migraine attack is generally considered to be arterial vasoconstriction causing cerebral ischemia and the aura, followed by vasodilation, causing the throbbing, pulsatile headache. The contribution of meningeal and large cerebral vessels is debated. Alterations in cerebral blood flow can be measured during an acute attack, and CT scan may demonstrate localized cerebral edema. The aura depends on the vessel causing ischemia; visual auras, for example, are caused by spasm of the retinal or occipital arteries. The scalp arteries may be tender and appear dilated during the headache.

Children with migraine frequently have perfectionistic, hypermature, striving personalities. Attacks may be triggered by (1) no apparent cause, (2) emotional stress (school exams or family problems), (3) nonemotional factors (minor head trauma, fatigue), and (4) dietary factors (chocolate and cheese). A positive family history of migraine is elicited in over half of the patients.

Diagnosis and Treatment

Since there is no specific test, diagnosis of migraine must rest on a good description of the attacks, on family history, and on a negative physical examination including blood pressure, optic fundi, ears, and paranasal sinuses, on auscultation for cranial bruits, and on neurologic examination. In cases of complicated migraine, in which focal signs are prominent or the diagnosis is not clear, EEG and CT scan may be helpful.

The most common cause of headache in childhood is anxiety or depression. Therefore, a careful history concentrating on psychosocial forces, particularly in the home, is vital. This may uncover psychological triggering events to migrainous attacks, or precipitants of depressive headaches.

Drug therapy for common and classic migraine is straightforward when salicylates have not provided adequate relief or when attacks are too short for any drug to be effective. Only severe, frequent attacks should be treated with agents other than salicylates.

Ergot preparations such as ergotomine/caffeine (Cafergot) tablets cause vasoconstriction counteracting the vasodilatory headache and are thereby useful in treating acute attacks. In order to be effective, the tablet should be taken at the onset of symptoms, and may be repeated once after 30 minutes. If vomiting precludes oral ergot, it is available as a rectal suppository for younger children and a sublingual preparation for older children. It is contraindicated in complicated migraine, since it may accentuate a focal deficit.

In contrast to ergot preparations which are given during the acute attack, daily administration of propranolol (Inderal) or phenytoin may be effective prophylaxis. A prophylactic drug should be periodically withdrawn to determine whether it is still necessary.

Frequently parents are more concerned about migraine than the child due to the widespread misbelief that a child cannot have headaches without serious intracranial pathology. In this situation, the physician's identification of migraine and reassurance are usually more therapeutic than any medication.

SYNCOPE

Syncope (fainting) is the most common paroxysmal disorder, so common that virtually everyone has fainted or at least felt faint. It results from transient cerebral ischemia or hypoxia. Fainting is often misdiagnosed as a seizure even though a careful history usually indicates the correct diagnosis. On the other hand, unwitnessed seizures, brief major motor seizures, or akinetic seizures may be erroneously attributed to fainting, especially when the full history is not available.

The typical vasovagal syncope (1) is nearly always precipitated by stress or excitement, such as minor injury or an emotionally startling experience, (2) is found when the patient is upright and aborted by lowering the head, (3) begins gradually with lightheadedness (the "I'm going to faint" sensation) and pallor, (4) results from temporary loss of vasomotor tone with bradycardia or even asystole, and (5) is typically associated with normal physical examination, ECG, and EEG. In a prolonged faint there can be brief tonic and clonic convulsive movements due to transient cerebral hypoxia which tends to cause confusion with epileptic seizures. Important reasons to differentiate vasovagal syncope from epilepsy include the nonresponsiveness of syncope to anticonvulsants and the serious implications of a misdiagnosis of epilepsy. More serious types of syncope must be excluded such as cardiac arrhythmia, anemia, hypoglycemia, drug side-effects, peripheral neuropathy, and anomalies of the heart or great vessels.

In cases of straightforward vasovagal syncope, there is virtually no likelihood of cerebral damage and the neurologic prognosis is excellent. Therefore, therapy consists mainly of reassurance along these lines and advice to abort impending attacks by lowering the head.

BREATH-HOLDING SPELLS

Breath-holding is common in infants and toddlers and can be frightening to the inexperienced parent. All infants may hold their breath briefly during crying, but about 5% of all children 6 to 24 months of age have *cyanotic breath-holding spells* in which they cry briefly, arrest breathing in expiration and do not inhale, turn blue or pale and lose consciousness for several seconds. If apnea persists for 30 seconds or longer, there are likely to be several clonic jerks of the extremities. Crying always has a precipitating event, such as frustration or a minor injury. Loss of consciousness and brief convulsive features result from hypoxia, although the mechanisms causing the hypoxia and cyanosis are less well established; among those suggested are glottic closure, diminished cardiac output, increased oxygen utilization, and right-to-left shunting.

In most instances breath-holding attacks begin between 6 and 18 months of age, occur at irregular intervals of days or weeks and are outgrown by 4 years of age. About 30% have one to several attacks per day. In spite of this considerable frequency of attacks the prognosis is excellent; these children are nearly always neurologically normal and do not suffer secondary central nervous system damage including epilepsy.

The diagnosis of breath-holding spells is based upon the characteristic history. If cyanosis accompanies an epileptic seizure, the seizure begins before the cyanosis appears. In breath-holding spells, the reverse is true. In the majority of cases the breath-holding becomes manageable as soon as the benign nature of the condition is explained to the parents, and the child's subsequent neurologic and emotional development proves to be normal. The attacks do not respond to anticonvulsants, often prescribed because of an erroneous diagnosis of seizure disorder.

In some severe cases, the breath-holding is aggravated by parental overindulgence occasioned by fear of triggering more attacks or by serious parental psychiatric problems resulting in anxiety or frustration in the child. In these cases, psychotherapy may be necessary.

PAROXYSMAL VERTIGO

Benign paroxysmal vertigo of childhood consists of frequent brief attacks of dizziness and inability to stand during which the child becomes frightened and pale and attempts to lie or sit down before he falls. On examination during an attack, the child is alert and is likely to exhibit nystagmus, vomiting, pallor, and sweating. The disorder is self-limited and usually disappears within a few months to a year. Functional vestibular abnormalities arise, often demonstrable by electronystagmography with caloric stimulation of the ears.

Unfortunately, some children cannot describe what they mean by dizziness. In these instances the associated features may be of greater diagnostic value, for example, fright or pain inducing loss of consciousness in vasovagal syncope as opposed to sudden inability to stand with preservation of consciousness in typical attacks of benign paroxysmal vertigo.

Dizziness is such a commonly used term by children and adults that suggestions on how to evaluate this symptom are in order. Usually when patients say they are dizzy, they imply a lightheaded, presyncopal sensation; this should generally be evaluated as a syncope problem. Patients also use dizziness to describe vertigo, that is, the illusion of movement of either the patient or the environment. Diagnostically, it is important to try to establish whether the patient is describing lightheadedness as opposed to "true" vertigo. Although establishing the illusion of movement is very important, the nature of the sensation such as spinning, rocking, or falling is of relatively small diagnostic value. Vertigo can be a component of syncope, but when it is the outstanding symptom the patient usually requires more extensive diagnostic investigation because vertiginous attacks can also arise from temporal lobe seizure foci and posterior fossa tumors. Appropriate investigations include otologic and neurologic consultations, audiogram, electronystagmogram, EEG, CT scan, and auditory (brain stem) evoked responses.

BIBLIOGRAPHY

Seizures

Browne TR: Valproic acid. New Engl J Med 302:661, 1980

Carter S: Management of difficult seizure problems. Brain and Development, 3:80, 1978

Kutt H, McDowell F: Clinical Neuropharmacology. Monographs in Clinical Pharmacology No. 4. New York, Churchill-Livingstone, 1979

Shorvon SD, Reynolds EH: Reduction in polypharmacy for epilepsy. Brit Med J 2:1025, 1979

Williams DT, Gold AP *et al*: The impact of psychiatric intervention on patients with uncontrolled seizures. J Nerv Ment Dis 167:626, 1979

Important sources regarding seizure management.

Menkes JH: Textbook of Child Neurology, 2nd ed, Chapter 11. Philadelphia, Lea & Febiger, 1980

Schmidt RP, Wilder BJ: Epilepsy. Contemporary Neurology Series No. 2. Philadelphia, FA Davis, 1968

Livingston S: Comprehensive Management of Epilepsy in Infancy, Childhood and Adolescence. Springfield, Ill, CC Thomas, 1972

These books provide further information and references on seizures and other paroxysmal disorders.

Weisberg LA *et al*: Cerebral Computed Tomography. Philadelphia, WB Saunders, 1978

Excellent general reference on CT scanning including findings in patients with seizures.

Neonatal Seizures

Fenichel GM: Neonatal Neurology, Chapter 2. New York, Churchill-Livingstone, 1980

Rose AL, Lombroso CT: Neonatal seizure states. Pediatrics 45:404, 1970

These describe well the special characteristics of neonatal seizures.

Febrile Convulsions

Consensus Development Panel on Febrile Seizures, NIH 1980: Febrile seizures: Long term management of children with fever-associated seizures. Pediatrics 66:1009, 1980

Freeman JM: Febrile seizures: a consensus of their significance, evaluation and treatment. Pediatrics 66:1009, 1980

Nelson KB, Ellenberg JH: Predictors of epilepsy in children who have experienced febrile seizures. New Engl J Med 295:1029, 1976

These articles summarize current concepts of febrile convulsions.

Status Epilepticus

Aicardi J, Chevrie JJ: Convulsive status epilepticus in fants and children. Epilepsia 11:187, 1971

Celesia GG: Modern concepts of status epilepticus. JAMA 235:1571, 1976

Cloyd JC *et al*: Status epilepticus, the role of intravenous phenytoin. JAMA 244:1479, 1980

These articles review current concepts of status epilepticus and its therapy.

Other Paroxysmal Disorders

Menkes JM: Textbook of Child Neurology, 2nd ed. Philadelphia, Lea & Febiger, 1980

Prensky AL: Migraine and migrainous variants in pediatric patients. Pediatr Clin North Am 23:461, 1976

Sources for further reading about migraine, syncope, breath-holding, and paroxysmal vertigo.

Serious Infections

33

Julia A. McMillan

The infections discussed in this chapter are especially important because they can kill or permanently damage normal children. Chapter 34 discusses other infections which are much less likly to cause death or permanent damage.

EPIGLOTTITIS

Epiglottitis is one of the most serious emergencies of the potentially fatal infections of children It occurs most frequently in children 2 to 5 years of age, but has been reported in every age group, including newborn infants and adults. Typically, the epiglottis, along with the entire upper larynx, is very red and edematous.

Epiglottitis also has been called supraglottic laryngitis. Usually it can be distinguished on clinical grounds from subglottic laryngitis or "croup," which is discussed in the next chapter. Epiglottitis is usually caused by *Hemophilus influenzae*, type B.

Inspiratory stridor, a crowinglike sound, is the hallmark of high respiratory obstruction and is seen in epiglottitis, as well as in croup, foreign body, or other high respiratory obstructions. Because of the severity of the upper airway obstruction in epiglottitis, an emergency airway is often needed yet often attempted too late and under unfavorable conditions.

Typically, the child is previously normal and has not had past episodes of croup. The parent may telephone to report fever and cough, but it is the hoarseness, the muffled or guttural voice, and the unwillingness to speak that should be recognized by the physician or nurse as potentially serious symptoms. The course of the illness is marked by changes which occur in a matter of hours, rather than days. The parents should bring the child directly to the office or emergency room if they recognize anxiety (probably secondary to hypoxemia) or if the child appears seriously ill.

On physical examination, the child, usually of preschool age, often appears anxious and acutely ill. The sternum may sink in on inspiration. The child sits and barely moves, leaning forward with the chin up to allow a maximum airway. Auscultation shows decreased breath sounds. Drooling indicates difficulty with swallowing. Restlessness, like anxiety, suggests hypoxia and impending respiratory arrest. Direct visualization of the epiglottis by gagging the child with a tongue blade should not be attempted if the child appears seriously ill or requires restraint in the supine position, since this may produce aspiration of secretions and additional laryngospasm and edema. High fever is usually present, somewhere in the range of 104°F (40°C). Tachypnea is proportional to hypoxemia; cyanosis is a late sign.

Diagnosis and Treatment

The physician should try to distinguish epiglottitis from subglottic laryngitis (croup), although this is not always as easy as is sometimes implied. Unnecessary restraint and manipulation, such as might be necessary for laboratory tests, should be avoided if the child appears seriously ill. If the patient appears likely to need an airway soon, both an anesthesiologist and an otolaryngologist should be summoned immediately.

If the patient does not appear seriously ill, a white blood count and differential, and lateral neck radiograph should be obtained. Leukocytosis is typically present. The lateral radiograph of the soft tissues of the neck may reveal unsuspected supraglottic obstruction in early or doubtful cases, but is not necessary or advisable in seriously ill patients. A chest film can be obtained at the time of the lateral neck examination. It is usually normal, and is useful primarily to exclude a foreign body. After an airway is provided by intubation or tracheotomy, a chest film is useful to show the location of the tip of the tube.

A blood culture usually reveals bacteremia with *H. influenzae* after 24 hours. However, the seriously ill patient should not be restrained for a blood culture until an airway is assured. If epiglottitis is suspected, a physician should always accompany the patient and should be prepared to intubate or to ventilate the patient with a bag and mask if respiratory arrest suddenly occurs.

Treatment Plan

Often a patient with epiglottitis has endotracheal intubation or tracheotomy before a detailed note is written. However, a flow sheet should be begun as soon as the patient is seen. Respiratory rate and effort, pulse, and general appearance (anxious, restless, breathing carefully and deliberately) should be recorded. Restraining the patient in the supine position for blood pressure or venipuncture (as for blood gases) usually aggravates the illness, and should not be done unless an adequate airway is present. If possible, a parent should be continuously present to comfort the child. Mist apparently has a soothing effect on the inflamed larynx. Oxygen should be used to lessen the hypoxemia. The patient should always be attended and accompanied by a person capable of providing intubation or assisted ventilation with a bag and mask.

At this time, either nasotracheal intubation or tracheotomy are acceptable methods for providing an airway in epiglottitis. The method used depends on the availability of an anesthesiologist or otolaryngologist and medical and nursing personnel experienced and skillful in management of each method.

Antibiotics effective against *H. influenzae* should be given, although this has a lower priority than an emergency airway, if one is needed. A single intramuscular injection of a corticosteroid, such as dexamethasone, may sometimes lessen edema and "buy time" before an airway can be achieved, particularly en route to the hospital from the doctor's office or patient's home. However, routine use of corticosteroids has been shown to be of no statistical value in prospective, placebo-controlled studies of subglottic laryngitis.

ACUTE PNEUMONIA SYNDROMES

Classification

Pneumonias can be classified into syndromes using the variables of type of onset, course, severity, radiologic appearance, and presence of underlying disease. The onset can be acute, subacute, or chronic; progressive or improving; recurrent or a first episode. It can also be classified as mild, moderate, or severe, as estimated by clinical observations, or by quantitation of respiratory acidosis and hypoxemia.

On the basis of the chest film, pneumonia can be classified as lobar, segmental, subsegmental, lobular, interstitial, perihilar, or miliary. Combinations of these forms may occur. Additional anatomic features may be present such as pleural thickening, effusion, cavitation, pneumatoceles, and pneumothorax.

Pneumonia can occur in healthy persons with no known underlying disease, it may be secondary to events such as aspiration or stasis, or it may be concurrent with underlying diseases such as cystic fibrosis of the pancreas or a malignancy.

Etiology

Most acute pneumonias are caused by infectious agents. These agents include viruses, bacteria, mycoplasmas, mycobacteria, and fungi. Unfortunately, etiologic diagnoses are not so easy to determine nor so accurate as is sometimes implied, and conclusive evidence of the etiology is not obtained in most cases. The most frequent etiologic diagnoses associated with various acute pneumonia syndromes are listed in Table 33-1.

It is useful to give a descriptive diagnosis for the primary diagnosis or statement of the problem, using variables listed in Table 33-1. The etiologic diagnosis can then be expressed as a probability, along with a statement of other reasonable possibilities. Examples of such preliminary clinical and probable etiologic diagnoses include: acute

Table 33-1. Acute Pneumonia Syndromes

Problem Pattern	Most Frequent Etiologies
Lobar, segmental, spherical pheumonias; or pneumonia with effusion	*S. pneumoniae* *H. influenza*, if preschool *S. aureus*, if less than 1 y ear old
Bilateral interstitial pneumonia; or mild subacute pneumonia witn minimal infiltrates	*M. pneumoniae* or adenovirus, if school age Respiratory syncytial virus, if infant (2 years of age) *H. influenzae*, if preschool
Cold agglutin positive pneumonia	*Mycoplasma pneumoniae* or adenovirus
Fulminating pneumonia	Influenza virus, if during outbreak *M. pneumoniae*, if sporadic Chickenpox or measles, if immunosuppressed
Pneumonia complicating other diseases Cystic fibrosis	*S. aureus* *P. aeruginosa*
Immunosuppressed state or malignancy	*S. aureus* *P. aeruginosa* *Pneumocystis carinii* *C. albicans*, tuberculosis, systemic mycoses
Pneumonary infiltrates with eosinophilia (PIE syndrome)	Unknown Asperigillosis Ascariasis
Miliary pneumonias	Tuberculosis Unidentified causes, presumed to be viral
Nodular pneumonias	Disseminated bacteremias usually *S. aureus* Disseminated fungemias, usually *H. capsulatum*

lobar pneumonia—probably pneumococcal; severe bilateral interstitial pneumonia—probably due to influenza virus; recurrent right middle lobe pneumonia—probably pneumococcal or consider partial bronchial obstruction; right upper lobe pneumonia with cavitation—probably tuberculosis; bilateral interstitial pneumonia—complicating acute leukemia—probably *Pneumocystis carinii.*

Acute Lobar or Segmental Pneumonia

Acute lobar or segmental pneumonia sometimes has been called typical pneumonia, in contrast to atypical pneumonia, discussed later. The following characteristics can be considered typical. Significant fever of >102°F (39°C) is usually present. Chills are frequently noted in older children and adults. Often there is a toxic appearance, described as acutely ill, anxious, and distressed. Definite chest signs are usually present and lateralized. These include consolidation as defined by dullness to percussion, decreased breath sounds, increased fremitus, and sometimes bronchophony. Fine end-inspiratory rales are often present.

Pleuritic pain or laterlizing differences in inspiratory expansion may be noted. Older children may fail to breathe deeply when asked to do so, or they may complain of pain and cough when they do breathe deeply. Shallow breathing (splinting) is sometimes the only sign suggesting that a child with high fever may have pneumonia. Grunting may be noted in infants or young children. *Pleurisy* is often used as a lay term or as an older medical term for pleuritis or pleural pain. *Pleurodynia* refers to pleuritic pain without pneumonia or pleural effusion and is characteristically caused by Coxsackie B virus.

In typical pneumonia, the chest radiograph shows a dense infiltration. It may appear segmental, lobar, or even spherical, but does not have multiple or diffuse "thin" infiltrates. Response to penicillin is often dramatic, with the temperature falling from the range of 104°F (40°C) to about 98°F (36.7°C) within 8 to 12 hours after the first dose of penicillin. The temperature often stays at a normal level.

Atypical Pneumonia Syndromes

Criteria for atypical pneumonia are the opposite of those for typical lobar pneumonia. The following features are usually regarded as "atypical."

Subacute Onset. The subacute onset is gradual, with cough for several days before the patient seeks medical attention. Chills, fever, and toxicity are minimal or absent.

Prominent Extrapulmonary Features. Headache, sore throat, and pharyngeal exudate are often present and more prominent than the nonproductive cough or dyspnea.

Minimal or Disparate Chest Signs. Rales may be bilateral or localized, but there is often a disparity between auscultatory and radiologic findings. The chest radiograph often shows more extensive involvement than the clinician hears and in different locations than suspected. Sometimes the radiologic findings are minimal when the patient is cyanotic, with an alveolar-capillary diffusion block. Hypoxemia secondary to the diffusion block may produce a more rapid respiratory rate than might be expected from the minimal involvement by chest radiograph.

Chest Infiltrate, Not Lobar or Segmental. The infiltrate is patchy, or mottled, with varying degrees of density, without a single dense area of consolidation. There may be a wedge-shaped or linear infiltrate, or a bilateral interstitial infiltrate.

No Clinical Response to Penicillin

No Significant Leukocytosis

Slow Course. The patient improves gradually and sometimes has a prolonged convalescence.

Exclusion. There are a number of other clinical patterns of pneumonias that are not typical of lobar pneumonia that can be excluded from the group of atypical pneumonia because of distinctive features. Most of these acute pneumonia syndromes are listed in Table 33-1: progressive or fulminating pneumonia, pulmonary infiltrates with eosinophilia, miliary or multiple nodular pneumonia, and bronchiolitis with minimal pneumonia.

Classification of Atypical Pneumonia Syndromes. Various classifications can be used to describe atypical pneumonias. "Non-bacterial pneumonia" is a term used sometimes. This has the disadvantage of implying that bacterial causes have been excluded, when this can rarely be done with certainty. "Nonbacterial" is a conclusion usually based on such observations as failure to respond to penicillin therapy, absence of leukocytosis, and sparse infiltrate.

"Cold agglutinin-positive pneumonia" is a diagnosis sometimes used, although many atypical pneumonias are not associated with cold agglutinins. Cold agglutinin-positive pneumonia should not be equated with mycoplasmal pneumonia. In children, many cold agglutinin-positive pneumonias are not associated with serologic evidence of *Mycoplasma pneumoniae* infection, and some patients with mycoplasmal pneumonia do not have positive cold agglutinins, even when studied serially.

Mycoplasmal pneumonia should not be used as a syndrome diagnosis without laboratory proof of etiology, since many atypical pneumonias are not caused by *M. pneumoniae.* Furthermore, it is not possible to distinguish mycoplasmal pneumonia from other atypical pneumonias on clinical grounds.

In summary, it is useful to preserve the definition of atypical pneumonia as a clinical-radiologic one, recognizing that the syndrome can be caused by a number of specific agents. However, it is useful to specify the features of the pneumonia which are atypical (usually the subacute course) and to add an additional descriptive diagnosis, using available objective information. Examples of useful working diagnses include: (1) cold agglutinin-positive pneumonia, (2) subacute pneumonia with bilateral interstitial infiltrates, (3) subacute pneumonia with patchy pneumonitis of both lower lobes, (4) right upper lobe pneumonia, unresponsive to penicillin.

Pneumonia with Effusion

When a pleural effusion is associated with an acute segmental or lobar pneumonia, pleural fluid should be obtained by thoracentesis. Gram stain and culture usually reveal *Staphylococcus aureus* in infants or children whose pneumonia has progressed while receiving parenteral penicillin. *Streptococcus pneumoniae* was formerly the most common cause, but is less common since penicillin has been used so widely. *H. influenzae* is occasionally a cause of purulent pleural effusion (empyema) in preschool children.

When the pleural effusion is small and is associated with a mild, subacute pneumonia, the cause is more likely to be *Mycoplasma pneumoniae.* Thoracentesis to obtain fluid may not be necessary if the illness is mild or if testing for cold agglutinins is positive.

Progressive or Fulminating Pneumonias

Progressive pneumonia can be defined as pneumonia that becomes worse radiologically and clinically, in spite of antibiotic therapy which should be effective against the presumed etiologic agent. In this situation the physician should consider penicillin-resistant staphylococci or gram-negative rods, including *Klebsiella* or *Pseudomonas aeruginosa*, and change antibiotic therapy to treat these possibilities. However, progressive pneumonia can be caused by nonbacterial infections or even a malignancy.

Fulminating pneumonia can be defined as a severe bilateral pneumonia, with an unusually rapid progression, clinically or radiologically, over a period of 24 to 48 hours. Usually, fine moist inspiratory rales are heard in all lung fields, and the patient may be suspected of having acute pulmonary edema. Possible etiologies include influenza virus and *M. pneumoniae* (Table 33-1). Oxygen is a very important part of therapy

Pneumonia Complicating Other Diseases

In some persons with acute or chronic diseases, particular etiologic agents or anatomic types of pneumonia are found more frequently than in healthy individuals. Cystic fibrosis and acute leukemia are examples of this situation.

Cystic Fibrosis of the Pancreas. Chronic and recurrent bacterial pneumonias are a frequent complication of cystic fibrosis of the pancreas. The common etiologic agent is *S. aureus* or *P. aeruginosa*. Staphylococcal empyma is unusal in patients with cystic fibrosis, except in the first year of life.

Malignancy or Immunosuppression. Patients with malignancies such as leukemia, or patients receiving immunosuppressive therapy, for example, after organ transplantation, have special risks for organisms rarely associated with pneumonia in normal persons. *Pneumocystis carinii* is a parasite that can cause pneumonia in this group of patients. Fever, marked tachypnea, cyanosis, and bilateral diffuse alveolar densities are found characteristically.

Pulmonary Infiltrates with Eosinophilia (PIE Syndrome)

PIE syndrome diagnosis is now used to include all of the variable clinical patterns with any type of pulmonary infiltrate and eosinophilia of the peripheral blood. Löffler's pneumonia (Löffler's syndrome) was the term formerly used for this pattern. Löffler originally described transitory infiltrates with few symptoms and a benign course, but the syndrome has been expanded in common usage to include illnesses with severe symptoms and a prolonged course.

In some cases, the pulmonary infiltrates are caused by trapping of worm larvae in the smaller blood vessels of the lung. In other cases, both the pulmonary infiltrates and the blood eosinophilia appear to be a hypersensitivity phenomenon (*e.g.*, during desensitization to poison ivy).

Miliary and Nodular Pneumonias

Miliary refers to the size of a millet seed. *Miliary* or *nodular pneumonia* is an anatomic diagnosis based on a chest radiograph that shows multiple circular densities. In general, miliary refers to small densities (usually about 2 mm in diameter) and nodular refers to larger densities (usually about 6 mm or more in diameter). For convenience, the general term nodular is used to include finely nodular and coarsely nodular disseminated patterns.

In experimental miliary tuberculosis in rabbits, using bovine tubercle bacilli, the miliary lesions become visible about 3 weeks after the intravenous injection. Relatively evenly distributed densities of the same size result from a gradual release into the blood of small particles of infectious agents. If dissemination of bacteria or emboli to the lung occur irregularly, it usually produces larger densities with more focal involvement of some parts of the lungs.

Acute Noduar Pneumonia. The possible etiologies of acute nodular pneumonia include miliary tuberculosis, multiple septic emboli, and disseminated fungus diseases. Other infectious causes, such as a virus, or noninfectious causes, such as acute pulmonary edema, should be considered.

ACUTE NEUROLOGIC SYNDROMES

Acute infection of the central nervous system is the most likely cause of a febrile illness with manifestations of central nervous system involvement (Table 33-2). Bulging fontanelle, headache, or vomiting suggest the presence of increased intracranial pressure. Stiff neck, or crying when handled, suggests meningeal irritation. Papilledema is unusual in any of the acute neurologic infections, but should be excluded before doing a lumbar puncture. If marked papilledema is present, chronic increased intracranial pressure is likely to be present, and lumbar puncture should be avoided because it might result in downward movement of the brain stem into the spinal canal, with compression of the vital centers, and death.

Table 33-2. Manifestations of CNS Infections

Sign or Symptom	Possible Etiology
Headache Vomiting Bulging fontanel	Increased CSF pressure
Stiff neck	Meningeal irritation
Crying when handled Disturbed consciousness (Lethargy, irritability)	Brain involvement
Fever	Infection

A change in consciousness, such as confusion or disorientation, is an alarming sign that suggests a disturbance of cerebral cortical function, probably caused by cerebral hypoxia, inflammation, or edema.

These general signs of an acute CNS infection described in Table 33-2 should be regarded as indicating a medical emergency until proved otherwise; they should indicate to the physician the necessity of a lumbar puncture. The illness can then be classified as a particular anatomic syndrome on the basis of both the clinical and spinal fluid findings (Table 33-3).

Purulent Meningitis. Purulent meningitis is best defined by a cerebrospinal fluid (CSF) that is cloudy and contains more than 1000 neutrophils/mm^3. Regardless of whether bacterial etiology is proved by culture, purulent meningitis is almost always bacterial. When the term meningitis is not further modified, it usually means prulent or bacterial meningitis.

Nonpurulent Meningitis (Aseptic Meningitis Syndrome). Nonpurulent meningitis is best defined on the basis of a CSF cell count of about 10 to 500 leukocytes, usually predominantly lymphocytes. Patients with CSF cell counts in the intermediate range of 500 to 1000 leukocytes can usually be classified tentatively as either presumed bacterial meningitis or aseptic meningitis syndrome on the basis of CSF cell count differential, glucose, protein, Gram's stain, and state of consciousness.

Acute Encephalitis. Acute encephalitis is best defined as an acute illness, with a severe and nontransient disturbance of consciousness and a CSF cell count characteristic of nonpurulent meningitis. Ordi-

TABLE 33-3. Classification of Acute Neurologic Syndromes (Usually Infectious)

Syndrome	Spinal Fluid Findings: Leukocytes (per mm^3)	Protein (mg/dl)	Glucose (mg/dl)	State of Consciousness
Purulent meningitis	>1000 (Mostly polys)	>100 (high)	<30 (low)	Variable
Nonpurulent meningitis (Aseptic meningitis syndrome)	10–500 (Mostly lymphs)	Variable	Variable	Usually normal
Encephalitis	10–1000 (Mostly lymphs)	Normal	Normal	Severely disturbed
Encephalopathy	Normal (<10)	Normal	Normal	Severely disturbed

narily, the number of cells is less than 500, and rarely exceeds $1000/mm^3$.

A disturbance of consciousness should be considered nontransient if it persists for more than 8 hours and should be distinguished from febrile delirium, which occurs only at the time of a high fever.

Acute Encephalopathy. Acute encephalopathy is best defined as the acute onset of severe and nontransient disturbance of consciousness and a normal CSF cell count (<10 leukocytes/mm^3).

Other manifestations of brain disease, such as convulsions and abnormal focal neurologic signs, are variably present. Thus, encephalopathy has the same clinical pattern as encephalitis, but a normal CSF cell count. This distinction between encephalitis and encephalopathy is a useful one, because the causes of encephalitis are usually infectious or postinfectious, whereas the causes of encephalopathy are usually toxic, metabolic, or vascular.

Meningismus. The term "meningismus" should not be used unless the spinal fluid is normal and the patient has a stiff neck due to local or reflex irritation. Streptococcal pharyngitis and pneumonia are frequent causes of meningismus. Acute juvenile rheumatoid arthritis and tetanus are uncommon causes.

Benign Intracranial Hypertension. Benign intracranial hypertension is defined by increased CSF pressure, as manifested by a bulging fontanelle or papilledema, with infection, tumor, sinus thrombosis, and obstruction of the ventricular system specifically excluded. It can be produced by tetracycline therapy, early congestive heart failure, or hypervitaminosis A.

Meningoencephalitis. The term "meningoencephalitis" has the disadvantage of failing to identify patients who should be diagnosed as having "encephalitis," a disease distinguished by severe cerebral signs and high probability of brain damage. A severe and persistent disturbance of consciousness (at least 8 hr) is an early and relatively reliable indication of a poor prognosis. Nonpurulent meningitis and acute encephalitis also differ in probable etiologies, another reason to try to avoid lumping them together as "meningoencephalitis."

Purulent Meningitis

Definitions. Purulent meningitis is a medical emergency. Early intensive therapy is essential to prevent brain damage or death. Typically, purulent meningitis is manifested by clinical signs of acute neurologic infection and cloudy spinal fluid. Usually, the CSF has more than 1000 leukocytes/mm^3, with a predominance of neutrophils, a low CSF glucose (often 0 to 10 mg/dl), and an elevated CSF protein (usually more than 100 mg/dl). Some patients with early or partially treated bacterial meningitis may have cell counts, glucose, and protein which are in the same range as those found in nonpurulent meningitis (aseptic meningitis syndrome). Therefore, it is more practical to use the term purulent or nonpurulent meningitis as a preliminary diagnosis.

Ventriculitis may occur without meningitis, particularly if the CSF flow is obstructed. This is most likely to occur as a complication of neurosurgical shunting operations for hydrocephalus; ventriculitis is discussed later in this chapter.

Mechanisms. The lowered CSF glucose concentration is the result of defective glucose transport into the CSF and increased utilization of glucose in the brain. The CSF glucose also depends on the blood glucose concentration. Thus, a simultaneous blood glucose determination is usually obtained to help interpret the CSF glucose. A CSF glucose less than 40% of the blood glucose is usually abnormally low.

The elevated CSF protein is due to inceased permeability of the blood-CSF barrier, allowing plasma proteins to enter the CSF. An active exudation of serum protein into the CSF occurs and at autopsy a thick exudate can usually be seen covering the meninges.

Possible Etiologies. Most purulent meningitis is caused by *Hemophilus influenzae, Neisseria meningitidis,* or *Streptococcus (Diplococcus) pneumoniae.* The probability of these three agents depends on the age of the patient: between 1 month and 5 years of age, *H. influenzae* accounts for more than half; between 5 years and 30 years of age, the meningococcus accounts for more than half; and after 30 years of age, the pneumococcus accounts for more than half of the cases.

In the first 30 days of life, the most common causes of purulent meningitis are enteric bacteria (such as *E. coli*) and the group B streptococcus. Other bacteria which rarely cause meningitis, except in the newborn period, include *Listeria monocytogenes* and *Staphylococcus aureus.*

Early Clinical Diagnosis. In young infants, it is important to do a lumbar puncture and examine the spinal fluid whenever the neck is questionably stiff or the anterior fontanelle is questionably bulging, even if the patient does not appear severely ill. Disturbed consciousness (lethargy, irritability) and crying when handled are especially important symptoms suggesting early meningitis, since a stiff neck may be absent or appear late in young infants. A convulsion which occurs in a child with fever should not be diagnosed as a simple febrile convulsion unless a lumbar puncture reveals a normal CSF.

Emergency Treatment (Before Lumbar Puncture). In rare cases, meningitis is so severe that supportive therapy should be begun before the diagnostic studies. For example, in patients with meningococcemia, suspected because of hypotension and purpura, a good intravenous route should be obtained and treatment of shock begun before doing a lumbar puncture. Meningococcemia may occur without meningitis, and the early treatment of septic shock is more important than determining whether meningitis is present. Patients with evidence of life-threatening brain swelling should be treated with mannitol before a lumbar puncture is done.

Spinal Fluid Examination. Complete examination of the CSF should be done in order to detect any abnormality that may be helpful in the diagnosis. A Gram-stained smear should be examined even when few or no white blood cells are found, but can lead to error when a few organisms are found that may have originated on the slide or in the stain. It does detect the rare instances in which many organisms are found in spinal fluids without many white blood cells, as may occur in pneumococcal meningitis. The meningococcus is the organism most frequently missed on smear but found on culture, and *H. influenzae* is often misinterpreted on the smear as another organism. Therefore, if the smear is not typical, and the child is less than 12 years old, ampicillin and chloramphenicol therapy are used for treatment of purulent meningitis until the culture results are available.

Glucose and protein should be determined and are especially valuable in nonpurulent meningitis (see Table 33-3).

Therapy should not be delayed until the results of spinal fluid examinations are available, if the fluid appears cloudy. As soon as the CSF is recognized to be grossly purulent (cloudy, like diluted milk), a bolus of intravenous ampicillin (one-fourth the total daily dose) should be given. If there is likely to be a delay in starting the infusion, the ampicillin should be injected into an antecubital vein, or intramuscularly if an intravenous route is not quickly obtained.

Nonpurulent Meningitis

Definitions. Nonpurulent meningitis can be separated from the other syndromes of presumptive CNS infections by the absence of severe cerebral manifestations, such as a severe disturbance of consciousness, and by a spinal fluid cell count in the range of 10 to 500 leukocytes/mm^3 (see Table 33-3). Aseptic meningitis syndrome, serous meningitis, benign lymphocytic meningitis, nonparalytic poliomyelitis, viral meningitis, and meningoencephalitis are terms with similar meanings. However, "nonpurulent meningitis" or "aseptic meningitis syndrome" is the most useful preliminary diagnosis for this syndrome, since it emphasizes the possibility of a number of different causes.

Importance of CSF Glucose. A decreased CSF glucose concentration is usually present in purulent meningitis but often has little more than supportive diagnostic value since the purulent spinal fluid already indicates the presumptive diagnosis of bacterial meningitis. A lowered glucose suggests severe brain involvement, and in nonpurulent meningitis, a low CSF glucose is correlated with a more chronic infection or more serious etiologic agents, such as tuberculosis. Therefore, in patients with nonpurulent meningitis, a decreased CSF glucose has special diagnostic value. It is useful to divide nonpurulent meningitis into two subgroups: nonpurulent meningitis with a decreased CSF glucose and nonpurulent meningitis without a decreased CSF glucose. A lowered CSF glucose can be conservatively defined as a CSF glucose less than 40% of the blood glucose, or less than 40 mg/dl, if the blood glucose is not known. It is important to measure the blood glucose concentration as well as CSF glucose in order to interpret the CSF glucose as a percentage of the blood sugar.

An elevation of CSF protein concentration is often present when there is a decreased CSF glucose. However, a slightly elevated protein may be a result of laboratory variability or may come from slight bleeding during the procedure of lumbar puncture.

Nonpurulent Meningitis with Low Glucose

Tuberculous Meningitis. Three factors are especially important in evaluating suspected tuberculous meningitis: tuberculin test, chest roentgenogram, and exposure history. If the intermediate-strength tuberculin test is negative, the chest roentgenogram is normal, and there is no history of exposure to tuberculosis, then tuberculous meningitis is unlikely.

A second lumbar puncture and CSF examination should be done if the CSF glucose is borderline low on the first examination. This is very useful because during the course of untreated tuberculous meningitis there is almost always a progressive fall in the glucose, a rise in the protein, and a continuation of the CSF lymphocytosis.

Partially Treated Bacterial Meningitis. Decreased CSF glucose may be present if the patient has been receiving an antibiotic for several days and has an unrecognized bacterial meningitis. In this situation, the protein is often elevated. Since the prior antibiotic therapy often prevents recovery of the infecting organism on culture, the frequency of partially treated bacterial meningitis as a cause of this syndrome is unknown. However, the pattern of CSF findings is seen often enough on the 48- to 72-hour follow-up examination of a patient treated for a known bacterial meningitis that a partially treated unrecognized bacterial meningitis should always be considered.

The following are rare causes of nonpurulent meningitis with low glucose:

Meningeal Neoplasm. Low cerebrospinal fluid glucose may occur in neoplastic meningitis, but the cells are usually predominantly neutrophils in this exceedingly rare disease.

Cryptococcal Meningitis. Cryptococcal meningitis is a rare cause of nonpurulent meningitis with low glucose and a high protein reading, and typically occurs in a compromised host. The budding yeast forms can usually be seen in an India ink preparation of the CSF. It often grows out in a few days on most of the solid media usually used for the culture of *Mycobacterium tuberculosis.* A latex agglutination test, using CSF, may be of diagnostic value. Other fungal diseases, such as histoplasmosis or coccidioidomycosis, may resemble cryptococcal meningitis. It is important to detect fungal causes of nonpurulent meningitis because therapy with amphotericin B is often lifesaving.

Mumps. Aseptic meningitis due to mumps virus has been shown to be associated occasionally with slightly decreased CSF glucose concentration.

Lymphocytic Choriomeningitis. CSF glucose may be slightly decreased in nonpurulent meningitis caused by this virus.

Amebic Meningitis. Low glucose and high protein are produced by amebic meningitis, but the cells usually are predominantly neutrophils in this exceedingly rare disease.

Nonpurulent Meningitis with Normal Glucose

Viral Meningitis. Viruses are the most common causes of nonpurulent meningitis with normal glucose, but are not the only cause. In three large series with viral cultures of patients with aseptic meningitis syndrome, the most common viral causes were Coxsackie virus (about 20%–50%); ECHO virus (about 10%–15%); and mumps virus (about 5%–15%).

In the United States, coxsackieviruses and echoviruses characteristically are found in the summer and fall, but echoviruses may be found all year. A history of exposure to mumps should be sought, and close examination for parotid enlargement should be performed. The above viruses can often be recovered on culture in a virus diagnostic laboratory; therefore, viral cultures of throat, rectum, and CSF should be done if facilities are available.

Serologic tests can be carried out for a number of viruses, including mumps, California encephalitis, lymphocytic choriomeningitis, eastern equine encephalitis, western equine encephalitis, and St. Louis encephalitis viruses. However, other than mumps, these viruses are relatively uncommon in the United States, except for occasional localized outbreaks. Pet hamsters or mice can be sources of lymphocytic choriomeningitis virus infection. These antibody studies require the study of two sera, the first obtained as soon as possible after the onset and the second obtained 3 to 6 weeks later.

Poliovirus infection is a rare cause of aseptic meningitis syndrome in the United States. However, poliovaccine virus can also be recovered as a coincidental finding unrelated to aseptic meningitis. Therefore, a history of past immunization or recent exposure to poliovaccine should always be sought in patients with aseptic meningitis syndrome. Arbovirus infection was demonstrated in about 1% of patients studied with aseptic meningitis, in one study; but arboviruses are more likely to be associated with a clinical diagnosis of encephalitis. Herpes simplex virus is recovered from the throat in about 1% of patients but this usually is coincidental.

Unknown Etiology. About 30% to 50% of patients with nonpurulent meningitis have negative cultures and negative serologic studies for viruses.

Partially Treated Bacterial Meningitis. Bacterial meningitis that has been partially treated can be a cause of nonpurulent meningitis with a normal CSF glucose, but the frequency of this etiology is unknown. Observation of CSF cell count, glucose, and protein during antibiotic therapy of proven bacterial meningitis shows that the range of these values overlaps that of viral meningitis. However, the mean CSF glucose of many patients is often normal after a few days of appropriate antibiotic therapy. The mean CSF protein is usually still elevated at this time.

Conclusive evidence that the preceding antibiotic therapy can sometimes modify the CSF findings, resulting in a nonpurulent meningitis with normal CSF glucose and protein can be seen in individual case histories. Occasionally, patients have been observed after some antibiotic therapy and have discontinued antibiotics. Relapse has then occurred within a day or two, with more typical findings of a bacterial meningitis with a positive culture. The recovery of the bacterial pathogen from spinal fluid or blood in patients with prior antibiotic therapy and spinal fluid findings of a nonpurulent, lymphoctic meningitis with normal glucose and protein clearly establishes partially treated bacterial meningitis as one of the causes of the "aseptic meningitis syndrome." Part of the confusion can be explained by the variation in the definition of aseptic meningitis. Recently, the terms purulent and nonpurulent appear to be used more frequently and have the advantage of avoiding the etiologic implications of the term "aseptic."

Leptospirosis. Leptospirosis was the cause of about 4% of 430 cases of aseptic meningitis in one study. Clues to this diagnosis include the presence of conjunctival effusion, muscle pain, tenderness, and a rash. Jaundice, tender liver, microscopic hematuria, pyuria, and proteinuria may also be present.

Brain Abscess. The CSF protein may be elevated, but the CSF glucose is not lowered in a brain abscess. Increased intracranial pressure and lateralized neurologic signs suggest this diagnosis. Computerized brain scan techniques are useful in confirming and localizing a mass.

Acute Encephalitis

Acute encephalitis is defined earlier in this chapter, and is characterized by a severe disturbance of consciousness and CSF lymphocytosis. Outbreaks of acute encephalitis are typically caused by an arbovirus, such as California encephalitis virus or St. Louis encephalitis virus. Often there is no etiology found for sporadic cases of encephalitis, although occasionally herpesvirus hominis can be shown to be the cause.

No specific treatment is effective for any viral encephalitis, except that new antiviral agents are being investigated currently for treatment of herpesvirus encephalitis and may prove effective.

Acute Encephalopathy

The CSF is often normal in acute encephalopathy. There may be an elevated CSF protein associated with lead encephalopathy. In acute encephalitis, the spinal fluid cell count reveals a lymphocytosis. Distinguishing between these two syndromes is clinically important, because specific therapy is often possible for an acute encephalopathy.

The possible etiologies of an acute encephalopathy include trauma (particularly head injury), poisoning (such as lead, carbon monoxide, acohol, or other drugs), metabolic disorders (such as diabetic acidosis, uremia, or hypoglycemia), and circulatory disorders (such as hypertension or water intoxication). Infectious causes (such as viral hepatitis or cerebral malaria) rarely are associated with the presence of CSF pleocytosis.

Infected Neurosurgical Shunts

In patients with hydrocephalus, a shunt (plastic tubing with a valve) is often placed between a lateral ventricle of the brain and the peritoneal cavity. These shunts may act as a foreign body and provide a place for bacteria to lodge during a transient bacteremia. Shunt infections typically occur months after the operation to insert the plastic tubing, but occasionally occur in the immediate postoperative period.

Shunt infections have many features in common with subacute bacterial endocarditis. The infection is often caused by a low virulence microorganism such as *Staphlococcus epidermidis*. Fever is prominent, but systemic toxicity is uncommon. It is important to obtain proper specimens and to obtain the organism for susceptibility testing. The infection may involve only the peritoneum, distal tubing, or valve; but if the ventricles are infected, the bacteria are transmitted through the tubing to the peritoneal cavity.

The infection should be treated with a bactericidal antibiotic, and concentrations adequate to kill the organism must be obtained in the CSF. An antibiotic may be injected easily into the ventricle if a reservoir has been inserted with the tubing. Occasionally, high doses of antibiotics given systemically and intraventricularly may cure an early infection, but usually the tubing must be removed.

MENINGOCOCCEMIA, HIGH FEVER, AND SEPTIC SHOCK

Meningococcemia

Meningococcemia is a life-threatening emergency which can produce death a few hours after onset in a previously normal person. Meningococcal disease occurs most frequently in infants and small children, although a smaller peak in frequency occurs in young adults, primarily because of outbreaks in military bases among new recruits (Fig. 33-1).

Meningococcemia is typically manifested by high fever, septic shock, and disseminated intravascular coagulation. Each of these features will be discussed in the con-

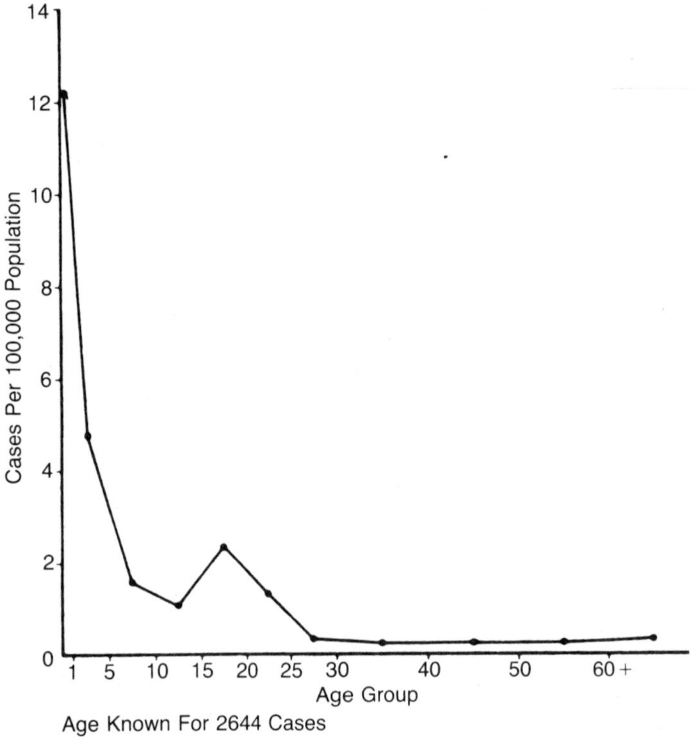

Fig. 33-1. Meningococcal disease attack rates by age group USA-1969. (Moffet HL: Clinical Microbiology, p 77. Philadelphia, JB Lippincott, 1975)

text of other possible causes, since a number of other diseases can resemble acute meningococcemia. Purulent meningitis is often present with meningococcemia, and is discussed in the preceding section.

High Fever

A common problem in children, high fever is only rarely a manifestation of bacteremia, but bacteremia should always be considered. The patterns and most frequent etiologies of acute fever syndromes are shown in Table 33-4.

Symptoms. Children themselves rarely have complaints related only to fever, but headache or vomiting may occur concurrently. The parents may note hot skin or may have detected the fever by taking the child's temperature.

The state of consciousness is the most important symptom related to high fever. Decreased alertness, lethargy, or irritability should raise the question of a serious illness; whereas an active, alert, playing child is unlikely to have a serious cause of high fever. A petechial or purpuric rash is not likely to be the presenting complaint in meningococcemia because it is typically preceded by other symptoms, particularly high fever. If a generalized petechial or purpuric rash is one of the presenting symptoms, the patient is either seriously and nearly fatally ill with bacteremia and disseminated intravascular coagulation, or else he has a noninfectious cause of the rash, such as thrombocytopenic purpura or anaphylactoid purpura.

Objective Findings. The general appearance and the vital signs are the most important objective observations and should be evaluated immediately on examination of the child with high fever. The blood pressure may not be obviously low when the child is first seen, but the blood pressure cuff should be left in place for further determinations

TABLE 33-4. Acute Fever Syndromes

Problem Pattern	Most Common Etiologies
Fever without localizing signs (including normal urine microscopic)	
With hypotension, petechiae, or seriously ill appearance	Septicemia, especially meningococcemia
With marked leukocytosis, in preschool child, not seriously ill	"Occult" bacteremia, especially pneumococcal or salmonella
Without marked leukocytosis, not seriously ill	Echovirus or coxsackievirus Roseola syndrome, if infant. Group A streptococcus Parainfluenza virus
Fever with upper respiratory symptoms and signs	(See Influenzalike illness and Table 34-6)

and to establish a trend for the blood pressure. The pulse should also be taken several times during the initial observation period to see whether there is any trend.

The general appearance of the child is extremely important, but too often is described poorly. The observations useful in describing the general appearance of a febrile child need to be emphasized. Anxiety may be manifested by an anxious facial expression. Usually the skin is warm and flushed. Occasionally, the child appears pale because of cutaneous vasoconstriction. Lack of spontaneous activity and lack of interest in the surroundings, particularly the parents, indicate a decreased alertness. More severe depression of consciousness may be manifested by lethargy or staring. Irritability or persistent crying after minimal stimulation suggests cerebral involvement and possibly meningitis.

Assessment. Several major decisions need to be made in the assessment of the child with high fever. In general, the younger the child, the more cautious the physician must be. The first consideration is whether the child has a bacteremic disease. If a child appears seriously ill or has a decreased state of consciousness or meningeal signs, a lumbar puncture is indicated, as already discussed. If a petechial or purpuric rash or hypotension is found along with the high fever, a blood culture should be obtained as an intravenous route is established, and intravenous antibiotics (usually including ampicillin) should be begun. The pulse, blood pressure, and general appearance should be closely monitored.

If the evaluation is negative for meningeal signs, petechial rash, hypotension, and focal areas of pain or tenderness, and the child's general appearance is good, bacteremia or meningitis is unlikely. If the physical examination and urinalysis are normal, the patient should be classified as having "undiagnosed fever" or "fever without localizing signs." The diagnostic plan can then be more deliberate and logical. In children who do not appear sick and who have a negative physical examination, only observation may be indicated. A urinalysis should be done to look for pyuria or bacteriuria. A throat culture for group A streptococci is usually indicated. In some patients, evaluation should include a white blood count with differential and a chest film.

The most common course of fever without localizing signs is either recovery without a specific etiologic diagnosis or development of specific localizing signs of an infection (such as pneumonia, otitis media, or "viral rash"). Occult pneumococcal bacteremia is an uncommon cause of high fever. It typically occurs in preschool children, with high fever, marked leukocytosis (over 20,000 with a left shift), and only minimal upper respiratory symptoms.

Recently, the use of blood cultures in young children with high fever and marked leukocytosis has been advocated to detect bacteremia, especially occult bacteremia. The disadvantages include the expense, the detection of skin contaminants such as *Staphylococcus epidermidis*, and the absence of clear evidence that this helps the clinician in the management of the child. Selective use of blood cultures in outpatients is still being investigated as a potentially helpful procedure. Currently, it is advocated by some, but is done by very few clinicians in private practice.

Septic Shock

Parents report that the complaints which precede septic shock typically include high fever, a general appearance of being seriously ill, and later possibly a petechial or purpuric rash. Usually the child who appears anxious with warm and flushed skin is in septic shock ("warm shock"). Later, the skin of the hands or feet may be cold. The entire skin should be examined for petechiae. The patient should be examined carefully for signs of meningeal irritation.

High fever and tachycardia (which usually accompanies fever) should stimulate the physician (or nurse or nurse's aide) to take the child's blood pressure. A low or falling blood pressure in this context should be presumed to indicate septic shock.

Treatment. Almost all authorities agree that a rapid infusion of intravenous fluids is indicated to increase plasma volume. Beyond this, treatment is controversial. Most authorities recommend adrenal corticosteroids—not because of adrenal insufficiency (which is not present)—to counteract peripheral vascular disturbances and protect inadequately perfused cells. A recent prospective controlled study in adults indicated that a corticosteroid was clearly more effective than a placebo in septic shock.

Disseminated Intravascular Coagulation (DIC)

Disseminated intravascular coagulation (DIC) is a serious and often terminal event in fulminating infections. Endotoxin release or tissue damage from the infection is the typical initial step that releases clotting factors which produce intravascular coagulation. The clotting factors become depleted so that DIC is clinically manifested by signs related to bleeding, rather than clotting.

The petechial or purpuric rash of meningococcemia is a manifestation of DIC. In meningococcemia, purpura is associated with a higher mortality than petechiae.

Oozing after a venipuncture may be the first sign noted. In meningococcemia, petechiae may be the first indication of DIC in a child with high fever. Sophisticated laboratory tests for DIC are sometimes available, but the smear of peripheral blood is readily available and typically shows decreased platelets and deformed erythrocytes (including burr cells, helmet cells, and other fragmented erythrocytes).

Usually, the presumptive diagnosis of DIC can be made by an experienced physician on the basis of fever, hypotension, and a petechial rash. Laboratory confirmation can be obtained later from blood obtained just before the physician began emergency therapy.

Treatment. The use of heparin is controversial. It is not useful in some diseases with DIC, such as hemolytic uremic syndrome. In meningococcemia, the data are conflicting. Heparin therapy corrected the coagulation disorder, but did not reduce mortality in most prospective studies in meningococcemia. However, heparin is recommended by some experienced clinicians. Replacement of coagulation factors is contraindicated because this increases the intravascular coagulation.

ACUTE BONE AND JOINT INFECTIONS

Orthopaedic infections can be classified into syndromes according to the anatomic area involved (Table 33-5).

TABLE 33-5. Bone and Joint Syndromes

Problem Pattern	Probable Etiologies
Cellulitis over an extremity or joint	Underlying arthritis or osteomyelitis
Osteomyelitis (diagnosed by tender bone)	*S. aureus* *Salmonella* if sickle cell disease
Septic arthritis (diagnosed by aspiration of joint)	*S. aureus* *H. influenzae*, if preschool child Gonococcus, if sexually active female Meningococcus, with signs of septicemia

Definitions

Acute arthritis is characterized by a warm, swollen, painful, erythematous joint or joints and can have causes other than infections. Purulent arthritis can be diagnosed when fluid containing many neutrophils is aspirated from a joint. In children, it is almost always caused by a bacterial infection, although the culture is not always positive. *Septic arthritis* implies bacterial arthritis, confirmed by culture. *Synovitis* can be defined as inflammation in a joint with sterile fluid and no preceding antibiotics. Usually the fluid is relatively clear and nonpurulent.

Osteomyelitis can be defined as infection of a bone. *Diskitis* is a term sometimes used to describe an inflammation of an intervertebral disk, often involving the adjacent vertebral bodies.

Cellulitis is inflammation (localized redness and warmth) of the skin and underlying soft tissue. Cellulitis over a bone or joint often is a manifestation of infection of the bone or joint.

Septic Arthritis

Septic arthritis is important because early diagnosis and proper treatment usually can prevent deformity or impaired function. A presumptive diagnosis of septic arthritis can often be made by immediate examination of the joint fluid, which is usually cloudy, with bacteria and segmented neutrophils seen on Gram's stain and a decreased glucose concentration. Moderately high fever, erythema over the joint, and exquisite pain on motion of the joint are usually present. The joint is typically held in the position of least pain (usually flexion).

Classification of Acute Septic Arthritis. *Acute Monarticular Arthritis.* Acute monarticular arthritis is characterized by rapid onset, usually with fever. When a child has fever with a single hot, tender, swollen joint, septic arthritis is the most likely diagnosis; joint aspiration is necessary. Cellulitis near a joint may resemble acute arthritis, but usually joint infection is not the cause of the cellulitis if the erythema is not distributed symmetrically around the joint. Diagnostic aspiration usually should be done if there is a reasonable suspicion of increased fluid in the joint. The risk of introducing bacteria from cellulitis into the joint is small compared with the risk of a delay in the diagnosis of septic arthritis.

Occasionally, a coagulation defect may be unrecognized until bleeding into a joint occurs after minor trauma and aspiration of the joint fluid reveals a hemarthrosis.

Acute Polyarticular Arthritis. Acute arthritis involving more than one joint in a child usually raises the question of acute rheumatic fever. However, septic arthritis can occasionally occur in more than one joint, particularly with staphylococcal bacteremia or during the newborn period.

Subacute Arthritis. Subacute arthritis can be defined as arthritis with gradual onset over several days or a week, with little or no fever and slow progression or recurrences of limitation of motion, tenderness, and swelling. The most likely infectious causes are partially treated septic arthritis or tuberculous arthritis. Rheumatoid arthritis, aseptic necrosis, or neoplasm should also be considered.

Importance. Subsequent growth of the child is likely to exaggerate any deformity caused by septic arthritis. Therefore, a suspected joint infection should be managed with diagnostic and therapeutic vigor. Diagnostic joint aspiration should be done promptly in acute monarticular arthritis when joint swelling or tenderness is recognized. Antibiotic treatment should be started after the joint fluid is aspirated, gram-stained, and sent for culture. Septic arthritis of the hip is especially urgent because destruction of the epiphysis or epiphyseal growth plate can result in unequal leg length or fusion of the joint, with severe gait disturbances.

Mechanisms. The blood supply to the head of the femur (or the humerus) is by way of the proximal metaphyseal (retinacular) arteries, which lie within the joint cavity. These vessels can be compressed by increased intraarticular pressure, with ischemia and destruction of the epiphyseal growth plate the result. Therefore, most orthopedic surgeons urge prompt open drainage followed by continuous irrigation for treatment of septic arthritis of the hip.

The action of proteolytic enzymes in pus—even when it is sterile—can destroy joint cartilage, the result being joint deformity and crippling. Therefore, preservation of joint cartilage is another reason for vigorous and continuous removal of pus from joint spaces.

Etiologies. *S. aureus* is the most common cause of septic arthritis. In preschool children, *H. influenzae* is the next most frequent cause. Less common etiologies include the group A streptococcus and pneumococcus. The gonococcus should be considered in sexually active females. Gram-negative enteric bacteria should be considered in the newborn period or in debilitated or compromised patients.

Treatment. A penicillinase-resistant penicillin should be given intravenously for septic arthritis, unless a Gram stain clearly indicates gram-negative rods. If a joint or blood culture reveals *H. influenzae* or a penicillin-susceptible organism, therapy should be changed to the appropriate antibiotic.

Acute Osteomyelitis

Osteomyelitis can be defined as any infection of a bone. Osteomyelitis usually is an acute illness. However, it occasionally is subacute, chronic, or recurrent—particularly when treatment has been delayed or is inadequate.

Acute Hematogenous Osteomyelitis. The child with acute hematogenous osteomyelitis typically has high fever and appears acutely ill. Young or newborn infants may be less febrile or less ill-appearing. There is marked redness, swelling, and tenderness over the involved bone, usually the tibia or femur. Marked leukocytosis with a neutrophilia is usually present, and the blood culture is usually positive for *S. aureus*.

Subacute Hematogenous Osteomyelitis. Brodie's abscess is a term sometimes used for a subacute pyogenic abscess of a bone, and typically occurs without fever or leukocytosis, even when the disease has not been modified by antibiotics. Subacute hematogenous osteomyelitis appears to have become more common in recent years, in part because of increased use of antibiotics. In one series, about one-third of children with osteomyelitis did not have fever over 100°F at the time of admission to the hospital. The fever and symptoms may also be modified by aspirin, and in some patients the infection becomes localized without antibiotic therapy. The organism is usually *S. aureus*. Treatment should be vigorous, just as for acute osteomyelitis.

Osteomyelitis can occur as an extension of an adjacent infection, such as overlying abscess, burns, and compound (open) fractures. Osteomyelitis can also occur after penetrating injuries. Puncture wounds of the foot may result in *P. aeruginosa* infection of soft tissue, bone, and especially cartilage. Typically, the patient improves the first day or so after the injury, then develops increased swelling, pain, and tenderness. Local pain is often significant, but fever and leukocytosis are usually mild or absent. Radiologic evidence of bone destruction usually is not seen for several weeks. Damage to the metatarsal joint is common, so that antibiotic therapy with gentamicin and surgical drainage is indicated when *P. aeruginosa* is cultured from a puncture wound of the foot.

Osteomyelitis can occur after inoculation of bone following operations, such as open reduction of fractures, craniotomies, or other operations involving bone. Gram-negative enteric bacteria also should be considered as possible infecting agents in these forms of osteomyelitis.

Mechanisms. Acute hematogenous osteomyelitis can occur in any bone, but the typical sites are the long bones (femur, tibia, humerus), near one end (the metaphysis), where the blood supply of the bone is most dense. However, the blood supply differs with different age groups and influences the clinical pattern, as described below, under age factors.

As pus forms and pressure increases within the metaphysis, the pus perforates the growth plate or the cortex, lifting up the periosteum. Periosteal elevation is not visible on radiograph until new bone is laid down and calcified, which takes at least 10 days.

Destruction of bone (lytic lesions) is usually not visible until about 1 to 3 weeks after onset of osteomyelitis. Radiologic signs of soft-tissue swelling, such as elimination of fascial planes, can be seen after a few days. However, this swelling also can be noted by examination of the patient. Thus, the diagnosis of acute hematogenous osteomyelitis *must be made on clinical grounds*, and antibiotic therapy must be begun before definitive bony changes can be seen by radiograph.

Age Factors. Over 85% of acute hematogenous osteomyelitis occurs in children 16 years of age or younger. In general, three age-related patterns can be distinguished for long bones.

1. The *infantile form* of acute hematogenous osteomyelitis typically occurs in patients less than 1 years of age. The infection usually spreads from the metaphysis to the epiphysis and joint, because the blood vessels of the shaft penetrate to the epiphysis. The periosteum is usually quickly perforated, and pus can often be aspirated from just below the skin. Epiphyseal growth centers may be damaged, with shortening of a limb if a long bone is involved.

2. The *childhood form* typically occurs in patients 1 to 15 years of age. The infection usually is localized to the metaphysis and does not penetrate to the epiphysis, because blood vessels do not penetrate the epiphyseal plate. Damage to the growth cartilage or joint is very rare.

3. The *adult form* typically occurs after 16 years of age. The growth cartilage has been resorbed, and the metaphyseal infection can penetrate to the epiphysis and joint. Chronic infection is more common in adults than in children.

Etiologies. *Staphylococcus aureus* is the most common cause of osteomyelitis in children. Species of *Salmonella* are a frequent cause in children with sickle-cell disease, but are not a consideration in those with sickle-cell trait or in normal persons.

Treatment. After at least one blood culture has been obtained, treatment of the child with osteomyelitis should be begun with a penicillinase-resistant penicillin, given intravenously. An operation to open the bone for drainage may be necessary in patients who are treated late or who do not respond well after 1 or 2 days of intravenous antibiotics.

Cellulitis

Cellulitis is defined as a localized inflammation of the skin, recognized by a localized area of redness and warmth. Fever may be present. *Erysipelas* is an older term for severe streptococcal cellulitis, with a sharply demarcated border. Lymphangitis is a thin line of redness, typically extending from an infected wound and following the lymphatic drainage up an arm or a leg.

The location of the cellulitis is very important. The descriptive diagnosis should always state the location, since there may be a serious infection underneath the cellulitis. The center point of the cellulitis may give a clue to the underlying disease (Table 33-6). The most important possible underlying diseases are osteomyelitis, septic arthritis, peritonitis, sinusitis, or deep wound infection.

Infectious Causes. Group A streptococcus is the most common cause of uncomplicated cellulitis in any location, including perianal cellulitis. The source of entrance of the organism may be a small wound that is not detectable. Severe necrotizing cellulitis or fasciitis is usually caused by beta-hemolytic streptococci, although other organisms may be found.

TABLE 33-6. Possible Causes of Cellulitis

Location	Possible Cause
Periorbital	Ethmoid sinusitis
Abdomen	Peritonitis
Extremity	Osteomyelitis or septic arthritis
Around a wound	Wound infection
Over an enlarged node	Adenitis or abscess
Perianal	Group A streptococci
Face (over cheek)	*Hemophilus influenzae* (in infant) *Staphylococcus aureus* (in newborn)
Over both tibia	Erythema nodosum
Over sacrum	Pilonidal cyst infection

Hemophilus influenzae is the typical cause of facial cellulitis in infants under 2 years of age. Periorbital cellulitis is usually secondary to ethmoid sinusitis and is also often caused by *H. influenzae.* It is rare for this organism to produce cellulitis of an extremity without involvement of an underlying joint, but underlying septic arthritis should always be considered. Typically, cellulitis due to *H. influenzae* has a purplish color, and may be mistaken for a bruise.

Cellulitis related to *S. aureus* is usually caused by underlying osteomyelitis or a wound infection. Facial cellulitis in a newborn infant can be a manifestation of underlying staphylococcal maxillary osteomyelitis.

Laboratory Approach. White blood count and differential suggest infection in most patients with an infectious cellulitis. A blood culture should be obtained before starting therapy. Needle aspiration of an area of cellulitis for Gram's stain and culture can be done. It is most likely to be useful if there is a bleb, or underlying abscess, elevated periosteum, or joint effusion.

Treatment. In most cases of simple cellulitis, group A streptococcus is the suspected cause, and parenteral penicillin and close observation are indicated. However, a penicillinase-resistant penicillin should be used if septic arthritis or osteomyelitis is suspected as the possible underlying cause of the cellulitis. In facial or orbital cellulitis, ampicillin is the drug of choice.

BIBLIOGRAPHY

Moffet HL: Pediatric Infectious Diseases: A Problem-Oriented Approach. Philadelphia, Lippincott, 1975

A detailed discussion of serious infections.

Epiglottitis

Battaglia JD, Lockhart DH: Management of acute epiglottitis by nasotracheal intubation. Am J Dis Child 129:334, 1975

A description of good success with intubation in one center.

Johnson GK, Sullivan JL, Bishop LA: Acute epiglottitis. Review of 55 cases and suggested protocol. Arch Otolaryngol 100:333, 1974

An excellent plan for management of epiglottitis.

Pneumonia

Dees SC, Spock A: Right middle lobe syndrome in children. JAMA 197:78, 1966

The importance of allergy in recurrent right middle lobe pneumonia.

Glezen WP, Denny FW: Epidemiology of acute lower respiratory disease in children. New Engl J Med 288:498, 1973

The frequency of various causes of pneumonia in children.

CNS Infections

Adair NV, Gauld RL, Smadel JE: Aseptic meningitis, a disease of diverse etiology: Clinical and etiologic studies on 854 cases. Ann Intern Med 39:675, 1953

The frequency of various causes of aseptic meningitis.

Converse GM, Gwaltney JM Jr, Strassburg DA, Hendley JO: Alteration of cerebrospinal fluid findings by partial treatment of bacterial meningitis. J Pediatr 83:220, 1973

Partially treated bacterial meningitis as a cause of "aseptic" meningitis.

Myers MG, Schoenbaum SC: Shunt fluid aspiration. An adjunct in the diagnosis of cerebrospinal fluid shunt infection. Am J Dis Child 129:220, 1975

A discussion of shunt infections.

Swartz MN, Dodge PR: Bacterial meningitis—a review of selected aspects. New Engl J Med 272:725–731, 779–787, 842, 847, 898–902, 954–960, 1003–1009, 1965

A very comprehensive review.

Fever, Sepsis, Shock

Dechovitz AB, Moffet HL: Classification of acute febrile illnesses in childhood. Clin Pediatr 7:649, 1968

A classification based on a study of cases.

Schumer W: Steroids in the treatment of clinical septic shock. Ann Surg 184:333, 1976

A discussion of the evidence favoring the use of steroids in shock.

Torphy DE, Ray CG: Occult pneumococcal bacteremia. Am J Dis Child 119:336, 1970

Fever and high white blood count can be due to this syndrome.

Bone and Joint Infections

Dich VQ, Nelson JD, Haltalin KC: Osteomyelitis in infants and children: a review of 163 cases. Am J Dis Child 129:1273, 1975

A good review of osteomyelitis.

Goetz JP, Tafari N, Boxerbaum B: Needle aspiration in *Hemophilus influenzae* type b cellulitis. Pediatrics 54:504, 1974

A description of the usefulness of direct needle aspiration in cellulitis.

Nelson JD, Koontz WC: Septic arthritis in infants and children: a review of 117 cases. Pediatrics 38:966, 1966

A good review of septic arthritis.

Common Infections

34

Julia A. McMillan

UPPER RESPIRATORY INFECTIONS

Upper respiratory infection (URI) is a vague diagnosis too often used by physicians who are capable of making a more precise diagnosis. Lay people are usually perfectly satisfied with the diagnosis of "URI," but the physician should be more specific. More accurate descriptive diagnoses the physician should consider are shown in the list that follows, and discussed sequentially in this chapter.

Alternatives to the Diagnosis of URI

Upper Respiratory Infections
- Common cold syndrome
- Purulent rhinitis
- Gingivostomatitis
- Pharyngitis (tonsillitis)

Pararespiratory Infections
- Acute otitis media
- Mastoiditis
- Sinusitis
- Cervical adenitis
- Parotitis

Influenzalike illness or Bronchitis (see Table 34-5)

Acute Fever Syndromes (see Table 33-4)

Common Cold Syndrome

The common cold syndrome is manifested by sneezing, watery nasal discharge, nasal obstruction, and no significant fever. The illness usually lasts a few days. Relief of symptoms can be obtained by a variety of over-the-counter or prescription medications, but a reasonable case can be made for simple therapy with rest, fluids, and appropriate doses of antipyretics as needed for discomfort.

Purulent Rhinitis

Purulent rhinitis is manifested by thick green or yellow-colored nasal discharge. It may be caused by sinusitis, a foreign body in the nose, or a self-limited infection of the nasopharynx. Excoriation around the nose suggests a group A streptococcal etiology, especially in a preschool child. A culture for group A streptococci is indicated if this organism is suspected. If found, it should be treated as described in the chapter on antibiotics.

Gingivostomatitis

Swollen red bleeding gums (gingivitis), ulcerations of the mucosa of the cheek (stomatitis), and ulcerations of the tongue (glossitis) are usually caused by *Herpesvirus hominis* (Herpes simplex virus). Vesicles, ulcers, and swelling of the lip (labiitis) or vesicles or ulcers on the face near the mouth or nose (rarely near the eye) or rarely, a pustule or ulcer of a sucked thumb or finger may also be seen.

There is no specific treatment for herpes stomatitis. The first infection in a young infant occasionally requires intravenous fluids because of fever, refusal to eat because of a painful mouth, and dehydration. Many local treatments have been recommended but none is truly needed. Many preventive measures, from vaccines to hypnosis, have been recommended, but prospective controlled studies have shown that all are of no value.

Pharyngitis

The patient suffering from pharyngitis may have obviously enlarged and reddened tonsils. A white or greenish yellow exudate may be present on the tonsils or fauces. However, some patients who complain of a sore throat may have only mildly injected tonsils. All children with pharyngitis should have a throat culture done to detect group A streptococci.

Streptococcal pharyngitis. Pharyngitis with a positive culture for beta-hemolytic streptococci is called streptococcal pharyngitis. The positive culture could be a coincidental finding in a child with a viral pharyngitis, but for practical purposes, the physician acts on this definition. About 5% of normal children have a positive throat culture. The physician should *not* obtain a throat culture unless there is sufficient suspicion of streptococcal disease so that the child can be treated appropriately.

Small numbers of group A streptococci in a child's throat may be due to a transient or convalescent carrier state; there is a rough correlation between number of streptococal colonies and the severity and significance of the illness. Therefore, semiquantitative estimates of numbers of colonies on a sheep blood agar plate (this can be done in a doctor's office) are more useful clinically than methods that can detect small numbers of organisms after growth in broth, which is sometimes done in fluorescent antibody methods.

Children with streptococcal pharyngitis as defined above should be treated with penicillin (or erythromycin if there is a penicillin allergy) as described in Chapter 36.

Nonstreptococcal Pharyngitis. Nonstreptococcal pharyngitis is defined as a red pharynx or tonsils with a negative culture for beta-hemolytic streptococci. The throat culture is especially useful in excluding group A streptococci as a cause of pharyngitis, so that the doctor can avoid unnecessary use of antibiotics.

The most common causes of nonstreptococcal exudative pharyngitis are adenoviruses in young children and infectious mononucleosis in older children (over 10 years of age). If ulcerations are present in the posterior pharynx, infection with herpes simplex or coxsackievirus (herpangina) should be suspected. Other viruses, such as parainfluenza virus, can cause pharyngitis. However, pharyngitis should not be confused with tracheitis, defined by cough and the child's pointing to the trachea, rather than to the tonsillar nodes, as the area of maximum discomfort. In addition, sore throat caused by a virus is often associated with cough, hoarseness, or conjunctivitis, with minimal evidence of focal disease of the pharynx.

Diphtheria is practically the only nonstreptococcal, bacterial cause of pharyngitis. It is very rare and usually has a membrane. Antitoxin therapy of diphtheria is more important than antibiotic therapy.

Gonorrhea is a rare cause of symptomatic pharyngitis in adolescents. The gonococcus can be detected in the pharynx only if a special medium is requested by the physician because of a clinical suspicion of the disease.

Infectious Mononucleosis. Severe nonstreptococcal pharyngitis is the typical manifestation of clinically apparent infectious mononucleosis in adolescents and young adults. Anterior and posterior cervical lymphadenopathy, splenomegaly, and atypical lymphocytes in the peripheral smear are often present. If the heterophile antibody of infectious mononucleosis is present (most conveniently detected by the Mono-Spot test), the patient is said to have heterophile-positive infectious mononucleosis, which is caused by infection with EB virus. Reference laboratories can study acute and convalescent sera for EB virus antibodies, but this is not necessary if a Mono-Spot test on a second serum is positive.

TABLE 34-1. Infectious Mononucleosis-Like Syndromes

Problem Pattern	Probable Etiologies
Heterophile-positive illnesses	
Pharyngitis, generalized lymphadenopathy or splenomegaly, atypical lymphocytosis	Infectious mononucleosis (EB virus infection)
Asymptomatic child	EB virus infection, possibly convalescent from months earlier
Heterophile-negative illnesses	
Pharyngitis, generalized lymphadenopathy or splenomegaly, atypical lymphocytosis	EB virus Rarely cytomegalovirus, or adenovirus
Generalized lymphadenopathy or splenomegaly, atypical lymphocytosis	EB virus Cytomegalovirus, adenovirus, or toxoplasmosis
Fever, atypical lymphocytosis	Adenovirus Unidentified agents Cytomegalovirus Viral hepatitis

Heterophile-Negative Infectious MononucleosisLike Illnesses. Children under 10 years of age usually have mild or asymptomatic infections with EB virus. Even when young children have infectious mononucleosislike illnesses, they rarely have a positive test for the heterophile antibody of infectious mononucleosis.

Heterophile-negative infectious mononucleosislike syndrome is a useful problem-oriented diagnosis if a patient has clinical features resembling infectious mononucleosis, atypical lymphocytosis, but a negative heterophile test. The possible causes of this syndrome are shown in Table 34-1. Reference laboratories can test paired sera for antibodies to EB virus (the most common cause of this syndrome), cytomegalovirus, or *Toxoplasma gondii.*

No specific treatment is available for infectious mononucleosis. Rare complications include rupture of the enlarged spleen, fata hepatitis, and pharyngeal airway obstruction. Therapy with corticosteriods is indicated when the patient appears to be in danger of these latter two complications. However, routine use of steroids for relief of symptoms in the uncomplicated patient is probably not justified.

PARARESPIRATORY INFECTIONS

Acute Otitis Media

The diagnosis and treatment of actue otitis media are controversial subjects for several reasons including the following:

1. Difficulties in visualization. Examination of the tympanic membranes often require adequate removal of ear wax. This is often difficult to do in young children, so that visualization of the tympanic membrane may be inadequate.
2. Difficulties in interpretation. Even when visualization of the tympanic membranes is adequate, interpretation may be difficult, especially for the physician without much experience with otitis media.
3. Differing definitions and terminology. In published studies, a variety of syndromes have been lumped into the category of acute otitis media, with few or no clinical subgroups.
4. Variable drainage. The drainage of the middle ear by the eustachian tube usually has not been considered in clinical studies. However, eustachian tube function is probably an important variable in the course of the illness. Relief of obstruction in an infected closed area has an important role in infections elsewhere and undoubtedly is important in otitis media.
5. Variable medical care. Social and economic differences appear to be involved in variations in results of studies of acute otitis media. Eskimos and native Americans have more severe and more frequent middle ear disease, presumably because they receive less adequate medical care. Studies based on children taken to an emergency room with fever and otalgia are not comparable to studies based on private practice in an office, in which asymptomatic middle ear effusions can be detected by a routine examination.

Controversy about otitis media will probably continue until these variables are clearly identified and controlled in prospective studies. Recognizing these difficulties is a first step in interpreting the literature about otitis media and should be remembered as one reads the rest of this section.

Clinical Diagnosis of Otitis Media

History. Middle ear effusions can be detected by pneumatic otoscopy in the routine examination of an asymptomatic child, but in many published series of acute otitis media, the child was brought to the physician because of ear pain (otalgia), nasal discharge, fever, or decreased hearing.

Otalgia. Ear pain can be a result of acute otitis media. Fluid in the middle ear may cause ear discomfort, with the infant "pulling at the ears." However, many patients with acute otitis media do not have ear pain, even before spontaneous perforation. Furthermore, ear pain in children has many causes other than otitis media, for example, otitis externa. Air pressure differences between the middle ear and the pharynx may be caused by temporary eustachian tube obstruction and can be associated with transient ear pain without otitis media.

Rhinitis. Nasal discharge, which is often purulent, is frequently found in association with otitis media.

Past Otitis Media. A history of previous otitis media often can be elicited in children with a current episode and is strong evidence for a recurrence. The history of a draining ear is also presumptive evidence of past otitis media in a patient who has not been seen before by the physician.

Fever. Acute otitis media often is associated with fever in the range of 101°, to 102°F (about 38°–39°C). Higher fever is unusual. Some children with acute otitis media have no fever. The true frequency of otitis media as a cause of fever has not been adequately studied. However, it is likely that many children with high fever and erythematous but mobile tympanic membranes are wrongly diagnosed as having acute otitis media.

Supine Swallowing. Feeding a supine infant by propping the bottle is a predisposing factor in acute otitis media. Nasopharyngeal secretions are pooled near the eustachian tube and are drawn into the middle ear by the negative pressure there, since swallowing opens the tube to equilibrate the pressure in the middle ear with the pressure of the nasopharynx, as can be demonstrated by the use of thin solutions of radiopaque media.

Hearing Loss. Sometimes hearing loss can be recognized by the parents of older infants and children. History of hearing loss is often more reliable than physical examination of a sick, irritable child. Decreased hearing is frequently associated with fluid in the middle ear.

Examination. The ear should be examined as thoroughly as possible before attempting to remove ear wax, since awkward attempts to remove wax sometimes make adequate removal and visualization more difficult. Suctioning is the most effective method of removing wax. A bent 14-gauge blunt needle attached by tubing to a trap and suction machine can be used and is especially useful for sticky wax.

Water irrigation may be useful if there is no perforation, and can be done by a nurse or aide using an ear syringe or a water-jet machine usually used for cleaning between teeth (Water Pik). The water-jet machine should be set at its lowest force, since perforation can occur at the highest force. Tools, such as a dull loop or a dewaxing speculum, can be used, but cotton swabs usually are not useful. Wax solvents followed by water irrigation or suction have been found useful by some physicians. However, severe local reactions to such solvents have been reported.

Appearance of the Tympanic Membrane. After the wax has been adequately removed, the tympanic membrane should be carefully examined. The color of the eardrum is normally gray or pink, but can be red, blue, or injected (prominent blood vessels). Tympanic membranes are often red in a crying infant. The drum normally appears thin and reflects the otoscope light. Diseased drums can appear dull or thick, with an absent light reflex. The drum can be bulging or retracted (atelectatic). Perforations, calcification, whitish exudate, or bullae may be noted on examination of the drum surface.

Mobility. The mobility of the drum should be tested because this is a very important guide to middle ear disease. The motion of the drum is observed while the examiner alternately puffs and sucks on a soft rubber tube attached to the otoscope head. The drum normally moves easily but moves poorly or not at all when fluid is present in the middle ear. An immobile drum usually indicates middle ear fluid. Rarely is an immobile drum caused by a rigid or scarred membrane or an undetected perforation. The redness of an eardrum may be only transient and may not indicate an infection if it is freely mobile.

Impedance Testing. Recently, impedance testing has been used for detection of middle ear fluid. The method is also useful for detection of perforations and for evaluation of hearing. Impedance testing has not yet been widely used in office practice, but eventually it will have more frequent use.

Hearing Tests. In children with ear infections, hearing should be tested using methods appropriate for the age of the patient.

Ear Puncture. The procedure of ear puncture is not widely used in office practice. However, the clinicians who have used this procedure in their office have made important contributions to knowledge about the diagnosis and treatment of otitis. This procedure has been particularly useful in defining the frequency of various microorganisms recovered from the middle ear. This procedure can be dangerous in inexperienced hands and should not be attempted by untrained persons.

Characteristics of Middle Ear Fluid. Middle ear fluid can be defined in accurate terms only if examined directly, which is possible if there is spontaneous perforation with drainage, or if ear puncture or myringotomy is done. The middle ear fluid may be purulent (cloudy, with many white blood cells), serous (clear, yellow, like serum), or mucoid (sticky, with threads of mucus) (See Table 34-2).

Definitions. Several definitions of acute otitis media have been used in published studies. Some studies define acute otitis media as an immobile, bulging, or dull drum, not necessarily abnormally red. Other studies define otitis media as an eardrum at least two-thirds of which is red, but do not mention mobility of the drum. Combinations of these definitions may have been used, without details to indicate different clinical subgroups. Thus, proper interpretation of published studies requires careful reading to determine the definitions used.

In order to obtain accurate date and to clarify the efficacy of treatment in future studies, it will be important to identify clinical subgroups of acute otitis media, as can be done with problem-oriented diagnoses.

Treatment. In most children, otitis media of recent or unknown onset is treated with an antibiotic even though some patients may have a sterile middle ear effusion. Ampicillin (or amoxicillin) is the antibiotic of choice for the child who is less than about 6 years of age. These drugs are effective against *Streptococcus pneumoniae* and beta-hemolytic streptocci, and are usually effective against *Hemophilus influenzae*. The emergence of ampicillin-resistant *H. influenzae* has prompted the use of other oral antibiotics including a new cephalosporin, cephaclor, for use in the younger child. Erythromycin and sulfa can be used if the child is allergic to penicillin. In older children, penicillin alone is usually used. Antibiotic therapy should continue for 10 days and the patient should be seen following treatment to verify that clinical response has been good.

TABLE 34-2. Acute Otitis Media and Draining Ears

Problem Pattern	Probable Etiologies
Draining Ears	
Perforated otitis media	*S. pneumoniae* Group A streptococcus
Otitis externa (swimmer's ear)	*P. aeruginosa* Other enteric bacteria
Acute Otitis Media	
If defined as "red ear drum"	Any febrile respiratory infection or crying
If defined as "immobile drum"	Eustachian tube dysfunction, possibly sterile, possibly bacterial
If defined as "red, bulging, dull, immobile drum"	*S. pneumoniae* *H. influenzae* Group A streptococcus

Oral decongestants are sometimes used to open the eustachian tube and promote drainage. There is no evidence that decongestants are helpful in the treatment of otitis media.

Acute Mastoiditis

Acute mastoiditis can be detected by clinical criteria without radiologic evidence of mastoid disease. Chronic mastoiditis can be detected by radiologic evidence of bony destruction, without any recent clinical findings.

The mastoid air cells communicate with the middle ear, and so the mastoid bone is usually involved to some degree in all purulent middle ear infections. Acute mastoiditis typically occurs when the purulent infection spreads to the mastoid in the absence of drainage through the eustachian tube or through perforation of the eardrum. It can be considered an abscess in which antibiotic therapy can aid in localization but which often requires surgical drainage.

Clinical Diagnosis. Acute mastoiditis should be suspected when there is pain behind the ear and tenderness on pressing the mastoid bone. The tympanic membrane looks abnormal and is often distorted. Perforation of the tympanic membrane with ear drainage may be present. In some cases, the skin overlying the mastoid is red and edematous, and the ear may be pushed forward by the swelling behind it. The ear canal may be narrowed by swelling. Radiologic examination of the mastoid may show destruction of the air cells, although this is often not present early in the disease.

Culture of ear drainage and blood is indicated and, if positive, may indicate a change from the initial therapy.

Treatment. Antibiotic therapy should be given by the intravenous route to prevent spread to the central nervous system and to aid in localization of the disease. If antibiotic therapy is begun early in the illness, ampicillin alone usually produces improvement in about 24 hours. Ampicillin is preferred for children because it is effective against *H. influenzae,* as well as the streptococcus and pneumococcus. In seriously ill patients or in patients in whom the disease was recognized late, both methicillin and chloramphenicol may be indicated if there is a concern for possible ampicillin-resistant *H. influenzae* or penicillin-resistant *S. aureus,* and insufficient time to watch for a clinical response to ampicillin.

Operative drainage of the mastoid area may be necessary, although it is usually not more urgent than in any other abscess. The patient's general condition should be stabilized. Intravenous ampicillin should be given preoperatively to aid localization and to prevent dissemination during operation. Early or mild mastoiditis often can be successfully treated without surgery.

Complications. Acute mastoiditis has become very rare in recent years because of early antibiotic treatment of otitis media. However, it still occurs and if untreated can extend to produce brain abscess or meningitis. Facial palsy or lateral sinus thrombosis are very rare complications.

Sinusitis

Acute purulent sinusitis can be defined as pus in a sinus cavity, for example, when pus is seen to appear at a meatus immediately after wiping the area or when pus is obtained on cannulation or puncture of a sinus. In many cases, acute sinusitis must be a presumptive diagnosis based on the clinical criteria described below. Chronic sinusitis is a presumptive diagnosis based on radiologic evidence of mucosal thickening. Purulent rhinitis can be a manifestation of acute purulent sinusitis.

Infection of a sinus cavity is usually secondary to obstruction of the meatus of the sinus, but the sinus must be developed enough to have a cavity to obstruct. Thus, the potential for sinus infection depends on the development and pneumatization of the various sinus cavities. The ethmoid sinuses are the first paranasal sinuses to develop. Ethmoid sinusitis may occur in an infant as early as 6 months of age, with most cases occurring between 1 and 3 years of age. Orbital cellulitis may occur as an extension of ethmoiditis and is discussed later in this chapter. Maxillary sinusitis is unlikely to occur before 5 years of age. Frontal sinusitis is uncommon before adolescence.

Predisposing Factors. Allergy is often a predisposing factor in sinusitis. Dental infections are a possible source of sinusitis in adults but very rarely in young children. Massive contamination of the sinus by bacteria with resultant sinusitis can occur from swimming underwater, from a foreign body in the nose, or from trauma. Viral infections as a cause of obstruction predisposing to sinusitis have not been studied adequately.

Clinical Diagnosis. Acute purulent sinusitis should be suspected when there is a purulent nasal discharge from the anterior nares or the posterior nasopharynx. Tenderness to pressure over the sinus, decreased transillumination, and localized pain are strongly indicative of sinusitis. Fever up to 101° or 102°F (38°-39°C) may be present. Nasal obstruction secondary to edema or purulent secretions may be present.

Radiologic demonstration of an air-fluid level usually indicates purulent sinusitis. Radiologic evidence of "clouding" or opacification of a sinus has usually been interpreted as evidence of past or present sinus disease.

Possible Etiologies. The bacteria recovered from patients with acute purulent sinusitis are the "normal flora" of the nose, (*Neisseria, S. epidermidis,* and *S. aureus)* and the common respiratory pathogens, (pneumococci, beta-stretococci and *H. influenzae).* More than one organism is often recovered. Enteric bacteria are less frequently recovered. Anaerobic bacteria, such an anaerobic streptococci, *Corynebacterium, Bacteroides,* and *Veillonella* are frequently recovered from sinuses of adults with chronic sinusitis, but they have not yet been shown to be important in sinusitis in children (see Table 34-3).

TABLE 34-3. Sinusitis, Orbital Cellulitis, Acute Conjunctivitis

Problem Pattern	Probable Etiologies
Acute sinusitis	Undetermined etiology, probably those listed below *S. pneumoniae,* beta hemolytic streptococci, *H. influenzae* in preschool children
Orbital cellulitis	Same as acute sinusitis
Acute conjunctivitis	
Purulent	*S. aureus,* if newborn *H. influenzae,* if preschool *N. gonorrhea* less common *Chlamydia*
Nonpurulent	Adenovirus Measles, if susceptible

Diagnostic Approach. Radiographs of the sinuses should be taken but should be interpreted with caution. Gram's stain and culture should be done if an adequate specimen can be obtained after wiping the meatal area. In one study, nasal cultures correlated with maxillary sinus puncture in about two-thirds of the patients.

Treatment. The most important part of therapy for sinusitis is to relieve the obstruction. This can be done by nasal vasoconstrictor drops or sprays for the first few days of acute sinusitis. Vasoconstrictors should not be used for prolonged periods. Antihistamines may be effective if allergy is a predisposing factor. Oral vasoconstrictors have not been studied in a controlled fashion.

Antibiotic therapy can be based on the Gram stain of pus obtained from near the meatus until culture results are available. In the absence of clear guidance from the Gram's stain, ampicillin is a reasonable choice, particularly for preschool children, so that effectiveness against *H. influenzae* is included. Clindamycin appears to be a reasonable choice for adults with chronic sinusitis presumably caused by anaerobes, but it has not yet been adequately studied in children. Penetration of some antibiotics into the sinuses has been studied; however, the clinical efficacy of various antibiotics has not been investigated adequately in a controlled study.

Irrigation of the sinuses may be indicated for some patients. Operative cannulation or puncture is very rarely necessary in children. Aspirin or codeine may be indicated for relief of pain.

Complications. Brain abscess, meningitis, or thrombosis of a major intracranial vessel are very rare complications of sinusitis. Orbital cellulitis is discussed in the following section.

Association With Older Diseases. Purulent otitis media sometimes occurs with purulent sinusitis. Bronchiectasis is often secondary to or associated with sinusitis. Kartagener's syndrome is the triad of sinusitis, bronchiectasis, and situs inversus, and it is usually suspected if the chest radiograph is properly labeled as to right or left side. Respiratory infections are the result of abnormal cilia.

Cystic fibrosis of the pancreas should be considered in patients with chronic sinusitis or nasal polyposis. Angiofibroma of the posterior nasopharynx occurs typically in adolescent boys and may produce refractory sinusitis because of obstruction.

Orbital Cellulitis

Orbital cellulitis (or periorbital cellulitis) is characterized by redness and edema of the eyelids and periorbital area of one or both eyes. Fever and leukocytosis are usually present. It is important that antimicrobial therapy for this disease be prompt and effective, because it may lead to loss of vision or extension into the central nervous system. Cellulitis of other areas of the face, particularly the cheek area, should be referred to as facial cellulitis, often caused by *H. influenzae* in infants, but not secondary to sinusitis.

Mechanisms. Orbital cellulitis is usually an extension of an infection. In young children, ethmoid sinusitis is the typical source of the infection in orbital cellulitis. A traumatic wound near the eye is occasionally a source of the infection. It is useful to distinguish these two sources, since penicillin-resistant staphylococcal infection is a significant hazard from traumatic cellulitis, whereas orbital cellulitis secondary to ethmoid sinusitis usually responds to intravenous ampicillin. Orbital cellulitis is rarely an extension of a sty or a pustule near the eye or of a dental abscess.

Clinical Diagnosis. Fever, redness, and swelling of the periorbital area indicate a presumptive diagnosis of orbital cellulitis. Other common findings include eye pain, headache, and purulent nasal discharge. In severe cases, there may be proptosis, limitation of eye motion, and decreased vision. Loss of retinal vein pulsation indicates thrombosis, but often the fundus cannot be adequately examined. Bilateral proptosis indicates cavernous sinus thrombosis. The use of computerized axial tomography has been found to be extremely useful in localizing the site and extent of the infection. The severity and toxicity of the illness may be modified by preceding oral antibiotics.

Differential Diagnosis. Purulent conjunctivitis can produce enough surrounding edema and erythema to resemble orbital cellulitis. Gonococcal conjunctivitis is particularly likely to be severe enough to resemble orbital cellulitis. Herpes simplex or vaccinia virus can produce cellulitis in the area of the pustules, which may occur near the eye. Secondary bacterial infection is often suspected because of the intense inflammatory reaction due to the virus. Vaccinia infections of the eye usually have a history of vaccination of the patient or a contact about a week before. Herpes simplex virus infections of the eye are usually associated with some evidence of gingivostomatitis.

Possible Etiologies. The reported series of cases of orbital cellulitis have not had enough positive blood cultures to give reliable information on the frequency of various bacterial causes. Nose or eye culture results are not conclusive. Presumably, the three bacterial agents which are the most frequent causes of otitis media are also the most frequent causes of orbital cellulitis secondary to sinusitis. *H. influenzae*, pneumococci, and beta streptococci and *S. aureus* are the most common bacteria recovered from a blood culture with the patient has ethmoid sinusitis as the source of the infection with no previous antibiotic therapy.

When the cellulitis is secondary to a wound, a nearby pustule or abscess, *S. aureus* is a frequent cause. Gram-negative enteric bacteria may also cause orbital cellulitis secondary to contaminated wounds.

Laboratory Approach. Pus should be gram-stained and cultured, whether found in a wound near the eye or exuding from the conjunctivae, or found as a nasal or posterior pharngeal discharge. The blood culture is positive in some cases and is therefore a useful procedure.

Treatment. Because of the severity of complications and the need for intravenous antibiotics, hospitalization is usually indicated for orbital cellulitis. Intravenous ampicillin is the antibiotic of choice if the source is sinusitis because the usual pathogens are susceptible to ampicillin. If the patient is seriously ill or has proptosis, intravenous oxacillin and chloramphenicol may be indicated since there is less time available to observe the clinical response of 18 hours of ampicillin therapy. Oxacillin or some other penicillinase-resistant penicillin should also be used if the child is less than 3 months old, if Gram's stain of pus from a wound indicates staphylococci, or if the infection is secondary to a wound and no satisfactory material is available from Gram's stain. Oxacillin should also be considered if there is no improvement after 12 to 18 hours of intravenous ampicillin. Gentamicin and oxacillin should be used initially if there has been a grossly contaminated penetrating wound. Chloramphenicol may be indicated in severe illness if ampicillin-resistant *H. influenzae* has been observed in the community.

If sinusitis is present, nasal vasoconstrictor sprays (0.25% phenylephrine) may be of value to shrink nasal mucosa and allow drainage through the meatus.

Pus may be present behind or adjacent to the globe or in the ethmoid sinus. Operative drainage by an ophthalmologist may be necessary if there is no response to adequate antibiotic therapy, particularly if visual acuity is decreased.

Complications. Since antibiotics have become available, complications are rarely seen with orbital cellulitis. Compression or stretching of the optic nerve can produce loss of vision. Exposure keratitis can occur if the proptotic eye is not protected. Cavernous sinus thrombosis with bilateral proptosis and ophthalmoplegia is an extremely rare complication of ethmoiditis. In the past, it usually was secondary to staphylococcal furuncles near the nose. The eye involvement is typically bilateral and the retinal veins appear engorged. Meningitis, septicemia, and death are extremely rare in this antibiotic era.

Cervical Adenitis or Adenopathy

Cervical adenitis is defined as enlarged, tender lymph nodes in the neck. The anterior cervical (tonsillar) nodes under the angle of the jaw are most frequently involved. Adenitis rarely occurs in the posterior cervical nodes (behind the sternocleidomastoid muscle).

Cervical adenopathy is distinguished from adenitis by the absence of tenderness or erythma over the node. Although many patients without evidence of local inflammation have an infection, noninfectious causes are more likely. It often occurs in the posterior cervical area.

Infectious Etiologies. There is overlap between the causes of cervical adenitis and cervical adenopathy, since the findings of tenderness or erythema may be made milder by previous antibiotic therapy, or by the partial immunity of the patient. Thus, group A streptococci, one of the most frequent causes of cervical adenitis, can also be a cause of cervical adenopathy.

Group A streptococci was found to be the most frequent cause of cervical adenitis in a recent series of children who had not received antibiotics; this was determined by culture of the organism from needle aspiration, by incision and drainage from the fluctuant nodes, or by evidence from antistreptolysin O titers. Sometimes beta-hemolytic streptococci are not recovered from the throat, even when recovered on needle aspiration of the node. Other recent studies have ranked beta-hemolytic streptococci second to *S. aureus* in frequency, regardless of prior antibiotic therapy.

Pneumococci, anaerobic peptostreptococci, or gram-negative rods rarely produce cervical adenitis, especially in young infants. Dental infections may be a predisposing factor for some unusual organisms, particularly anaerobes.

Infectious mononucleosis is a possible cause of cervical adenitis or adenopathy, especially in older children and adolescents. Anterior nodes associated with pharyngitis may be tender, but the enlarged posterior nodes are usually not tender. Splenomegaly is often present.

Atypical mycobacteria, previously called unclassified or anonymous mycobacteria, occasionally cause chronic cervical adenitis. Skin tests, using representative atypical mycobacterial antigens, can be compared with the reaction of a standard tuberculin test. In atypical mycobacterial diseases, the induration produced by an atypical antigen is larger than that produced by the standard tuberculin test. Culture of an atypical mycobacterium from the node is conclusive, but in one recent series only about one-third of children with the diagnosis based on skin tests had a positive culture. The mycobacterium can often be recognized as an atypical species on the basis of a yellow or orange color after only a few weeks, before growth is sufficient to allow metabolic differentiation from *Mycobacterium tuberculosis*. Some patients can be observed without therapy since the adenopathy often resolves spontaneously. If the node drains and forms a sinus tract, excision and therapy with rifampin is indicated.

Tuberculosis is now a rare cause of cervical adenitis in the United States. While awaiting the results of the culture, an excised cervical node reported as showing acid-fast bacilli and typical histologic findings of tuberculosis can be assumed safely to be an atypical mycobacterial infection.

Cat-scratch disease may produce enlarged nodes in the head or neck. Cat scratches are found in the majority of patients with cat-scratch disease. Fever over 101°F (38.3°C) occurs for about a week in about 25% of patients. A rash, conjunctivitis, or parotid enlargement may be noted. The enlarged regional lymph node is noted about 2 weeks after the scratch but may occur as late as 7 weeks or as early as 3 days after the scratch. Suppuration and liquefaction of the node occurs in 10% to 25% of cases.

Occasionally, toxoplasmosis is a cause of cervical adenopathy in the United States.

Diagnostic Approach. White blood count and differential may reveal a leukocytosis that implies a bacterial adenitis. Atypical lymphocytes suggest infectious mononucleosis, but rarely toxoplasmosis. A slide serologic test for infectious mononucleosis should be done. Serologic evaluation for histoplasmosis, coccidiomycosis, or toxoplasmosis may be indicated.

A tuberculin test is usually indicated in the case of a patient with cervical adenitis which does not respond to initial penicillin therapy and persists longer than 2 weeks. Equivocal reactions may be the result of cross-reactions from atypical mycobacterial infection, and skin testing with atypical mycobacterial antigens should then be done if antigens are available.

Chest radiograph is characteristically abnormal in tuberculous cervical adenitis but is usually normal in atypical mycobacterial adenitis. It may reveal mediastinal adenopathy if cervical adenopathy is caused by a neoplasm.

Needle aspiration or incision and drainage with Gram's stain and culture of the pus are often conclusive. Anaerobic culture of the pus may be useful. Smear and culture of the pus for acid-fast organisms should also be done in selected cases. Biopsy or excision of the node, with histologic examination, may reveal the granulomatous lesion of mycobacteria or a fungus, the sulfur granules of actinomycosis, or the eosinophilic histiocytes of toxoplasmosis. A skin test with cat-scratch antigen may be helpful if the antigen is available.

Treatment. Local warmth may be of value for symptomatic relief in mild cases of cervical adenitis. Penicillin is indicated initially for most patients with cervical adenitis because of the probability of beta-hemolytic streptococcal infection. Usually the nodes decrease gradually during penicillin therapy. If there is no improvement in 2 or 3 days, needle aspiration of the node should be considered, and antibiotic therapy should be changed to treat a penicillin-resistant staphylococcus. If there is still no decrease in the size in another 3 days, incision and drainage of the node will probably be necessary, and antibiotics may be stopped. When the mass becomes fluctuant, the abscess should be incised widely and the septae broken up, usually under general anesthesia.

Antituberculous chemotherapy and surgical excision are indicated if *M. tuberculosis* is found. Excision is sufficient for atypical mycobacterial adenitis, but rifampin is useful if there is a chronic draining sinus.

Complications. Torticollis (wryneck) may occur as a complication of cervical adenitis or peritonsillar infection. Occasionally it is mistakenly believed to be associated with dislocation of the cervical vertebrae.

Parotitis

Parotitis can be defined as enlargement of the parotid gland, accompanied by fever. Sometimes the parotid gland may appear to be enlarged, when in reality the tonsillar lymph nodes are enlarged. The clinician should try to distinguish cervical adenitis from parotitis by looking carefully at the anatomic location of the swelling. When the paratid gland is enlarged, the location of the swelling occurs both above and below the angle of the jaw, although dependent edema may result in slightly more swelling below. In contrast, when cervical nodes are enlarged, the center of the swelling is located below the jaw. Minimal parotid swelling can best be detected by seeing enlargement of the parotid area, rather than by palpation.

Several other findings are helpful in recognizing parotitis. Parotid enlargement may occur rapidly if the major ducts are obstructed. Parotitis is usually somewhat painful because of stretching of the capsule, and is made worse by foods which stimulate production of saliva. A bacterial infection, such as a cervical abscess, is tender to palpation, whereas parotitis is usually not tender, unless it is a suppurative parotitis.

Mumps *Versus* Parotitis. The word "mumps" originally referred to the swelling seen in epidemic parotitis. Mumps virus infection is the typical cause of parotitis, but parotitis is occasionally caused by other viruses. In addition, mumps virus often produces infection without parotitis. Therefore the word "mumps" should not be used as if parotitis and mumps virus infection were identical. The best diagnostic phrasing is "parotitis, probably due to mumps virus infection." Outbreaks of parotitis, or cases of parotitis that can be related to exposure to another person with parotitis, are almost always caused by mumps virus.

Possible Causes. As already mentioned mumps virus is the most common cause of parotitis. Classic mumps virus infection is painful parotitis, with enlargement of the parotid glands and fever. Edema of the openings of Stensen's ducts in the mouth can often be seen. The other salivary glands may also be enlarged. Edema of the neck or presternal area can occur in severe cases. Headache and vomiting may be very severe (see Table 34-4).

Parainfluenza virus is probably the second most common cause of acute parotitis. Very rare causes of parotitis include lymphocytic choriomengitis virus and coxsackie viruses. Presumably, other agents can cause parotitis, since infection with the previously mentioned viruses were excluded by laboratory results in a study of children developing parotitis months or years after being immunized with live mumps virus vaccine.

Staphylococcus aureus is the common cause of bacterial parotitis, and rarely occurs in the newborn period. Purulent material can often be expressed from the ducts. Postoperative suppurative parotitis is rare in children.

TABLE 34-4. Acute Parotitis and Cervical Adenitis

Problem Pattern	Probable Etiologies
Parotitis: parotid enlargement (mostly above angle of jaw), usually with fever	Mumps virus, if known exposure Parainfluenza virus Coxsackie virus Rarely lymphocytic choriomeningitis virus, bacterial parotitis
Cervical adenitis: fever or erythema and anterior cervical lymph node enlargement (below angle of jaw; in front of sternocleidomastoid muscle)	Group A streptococcus *S. aureus* Possibly anaerobic bacteria from mouth Infectious mononucleosis Rarely atypical mycobacteria, cat-scratch disease, toxoplasmosis

Persistent or Recurrent Parotid Enlargement. There is no laboratory confirmation of the widespread belief that mumps virus infection can produce parotitis more than once. However, parotitis with isolation of mumps virus in spite of past live mumps virus vaccine has been documented. A second episode of parotitis might result from a virus other than mumps, but several other possibilities should always be considered. These include parotid duct narrowing (sialostenosis), presumably secondary to past inflammation; drug hypersensitivity, such as to iodides; and swelling of the mandibular joint because of rheumatoid arthritis.

Complications of Mumps Virus Infection. The incidence of various complications of mumps has seldom been studied adequately in a prospective fashion. Some case reports of serious complications may in reality have been coincidental, since mumps parotitis was a frequent disease before vaccine was available.

Orchitis is a complication that occurs in about 10% to 20% of adult males with mumps parotitis, during outbreaks. Oophoritis appears to occur less frequently than orchitis; atrophy of the ovary apparently does not occur, presumably because the ovary is not surrounded by an inelastic tunica albuginea, as is the testis. Deafness is exceedingly rare. It apparently does occur, but there are no adequate data on the frequency of this complication.

Aseptic meningitis syndrome is very common but significant permanent neurologic sequelae are extremely rare. The patient may have severe headache and transient delirium, but brain involvement (encephalitis) is rare, if defined as a severe and persistent disturbance of consciousness with a CSF lymphocytosis. Death due to mumps virus infection is sometimes reported on death certificates and can occur as a complication of encephalitis; death due to mumps rarely has been documented by virus isolation, with exclusion of other causes. Pancreatitis is probably less common than is generally believed. The elevated serum amylase comes from the parotid gland rather than from the pancreas.

Very rare complications can include diseases which may have been coincidental. A causal relationship remains unproven for illnesses commonly listed as rare complications. Prospective studies of mumps infections in pregnancy have not indicated any adverse effect except an increased risk of abortion, although endocardial fibroelastosis in infancy appears to have a statistical association with a positive skin test for mumps. Other rare complications include arthritis, thyroiditis, myocarditis, facial paralysis, transient psychosis, thrombocytopenic purpura, and transverse myelitis. Diabetes mellitus in children has been suggested as a possible late sequela of mumps virus infection, but this has not been proved.

Laboratory Studies. Mumps virus is isolated relatively easily in laboratories equipped for virus isolation. The virus produces a typical cytopathic effect on rhesus monkey kidney cells, and hemadsorption occurs when guinea pig erythrocytes are added to the infected cell cultures.

Paired sera should be obtained if serologic studies for mumps virus antibody are desired. The complement fixation is usually done.

Serum amylase is elevated in patients with parotitis due to any cause. It may be useful as a laboratory guide to distinguish parotitis from cervical adenitis or other masses in the neck. However, amylase elevation is not specific for mumps parotitis. Amylase elevation persists a few days in some patients after the parotid swelling disappears, so that elevated amylase may indicate recent parotid gland disease. The elevation probably does not indicate pancreatitis, since it is proportional to the severity of parotitis rather than to the severity of abdominal pain.

Treatment. There is no specific treatment for mumps parotitis. Bed rest is of no proven value to prevent orchitis, which can occur in post-pubertal males. In one controlled study of orchitis, steroids were of no value in relief of pain, swelling, or tenderness, and apparently did not influence testicular atrophy on evaluation 6 months after infection. Aspirin or codeine and support of the scrotum usually provide some relief.

Prevention. The commercially available mumps skin-testing antigen appears to be relatively unreliable as a guide to immunity. Postpubertal males who have not had clinical parotitis should be given the attenuated mumps virus vaccine (see Chap 4 on immunization). The commercially available hyperimmune serum has not been proved to be of value in preventing mumps after exposure.

MIDDLE RESPIRATORY SYNDROMES

The phrase *middle respiratory infections* is not used often by physicians, but the concept is very useful. Infections of the middle and lower respiratory airways are as common and as important a cause of hospitalization and death in children as pneumonia syndromes. A patient's acute middle respiratory infections can be classified as laryngitis, bronchitis, bronchiolitis, and influenzalike illness. The distinction between bronchiolitis, asthmatic bronchitis, and acute bronchial asthma is also described below. Subglottic laryngitis, described below, should be distinguished from supraglottic laryngitis, a life-threatening infection described in Chapter 33.

Subglottic Laryngitis (Croup)

Croup is a syndrome with several possible causes, although it is usually viral. It is characterized by inspiratory stridor and a typical brassy cough, but the epiglottis is normal, whether visualized directly or outlined by lateral roentgenogram of the soft tissues of the neck. High fever, marked leukocytosis, a very ill appearance, and drooling suggest epiglottitis rather than subglottic laryngitis. Subglottic laryngitis is about 100 to 1000 times more common than epiglottitis. Epiglottitis requires an artificial airway in at least 50% of cases, whereas ordinary croup is rarely severe enough to require an airway, although it may be necessary in prolonged illnesses or in infants who become fatigued.

Croup is often referred to as *viral croup* because the typical cause is a virus, especially a parainfluenza virus. A foreign body or diphtheria is a rare cause of the croup syndrome. *Spasmodic croup* refers to an illness which tends to be recurrent in some children and is associated with laryngospasm, possibly precipitated by cold, allergens, aspiration of secretions, or a viral illness.

Mist and humidified oxygen are probably helpful in moderate to severe illnesses. Racemic epinephrine by aerosol is often used, but has not been proved to be of value in a controlled study. Antibiotics are probably not indicated, and they have not been adequately studied in a controlled study. However, antibiotics are often used if the patient has marked fever or leukocytosis. Observation of the patient for hypoxemia, as manifested by restlessness and anxiety, is important, because intubation or a tracheotomy may be needed if the patient becomes worse in spite of mist and oxygen.

Acute Bronchitis and Influenzalike Illness

Acute bronchitis and influenzalike illness are discussed together because of their similarity. Both illnesses are manifested by cough without clinical evidence of pulmonary involvement. It is useful to regard coarse inspiratory rhonchi which clear with coughing as essential for the diagnosis of bronchitis, but fever is usually moderate or absent (Table 34-5). In an influenzalike illness, headache, sore trachea, and moderate to high fever are usually present, but fatigue or myalgia is essential for the diagnoosis if fever is absent. Neither tachypnea nor inspiratory rales is found in either if these diseases are uncomplicated. Vomiting or diarrhea is usually absent, although lay persons often mistakenly refer to acute gastroenteritis as "the flu."

Bronchitis. Usually, a virus infection is the cause of bronchitis in children. Measles should be suspected in an unimmunized child with acute febrile bronchitis if conjunctivitis is prominent, since this is the typical clinical appearance of measles for a few days before the rash occurs. Whooping cough occasionally is manifested as acute bronchitis, with episodes of a stacatto cough, but the typical inspiratory whoop may not occur early in the illness or in young infants.

TABLE 34-5. Comparison of Influenzalike Illness and Acute Bronchitis

Symptom	Influenzalike illness	Acute Bronchitis
Cough	Prominent	Prominent
Muscle aches, fatigue	Prominent	Absent
Headache	Often present	Absent
Rhonchi which clear	Unusual	Typical
Usual fever pattern	Moderate to high	Moderate to absent
Rapid breathing	Absent	Absent

Parainfluenza virus, *Mycoplasma pneumoniae*, respiratory syncytial virus, and foreign body are important possible causes of acute bronchitis.

Influenzalike Illness. In a civilian outbreak, influenza virus is the usual cause. In sporadic cases, adenovirus, parainfluenza virus, and *Mycoplasma pneumoniae* are common causes, although the myalgia and fatigue are much less prominent than with influenza virus infection.

Laboratory Approach. Respiratory virus infections are identified most conveniently by antibody studies of paired sera, which are easily transportable. Most respiratory viruses can also be cultured in a reference laboratory, but the specimen must be obtained early in the illness and transported promptly.

Treatment. Muscle aches and fever are usually treated with aspirin or acetaminophen. Rest should be encouraged for patients with fatigue. Antibiotics are unnecessary, unless pneumonia, a rare complication, occurs.

Bronchiolitis, Asthmatic Bronchitis, and Asthma

The three syndromes, bronchiolitis, asthmatic bronchitis, and asthma, closely resemble each other. However, it is clinically useful to distinguish them (Table 34-6). In each syndrome there are tachypnea and expiratory obstruction. In severe expiratory obstruction, the breath sounds are decreased. In mild to moderate obstruction, the breath sounds are low-pitched and coarse, and wheezes are usually present.

Bronchiolitis. Bronchiolitis characteristically occurs in infants less than 2 years of age. After a few days of mild cough and rhinitis, the infant develops rapid respiration and is taken to a physician. The breath sounds may be decreased throughout or may be coarse, with coarse rales throughout. Chest radiographs show little or no pneumonia, but the diaphragms are low (air-trapping). The cause is usually viral, particularly respiratory syncytial virus. Treatment consists of humidified oxygen, although mechanical ventilation may be needed in extremely severe cases. Bronchodilators are generally of no value.

Asthmatic Bronchitis. Asthmatic bronchitis is the syndrome that the British

TABLE 34-6. Differentiation of Bronchiolitis, Asthmatic Bronchitis, and Asthma

Feature	Bronchiolitis	Asthmatic Bronchitis	Bronchial Asthma
Typical age	Less than 2 yr	1–4 yr	4 yr and older
Recurrences	Rare	Sometimes	Repeated
Presumed location	Bronchioles	Small bronchi	All bronchi
Response to epinephrine	Little or none	Variable	Usual
Differential auscultatory features	Coarse breath sounds, wheezes, rhonchi and occasionally rales	Wheezes, rhonchi	Musical wheezes
Usual etiology	RS virus	Viral infections	Allergens: inhalants, food, or infections

call "wheezy bronchitis." The child usually is about 1 to 4 years of age. Asthmatic bronchitis resembles the bronchiolitis syndrome, except that the child often has a history of one or two previous similar episodes. This syndrome can be considered an early or mild form of acute bronchial asthma precipitated by infectious bronchitis; it may not necessarily progress to the more typical pattern of acute bronchial asthma. The etiology is usually viral, including rhinoviruses, which in an ordinary host produce only the common cold.

Acute Bronchial Asthma. Acute bronchial asthma can usually be recognized after 2 years of age and is characterized by a history of repeated attacks of bronchospasm, relieved by epinephrine. In severe episodes unresponsive to epinephrine (status asthmaticus), hospitalization is indicated for humidified oxygen, corticosteroids, and intravenous high-dose theophylline (monitored by blood level, if possible). See Chapter 26.

COMMON EXANTHEMS

An *exanthem* is defined as a skin rash typically associated with fever. An enanthem is defined as lesions of the mouth associated with a skin rash. Exanthems are best classified by reference to the classic disease they most nearly resemble (e.g., measles, rubella, and chickenpox, Table 34-7.

TABLE 34-7. Probable Etiologies of Rash Syndromes

Problem Pattern	Probable Etiologies
Measleslike rashes	Measles virus, if susceptible Drug reactions
Rubellalike rashes	Rubella virus, if susceptible Ampicillin rash Adenovirus Echovirus or coxsackieviruses
Roseolalike rashes	Unknown etiology, presumably an unidentified virus Coxsackieviruses and echoviruses
Maculopapular exanthem (not like rashes above)	Echoviruses or coxsackievirus Unidentified causes
Rose spots	Typhoid fever Shigellosis Echo- or coxsackie viruses
Scarlet feverlike rashes	Group A streptococci *S-aureus* Drug reactions Erythema infectiosum involving cheeks Rarely, mucocutaneous lymph node syndrome (Kawasaki's disease)
Vesicular or pustular rashes	Chickenpox Gonococcal or other bacteremia Herpes zoster Herpes simplex Hand-foot-and-mouth disease (coxsackievirus) Stevens-Johnson syndrome
Petechial or purpuric rashes	Meningococcemia Rocky Mountain spotted fever Endocarditis, if petechial Anaphylactoid purpura Rarely, atypical measles Thrombocytopenia Adenoviruses Group A streptococci
Multiforme-urticarial rashes	Urticaria ("hives") Erythema multiforme *Mycoplasma pneumoniae*

Uses of the Word Rubella. The classification of rubella is illustrated best by the concept of a rubellalike rash. It is useful to distinguish the clinical diagnosis of a rubellalike rash from a laboratory-documented rubella virus infection. Rubellalike rash is a legitimate description of a rash and can be used as a problem-oriented syndrome diagnosis. Rubellalike illness is a descriptive diagnosis that implies that other typical features are present, such as lymphadenopathy and arthralgias. Rubella virus infection is a laboratory-confirmed etiologic diagnosis.

Rubella without further modification is a term that should be avoided, since it is not clear whether the word is being used as a problem-oriented descriptive diagnosis meaning a rubellalike rash, or a laboratory-confirmed etiologic diagnosis.

Classifications, Definitions, and Possible Causes. Table 34-8 lists a classification of rashes based on the typical or classic patterns.

URINARY INFECTIONS

Diagnosis

A presumptive clinical diagnosis of urinary tract infection can be made on the basis of typical clinical manifestations and pyuria, but a laboratory-confirmed diagnosis depends on the demonstration of significant bacteriuria. These characteristics need further definition.

Clinical Manifestations. Fever implies infection. In adults with a urinary infection, high fever (> 103°F, or > 39.5°C) usually indicates renal involvement. However, this is not the case with children, who may have high fever without renal involvement. Frequent or urgent urination implies bladder irritation. Burning on urination implies urethral irritation. Cloudy urine may be caused by bacterial growth in the bladder urine but may also result from precipitated solutes.

Foul-smelling urine implies bacterial growth; however, the patient may regard concentrated urine as foul-smelling. Suprapubic pain or tenderness implies bladder infection. Flank pain or tenderness implies kidney infection.

In infants and young children, symptoms may be absent, mild, or perhaps not even traced to the urinary tract. Therefore, a careful urinalysis should be done in a child with unexplained fever. Asymptomatic infections are detected in about 2% of school-age girls when screening cultures are done.

Pyuria. There is no widely agreed upon definition of pyuria, so that the upper limit of normal for leukocytes in the urine is defined by the laboratory or the physician doing the examination and is dependent on the method used. Usually, the number of leukocytes in the urine is more than the observer normally finds and can be clearly recognized as pyuria. Clumps or casts of white blood cells usually indicate pyuria. Pyuria can also be defined as more than 5 or 10 leukocytes per high-power field in the centrifuged sediment. Pyuria cannot be excluded by the microscopic examination of uncentrifuged specimens unless a large volume is examined quantitatively in a hemocytometer.

Microscopic Bacteriuria. Microscopic examination for pyuria also is useful for immediate recognition of the presence of bacteria. Experienced observers can usually give a semiquantitative estimate of the number of bacilli in the sediment, which usually correlates well with culture of the urine. Absence of bacteria in the centrifuged sediment does not exclude urinary infection, but rodlike bacteria can usually be seen in large quantities in the sediment if the culture is going to result in >100,000 bacteria/ml. A methylene blue-stain or Gram's stain of a drop of uncentrifuged urine is an equally accurate test for microscopic bacteriuria; some physicians prefer this method.

Microscopic bacteriuria with a negative culture may have several possible explanations. Most frequently, the bacteria seen are contaminants which are not detected by the typical bacteriologic media (*e.g.,* diphtheroids or vaginal lactobacilli). Artifacts and technical errors in collection and culture are much more likely explana-

TABLE 34-8. Clinical Patterns of Common Rashes

Illness	Type of Rash	Incubation Period	Length of Illness	Time of Year	Method of Diagnosis	Signs and Symptoms	Complications
Measles (rubeola)	Maculopapular	10–11 days	7 days	Winter/ Spring	Clinical characteristics; viral culture, serology	Fever, cough conjuctivitis, rash, Koplik's spots	Otitis media, pneumonia, encephalitis
Rubella	Faint maculopapular	16–18 days	3 days	Spring	Clinical characteristics; serology viral culture	Mild to asymptomatic illness. Cervical and postauricular nodes	Arthritis encephalitis, congenital infection
Roseola	Faint maculopapular	?10–15 days	3–4 days	Year-round	Clinical characteristics	Fever during the first 3 days then rash appears. Occurs in children 6 months to 3 years	Febrile seizures
Enterovirus	Maculopapular or vesicular	Variable	Variable	Warm months	Clinical characteristics; viral culture, serology	Fever, aseptic meningitis, pleurodynia, hand-foot-and-mouth disease, herpangina,	Only those related to the presenting syndrome

						gastroenteritis, and others. Any of these may be associated with rash	
Erythema infectiosum	Red cheeks, then maculopapular rash on the trunk	6–14 days	7 days	Year-round	Clinical characteristics	Fever, vomiting, sore throat, headache, rash. Tonsils and pharynx are edematous and red.	Rare; arthritis, pneumonia, encephalopathy, hemolytic anemia
Scarlet fever	Red, macular rash; feels like sandpaper	2–4 days	5–7 days	Late winter, early spring	Clinical characteristics; throat culture positive for group A streptococcus, serology	No symptoms except rash	Rheumatic fever and acute glomerulonephritis
Chicken pox (varicella)	Vesicular	14–16 days	7–10 days	Cold months	Clinical characteristics, viral culture, serology	Height of fever parallels severity of rash. Lesions appear in crops that progress from papule to vesicle to crust.	Secondary bacterial infection, encephalitis, pneumonia

tions than failure to grow a fastidious pathogen, such as an anaerobe.

Significant Bacteriuria. Quantitative culture of the urine ("colony counts"), is a significant advance in the study of urinary infections. In a clean voided urine >100,000 bacteria/ml usually indicates urinary infection. The difficulties with this figure of 100,000 do not lie with the accuracy of the counting, which is well within the capabilities of office bacteriology, but rather with the collection of the specimen. The value >100,000 bacteria/ml should not be taken as significant by itself, since it depends on the method used to collect urine as well as a number of other variables.

Preliminary Classification

Using the three factors—clinical manifestations, pyuria, and bacteriuria—it is possible to classify any patient into one of the following eight logical possibilities (Table 34-9). The use of such a preliminary diagnostic category aids the clinician by giving guidance toward making a more specific diagnosis. The logical preliminary diagnoses can have a number of possible etiologies.

Typical Urinary Infection. If all three features of clinical findings, pyuria, and significant bacteriuria are present, the illness is a typical urinary infection.

Suspected Urinary Infection Without Pyuria or Bacteriuria. Suspected urinary infection should be the preliminary diagnosis when there are signs and symptoms suggesting a urinary tract infection but no pyuria or significant bacteriuria. There are several possible causes of this pattern. Urethritis is a common cause. Recent or current chemotherapy that has suppressed cultural confirmation of the infection is one of the most frequent causes. Overhydration with rapid urine flow and frequent voiding of urine before bacteria can reach high concentrations is another cause.

Fastidious or anaerobic organisms causing a bladder or kidney infection is a rare cause of this pattern. However, *Hemophilus influenzae,* which will not grow on the plating media usually used for urine, should be considered a rare cause of this pattern. Suppression of bacterial growth by contamination of the urine with the disinfectant used to prepare the urethral area is also a very unlikely cause. Adenoviral cystitis is an uncommon cause of microscopic hematuria and pyuria

TABLE 34-9. Logical Combinations of Three Major Variable Observations in Urinary Infections

Diagnostic Classification	Clinical Findings Suggesting Infection	Pyuria	Bacteriuria
Typical urinary infection	+	+	+
Suspected urinary infection without bacteriuria	+	0	0
Presumptive urinary infection without bacteriuria	+	+	0
Probably urinary infection without pyuria	+	0	+
Asymptomatic bacteriuria and pyuria	0	+	+
Asymptomatic bacteriuria without pyuria	0	0	+
Asymptomatic pyuria	0	+	0
No bacterial urinary infection	0	0	0

(Moffet HL: Urinalysis and urine cultures in children. Urol Clin North Am *1*:387, 1974)

without bacteriuria. Polycystic kidney, with intermittent obstruction of infected portions of the kidney, is a possible cause of variable urinalysis or culture results.

Presumptive Urinary Infection Without Bacteriuria. Urethritis is probably the most frequent cause of urinary infection without bacteriuria. Gonorrhea and nongonococcal urethritis are discussed later in this chapter. Medications such as atropinelike drugs are an occasional cause of frequent urination. Unilateral pyelonephritis with complete ureteral obstruction is an unusual cause of this pattern.

Probable Urinary Infection Without Pyuria. Urinary infection without pyuria is uncommon, but may occur several days after the onset of an infection when pyuria has decreased. The urinalysis and urine culture should be repeated to clarify the situation if antibiotics have not been administered.

Asymptomatic Bacteriuria and Pyuria. Recent or current chemotherapy can cause suppression of signs and symptoms of urinary infection. It may also be due to poor technique in collecting a voided urine when there is no true urinary infection, particularly if there is a delay in inoculation of the specimen. This is especially likely in the presence of vaginitis or in an uncircumcised male unretracted foreskin.

Asymptomatic Bacteriuria Without Pyuria. Asymptomatic bacteriuria can occur several days or weeks after the onset of the infection, after the initial clinical manifestations and pyuria have disappeared. It can rarely occur after the suppression of symptoms and pyuria by inadequate chemotherapy. This pattern also can be caused by poor collection of a voided urine as previously described.

Asymptomatic Pyuria. There are many possible causes of asymptomatic pyuria, several of which are infectious. A bacterial urinary infection suppressed by chemotherapy may produce this pattern. Urethritis can be gonococcal, nonspecific, or chemical, as discussed below. Renal tuberculosis should also be considered.

Poor urine collection is a possible cause. Pyuria without infection often occurs after urethral instrumentation or bladder surgery. Noninfectious subacute or chronic renal disease can be associated with pyuria, but proteinuria, casts, and hematuria are often present. Fever in a patient with chronic renal disease may stimulate pyuria. Pyuria is also observed during convalescence from acute glomerulonephritis or toxic nephritis, but some hematuria is usually present. Extreme dehydration can also produce pyuria.

No Bacterial Urinary Infection. All three variables are negative in most normal children, provided there has been no recent chemotherapy.

Management

Chemotherapy. Sulfisoxazole or ampicillin is used most often to treat a first urinary infection (see Table 36-1), but nitrofurantoin is equally effective. Two weeks of therapy is usually adequate. A follow-up culture obtained about 1 week after stopping medication is essential to be sure there is no relapse. If a follow-up culture is positive, antimicrobial susceptibility tests should be obtained to guide selection of the drug used in the second course of therapy.

Urologic Evaluation. An intravenous pyelogram is probably advisable after the first urinary infection for males and females. It certainly is advisable in infants. More complete urologic investigation with a cystourethrogram and cystoscopy is advisable after the first infection in boys.

Other Therapy and Follow-up. Children with a recent urinary infection should have several follow-up urine examinations and cultures for one year, even if no abnormalities have been noted. Culture can be done easily using a quantitative loop in the physician's office. As an alternative, the parent can test the child's first voided urine in the morning with a dipstick type of chemical test.

Children with recurrent urinary infections and no anatomic abnormalities seem to be helped by prophylactic therapy with low-dose nitrofurantoin (Table 36-1) and extra oral fluids.

GENITAL INFECTIONS

Genital Ulcers

The general category of genital ulcers includes ulceration of the skin or mucosa on or near the external genitalia. A syphilitic chancre is a shallow ulcer about 1 to 2 cm in diameter, with hard, elevated edges. The chancre is painless if located on the genitalia but it may be painful if it is extragenital. It is overlooked easily if it is on the cervix or in the rectum. The incubation period between exposure and appearance of the chancre is 10 to 90 days (usually about 3 weeks).

Chancroid or soft chancre is a chancrelike ulcer caused by *Hemophilus ducreyi.* This disease is about as common as syphilis. The lesion begins as a papule or vesicle that later ruptures and leaves a shallow, painful ulcer. Most patients have two or more soft chancres. Later, there are large ulcers in the genital area with beefy red granulation tissue. The incubation period is 3 to 5 days.

Herpesvirus hominis infection in the genital area (herpes progenitalis) can result in small painful ulcerations. In children, genital herpes is not always spread by sexual contact.

Granuloma inguinale is a rare disease due to a gram-negative bacillus. The lesion begins as a nonpainful nodule that erodes to leave a beefy red exuberant granulation tissue. The incubation period is 1 to 12 weeks, usually about 7 weeks.

Other possible causes of genital ulcers include moniliasis, psoriasis, scabies, molluscum contagiosum, erythema multiforme, and simple friction ulceration.

Laboratory Approach. The Venereal Disease Research Laboratory (VDRL) test may not be positive when the syphilitic chancre first appears, but it usually becomes positive within a few weeks. The VDRL should be obtained as soon as the chancre is seen and repeated in about 3 weeks. Antisyphilitic therapy should be given as soon as the ulcer is seen by the physician, without waiting for the VDRL results.

All positive VDRL results should be confirmed in a reference laboratory by specific tests such as the fluorescent treponemal antibody absorption test (FTA-ABS), since biologic false-positive VDRLs are common in adolescents. False-positive FTA-ABS tests can also occur, so that this test should not be used for screening purposes.

Dark field examination of material from a chancrelike ulcer may reveal the spirochetes of syphilis, but dark field facilities with experienced observers are usually not available except where the disease is frequently seen. Gram's stain of the smear of a chancrelike ulcer may reveal rows and chains of gram-negative rods, characteristic of *Hemophilus ducreyi.* Special stains of a smear from crushed tissue preparations are necessary to demonstrate the oval Donovan bodies found in granuloma inguinale.

Treatment. Genital ulcers are best treated with an antisyphilitic regimen until follow-up serologic tests determine syphilis has been excluded. Syphilitic chancre in an adolescent or adult is conventionally treated by 2.4 million units of benzathine penicillin, given intramuscularly in two sites. Tetracycline 500 mg 4 times daily for 15 days is an alternative therapy for adults allergic to penicillin. Fever, malaise, and intensification of skin lesions (Jarisch-Herxheimer reaction) occur in many patients within 12 hours of the onset of therapy.

Chancroid responds to sulfonamides. Granuloma inguinale is treated effectively by tetracycline or erythromycin, but not by ampicillin. Treatment of herpes simplex lesions of external genitalia is currently controversial with no controlled studies showing benefit from any kind of therapy.

Inguinal Adenopathy

Enlargement of inguinal or femoral lymph nodes can be due to many causes unrelated to genital diseases and in children it is usually a result of infections of the leg. However, tender or suppurative nodes in a postpubertal person should raise the question of a genital infection. Lymphogranuloma venereum (LGV) caused by *Chlamydia lymphogranulomatosis* is rare. The first manifestation of disease is a tender inguinal node (bubo). Typically, the primary lesion, a small papule or erosion which occurs 1 or 2 weeks after exposure, is not noticed or reported. Then the bubo appears 2 to 4 weeks after exposure. The bubo may proceed to suppuration.

Syphilis and chancroid also may produce inguinal adenopathy and should always be considered because the primary ulceration may have been overlooked.

Laboratory Approach. The diagnosis of lymphogranuloma venereum can be confirmed by a skin test (Frei test), but determination of serum antibodies is more reliable. Syphilis should be excluded by a VDRL in sexually active persons with inguinal adenitis and should be repeated at monthly intervals for 3 months.

Treatment. Lymphogranuloma venereum can be effectively treated by a 21-day course of tetracycline or sulfonamides. Aspiration of fluctuant nodes is also helpful.

Urethritis

Urethritis is defined as redness of the urethra or pain in the urethra on voiding. It can be classified as purulent or nonpurulent, depending on the appearance of the discharge. Urethritis can also be classified as gonococcal or nongonococcal, according to the results of culture of the discharge. This is similar to the classification of pharyngitis as streptococcal or nonstreptococcal.

Purulent urethritis. The gonococcus usually causes purulent urethritis. It occurs most frequently in the male. Symptoms of gonorrhea in the male begin about 3 to 5 days after exposure. Urination is painful, and there is a yellow discharge. Fever is usually absent. Urethritis is more likely to be gonococcal if there is a spontaneous discharge. Because the symptoms are acute, the male seeks medical care within a few days of the onset. Gram's stain of the discharge is usually unequivocally positive for gram-negative diplococci, if the culture is going to be positive for the gonococcus.

In females, findings of urethritis are usually absent, and the gonococcal infection is more likely to cause cervicitis or salpingitis. Gonorrhea is one of the possible causes of painful urination with negative urine culture for the common urinary tract pathogens. Gonorrhea in females is often asymptomatic, but can spread to the endometrium and fallopian tubes. Dissemination with fever and arthritis may be the first sign of disease.

Bacteria other than the gonococcus are occasionally recovered from a purulent urethral discharge. Enteric bacteria, *S. aureus,* or streptococci are occasionally recovered, but the etiologic significance is not easily proved. It is rare for purulent urethritis to be caused by a species of *Acinetobacter* (formerly called *Mima polymorpha,* so named because of its ability to mimic the gonococcus by Gram's stain). Occasionally, nonpurulent urethritis can be caused by the same bacteria which usually produce a purulent urethritis.

Nonpurulent urethritis. There may be a number of causes of nonpurulent urethritis including gonorrhea, but usually a bacterial cause is not found. Nongonococcal nonpurulent urethritis is common in sexually active adolescents. Urethritis may also be caused by physical irritation. Some strains of mycoplasma, called T-strains for the tiny colonies, have been regarded as a possible cause of nongonococcal urethritis. However, recent studies indicate little or no role for mycoplasmas and a major role for chlamydiae.

Chlamydia, probably *C. trachomatis,* seem to be the common cause of nonpurulent urethritis. This disease has an incubation period of about 10 days and responds to tetracycline.

Trichomonas vaginalis is a protozoan which can cause urethritis in the male or female.

Vaginitis

Vaginitis can be defined as redness and exudate of the vaginal mucosa. Noninfectious causes predominate in prepubertal girls and include poor perineal hygiene, foreign bodies, and chemical irritants. Gonorrheal vaginitis can occur in prepubertal girls and should always be considered. The squamous epithelium of the postpubertal female is relatively resistant to infection by the gonococcus, so that vaginitis is rarely gonococcal in mature females.

The most likely infectious causes in postpubertal females include *Candida albicans* (moniliasis), *Trichomonas vaginalis,* and *Corynebacterium vaginale (Hemophilus vaginalis).* Bacteria other than the gonococci appear to account for nearly half of all cases of vaginitis in adult women. A purulent, copious gray discharge with a characteristic offensive odor is suggestive of *C. vaginale,* as has been demonstrated by inoculation of volunteers.

Candidiasis appears to account for the majority of cases of infectious vaginitis in children. Itching is prominent and the discharge is curdy. In prepubertal girls, beta-hemolytic streptococcus is also a possible cause. Shigella infection is a rare cause of vaginitis in prepubertal girls.

Laboratory Approach. A fresh wet preparation and Gram stain should be examined. Recent douching or menstruation can interfere with these studies. In one study, the wet mount preparation was inadequate, compared with culture, for candida or trichomonas. *Clue cells,* which are rounded epithelial cells with intracellular granules, suggest *C. vaginale.* Culture should be done to exclude gonococcus in all cases. Special techniques are necessary for candida, trichomonas, or *C. vaginale,* so that the laboratory should be informed when one of these organisms is suspected on the basis of clinical or microscopic evidence. Culture should be done if the wet preparation is negative.

Treatment. *Trichomonas* vaginitis is treated with metronidazole. *C. vaginale* vaginitis appears to respond to ampicillin, but it has not been studied in a controlled fashion. Triple-sulfa cream applied locally is also effective. *C. albicans* vaginitis can be treated with nystatin or miconazole cream.

Orchitis

The acute onset of swelling and pain in one or both testicles in a postpubertal boy suggests *acute orchitis,* but the clinician should consider noninfectious etiologies including trauma and torsion.

Epididymitis is a clinical diagnosis based on palpation that localizes the swelling and tenderness to the epididymis and not to the testicle. Urinary tract anomalies may be the underlying reason for acute epididymitis in prepubertal boys, and a urologic investigation should be carried out to look for such anomalies. Anaphylactoid purpura is another possible cause of epididymitis.

Mumps virus infection is an important and relatively common cause of orchitis and a rare cause of isolated epididymitis. Typically, the patient has parotitis and has had a known exposure to another person with parotitis. Before mumps vaccine was available, mumps was the most common cauuse of orchitis.

The prognosis for fertility after mumps orchitis is probably very good. In one study of 105 cases of testicular causes of infertility with bilateral testicular biopsy, only two patients had a histologic diagnosis of atrophy due to past mumps virus infection, and in these cases a history of mumps orchitis was needed to support the histologic diagnosis.

In a controlled study, cortisone did not have any favorable effect on mumps orchitis in terms of acute symptoms or testicular size 5 months later.

Coxsackie B virus has been recovered from a testicular biopsy of a patient with orchitis, confirming the etiologic relationship implied by the increased frequency of orchitis in patients with pleurodynia.

Infectious mononucleosis is rarely complicated by orchitis. Other infections which are rare causes of acute orchitis include the viruses of chickenpox, dengue, and lymphocytic choriomeningitis.

BIBLIOGRAPHY

General

Krugman S, Ward R, Katz SL: Infectious Diseases of Children. St. Louis, CV Mosby, 1977

An excellent source of information about common childhood diseases.

Moffet HL: Pediatric Infectious Diseases: A Problem-Oriented Approach. Philadelphia, JB Lippincott, 1975

A detailed discussion of infectious syndromes in children.

Upper Respiratory Infections

Andiman W.A: The Epstein-Barr virus and EB virus infections in children. J Pediatr 95:171, 1979

Discussion of clinical findings in children and methods of serologic diagnosis.

Barton LL, Feigin RD: Childhood cervical lymphadenitis: a reappraisal. J Pediatr 84:846, 1974

Cases proved by needle puncture.

Brunell PA, Brickman A, Steinberg S, Allen E: Parotitis in children who had previously received mumps vaccine. Pediatrics 50:441, 1972

Viral studies of this syndrome.

Moffet HL, Cramblett HG, Smith A: Group A streptococcal infections in a children's home. II. Clinical and epidemiologic patterns of illness. Pediatrics 33:11, 1964

Clinical details about streptococcal pharyngitis.

Moffet HL, Siegel AC, Doyle HK: Nonstreptococcal pharyngitis. J. Pediatr 73:51, 1968

Viral and serologic studies of nonstreptococcal pharyngitis.

Parrott RH, Wolf SI, Nudelman J, Naiden E, Huebner RJ *et al.*: Clinical and laboratory differentiation between herpangina and infectious (herpetic) gingivostomatitis. Pediatrics 14:122, 1954

Clinical distinctions between herpes simplex and herpangina.

Peter G, Smith AL: Group A streptococcal infections of skin and pharynx. N Engl J Med 297:311; 365, 1977

A helpful review of both types of streptococcal infections.

Polson AM: Gingival and peridontal problems in children. Pediatrics 54:190, 1974

Stomatitis is not necrotizing ulcerative gingivitis (trench mouth).

Taranta A, Moody, MD: Diagnosis of streptococcal pharyngitis. Pediatr Clin North Am 18:125, 1971

Laboratory studies for suspected streptococcal pharyngitis.

Townsend EH, Jr, Radebaugh, JF: Prevention of complications of respiratory illnesses in pediatric practice. A double-blind study. N Engl J Med 266:683, 1962

Lack of value of antibiotics in minor respiratory illnesses.

Otitis Sinusitis

Bernstein L: Pediatric sinus problems. Otolaryngol Clin North Am 4:127, 1971

A good review of sinusitis.

Paradise JL: Otitis media in infants and children. Pediatrics 65:917, 1980

An excellent review of otitis media.

The Child with a Limp

35

Walter W. Tunnessen, Jr.

Etiologic Classification of Limps in Childhood Causes of Painful Limps

I. Trauma
   Skin irritation from ill-fitting shoes
   Lacerations and foreign bodies
   Plantar warts
   Muscle bruising
   Ligament strains and sprains
   Fractures
   a. Toddlers fracture
   b. March or stress fractures
   Achilles tendinitis
   Ruptured Achilles tendon
   Subluxation of patella
   Battered child
   Following injections

II. Inflammation
   Toxic synovitis
   Septic arthritis
      Bacterial
      Viral
      Other
   Cellulitis; adenitis
   Reactive arthritis
      e.g., Yersinia pseudotuberculosis
         Campylobacter
   Osteomyelitis
   Juvenile rheumatoid arthritis
   Ankylosing spondylitis
   Acute rheumatic fever
   Henoch-Schönlein purpura
   Systemic lupus erythematosus
   Periarteritis nodosa
   Kawasaki's disease
   Allergic reactions (serum sickness
   Dermatomyositis
   Polymyositis
   Acute myositis (influenzal)
   Pyomyositis
   Inflammatory bowel disease
   Congenital infections (syphilis)
   Plasma cell hepatitis

III. Osteochondroses
   Legg-Calvé-Perthes disease
   Osgood-Schlatter disease
   Sever's disease
   Freiberg's disease
   Köhler's bone disease

IV. Bone and Cartilage Lesions
   Slipped capital femoral epiphysis
   Osteochondritis dissecans
   Chondromalacia patellae
   Larsen-Johansson disease
   Sinding-Larsen disease

V. Neoplastic Disorders
   Leukemia, lymphoma
   Malignant bone tumors
      Osteogenic sarcoma
      Ewing's sarcoma
      Metastatic neuroblastoma
   Benign bone tumors
      Osteoid osteoma
      Eosinophilic granuloma
      Nonossifying fibroma
      Fibrous dysplasia

VI. Hematologic and Nutritional Disorders
   Hemophilia
   Sickle cell anemia
   Phlebitis
   Scurvy
   Vitamin A intoxication

VII. Neurologic Disorders
   Diskitis
   Epidural abscess
   Guillain-Barré syndrome
   Herniated disk

VII. Miscellaneous Conditions
   Acute appendicitis
   Acute iliac adenitis
   Retroperitoneal masses

Etiologic Classification of Limps in Childhood
Causes of Nonpainful Limps

I. Neurologic Disorders
  - Flaccid paralysis
  - Spastic paralysis
  - Ataxia
    - Drug-induced
    - Acute cerebellar
    - Friedreich's
  - Spinal cord and column problems
    - Intraspinal masses
    - Diastematomyelia
    - Spondylosis

II. Muscle Disorders
  - Primary muscle diseases
  - Muscular dystrophies
  - Arthrogryposis

III. Joint Disorders
  - Joint stiffness and contractures
  - Joint instability
  - Congenital dislocated hip
  - Joint hyperextensibility
    - Pes planus
    - Ehlers-Danlos syndrome
  - Popliteal cyst

IV. Bony Deformities
  - Leg length discrepancies
  - Congenital coxa vara
  - Genu valgum
  - Torsional deformities
  - Blount's disease

V. Functional States
  - Hysterical reactions
  - Mimicry

A limp is a challenge to the examining physician—a problem-solving challenge that is often rewarded by a successful diagnostic effort. By applying careful investigative techniques, particularly a thorough history, a detailed physical examination, and considerable common sense, one may focus in on the perpetrator of the problem.

The most common causes of limps in children are presented in this chapter. A long list of "suspects," known in medical parlance as etiologic classifications, is presented in this chapter. Obviously all suspects are not indiscriminately incriminated in each case of limp; rather, the choices are narrowed to a workable few.

HISTORY

Is the limp painful or nonpainful; is it acute in onset, or has it been long-standing?

Most children are able to voice discomfort. At times the pain may be minimal and the child may not complain directly about it. The child's gait, however, often reveals the painful nature of the limp.

The more acute the onset of the limp, the more likely it is to be a result of trauma or inflammation. Therefore, a careful history about the duration of the problem must be obtained. A limp that has been present since the child started to walk obviously suggests congenital problems such as a dislocated hip or leg length discrepancy. The shorter the duration of the complaint, the more aggressive one should be to uncover a situation that may have resulted in injury.

The abdomen should be carefully examined for masses and organomegaly, and the back, particularly the vertebral column, carefully inspected for mobility and palpated for tenderness. Following examination of the chest, heart, head, and neck, the child should be asked to stand on one leg and then the other. The Trendelenburg test will reveal difficulties with the muscular support system of the pelvis. Normally when we stand on one leg the gluteal muscles support the pelvis to keep the opposite iliac crest level. When standing on a dislocated hip or in the presence of pelvic girdle muscle weakness, the iliac crest on the opposite side sags.

Following a careful history and physical examination, laboratory aids may be helpful in establishing a diagnosis or in providing evidence against other conditions that must be separated from the disorder being considered. The most frequently used aid in the evaluation of limps is the roentgenogram. Often the films are negative, but they are helpful in assuring that there are no fractures, dislocations, and they may even assure that there are no infections. A white blood count and sedimentation rate are often ordered, since they are nonspecific indicators of inflammation. Other laboratory tests, such as cultures and radionuclide scans, are obtained if indicated.

AGE AND DIAGNOSES

At certain ages some disorders are much more common than others. In the 1- to 3-year-old age group, the leading causes of limp are trauma, congenital hip dislocations, and monarticular juvenile rheumatoid arthritis. In the 4- to 8-year-old age group toxic synovitis of the hip and Legg-Calvé-Perthes disease are most prevalent, and in the 9- to 16-year-old group, slipped capital femoral epiphysis, Osgood-Schlatter disease, osteochondritis dissecans, and epiphyseal fractures are most likely (Table 35-1).

Children fall and sustain bruises and abrasions almost constantly during normal play. In fact, a child under the age of ten who has no bruises or scrapes on his lower legs must be an object of concern! A history of trauma will often be obtained, but one must be selective in picking out episodes that are significant. Perhaps there was a seemingly innocuous fall from a swing set or a tree limb the day before; or, a toddler's leg or foot may have been stuck in a chair spring and suddenly pulled free, resulting in a spiral fracture of the tibia, unapparent on roentgenograms for a week to ten days. The traumatic episode may not have been an acute injury at all. A new exercise or activity may have initiated the problem. Hip joint irritation may have resulted from lateral movements of the pelvic girdle associated with hitting a bucket of golf balls at a driving range or from raking lawns. During training, the cross-country runner may have developed a stress fracture of the 5th metatarsal.

Perhaps the limp has been a recurrent one. Have there been prior episodes, and, if so, did they follow any specific activities? The pain of chondromalacia patellae may recur after repetitive deep knee bends or squatting. A subluxable patella may present with recurrent episodes of acute knee pain followed by swelling. Can the child pinpoint the area of pain or discomfort? Locating the problem greatly reduces the types and numbers of disorders to be considered. Remember, however, that pain may be referred. Disorders affecting the hip may present as knee pain. Pain in the hip may be

TABLE 35-1. Important Causes of Limp by Age at Presentation

	1 to 3 Years	4 to 8 Years	9 to 16 Years
Trauma	Toddler's fracture Battered child	Muscle bruises	Stress fractures Ligamentous strains Subluxation of patella
Infection	Osteomyelitis Septic arthritis Cellulitis	Osteomyelitis Septic arthritis Adenitis	Osteomyelitis Septic arthritis Gonococcal
Other Causes	Juvenile rheumatoid arthritis Congenital dislocated hip	Toxic synovitis Legg-Calvé-Perthes disease	Osgood-Schlatter disease Slipped femoral epiphysis

referred from the spine, such as an intervertebral disk space infection (diskitis), or from an intraabdominal process, such as an acute iliac adenitis.

The limp may not be present constantly. Stiffness of joints upon arising in the morning or after periods of inactivity is frequently seen in juvenile rheumatoid arthritis. The limp associated with hyperextensible joints, particularly flat feet, may not become apparent until later in the day or after prolonged standing.

Systemic symptoms are important diagnostic clues. The presence of fever should direct attention to inflammatory and infectious disorders and away from traumatic causes of limp. Weight loss similarly should suggest the possibility of inflammatory, infectious, or neoplastic disorders.

The perinatal history may disclose evidence of a difficult delivery with trauma or anoxia resulting in cerebral palsy and a spastic gait. Developmental delay, particularly in motor skills, suggests the possibility of neurologic or muscle disorders. Inheritable disorders of muscles or the nervous system that may result in weakness, ataxia, or sensory deficits resulting in a limp should be sought in the family history. Reactions to drugs producing serum sickness or ataxia must be considered. A preceding muscular injection, such as an immunization, may have been forgotten.

The social history should also be reviewed. Family upheavals or discord may suggest the possibility of child abuse. Stressful situations at home or school may have led to an hysterical limp

PHYSICAL EXAMINATION

A limp cannot be considered simply a manifestation of lower extremity disease. The patient as a whole must be evaluated both historically and physically.

It is important to observe the child's gait unencumbered by clothing or examination gowns. A small room is not enough space to evaluate the gait. A hallway at least 20 feet long is required. It may be necessary to have the child run in order to exaggerate the limp.

A normal gait is usually graceful and fluid, although many persons have characteristic gaits that allow them to be picked out of a crowd. Painful limps are generally associated with an *antalgic* gait (against pain). The child with an antalgic gait takes short steps on the affected side, bearing as little weight as possible on that extremity. Nonpainful limps come in a variety of forms. A shortened extremity may cause the child to toe walk or lurch toward that side, but so may a child with spastic cerebral palsy or a flexion contracture of a knee. A waddling gait may be produced by bilateral congenitally dislocated hips or pelvic girdle muscle weakness. The ataxic gait is broad-based and unsteady.

Observation of the child's gait often helps in focusing on the etiology of the limp, but better definition and confirmation are afforded by close inspection and palpation. A simple but often neglected clue is the general appearance: Does the child look sick? Does the skin provide any clues? The rash of the systemic form of juvenile rheumatoid arthritis is macular, pink, and fleeting. Serum sickness is associated with urticarial lesions, Henoch-Schönlein purpura with purpuric or petechial lesions, and dermatomyositis with papular, erythematous, scaly eruptions over elbows, knees, and knuckles. Are there localized areas of erythema or swelling? The extremities, both upper and lower, should be palpated carefully. The detection of subtle changes in temperature, swelling, or pain may pay large diagnostic dividends.

Each joint should be put through its full range of motion. One may use their own joint mobility, providing it is normal, as a comparison. Pain on motion of an extremity or of a particular joint must be noted. Muscle strength is evaluted during these movements and the circumferences of the thighs and calves compared. A diminution in muscle mass occurs rapidly if the extremity is not used normally. Leg length should be measured, using the distance from the anterior superior iliac spine to the medial malleolus.

PAINFUL LIMPS

Trauma

Episodes of trauma are the most common causes of limps. The trauma may range from a simple muscle bruise, to ligamentous strains and sprains, to bone fractures. The onset of a limp associated with trauma is usually acute, and the site of pain often can be pinpointed by the patient or during the physical examination.

Battered Child. Unusual injuries or skin lesions compounded by conflicting or inappropriate accompanying explanations should raise the suspicion of child abuse.

Toddler's Fracture. Toddler's fracture is an undisplaced fracture of the tibia, usually the result of a sudden twisting pull on the toddler's leg. The fracture usually is not visible on roentgenograms for seven to ten days, thereby confounding the correct diagnosis.

Subluxation of Patella. Sudden lateral displacement of the patella followed by pain and subsequent swelling of the knee most frequently occurs in preadolescent girls. The patella usually is not dislocated when the child is examined, but once the knee swelling has subsided the excessive mobility of the patella can be tested by pushing it cephalad and laterally. If the patella is subluxable, this procedure will result in apprehension and guarding by the child—the patellar apprehension test.

Inflammation

Included in this important group of disorders are infectious causes of limp such as osteomyelitis, septic arthritis, and cellulitis. Any single swollen, tender joint should be considered infected until proven otherwise by removal of joint fluid for examination and culture. Other important disorders to consider in this group include the following:

Toxic Synovitis. Toxic synovitis is a common cause of hip pain in children is acute in onset and usually transient. It occurs most frequently in 4- to 8-year-olds. Decreased flexion and rotation associated with pain are found on examination. Trauma, upper respiratory infections, and allergic responses have been suggested as causes of synovitis. Toxic synovitis of the hip must differentiated primarily from septic arthritis and Legg-Calvé-Perthes (LCP) disease. Roentgenograms may show a distended hip joint capsule or LCP. Children with toxic synovitis of the hip may develop LCP over the subsequent 6 to 12 months.

Juvenile Rheumatoid Arthritis (JRA). Three presentations of JRA are recognized. The most common is a chronic polyarthritis involving six or more joints. Hand involvement is common in this type of the disease. The systemic form of JRA is characterized by high spiking fevers, a fleeting macular rash, anemia, and neutrophilia. The pauciarticular form of JRA involves five or fewer joints and has the best prognosis. Monarticular (one joint) involvement is not uncommon. Inexplicably, children, particularly girls under the age of 5 years with positive antinuclear antibody titers, are at greatest risk for the development of an insidious, chronic inflammation of the eye in this form of JRA with the most benign joint involvement.

Diagnosis of JRA is one of exclusion. There are no confirmatory diagnostic tests. The rheumatoid factor, present in 85% of adults with rheumatoid arthritis, is found in only 15% of children with this disease. Morning stiffness is a common finding.

Osteochondroses

Avascular necrosis of various epiphyses in the lower extremities produce characteristic clinical pictures that should be readily recognized (Table 35-2).

Bone and Cartilage Lesions

Slipped Capital Femoral Epiphysis. Displacement of the femoral head on the neck of the femur usually occurs insidiously. Pain is usually mild located in the groin or referred to the anteromedial aspect of the thigh. Diminished internal rotation, flexion, and abduction of the involved hip is found. Males, usually between 11 and 15 years, are affected 2 to 5 times more frequently than females. Half of the males with a slipped femoral epiphysis are overweight and have a female type of body fat distribution. Roentgenograms will confirm the slippage.

Osteochondritis Dissecans. The knee is the joint most frequently affected by osteochondritis dissecans. A piece of cartilage separates most commonly from the medial femoral condyle causing mild recurrent arthralgia, unexplained joint effusions, and occasional episodes of knee-locking. The knee pain usually can be pinpointed by the child. Males in the 8- to 15-year range are more commonly affected than females.

Chondromalacia Patellae. Scoring of the cartilaginous surface of the patella may produce an antalgic gait, but more commonly results in an annoying aching of the knees. Crepitation on movement of the relaxed patella over the knee joint and acute knee pain as the patella is forced to slide against the knee joint as the thigh muscles are contracted occur.

Neoplastic Disorders

Leukemia or lymphoma may be characterized by leg pain and limp or may mimic rheumatoid arthritis with joint swelling and pain. Anemia and thrombocytopenia are important clues to these disorders. Osteogenic sarcoma, metastatic bone lesions, and osteoid osteomas are usually visible on roentgenographic examination. The complaint of localized bone pain should always be thoroughly examined for these disorders.

Acute Adenitis

Inflammation of iliac or inguinal nodes may irritate the hip joint capsule and cause pain and limp. Careful, deep palpation of the lower quadrants of the abdomen along the iliac crest and inguinal ligament are necessary to detect iliac adenopathy.

TABLE 35-2. Osteochrondroses—Avascular Necroses

Disease	Involved Bone	Typical Age	Sex	Symptoms
Legg-Calvé-Perthes	Femoral head	4–8 yr	M 5:1	Pain may be referred to knee
Osgood-Schlatter	Tibial tubercle	11–15 yr	M	Tenderness present
Sever's	Os calcis	8–12 yr	M	Painful heel syndrome
Köhler's	Tarsal navicular	3–6 yr	M	
Freiberg's	Second metatarsal	teens	F	

NONPAINFUL LIMPS

Neurologic Disorders

A variety of neurologic disorders can produce an abnormal gait or limp. The circumduction swing of the leg in a child with a hemiplegia or the jerky, stiff gait of spastic cerebral palsy are two easily recognizable gait disturbances. Ataxia from a variety of causes produces a broad-based unsteady gait.

Muscle Disorders

In most cases of primary muscle disease, delayed developmental milestones and hypotonia will have prompted medical consultation rather than an abnormal gait. Children with sex-linked muscular dystrophy, however, may first present with parental concern about a waddling gait. Pseudohypertrophy of the calf muscles and a positive Gower's sign (child climbs up his own body to attain a standing position) suggest this diagnosis.

Joint Disorders

Congenital Dislocated Hip (CDH). Occasionally, cases of CDH escape detection in the neonatal period. The child with a unilateral dislocated hip stands as if the affected leg is shortened. The pelvis dips toward the opposite side when the child walks. Limited abduction and internal rotation are found on examination of the hip. If both sides are dislocated, a waddling gait is produced. Roentgenograms of the hips confirm the diagnosis.

Bony Deformities

Leg Length Discrepancy. One leg may be congenitally shorter than the other, resulting in a shifting type of gait. If the discrepancy is large, the child may toe walk on the shortened side. The apparent short extremity may be the normal-sized one in the child with hemihypertrophy. Leg lengths should be measured from the anterior superior iliac spine to the medial malleolus.

The duration of the limp, the age of the child, the presence or absence of systemic symptoms, as well as consideration of disorders occurring most frequently, all help in narrowing the diagnostic choices to consider in the child with a limp.

BIBLIOGRAPHY

Illingworth CM: 128 limping children with no fracture, sprain, or obvious cause. Clin Pediatr 17:139, 1978

A discussion of the causes of limps in a series of children presenting to an emergency room.

Jacobs BW: Synovitis of the hip in children and its significance. Pediatrics 47:558, 1971

Worthwhile and informative information about the most common cause of hip pain in children.

Salter RB: Gait disturbances and limp in childhood. In Green M, Haggerty RJ, (eds): Ambulatory Pediatrics, pp 232-236. Philadelphia, WB Saunders, 1968

A general overview of the limping child.

Singer J: Evaluation of acute and insidious gait disturbance in children less than five years of age. Adv. Pediatr 26:209, 1979

A step-by-step evaluation of the child with a limp.

Principles of Antimicrobial Therapy

36

Julia A. McMillan

Recommendations about antimicrobial therapy are based on past studies of the usual susceptibilities of the various microorganisms, the pharmacology of the antimicrobial agents, and clinical studies of the treatment of human infections. Many review articles and textbooks deal with these principles in detail and in depth. The purpose of this chapter is to provide a simple introduction to these principles and to indicate some special differences in the pediatric age group.

DECIDING TO USE ANTIBIOTICS

The severity of the illness is an important factor in deciding whether to use an antibiotic. A child with a small skin abscess usually does not need to be treated with an antibiotic in addition to incision and drainage; but a large skin abscess, poorly localized, with surrounding erythema usually should be treated with an antibiotic.

Young age or underlying host disease often influence the clinician to use an antibiotic as an exception to the general rule. For example, a small skin abscess in a newborn infant should be treated with an antibiotic because of the newborn's poorer resistance.

The patient's cooperation is another important factor. In some situations in which the patient is unlikely or unable to return for medication or to fill a prescription, antibiotic therapy may be used if a delay would ordinarily be made for culture or reexamination. For example, intramuscular benzathine penicillin may be appropriate in an emergency room for a child with exudative pharyngitis before results of the throat culture for beta-hemolytic streptococci are known, if follow-up contact is unlikely. If the patient's clinical picture is most consistent with viral disease, antibiotics should, of course, be withheld.

SELECTING AN ANTIBIOTIC

Careful assessment of the type and severity of clinical illness is important in choosing an antibiotic. The age of the patient is also a critical factor in determining the therapeutic agent and the route of administration. In the newborn infant, almost any sign of infection requires careful evaluation including cultures of the blood, urine, and CSF. The antibiotics selected for this vulnerable patient must be effective against the most common pathogens in the newborn, and usually they should be administered intravenously so that effective serum concentrations may be achieved as quickly as possible.

In the older child, clinical signs and symptoms may prove to be more useful in determining the selection of antibiotics. The child with otitis media or pneumonia may be treated, at least initially, with the antimicrobial agent or agents known to eradicate the likely pathogens causing the specific clinial disease.

The Gram stain may be helpful in determining the initial antibiotic therapy. Pus should always be Gram-stained to provide a preliminary guide to the likely organism involved. Often, however, there is no material available for the Gram stain, or the clinical condition is serious enough that therapeutic choice should not depend upon the staining characteristics of the organism (*e.g.,* in meningitis). When the Gram stain is not helpful, the initial choice of an antibiotic must depend upon the clinical clues. Culture and susceptibility testing determine the appropriateness of that choice.

Table 36-1 lists the recommended choices of antibiotics in selected clinical situations according to the age of the patient. Guidelines for selection of antibiotics in children change periodically as new information is accumulated regarding drug toxicities and bacterial susceptibility. Pediatric journals and the *Medical Letter on Drugs and Therapeutics* should be consulted for the most current information. The *Physicians Desk Reference* is updated annually and is another useful source of drug information.

Convenience and cost are factors involved in selection of an antibiotic if all other considerations are equal.

PHARMACOLOGIC PRINCIPLES

The effectiveness of orally administered antibiotics depends upon the degree with which they are absorbed from the gastrointestinal tract. Concomitant ingestion of food decreases subsequent serum levels of some oral antibiotics. Parents should be advised to give oral ampicillin and any of the oral cephalosporins on an empty stomach. Simultaneous ingestion of food does not affect the absorption of ampicillin, erythromycin, chloramphenicol, or clindamycin.

Excretion and inactivation of antibiotics in newborn infants deserve some special consideration. In the first week of life, conjugation and excretion by the immature liver is limited, so that chloramphenicol blood levels may increase to toxic levels and produce vascular collapse and death (gray syndrome). Because of this possibility, chloramphenicol is not used in the newborn period, except in special situations in which it is clearly a superior drug and when blood levels can be monitored.

The renal excretion of many drugs is decreased in the first week of life, so that recommended dosages are decreased, especially in the case of aminoglycosides such as gentamicin. In low birth weight infants, renal and hepatic functions are even more decreased than in full term infants, so that even lower dosages, based on past pharmacologic studies, are recommended. The current *Physician's Desk Reference,* or the package circular, can also be consulted for appropriate antibiotic doses for newborn infants and for children with renal or hepatic disease.

In children, intramuscular injections are often limited by the muscle size of young infants or patients with muscle atrophy. In some diseases, intramuscular injections might interfere with observation of the function of the leg (*e.g.,* in paralysis or osteomyelitis). Skin diseases, particularly burns, limit muscles available for injection. Inaccurately placed injection into the gluteal area can cause sciatic nerve palsy, particularly in young children. Excessive injections into the anterior thigh can cause quadriceps-femoris contractures in infants. Use of 1½-inch needles in the lateral thigh of infants can cause thrombosis of the femoral artery. If the lateral thigh is injected in small infants,

TABLE 36-1. Recommended Antibiotic Therapy for Selected Pediatric Infections

Clinical Diagnosis	Typical pathogen(s)	Antibiotic(s)
Newborn		
Skin infections	Staphylococcus	Nafcillin with or without gentamicin for synergy
Omphalitis	Staphylococcus, gram-negative rods	Nafcillin with an aminoglycoside
Sepsis/meningitis	Group B streptococcus Gram-negative rods	Ampicillin with an aminoglycoside
Urinary tract infection	Gram-negative rods	Ampicillin with or without an aminoglycoside
Minor Illness in Older Children		
Streptococcal pharyngitis	*Streptococcus*	Penicillin, oral or IM, or erythromycin, oral
Otitis media	*H. influenzae* Pneumococcus *Streptococcus*	Ampicillin, oral, or Cefaclor, oral, or Pediazole (erythromycin plus sulfisoxazole), oral
Urinary tract infection	*E. coli* and other gram negative rods	Ampicillin or sulfisoxazole, oral
Skin or wound infection	Staphylococcus Streptococcus	Dicloxacillin, oral
Pneumonia	Pneumococcus	Penicillin, oral
Cellulitis	Staphylococcus Streptococcus	Dicloxacillin, oral
Cervical adenitis	Staphylococcus Streptococcus	Dicloxacillin, oral
Major Illness in Older Children		
Pneumonia	Pneumococcus *H. influenzae*	Ampicillin, IV
Urinary tract infection	Gram-negative rods	Ampicillin or an amino-glycoside, IV
Epiglotitis	*H. influenzae*	Ampicillin or chloramphenicol, IV
Facial cellulitis	*H. influenzae*	Ampicillin or chloramphenicol, IV
Orbital cellulitis	*H. influenzae* Staphylococcus Streptococcus	Ampicillin or chloramphenicol along with nafcillin, both IV
Bone and joint infection	Staphylococcus Streptococcus	Nafcillin, IV
Sepsis	Pneumococcus *H. influenzae* Streptococcus Staphylococcus Gram-negative rods	Chloramphenicol and/or ampicillin, IV
Meningitis	*H. influenzae* *N. meningiditis* Pneumococcus	Chloramphenicol and/or ampicillin, IV. NOTE. The cephalosporins do not reach the CNS in concentrations high enough to treat meningitis.

a 1-inch needle should be used and inserted obliquely into the muscle mass. If anatomic landmarks and proper direction of the needle perpendicular to the surface are carried out, the gluteal area can be used in chldren over 2 years of age who have developed their gluteal muscles by walking.

TOXICITY AND SIDE-EFFECTS

Usually, an antibiotic should be discontinued at the first clinical or laboratory sign of a known associated toxic effect. Toxic effects that are especially important in children are shown in Table 36-2.

ANTIBIOTIC DOSAGE FOR CHILDREN

As the size of children varies, so does the proper dosage of antibiotics. Although body surface area measured in meters squared gives the best estimate of the appropriate dosage, most calculations are based on weight alone. For the aminoglycosides and chloramphenicol, suggested doses must be verified by serum levels determined following the initiation of therapy. The serum concentration required for adequate antibacterial effect is very close to the toxic concentration for these drugs, and the determination of serum concentrations allows optimal therapy without undue risk.

When there is doubt about the effectiveness of an antibiotic because of suspected antibiotic resistance of the pathogen, laboratory evaluation may be helpful. The mean inhibitory concentration (MIC) and mean bactericidal concentration (MBC) determine the smallest concentration of the antibiotic necessary to prevent growth (MIC) and to kill (MBC) the organism. The results of these tests may be compared with

TABLE 36-2. Most Common Adverse Effect of Antibiotics in Infants and Children

Antibiotics	Adverse Effects
Penicillin*	Allergic reaction, renal and CNS toxicity in very high doses
Ampicillin	Rash, GI upset, CNS irritation in large doses
Semisynthetic penicillins (*e.g.*, dicloxacillin, nafcillin)	Nephritis, bone marrow suppression, liver enzyme elevation
Aminoglycosides† (gentamicin, tobramycin, amikacin, kanamycin)	Renal and ototoxicity
Cephalosporins‡	Same as penicillins
Chloramphenicol	Aplastic anemia (rarely), transient bone marrow suppression, gray syndrome in newborns.
Tetracycline	Teeth staining. A problem during fetal life and as long as teeth are developing. Should not be prescribed for pregnant or nursing women.
Erythromycin	GI disturbance, allergic reactions, hepatic dysfunction with estolate form
Clindamycin	Enterocolitis
Trimethoprim	Bone marrow suppression
Sulfonamides	Hyperbilirubinemia in newborns, renal, hepatic, bone marrow, and cutaneous reactions in older children
Rifampin	GI upset, CNS disturbances, bone marrow suppression. May cause reddish color of urine, tears, and other body fluids.
Isoniazid	Hepatitis and neuropathy—much less common in children than in adults

*The penicillins, including ampicillin and the semisynthetic forms, inhibit the synthesis of bacterial cell walls. Modification of the basic structure has given rise to antibiotics that are effective against gram-negative as well as gram-positive organisms (*e.g.*, ampicillin) and to agents that are able to resist enzymatic degradation by beta-lactamases (*e.g.*, semisynthetic penicillins including nafcillin, methicillin, oxacillin, dicloxacillin).

†The aminoglycosides inhibit bacterial protein synthesis. This is a growing group of antibiotics that is most active against gram-negative organisms. They are not well absorbed from the gastrointestinal tract and must be given parenterally.

‡The cephalosporins resemble the penicillins in structure, but are relatively resistant to the action of beta-lactamase. This is a large and increasing group of antibiotics that are active against a variety of gram-negative and gram-positive organisms. Some cephalosporins are well absorbed from the gastrointestinal tract, but others must be given parenterally.

TABLE 36-3. Dosages for Antibiotics Commonly Used in Pediatrics

Antibiotic	Dose	Interval	Comment
Penicillin G	25–50 mg/kg/d, oral 200,000 to 300,000 units/kg/d, IV	q 6 hr q 3 hr	Same dose for penicillin V
benzathine	50,000 units/kg IM	1 dose	
procaine	25,000 to 50,000 units/kg/d IM	q 12–24 hr	
Ampicillin	50–100 mg/kg/d	q 6 hr	Amoxicillin is a derivative of ampicillin and is better absorbed. It may be given q 8 hr.
Nafcillin	200–400 mg/kg/d, IV	q 4 hr	Same dose for oxacillin and methicillin
Dicloxacillin	25–50 mg/kg/d, oral	q 6 hr	Cloxacillin has the same spectrum, but the dose must be doubled.
Erythromycin	20–40 mg/kg/d, oral	q 6 hr	
Carbenicillin	30–50 mg/kg/d, oral 400–600 mg/kg/d IV	q 6 hr q 6 hr	Should be used in combination with an aminoglycoside for treatment of infection due to Pseudomonas aeruginosa.
Cefaclor	40–60 mg/kg/d, oral	q 6–8 hr	
Cefazolin	50–100 mg/kg/d IV	q 6 hr	The same dose may be used for cefoxitin, cephaloradine, cephalothin, cephapirin.
Cephalexin	25–50 mg/kg/d, oral	q 6 hr	
Chloramphenicol	50–100 mg/kg/d, oral or IV	q 6 hr	
Clindamycin	10–25 mg/kg/d, oral 20–40 mg/kg/d, IV	q 6 hr q 6 hr	
Gentamycin	3–7.5 mg/kg/d, oral or IM	q 8 hr	Same dose for tobramycin
Isoniazid	10–20 mg/kg/d, oral	q 12–24 hr	It is not necessary to use supplemental pyridoxine in children.
Kanamycin	15–30 mg/kg/d, IV	q 8 hr	Same dose for amikacin
Sulfisoxazole	120–150 mg/kg/d, oral	q 6 hr	
Ticarcillin	200–300 mg/kg/d	q 6 hr	Used with aminoglycoside to treat *Pseudomonas aeruginosa*.
Trimethoprim-sulfamethoxazole	6–12 mg TMP/30–60 mg SMX/kg/d, oral	q 12 hr	For treatment of *Pneumocystis carinii* pneumonia, this dosage should be increased to 20 mg TMP/100 mg SMX/kg/d divided q 6 hr.

the serum concentrations achieved in the patient. The serum bactericidal titer (SBT) is another useful test of antibiotic effectiveness. Serum samples are obtained from the patient after a dose of antibiotic has been given. The organism isolated from the patient is then incubated with dilutions of the serum, and the dilution at which the organism is killed is the SBT.

Table 36-3 lists the dosages of antibiotics that are frequently used for children. Dosages for the newborn are not included, since the recommendations for antibiotics in the newborn are constantly being revised.

BIBLIOGRAPHY

Eichenwald HF, McCracken GH: Antimicrobial therapy in infants and children: a review of antimicrobial agents and therapy of infectious conditions. J Pediatr 93:337, 1978

A recent review article.

Evans WE, Feldman S, Barker LF, *et al:* Use of gentamicin serum levels to individualize therapy in children. J. Pediatr 93:133, 1978

Review of methods of obtaining and interpreting gentamicin serum concentrations.

Grossman ER, Walcheck A, Freedman H: Tetracycline and permanent teeth: the relation between dose and tooth color. Pediatrics 47:567, 1971

A description of tooth staining by tetracycline.

Kagan BM: Antimicrobial Therapy. Philadelphia, WB Saunders, 1974

An excellent general reference.

Klein JO: Current usage of antimicrobial combinations in pediatrics. Pediatr Clin North Am 21:443, 1974

Discussion of combinations of antibiotics.

Levine BB: Skin rashes with penicillin therapy: current management. New Engl J Med 286:42, 1972

Discussion of ampicillin rashes.

Moffet HL: Pediatric Infectious Diseases: A Problem-Oriented Approach. Philadelphia, JB Lippincott, 1975

Chapter 21 is a more detailed discussion of principles and individual antibiotics.

Nelson JD: Pocketbook of Pediatric Antimicrobial Therapy. Waco, Texas, Hill Printing and Stationery Co., 1979-80

A very useful list of recommended dosages.

Sutherland JM: Fatal cardiovascular collapse of infants receiving large amounts of chloramphenicol. Am J Dis Child 97:761, 1959

A description and discussion of the gray syndrome.

Poisoning

37

Frank A. Oski

Accidents, drownings, and poisonings are the leading causes of death in children between the ages of 1 and 16 years. Almost 1000 deaths per year occur from poisoning in children under 5 years of age; most of these are preventable.

In many instances of poisoning, parental negligence is largely responsible. In close to three-quarters of all poisonings in childhood, there is some evidence of disruption in the household. These include one-parent homes, mother-father strife, a recent move, an illness in a member of the household, or the presence of visitors in the home that have altered normal routines. In every instance of poisoning, a careful social history should be obtained. Help should be provided for the family in dealing with the basic problem that may have been directly or indirectly responsible for the child's ingestion.

Poisoning, either acute or chronic, should always be suspected when there has been a change in a child's state of consciousness or pattern of behavior.

Parental counseling is the best way to prevent poisoning in the home. When parents have children 6 to 9 months of age, they must be urged to poison-proof their homes. The creeping infant or toddler can gain access to many dangerous items. Some simple instructions should include:

1. Keep all drugs, pesticides, and potentially poisonous household chemicals out of the reach of children and away from all foods.
2. Do not store poisons or inflammable materials in food containers or bottles.
3. Lock up all dangerous substances.
4. Never tell children that their medicine is "candy" to induce them to take it. They may remember this later and innocently eat it.

The principles of management of poisonings include:

1. Identification of the drug or chemical as quickly as possible
2. Evacuation of the poison from the stomach, except where contraindicated
3. Administration of a specific, or nonspecific, antidote if available
4. Symptomatic and supportive therapy, as necessary.

IDENTIFICATION OF THE DRUG OR CHEMICAL

Usually the ingested material can be identified by a careful history. Information regarding the specific ingredients in a commercial preparation should be available from a product label, a manufacturer, or a poison information center.

The 12 most common causes of poisoning in the pediatric age group in order of frequency are: aspirin, diazepam, acetaminophen, vitamins, isopropyl alcohol, Dimetapp, Desitin, flurazepam hydrochloride, hydrogen peroxide, penicillin, Percodan, and phencyclidine hydrochloride. In children under 5 years of age, the most common sources of poisoning are aspirin, vitamins, and acetaminophen. Over 60% of all overdoses occur in children under 5 years of age and approximately one-fourth of these accidents produce symptoms in the child.

Always attempt to determine as rapidly as possible what and how much was taken. Assume that the largest estimated amount was consumed when planning therapy. All vomitus, urine, and containers should be saved to assist in identification of the poison when its identiy cannot be established.

Clues to the nature of the poison can be obtained from the physical examination. Burns on the lip, mouth, or tongue, difficulty in swallowing, or excessive salivation suggest that a corrosive substance has been ingested. A gasoline odor on the breath or clothing should suggest that a petroleum distillate has been swallowed.

Combinations of signs and symptoms that suggest specific types of poisons are listed in Table 37-1. See list for description of emergency symptoms and signs.

REMOVAL OF THE POISON

Emesis should be induced following poisoning except when the material ingested is a corrosive or a petroleum distillate, or when the patient is comatose, convulsing, or already vomiting bloody material.

Emesis is induced by the administration of 5 ml syrup of ipecac followed by the administration of 6 to 8 oz water. If no vomiting occurs within 15 minutes, the ipecac may be safely repeated in patients over 5 years of age.

If emesis has not occurred, gastric lavage should be performed. In comatose patients, lavage should not be attempted unless proper protection has been provided for the airway with an endotracheal tube to prevent aspiration. The patient should be placed on his left side, with his head hanging over the table during lavage. The contents of the stomach should be aspirated before lavage is instituted.

TABLE 37-1. Symptom Complexes Suggestive of Specific Poisons

Symptoms and Signs	Possible Poison
Agitation, hallucinations, dilated pupils, bright red color of the skin, dry skin, and fever	Atropinelike agents, LSD
Marked activity, tremors, headache, diarrhea, dry mouth with foul ordor, sweating, tachycardia, arrhythmia, dilated pupils	Amphetamines
Slow respirations, pinpoint pupils, euphoria, or coma	Opiates
Salivation, lacrimation, urination, defecation, meiosis, and pulmonary congestion	Organic phosphates or poison mushrooms
Sleepiness, slurred speech, nystagmus, ataxia	Barbiturates or tranquilizers
Hyperpnea, fever, and vomiting	Salicylates
Oculogyric crisis, ataxia, and unusual posturing of head and neck	Phenothiazines
Lethargy, cerebellar sign agitation, miosis salivation, insensitivity to pain, seizures	Phencyclidine

Gastric lavage becomes mandatory if ipecac does not induce vomiting. Ipecac left in the stomach is an irritant, and when absorbed, it is a cardiac toxin capable of producing conduction disturbances and myocarditis.

ANTIDOTES

Many drugs are adsorbed by activated charcoal. Charcoal should never be given before or with ipecac because it will adsorb the ipecac and render it ineffective. The administration of 2 tbsp activated charcoal in 8 oz water should follow emesis or lavage when dealing with drugs for which charcoal is a useful antidote (see list). Specific antidotes are described in Table 37-2.

SUPPORTIVE THERAPY

The goal of supportive therapy is to maintain the patient in a satisfactory condition until normal renal and hepatic function rids the body of the offending agent. Therapy may include respiratory support, treatment of shock, correction of fluid losses, correction of anemia or coagulation disturbances, treatment of seizures, and treatment of renal or hepatic failure. Attention to detail is required in the event of poisoning in order to save the patient's life and reduce morbidity.

Drugs and Other Agents Adsorbed by Activated Charcoal

Amphetamines	Morphine
Antipyrine	Muscarine
Aspirin	Nicotine
Atropine	Opium
Barbiturates	Parathion
Camphor	Penicillin
Cantharides	Phenol
Chlorpheniramine	Phenolphthalein
Cocaine	Primaquine
Colchicine	Propoxyphene
Digitalis	Quinine
Diphenylhydantoin	Salicylates
Glutethimide	Sulfonamides
Iodine	Strychnine
Ipecac	

TABLE 37-2 Poisons and their Specific Antidotes

Poison	Antidote
Arsenic, bismuth, chromium, cobalt, copper, iron, lead, magnesium, radium, selenium, and uranium	BAL
Lead, mercury, copper, nickel, zinc, cobalt, beryllium, and manganese	EDTA
Cyanide	Sodium nitrite
Narcotics	Naloxone (Narcan)
Warfarin, dicumerol	Vitamin K_1
Ferrous sulfate	Deferoxamine
Methanol, ethylene glycol	Ethanol
Insecticides that are cholinesterase inhibitors	Atropine
Amphetamines	Chlorpromazine
Phenothiazines	Diphenhydramine
Carbon monoxide	Oxygen
Nitrite-induced methemoglobinemia	Methylene blue

Emergency Symptoms and Signs That may be Encountered in Poisoning

Ataxia
- Alcohol
- Barbiturates
- Bromides
- Carbon monoxide
- Diphenylhydantoin
- Hallucinogens
- Heavy metals
- Organic solvents
- Phencyclidine
- Tranquilizers

Convulsions and muscle twitching
- Alcohol
- Amphetamines
- Antihistamines
- Boric acid
- Camphor
- Chlorinated hydrocarbon insecticides (DDT)
- Cyanide
- Lead
- Organic phosphate insecticides
- Phencyclidine
- Plants (lily-of-the-valley, azalea, iris, water hemlock)
- Salicylates
- Strychnine
- Withdrawal from barbiturates, benzodiazepines (Valium, Librium), meprobamate

Coma and drowsiness
- Alcohol (ethyl)
- Antihistamines
- Barbiturates and other hypnotics
- Carbon monoxide
- Narcotic depressants (opiates)
- Salicylates
- Tranquilizers

Paralysis
- Botulism
- Heavy metals
- Plants (coniine in poison hemlock)
- Triorthocresyl phosphate

Pupils

Pinpoint
- Mushrooms (muscarine)
- Narcotic depressants (opiates)
- Organic phosphate insecticides
- Phencyclidine

Dilated
- Amphetamines
- Antihistamines
- Atropine
- Barbiturates (coma)
- Cocaine
- Ephedrine
- LSD
- Methanol
- Withdrawal (narcotic depressants)

Nystagmus on lateral gaze
- Barbiturates
- Minor tranquilizers (meprobamate, benzodiazepine)

Pulse rate

Slow
- Digitalis
- Lily-of-the-valley
- Narcotic depressants

Rapid
- Alcohol
- Amphetamines
- Atropine
- Ephedrine

Respiratory alterations

Rapid
- Amphetamines
- Barbiturates (early)
- Carbon monoxide
- Methanol
- Petroleum distillates
- Salicylates

Wheezing & pulmonary edema
- Mushrooms (muscarine type)
- Narcotic depressants (opiates)
- Organic phosphate insecticides
- Petroleum distillates

Slow or *Depressed*
- Alcohol
- Barbiturates (late)
- Narcotic depressants (opiates)
- Tranquilizers

Paralysis
- Organic phosphate insecticides
- Botulism

Emergency Symptoms and Signs That may be Encountered in Poisoning *(Continued)*

Mouth
- *Salivation*
  - Arsenic
  - Corrosive
  - Mercury
  - Mushrooms
  - Organic phosphate insecticides
  - Phencyclidine
  - Thallium
- *Dryness*
  - Atropine
  - Amphetamines
  - Antihistamines
  - Narcotic depressants

Breath odor
- Acetone: acetone, alcohol (methyl, isopropyl), phenol, salicylates
- Alcohol: alcohol (ethyl)
- Bitter almonds: cyanide
- Coal gas: carbon monoxide
- Garlic: arsenic, phosphorus, organic phosphate insecticides, thallium
- Oil of wintergreen: methyl salicylate
- Petroleum: petroleum distillates
- Violets: turpentine

Skin color
- *Jaundice* (hepatic or hemolytic)
  - Aniline
  - Arsenic
  - Carbon tetrachloride
  - Castor bean
  - Fava bean
  - Mushroom
  - Naphthalene
  - Yellow phosphorus
- *Cyanosis*
  - Aniline dyes
  - Carbon monoxide
  - Cyanide
  - Nitrites
  - Strychnine
- *Red Flush*
  - Alcohol
  - Antihistamines
  - Atropine
  - Boric acid
  - Carbon monoxide
  - Nitrites

Violent emesis often with hematemesis
- Aminophylline
- Bacterial food poisoning
- Boric acid
- Corrosives
- Fluoride
- Heavy metals
- Phenol
- Salicylates

Abdominal colic
- Black widow spider bite
- Heavy metals
- Narcotic depressant withdrawal

BIBLIOGRAPHY

Arena J: Poisoning—treatment and prevention. JAMA 232:1272, 1975

A review of the common causes of poisoning in children with suggestions for prevention.

Kaye S: Bedside toxicology. Pediatr Clin North Am 17:519, 1970

Helpful clues to the establishment of prompt diagnosis in the poisoned patient.

Mofenson HC, Greensher J: The unknown poison. Pediatrics 54:336, 1974

This article provides the reader with clues to the interpretation of physical findings which may point to the poison ingested by the patient.

Saracino M, Flowers J, Lovejoy FH, Jr: The epidemiology of poisoning from drug products. Am J Dis Child 134:763, 1980

This article is a study of the common offenders and provides a perspecitve on the nature of the problem.

The Newborn

38

Margaret L. Williams

Understanding normality and, therefore, abnormality in a newborn infant rests on a view of him or her individuality within a circumscribed age frame—already a product of several months' growth and development but still far from the maturity that will allow survival without considerable manipulation of the environment. Evaluation of physical findings, recognition of aberrations from the norm, and maneuvers in providing physical care all must be based on a knowledge of the normal progression of fetal to neonatal adaptation. This process, encompassing enormously rapid change, nevertheless produces a human being in whom every system has certain predictable immaturity; these "normal" peculiarities have significant impact on the infant's state of well-being. It is against this background that neonatal care must be considered.

INTRAUTERINE RISK

Assessment of risk during pregnancy can identify before delivery as many as 50% of infants who will have difficulty in the newborn period. An additional 30% of such infants are identifiable by a second assessment of risk during labor. These statistics stress the importance of obstetrical information in understanding the newborn's condition. Although formal risk assessment encompasses the evaluation of a large number of factors, the following broad categories of prenatal risk should be investigated for each birth:

Preexisting Maternal Disease. Although any serious illness in the mother confers risk on the fetus, the presence of diabetes, chronic hypertension, renal or significant cardiac disease are most often associated with unfavorable outcome of the fetus. In addition, history of familial illness, not necessarily expressed in the mother, may be of great importance.

Difficulty in Previous Pregnancies. Rh sensitization, a previous fetal or neonatal death, low birth-weight infant, or an infant with a major anomaly or with neurologic damage, statistically increase risk for the present infant.

Maternal Habitus and Life Style. Maternal age less than 17 years and greater than 35 years, shortness of stature, deficient diet, heavy smoking, intake of alcohol and poor socioeconomic status may compromise fetal well-being.

Morbidity in Present Pregnancy. Increased risk to the fetus is present with multiple pregnancies, evidence of poor fetal growth, third trimester bleeding, toxemia, hydramnios, Rh sensitization, and premature rupture of the membranes.

Premature Delivery. Neonatal mortality and morbidity are directly related to degree of prematurity. For this reason, knowledge of fetal maturity is important when early labor occurs spontaneously and particularly when circumstances dictate early delivery. Estimates of maturity based on clinical data including uterine size, which is often variable, time of maternal perception of fetal movement (18-20 weeks' gestation), and time when the fetal heart becomes audible (apparently 20 weeks) are not always accurate. Radiographic demonstration of bone maturity is also not generally helpful since calcification of epiphyses occur over a wide gestational range although the absence of the distal femoral epiphysis at birth does connote prematurity. Sonograhic measurement of the biparietal diameter of the fetal head between the 16th and 28th weeks of gestation probably represents the current most accurate assessment of maturity; however, this method is not reliable in later pregnancy.

Direct evidence of lung maturity is obtained from the lecithin-sphingomyelin ratio of fluid obtained ay amniocentesis. A value of 2.0 or above generally indicates maturity with resultant protection from the neonatal respiratory distress syndrome, while ratios of less than 1.5 are associated with immaturity and high risk of disease.

Prepartum and Intrapartum Risk. Significant jeopardy to the infant is associated with any situation in which uterine blood flow is decreased or fetoplacental integrity is impaired. These occur frequently in maternal toxemia, placenta previa and abruptio and in cord prolapse. Premature rupture of the membranes may lead to infection of the infant. Fetal compromise may be suspected by decrease in materanl urinary estrogens and by the occurrence of abnormalities in fetal heart rate and variability demonstrated by monitoring either before the onset of labor or during labor itself. The recognition of intrauterine hypoxia is essential information in caring for the newborn.

THE NORMAL NEWBORN

In the majority of births, the baby makes his way down the birth canal with no more serious difficulty than minor compression of the head. He enters a world of air and light, is separated from his intrauterine supply of oxygen and nutrients, takes a first breath, alters his circulation to increase pulmonary blood flow from 10% to 50% of the total cardiac output, and is ready for extrauterine life within minutes of birth. This transitional human being is covered with vernix (white cheesy material) and appears dusky but rapidly turns pink or red. First breaths are irregular but interspersed with lusty crying and the expulsion of much fluid from the upper airway. Tachycardia is present. In 15 to 30 minutes, a calmer, regular respiration is established, the heart rate drops and the infant falls asleep.

A complete examination should be conducted soon after birth. Alteration of usual adult examination techniques to avoid crying facilitates the procedure and serves to highlight findings unique to the infant. The following order is useful. The examination outlined here is generally geared to the full-term newborn infant who has no immediate indication of illness. Other specific physical signs will be discussed in a following section on the problem infant.

Total Inspection of Undressed Infant

Examination of the undressed infant should include assessment of the following:

Activity and Muscular Tone. The normal full-term infant lies with all limbs flexed and has much spontaneous vigorous movement.

Color. The skin is normally pink with some duskiness of lips, perioral area, or nails. Meconium staining of the skin, cord, and nails may indicate postmaturity or other intrauterine compromise. Other abnormalities to be noted include pallor, central (body) cyanosis, and jaundice, best evaluated by inspect skin blanched by fingertip pressure.

Skin Lesions. Pale wheals or papules with red bases, the so-called erythema toxicum are insignificant, but pustular, morbilliform or petechial rashes are of importance. The skin may be excessively dry, scaly, or cracked; this usually represents postmaturity.

Umbilical Cord. One vein and two arteries should be identified. A single umbilical artery correlates with the presence of other congenital anomalies, often renal. A halo of erythema on the abdominal skin around the cord or a red line extending cephalad from the umbilicus is indicative of omphalitis.

Examination of Chest

Contour. The normal infant chest is relatively flat: that is, the width is greater than the depth. An increased anterior-posterior diameter is generally indicative of air-trapping. Anterior bulging may be bilateral, unilateral (cardiac enlargement, diaphragmatic hernia), associated with a high diaphragm (diaphragmatic paralysis) or with a low diaphragm (overexpansion). Retraction or the pulling in of soft tissues suprasternally, subcostally, or intercostally denotes respiratory obstruction. Depression of the sternum may be a primary anatomic abnormality or may be secondary to the retraction. Other indications of compromised respiratory function to be checked at this time include flaring of the alae nasi and audible expiratory grunting.

Respiratory Rate. Normal respiratory rate in a quiet infant should not exceed 60 breaths per minute. Irregularity of rate may occur. Some infants show periodic breathing, and the duration of the apnea should be noted along with observation of related bradycardia or color change.

Lungs. Percussion is generally of little value, although hyperresonance may be present with a massive pneumothorax. Evaluation of air entry by auscultation is easier in an infant than an adult and can generally be correlated with adequacy of ventilation. Directly after birth, there are many adventitial sounds in the chest but persistence of rales, rhonchi, or wheezes at 3 to 4 hours of age are suggestive of disease.

Heart. The point of maximum impulse of the heart is much closer to the sternum in an infant than an adult, due to the anterior position of the predominant right ventricle. Percussion of heart size is unrewarding but careful auscultation for murmurs along the left sternal border, in the pulmonic area and at the apex is important. Thrills are rarely felt. Cardiac rate of the quiet infant lies between 110 and 160, but is extremely variable with agitation. Brachial and femoral pulses should be palpated. If the latter are decreased or absent, blood pressure should be measured in both upper and lower extremities to rule out coarctation of the aorta.

Examination of Abdomen

Contour. Distention is an important symptom in infants, denoting possible intestinal obstruction, infection, or food intolerance. A scaphoid abdomen may indicate displacement of abdominal organs as in diaphragmatic hernia.

Organ Size. The liver edge is generally right at the costal margin. Liver enlargement should be evaluated in terms of the position of the diaphragm. The spleen is rarely felt but a palpable tip is not abnormal. Both kidneys are usually palpable as 3.5 to 5.0 cm-long masses and are best felt by bimanual palpation. The presence of a palpable bladder should be noted and its disappearance at the time of the next voiding carefully checked. The anal opening should be observed for position, patency, and normal surrounding rugation.

Examination of Head and Neck

Contour of Head. Mean head circumference in a normal full-term infant is 35 cm with a range of 33.5 to 37.0 cm. Percentile distribution of circumference is available for each gestational age. Although there is great variation in the size of the fontanelles and the width of the sutures in newborns, excessively large fontanelles may indicate poor bone development as in intrauterine malnutrition, hypothyroidism, or osteogenesis imperfecta. Bulging of the fontanelle or sutures suggests increased intracranial pressure.

The compression of vaginal delivery can cause marked molding of the skull. Freely movable cranial bones can override one another at the suture lines causing considerable distortion of the head contour. In a full-term infant, overriding of bones at the sutures should disappear within the first few days but in small prematures, particularly those with poor growth, it may be palpable for weeks.

With signs of trauma, careful palpation of the skull should be carried out to detect possible fractures. These may appear as depressions or crepitation may be palpated. Occasionally a "ping-pong" sensation is detected, usually near the suture lines. This also may represent a fracture or merely poor calcification. Thickened edematous tissue over the head—so-called caput succedaneum—may result from presentation of scalp through the cervix in advance of the bony skull. More localized fluctuant swelling overlying a single cranial bone represents subperiosteal bleeding or cephalhematoma which is self-limiting and should not receive treatment. Occasionally, bleeding occurs outside the periosteum which will track down through the soft tissues and may be extensive enough to lead to anemia.

Face. Distinctive or bizarre facial features such as widely spaced or slanting eyes, low-set ears or underslung mandible should be noted, as should nerve weakness. Facial palsies due to 7th nerve damage are common and fortunately are generally transient. They usually occur from peripheral compression of the nerve *in utero* or by forceps, and involve both the lower face and the forehead. Facial palsies may originate in the central nervous system and then involve only the lower face. Easily confused with nerve weakness is hypoplasia of the depressor muscle of the mouth.

Eyes. Periorbital edema is often present at the first examination, the result of silver nitrate prophylaxis administered in the delivery room. Subconjunctival hemorrhages may be present, particularly with long labor or vertex delivery. Of more ominous significance is hyphema, or the presence of blood in the anterior chamber, which may be visible as a fluid level when the child is erect. Despite the difficulty in examining the eyes during the first day of life, it is important to inspect the pupil for cataracts and the cornea for clouding of congenital glaucoma. Accomodation of the pupils to light can be demonstrated, although there is a tendency for the pupils to stay contracted. The pupillary-iris boundaries should be identified to rule out aniridia. Minimally, the red reflex from the eye grounds should be observed, although a more meticulous examination of the retina is best postponed.

Extraocular movements may not be well coordinated in the first days of life and varying degrees of strabismus are often present. Identification of true 6th nerve paralysis is importnat and can be gauged by the ability of the eye to travel laterally as the head is moved in the opposite direction (doll's eye maneuver).

Ears, Nose, Throat. Routine examination of the ears can be limited to inspection of the pinna for abnormalities and the determination that external ear canals are present. If distortion of the nose or face is apparent, careful palpation for fractures is important. Examination of the mouth includes inspection of the gums on which cysts, ranging from small mucosal tags to hard bony masses, or teeth may be present. The hard palate should be palpated as well as inspected for clefts. Clefts may occur with or without clefting of the lip and may involve only the posterior palate. The presence of high arching of the palate with or without a cleft can be a clue to other developmental abnormalities. With the use of a tongue blade, the oropharynx can be seen easily and potentially obstructive cysts are occasionally detected.

Neck. Marked shortening of the neck due to missing cervical vertebrae is generally obvious. Redundancy of the skin of the neck has pertinence in defining syndromes such as gonadal dysgenesis (Turner's). Several types of cysts (thyroglossal, branchial cleft) present as neck masses both in the midline and laterally. The thyroid itself may be enlarged.

Examination of Extremities and Trunk

Clavicles. Crepitation is usually the only physical sign of clavicular fracture in the first day's examination but rapid callous formation permits palpation of a mass by the third day. A hint that a fracture may be present is determined by unilateral restriction of arm extension in the Moro reflex.

Upper Extremity Function. Unilateral restriction or absence of extension in a Moro reflex or mere inequality in the random movements of the arms may signal peripheral nerve damage resulting from brachial plexus injury. The most common form is Erb's palsy, in which the affected arm hangs limply with internal rotation at the shoulder and pronation of the lower segment. Various modifications of this injury can be seen, depending on the cervical nerve roots affected; an effort should be made to analyze the actual areas and degree of deficit.

Hands and Feet. Extra digits can occur as small pediculated appendages, usually without bone, or as perfectly formed 6th fingers or toes. Webbing, particularly of the toes, is a common anomaly. With abnormality of hand structure it is important to evaluate the position and function of the thumb in terms of its ability to oppose the fingers. A simian (single transverse) crease on the palms is important to note because of its association with chromosoaml abnormalities. However, it is seen unilaterally in 4% of normal persons.

Hips. Congenital hip dysplasia is suspected when abduction at the hips is limited or produces a pronounced click as the head of the femur moves out of the acetabulum. Many minor clicks without a sense of displacement occur with the same maneuver and are not significant. These generally disappear by one week of age but the click of congenital dysplasia continues and requires evaluation by an orthopaedist.

Examination of Genitalia

In the male, the presence of both testes in the scrotum or canals should be ascertained. On examination of the penis, the position of the urethral meatus should be noted, although this is sometimes difficult in a noncircumcised child. With any visible abnormality of the foreskin, it is imperative to determine the position of the urethral orifice by observation of the child voiding. Circumcision should be delayed if any abnormality is present.

In the female, the presence of a vaginal opening should be assured. Mucosal tags frequently present from the orifice and are generally insignificant; in contrast, bulging of the imperforate hymen with accumulated blood or mucus needs correction.

Immediate attention should be given to any ambiguity of the genitalia. Microphallus, clitoral enlargement, bifid scrotum, or partial fusion of the labia should trigger rapid determination of the infant's sex and evaluation of potential management.

Neurologic Evaluation

Complete evaluation of motor and sensory function of a newborn demands subtle testing and correlates erratically with later neurologic or cognitive development. Indication of generally intact neuromuscular function can be obtained through the following observations:

Tone. Tone is best judged by extending flexed extremities and observing recoil.

Strength. Strength is observed as equal spontaneous movements of extremities and resistance of manipulation, ability to raise head when pulled to sitting position, ability to extend head to level of body when suspended in prone position, ability to place feet firmly on flat surface and "step" ahead.

Mass Reflex. The best known mass reflex is Moro's reflex, which involves extension and then flexion of the arms when an infant is startled. It is most easily elicited by the examiner dropping the baby's head into his other hand. The extent of Moro's reflex depends on maturity of the infant.

Reflex Coordination. Evaluate grasping, rooting, withdrawing of an extremity from pin prick.

Vision. With enough patience, momentary focusing or even following by the eyes can be observed in almost every quiet, awake full-term infant.

Hearing. Hearing is present in the newborn but hard to demonstrate without sophisticated electronic equipment.

GENERAL CARE OF THE NEONATE

Delivery Room

Throughout the United States and much of the rest of the world, a standardized scoring system is used to evalute an infant's condition in the immediate postpartum period. The Apgar score, which is most frequently recorded at 1 and 5 minutes of age, assigns values of 0 to 2 for each of five physical findings: pulse, respiration, color, tone, and reflex irritability (Table 38-1). The *sum* of these scores is used as an index of well-being; thus scores 8 to 10 reflect a healthy infant, 4 to 7 an infant with suspicious signs of difficulty, and 0 to 3, an infant in need of immediate resuscitation. The 1-minute Apgar score indicates the degree of asphyxia present while the 5-minute score correlates more closely with mortality and morbidity in the newborn period and to some extent with long-range outcome.

The immediate needs of the typical healthy infant in the first minutes of life include gentle removal of oral and nasal secretions by bulb suction, towel drying to reduce heat loss through evaporation and the provision of a source of warmth. Prophylaxis against gonorrheal ophthalmia is adminis-

TABLE 38-1. The Apgar Score

	0	1	2
Heart rate	Absent	Less than 100/min	More than 100/min
Respiratory effort	Absent	Slow irregular	Strong cry
Muscle tone	Limp	Some flexion of extremities	Good flexion, active motion
Reflex irritability (when feet stimulated)	No response	Some motion	Cry
Color	Blue, pale	Body pink, extremities blue	Completely pink

tered by the instillation into the eyes of a 1% solution of silver nitrate or an antibiotic solution as prescribed by individual State laws. The most generally used antibiotics are tetracycline, 1.0% solution, and erythromycin, 0.5% ointment. Silver nitrate instillation is usually followed in 1 minute by a water flush but the value of flushing is disputed. In most maternity services, 1.0 mg of vitamin K is routinely administered intramuscularly to relieve the physiologic deficiency of vitamin K-dependent coagulation factors. Appropriate identification procedures, preferably fingerprinting, plus recording of data on a bracelet attached to the baby, must be completed before the child leaves the delivery room.

The baby with a low Apgar score needs medical support which may amount only to brief suctioning by catheter and provision of an enriched oxygen environment or may include full-scale resuscitative efforts. In the latter instance, successive steps include the establishment of a clear airway, a short trial of positive pressure ventilation with 100% oxygen by bag and mask, intubation of the trachea to ensure more adequate ventilation and, if necessary, cardiac massage. A glucose infusion is started and, if the infant is profoundly hypoxic or has circulatory failure, sodium bicarbonate is administered while positive pressure ventilation is continued. Throughout the procedure, careful attention is paid to keeping the child warm.

Nursery

On admission to the nursery, a full-term infant is weighed and temperature, pulse, and respirations recorded. He is warmly wrapped and placed in a crib. If the rectal or axillary temperatue is less than 36.0°C (96.8°F), the baby should be placed on a radiant warmer or in an incubator and the temperature checked every 30 minutes until it reaches 36.5°C (97.7°F).

Many mothers choose to nurse their babies in the Delivery Room and this should be allowed if the child is vigorous and can be kept warm. In the nursery feedings can be instituted at any time but the frequent persistence of excessive upper airway mucus in the first few hours make a 4-hour delay expedient as a routine. Depression or respiratory difficulty is cause to delay feedings further, but some type of fluid administration should be started by 12 hours.

Sterile water is offered to the infant first and if this is taken without difficulty, milk feeding can be initiated. The current evidence that human milk is the most appropriate feeding for an infant imposes a responsibility on the physician to actively recommend breast-feeding to mothers. It is obvious that this attitude should be modified if there is a physical or emotional reason for the mother to reject nursing, but there is little justification now for statements that formula is "just as good and easier." If formula is to be used, any of several proprietary products containing 20 calories per ounce and 1.5% to 1.7% protein is adequate. Iron-fortified formulas are well tolerated and are recommended. All the commercial formulas provide sufficient vitamins when they are fed in quantities that meet the infant's caloric requirements. Infants fed human milk may require a vitamin D supplement.

The only routine laboratory work to be recommended is blood typing and direct Coombs' testing of infants whose mothers are Rh negative. Some physicians believe similar routine testing (with indirect Coombs') is warranted on infants of mothers with blood type O, particularly in predominantly black populations.

During the physician's daily visits to the infant in the nursery, the following data should be reviewed: temperature, weight, intake, voiding, and stooling. The presence of hypothermia, duskiness, lethargy, poor feeding, vomiting, distention, or jaundice should be noted and appropriate investigation instituted. Observations of the mother-infant relationship and discussion with both parents of their fears and expectations can be extremely valuable to both the family and the physician. With the current trend toward early discharge, it is particularly important to make an early appraisal of any potential problem, physical or emotional, and to ensure safeguards against increasing difficulty after discharge.

HIGH-RISK INFANT

The spectrum of neonatal disease is as wide as that of older persons, but many newborn problems either relate to antenatal adversity or reflect their immature physiologic status. Of necessity the following descriptions of neonatal abnormality are brief but deal with the six most common areas in which problems arise. An attempt is made to focus on the observations needed for physicians to recognize and identify illness and to initiate appropriate management.

Low Birth Weight

Infants weighing less than 2500 g at birth are generally designated as "low birth weight" but in no way represent an homogeneous group. Any given birth weight may primarily reflect prematurity or may represent a low rate of growth *in utero*. The terms "appropriate for gestational age" (AGA) and "small for gestational age" (SGA) are used to state this difference. Since intrauterine growth retardation can occur at any time during pregnancy, both premature and full-term babies can be SGA. Prematurity is usually defined as gestational age of less than 37 weeks, while intrauterine growth retardation is variously defined as weight less than the 10th percentile or less than two standard deviations from the mean for gestational age. *In utero* development, both anatomic and physiologic, occurs in a reasonably predictable sequence; thus, an analysis of characteristics of a newborn infant can be used to calculate gestational age if date of delivery cannot be estimated by other means. This scoring system, designed by Capurro *et al* as a simplified modification of the Dubowitz assessment, is shown in Figure 38-1. Statistical charts such as the Lubchenco intrauterine growth curves are available (Fig. 38-2); these charts relate gestational age to weight, length, and head circumference on a percentile basis, thus allowing identification of the given infant as AGA, SGA, or even LGA (large for gestational age).

The division of low birth weight infants into AGA or SGA categories is useful

	A.	VARIABLES					
B. SOMATIC AND NEUROLOGICAL	SOMATIC	Nipple formation	Nipple barely visible: no areola 0	Well-defined nipple: areola <0.75 cm 5	Areola stippled not raised >0.75 cm 10	Areola raised >0.75 cm 15	
		Skin texture	Thin, gelatinous 0	Thin and smooth 5	Smooth, medium thickness, superficial peeling 10	Slight thickening, superficial cracking & peeling of hands & feet 15	Thick and parchment like 20
		Ear form	Pinna flat & shapeless 0	Incurving of part of edge 8	Partial incurving of whole of upper pinna 16	Well-defined incurving of pinna 24	
		Breast size	No breast tissue 6	Diameter <0.5 cm 5	Diameter 0.5 - 1 cm 10	Diameter >1 cm 15	
	K = 204 days	Plantar creases	No creases 0	Faint red marks over anterior 1/2 5	Definite red marks over anterior 1/2, indentations over anterior 1/3 10	Indentations over anterior 1/2 15	Deep indentations over more than anterior 1/2 20
		Scarf Sign	 0	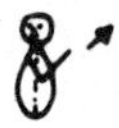 6	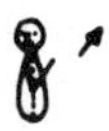 12	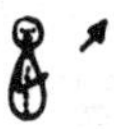 18	
K = 200 days		Head lag	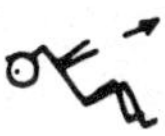 0	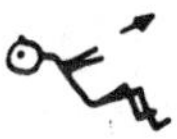 4	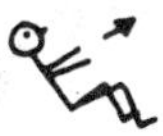 8	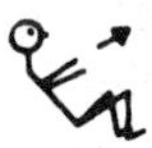 12	

Fig. 38-1. Scoring system for estimation of gestational age. (Capurro H, Konichezley S, Fonseca D, Caldeyro-Barcia R: A simplified method for diagnosis of gestational age in the newborn infant. J Pediatr 93:120, 1978)

because of the marked differences in their neonatal problems. The true premature infant suffers most often as a result of immature respiratory function, poor weight gain, infections, apnea, jaundice, necrotizing enterocolitis, and intracranial hemorrhage. The infant with intrauterine deprivation, on the other hand, rarely has evidence of the respiratory distress syndrome but frequently has birth asphyxia, hypoglycemia, seizures, and a high incidence of congenital anomalies.

Respiratory Abnormality

The highest mortality in the first month of life is associated with the respiratory distress syndrome (RDS) or hyaline membrane disease in premature infants. The pathogenesis of this condition is instability of the terminal airways and alveoli resulting from deficiency of the phospholipid-lining substance, surfactant, which ordinarily functions to reduce surface tension. For this rea-

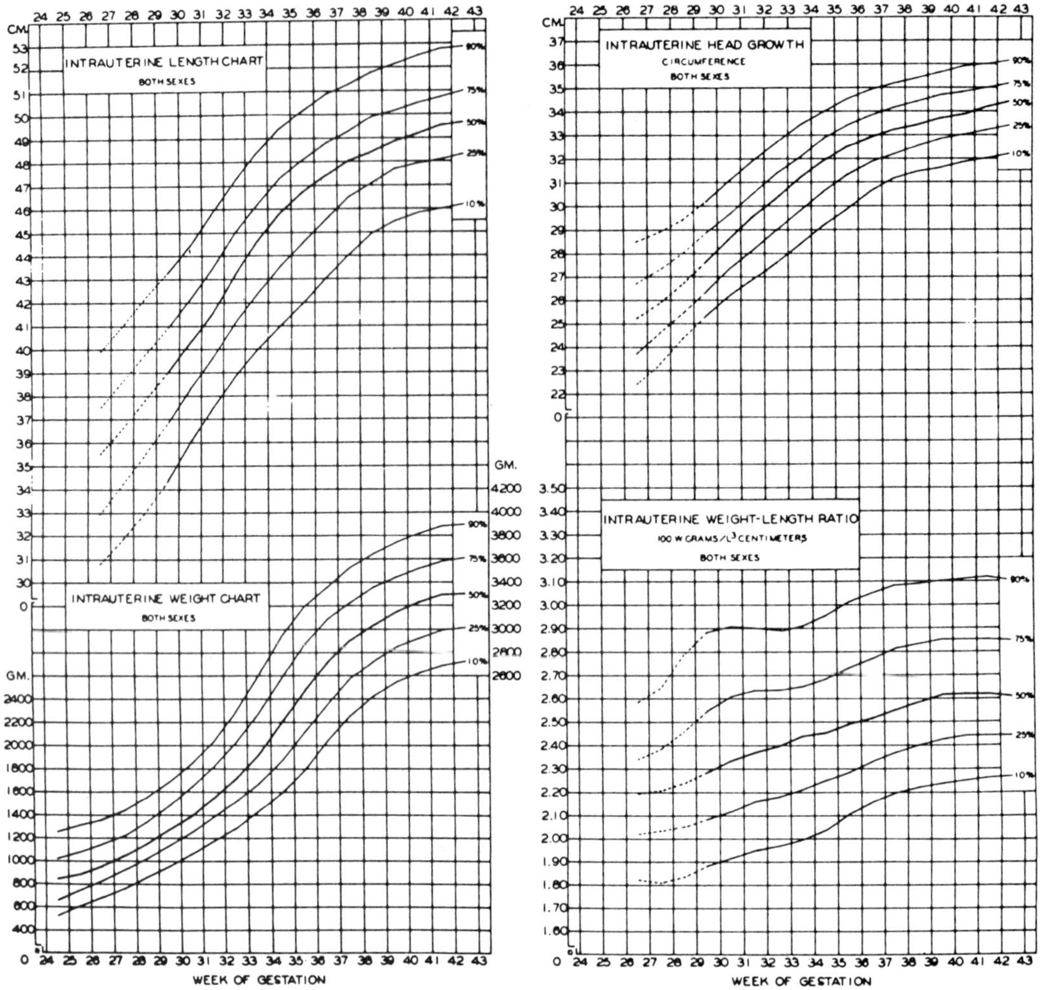

Fig. 38-2. Colorado intrauterine growth charts. (Lubchenco LO, Hansman C, Boyd E: Pediatrics 37:403, 1966)

son, lung compliance is reduced. Additionally there is a marked decrease in lung perfusion and a large right-to-left shunt of blood, both extra- and intrapulmonary. The imbalance in ventilation and perfusion severely compromises gas exchange.

The infant with RDS generally has a gestational age of less than 37 weeks and often has a history of perinatal difficulty, frequently of fetal distress. Apgar scores are often, but not always, low. Respiratory distress may develop directly after birth or more slowly over the course of 6 to 8 hours. Flaring of the alae nasi, expiratory grunting, retraction, tachypnea, or cyanosis are seen. The typical radiologic appearance of the chest is one of homogeneous reticulogranular density with air bronchograms. Blood gases show a mixed metabolic and respiratory acidosis and a low PaO_2. Current therapy involves the use of increased oxygen concentrations, constant distending pressure

(CPAP), and when necessary, ventilation by respirators. The course may vary from 72 hours to weeks depending on the occurrence of complications such as pneumothoraces, intracranial hemorrhage, persistent patency of the ductus arteriosus, and chronic lung disease secondary to high oxygen and positive-pressure ventilation.

In contrast to the premature infant, the asphyxiated full-term or postmature infant may suffer meconium aspiration as the result of intrauterine gasping of meconium-contaminated amniotic fluid. The problem can be minimized by rapid removal of meconium from the nasopharynx directly after birth. Infants who have aspirated meconium have overinflated chests and irregular breathing with many auscultatory adventitial sounds. Chest radiographs show nonhomogeneous coarse density, and blood gases demonstrate marked hypoxia with accompanying acidosis. The course is variable, some chests clearing in 48 hours and others taking several days. The most frequent complication is pneumothorax.

Prenatal asphyxia may also be responsible for the syndrome of persistent fetal circulation or persistent pulmonary hypertension in which the pulmonary arterioles remain constricted after birth, causing marked right-to-left shunting with venous admixture of blood and failure of oxygenation.

Other respiratory diseases occurring in a newborn population include a group of moderately benign conditions, two of which are transient tachypnea of the newborn and the so-called type II respiratory distress syndrome. Each of these mimics RDS in symptoms and blood gas abnormalities, but the radiograph appearance differs and the diseases are mild and limited in duration. Of much more serious nature are the congenital pneumonias; presently, the most frequent is that caused by group B beta-hemolytic streptococcus. The radiographic appearance and symptoms are easily mistaken for RDS and the mortality rate is approximately 50%. Finally, major confusion can exist in the differential diagnosis of respiratory and cardiac disease.

Congenital Heart Disease

Severe congenital cardiac anomalies may cause symptoms shortly after birth or at variable periods from hours to weeks thereafter. Presenting symptoms are usually cyanosis and/or respiratory distress from pulmonary disease. Differentiation can be attempted by the administration of supplemental oxygen which will generally increase PaO_2 in pulmonary disease but not in cardiac.

The customary signs of cardiac failure in a newborn are tachypnea, hepatic enlargement, and increasing heart size. Peripheral edema is less common but ominous. In terms of frequency, cardiac failure is most often seen in premature infants who have persistence of the ductus arteriosus. Infants with ventricular septal defects rarely have difficulty in the immediate newborn period, although they may have audible murmurs. Of the serious anomalies, transposition of the great vessels and hypoplastic left heart are most common.

Preliminary investigation of cardiac status includes auscultation of murmurs, detection of signs of cardiac failure, evaluation of the heart size, and pulmonary vasculature by chest radiograph and analysis of the EKG. More definitive diagnosis can be approached by echocardiography and cardiac catheterization.

Infection

The poor immunologic defenses of the newborn, particularly the premature infant, lead to a high incidence of infection in this age group. The responsible bacterial pathogens vary from decade to decade with the current offenders being primarily group B beta-hemolytic streptococcus and *Escherichia coli.* Coagulase-positive *Staphylococcus aureus* still poses a threat as a nosocomial agent but to a diminished degree compared with that of previous decades. *Listeria monocytogenes,* enterococci and *Pseudomonas aeruginosa* infections also occur frequently in newborns.

The common route of infection is by ascending vaginal organisms invading the uterine cavity following premature rupture of the membranes. With ruptured membranes, the incidence of infection increases rapidly beyond 24 hours; infection also appears to correlate with the stress of labor. Any infant who is not delivered within a 24-hour period postrupture should be checked for infection and investigated by blood culture, white blood cell count, and differential.

The common infection of the neonate is septicemia without a localized site, although meningitis and pneumonia occur frequently. Sepsis presents with nonspecific symptoms: lethargy, poor feeding, hypothermia, distention, or vomiting. These alterations in behavior should be investigated with cultures of blood, spinal fluid, and urine, and the differential blood smear should be observed for leukopenia or the presence of band forms. Absolute neutrophil counts of less than 1500 per cu mm or absolute band counts of more than 1500 in the first 5 days of life or 500 thereafter are very suggestive of infection. Initiation of antibiotic therapy is indicated after cultures are obtained where suspicion of infection exists. With the present threat of streptococcal pneumonia, initiation of therapy is probably justified in all infants with respiratory distress resembling hyaline membrane disease radiologically. A combination of ampicillin with an aminoglycoside is effective in most neonatal infections. If cultures are negative at 72 hours, the antibiotic therapy may be discontinued.

A group of nonbacterial agents including syphylis, *toxoplasma gondii,* cytomegalovirus, and rubella and herpes simplex (STORCH) cause serious intrauterine infections which may be responsible for congenital malformations. Hepatosplenomegaly, cerebrospinal fluid pleocytosis, and thrombocytopenia are the common presenting features.

Jaundice

Hyperbilirubinemia occurs frequently in the first days of life and stems from multiple etiologies. Its danger lies in its potential to cause central nervous system damage or kernicterus, but the level of serum bilirubin that is damaging varies with the maturity of the infant, the day of life, the partition between indirect and direct bilirubin, and other factors such as oxygenation, pH, and circulating substances interfering with albumin-bilirubin binding.

Investigation of the cause of jaundice is directed by the circumstances under which it appears. Thus, on the first day of life the possibility of a hemolytic process due to isoimmune sensitization is high, while jaundice that does not appear until the third day probably represents the physiologic inability of the immature liver to cope with the normal increased breakdown of red cells. Infection is a common cause of jaundice at any time during the neonatal period. Serum bilirubin levels above 12 mg/dl cannot be considered normal in a full-term infant, and an etiologic factor should be sought. Premature infants develop higher levels of physiologic jaundice but the cause of jaundice still merits careful investigation. A list follows, showing a standard scheme of investigation of hyperbilirubinemia based on the day of life that jaundice is seem.

Current management of hyperbilirubinemia consists of phototherapy and exchange transfusion at bilirubin levels where the central nervous system is endangered.

Schema for Diagnosis of Neonatal Jaundice

Jaundice appearing on first day of life

Known Rh sensitization
- Cord blood: type, Rh, direct Coombs' test, hemoglobin, and bilirubin
- Infant blood: CBC with smear, hemoglobin, and bilirubin at 2–4 hours

Unexpected jaundice
- Type, Rh, direct and indirect Coombs', bilirubin, CBC with smear, reticulocyte count
- If history or clinical evidence of infection: cultures of blood, urine, CSF
- If suggestive evidence of intrauterine (STORCH) infection: lgM, VDRL, viral titers, platelets

Jaundice appearing on second day
- Studies as in section above (unexpected jaundice)
- RBC enzymes (G6PD, pyruvate kinase)
- Physical examination for hemotomas, concealed hemorrhage, or signs of infection
- Review of hydration, intake, weight, urine-specific gravity

Jaundice appearing on third day with indirect bilirubin greater than 12 mg dl in full-term infant
- Study as in section above (unexpected jaundice): Include lgM even without evidence of STORCH infection.
- Check for concealed hemorrhage.
- Check hydration.

Persistent jaundice after third day
- Carboxyhemoglobin to define hemolysis
- Urinalysis and urine culture
- Appropriate studies to rule out galactosemia, hypothyroidism, aminoaciduria lgM, viral titers
- Consider temporary cessation of breast-feeding to note response of bilirubin level

Persistent jaundice with increased direct bilirubin
- CBC and blood culture
- Liver function studies
- α-1-antitrypsin
- STORCH serologies, VDRL
- Vitamin E absorption test

Metabolic Disorders

The most common metabolic abnormality in the newborn is hypoglycemia. Blood sugar at birth is approximately 70% of maternal glucose concentration but the level falls over the first 2 to 3 hours with stabilization in the full-term infant at concentrations of 45 to 60 mg/dl. With feedings, levels increase to 55 to 70 mg/dl at which they remain for the first week. Blood sugar concentrations of less than 30 mg/dl can be considered hypoglycemia. Low birth weight infants have larger decreases in blood glucose than term infants and often have concentrations as low as 20 mg/dl at 2 to 4 hours.

Symptoms of hypoglycemia in the neonate include limpness, high-pitched cry, apnea, cyanosis, twitching, and occasionally convulsions or coma. However, there is poor relationship between symptomatology and blood sugar level, and it is not unusual to find entirely asymptomatic infants with glucose levels less than 20 mg/dl. For this reason it has become common nursery practice to make measurements of blood glucose in capillary blood at frequent intervals in all infants at risk of hypoglycemia.

High-risk groups include infants of diabetic mothers, infants with intrauterine growth retardation, premature infants, and those who have suffered birth asphyxia, respiratory distress, infection, cold stress, or other serious disease. In the case of the infant of a diabetic mother, the hypoglycemia results from hyperinsulinism generated in response to the mother's hyperglycemia, while in small-for-date infants the hypoglycemia is probably related to decreased liver glycogen stores or defective gluconeogenesis. The mechanism of the other secondary hypoglycemias is not clear.

There is little doubt that uncorrected symptomatic hypoglycemia can have permanent sequelae, but confusion exists regarding the danger of unsymptomatic hypoglycemia. It appears prudent to attempt correction of any blood sugar less than 40 mg/dl by intravenous infusion of 10% to 25% glucose or by the use of glucagon. As a routine, infants at risk of hypoglycemia should be fed early.

A second metabolic problem that occurs with some frequency is hypocalcemia. This can be defined as serum calcium less than 7.0 mg/dl and is seen most often in premature infants, infants of diabetic mothers, and infants with birth asphyxia. Symptoms are quite variable and include rapid, shallow respirations, apnea, duskiness or pallor followed by increasing agitation, tachycardia and finally, flaccidity. The carpopedal spasm, Chvostek's sign and stridor of classic tetany are generally absent.

Treatment by intravenous infusion of 0.2 ml of 10% calcium glucomate per kg per hr is effective.

Congenital Anomalies

Major congenital defects occur in approximately 2% of all live births and can involve every organ system of the body. Many are life-threatening, some interfere with growth or development, and others are cosmetically disastrous. Anomalies involving several systems, often appearing in a recognizable constellation, suggest the presence of a chromosomal abnormality, the most common of which is trisomy 21 or Down's syndrome. When suspicion of chromosomal aberration exists, a karyotype should be obtained in the immediate newborn period.

Congenital defects constitute the bulk of neonatal surgical emergencies including problems of the airway (choanal atresia, laryngeal webs), lungs (diaphragmatic hernia), gastrointestinal tract (tracheoesophageal fistula, intestinal atresia), and genitourinary tract (urethral obstruction, hydronephrosis). Early recognition of the problem is in most cases essential to adequate correction.

Investigation of etiology of anomalies is a later but important facet of their management. A search for the presence of teratogenic factors in pregnancy should be made. Particular care must be taken to detect any indication of inheritable abnormality; in these cases, genetic counseling should be made available. The physician who cares for a newborn infant with anomalies is responsible for starting the long-term planning process necessary for successful future development.

CONCLUSION

Over the past 20 years, reduction on the order of 30% has taken place in neonatal mortality with the greatest decrease in the category of the small premature infant. Progress continues with attention now being focused both on intensive care of catastrophic illness and the subtler issues of optimal nutrition, growth, stimulation, and maternal-infant relationships. The new area of infant care during transport has arisen as a result of regionalization of perinatal facilities for the high-risk infant and mother.

The final results of neonatal care are hard to quantitate since outcome is measurable over a lifetime. Recent studies of development of low birth weight infants are generally optimistic, with a decreasing number of major handicaps reported. However, the incidence of behavioral aberrations in this group continues to be high. Further improvement will rest not only on increased understanding of fetal and neonatal physiology but also on expansion of the availability of perinatal care.

BIBLIOGRAPHY

Avery ME, Fletcher BD: The Lung and its Disorders in the Newborn Infant. Philadelphia, WB Saunders, 1974

Contains good chapters on normal lung development and neonatal respiratory function as well as comprehensive discussion of all types of pulmonary abnormality in the newborn period.

Capurro H, Konichezky S, Fonesca D, Caldeyro-Barcia R: A simplified method for diagnosis of gestational age in the newborn infant. J Pediatr 93:120, 1978

Presents a scoring system for physical findings which allows estimation of gestational age.

Cook LN: Intrauterine and extrauterine recognition and management of deviant fetal growth. Pediat Clin North Am 24:431, 1977

A good description of fetal growth retardation and the SGA baby.

Effer SB: Biochemical and biophysical indices of fetal risk. Clin Perinatol 1:161, 1974.

Reviews laboratory data used to delineate risk in a fetus.

Klaus MH, Fanaroff AA: Care of the High-Risk Neonate. Philadelphia, WB Saunders, 1979

A thoroughly readable text covering common illnesses of the newborn period. Has a particularly good section on congenital heart disease.

Standards and Recommendations for Hospital Care of Newborn Infants. Evanston, Ill, American Academy of Pediatrics, 1977

Recently published guidelines for delivery of newborn care.

Index

Numerals followed by an "f" indicate a figure, "t" following a page number indicates a table.